KAPLAN

MCAT®
Biochemistry Review
2027–2028

Edited by Alexander Stone Macnow, MD

ACKNOWLEDGMENTS

Editor-in-Chief, 2027–2028 Edition
M. Dominic Eggert

Contributing Editors, 2027–2028 Edition
Ae-Ri Kim, PhD; Elizabeth Minten, MD PhD; Gregory J. Riviello, MA; Christopher Vestuto

Prior Edition Editorial Staff: Elisabeth Fassas, MD MSc

Published by Kaplan North America, LLC
1515 West Cypress Creek Road
Fort Lauderdale, Florida 33309

Printed in India.

ISBN: 979-8-3497-0107-8

10 9 8 7 6 5 4 3 2 1

TABLE OF CONTENTS

THE *KAPLAN MCAT REVIEW* TEAM

Alexander Stone Macnow, MD
Editor-in-Chief

Tyra Hall-Pogar, PhD
Editor

Samer T. Ismail
Kaplan MCAT Faculty

Bela G. Starkman, PhD
Editor

Kelly Kyker-Snowman, MS
Kaplan MCAT Faculty

Joshua D. Brooks, PhD
Kaplan MCAT Faculty

Christopher Lopez
Kaplan MCAT Faculty

Alisha Maureen Crowley
Kaplan MCAT Faculty

M. Dominic Eggert
Editor

Faculty Reviewers and Editors: Elmar R. Aliyev; James Burns; Jonathan Cornfield; Brandon Deason, MD; Nikolai Dorofeev, MD; Benjamin Downer, MS; Colin Doyle; Christopher Durland; Marilyn Engle; Eleni M. Eren; Raef Ali Fadel; Elizabeth Flagge; Adam Grey; Justine Harkness, PhD; Scott Huff; Ae-Ri Kim, PhD; Elizabeth A. Kudlaty; Ningfei Li; John P. Mahon; Matthew A. Meier; Nainika Nanda; Caroline Nkemdilim Opene; Kaitlyn E. Prenger; Uneeb Qureshi; Derek Rusnak, MA; Kristen L. Russell, ME; Michael Paul Tomani, MS; Nicholas M. White; Kerranna Williamson, MBA; Allison Ann Wilkes, MS; and Tony Yu

Thanks to Kevin Anderson; Rebecca Anderson; Jeff Batzli; Jurre Blom; Hari Priya Chandran; Eric Chiu; James Coleman; Deepika Devan; Tim Eich; Samantha Fallon; Tyler Fara; Owen Farcy; Dan Frey; Robin Garmise; Rita Garthaffner; Joanna Graham; Allison Gudenau; Allison Harm; Beth Hoffberg; Aaron Lemon-Strauss; Keith Lubeley; Diane McGarvey; Leonard Mendoza; Petros Minasi; Elizabeth Minten, MD, PhD; Beena P V; John Polstein; Deeangelee Pooran-Kublall, MD, MPH; Andrea Repole; Rochelle Rothstein, MD; Larry Rudman; Tor Sanden; Srividhya Sankar; Sylvia Tidwell Scheuring; Carly Schnur; Aiswarya Sivanand; Todd Tedesco; Karin Tucker; Bonnie Wang; Lee Weiss; Christina Wheeler; Kristen Workman; Amy Zarkos; and the countless others who made this book possible.

GETTING STARTED CHECKLIST

Getting Started Checklist

- [ ] Register for your free online assets: if you bought this book new as part of a set, scan the QR code on the front of the book set's slipcase and enter the unique code there; if you bought this book separately, instead go to **www.kaptest.com/moreonline**.
- [ ] Create a study calendar that ensures you complete content review and sufficient practice by Test Day!
- [ ] As you finish a chapter and the online practice for that chapter, check it off on the table of contents.
- [ ] Register to take the MCAT at **www.aamc.org/mcat.**
- [ ] Set aside time during your prep to make sure the rest of your application—personal statement, recommendations, and other materials—is ready to go!
- [ ] Take a moment to admire your completed checklist, then get back to the business of prepping for this exam!

PREFACE

And now it starts: your long, yet fruitful journey toward wearing a white coat. Proudly wearing that white coat, though, is hopefully only part of your motivation. You are reading this book because you want to be a healer.

If you're serious about going to medical school, then you are likely already familiar with the importance of the MCAT in medical school admissions. While the holistic review process puts additional weight on your experiences, extracurricular activities, and personal attributes, the fact remains: along with your GPA, your MCAT score remains one of the two most important components of your application portfolio—at least early in the admissions process. Each additional point you score on the MCAT pushes you in front of thousands of other students and makes you an even more attractive applicant. But the MCAT is not simply an obstacle to overcome; it is an opportunity to show schools that you will be a strong student and a future leader in medicine.

We at Kaplan take our jobs very seriously and aim to help students see success not only on the MCAT, but as future physicians. We work with our learning science experts to ensure that we're using the most up-to-date teaching techniques in our resources. Multiple members of our team hold advanced degrees in medicine or associated biomedical sciences, and are committed to the highest level of medical education. Kaplan has been working with the MCAT for over 50 years and our commitment to premed students is unflagging; in fact, Stanley Kaplan created this company when he had difficulty being accepted to medical school due to unfair quota systems that existed at the time.

We stand now at the beginning of a new era in medical education. As citizens of this 21st-century world of healthcare, we are charged with creating a patient-oriented, culturally competent, cost-conscious, universally available, technically advanced, and research-focused healthcare system, run by compassionate providers. Suffice it to say, this is no easy task. Problem-based learning, integrated curricula, and classes in interpersonal skills are some of the responses to this demand for an excellent workforce—a workforce of which you'll soon be a part.

We're thrilled that you've chosen us to help you on this journey. Please reach out to us to share your challenges, concerns, and successes. Together, we will shape the future of medicine in the United States and abroad; we look forward to helping you become the doctor you deserve to be.

Good luck!

Alexander Stone Macnow, MD
Editor-in-Chief
Department of Pathology and Laboratory Medicine
Hospital of the University of Pennsylvania

BA, Musicology—Boston University, 2008
MD—Perelman School of Medicine at the University of Pennsylvania, 2013

ABOUT THE MCAT

Anatomy of the MCAT

Here is a general overview of the structure of Test Day:

Section	Number of Questions	Time Allotted
Test-Day Certification		4 minutes
Tutorial (optional)		10 minutes
Chemical and Physical Foundations of Biological Systems	59	95 minutes
Break (optional)		10 minutes
Critical Analysis and Reasoning Skills (CARS)	53	90 minutes
Lunch Break (optional)		30 minutes
Biological and Biochemical Foundations of Living Systems	59	95 minutes
Break (optional)		10 minutes
Psychological, Social, and Biological Foundations of Behavior	59	95 minutes
Void Question		3 minutes
Satisfaction Survey (optional)		5 minutes

The structure of the four sections of the MCAT is shown below.

Chemical and Physical Foundations of Biological Systems	
Time	95 minutes
Format	• 59 questions • 10 passages • 44 questions are passage-based, and 15 are discrete (stand-alone) questions. • Score between 118 and 132
What It Tests	• Biochemistry: 25% • Biology: 5% • General Chemistry: 30% • Organic Chemistry: 15% • Physics: 25%

Critical Analysis and Reasoning Skills (CARS)	
Time	90 minutes
Format	• 53 questions • 9 passages • All questions are passage-based. There are no discrete (stand-alone) questions. • Score between 118 and 132
What It Tests	Disciplines: • Humanities: 50% • Social Sciences: 50% Skills: • *Foundations of Comprehension: 30%* • *Reasoning Within the Text: 30%* • *Reasoning Beyond the Text: 40%*
Biological and Biochemical Foundations of Living Systems	
Time	95 minutes
Format	• 59 questions • 10 passages • 44 questions are passage-based, and 15 are discrete (stand-alone) questions. • Score between 118 and 132
What It Tests	• Biochemistry: 25% • Biology: 65% • General Chemistry: 5% • Organic Chemistry: 5%
Psychological, Social, and Biological Foundations of Behavior	
Time	95 minutes
Format	• 59 questions • 10 passages • 44 questions are passage-based, and 15 are discrete (stand-alone) questions. • Score between 118 and 132
What It Tests	• Biology: 5% • Psychology: 65% • Sociology: 30%
Total	
Testing Time	375 minutes (6 hours, 15 minutes)
Total Seat Time	447 minutes (7 hours, 27 minutes)
Questions	230
Score	472 to 528

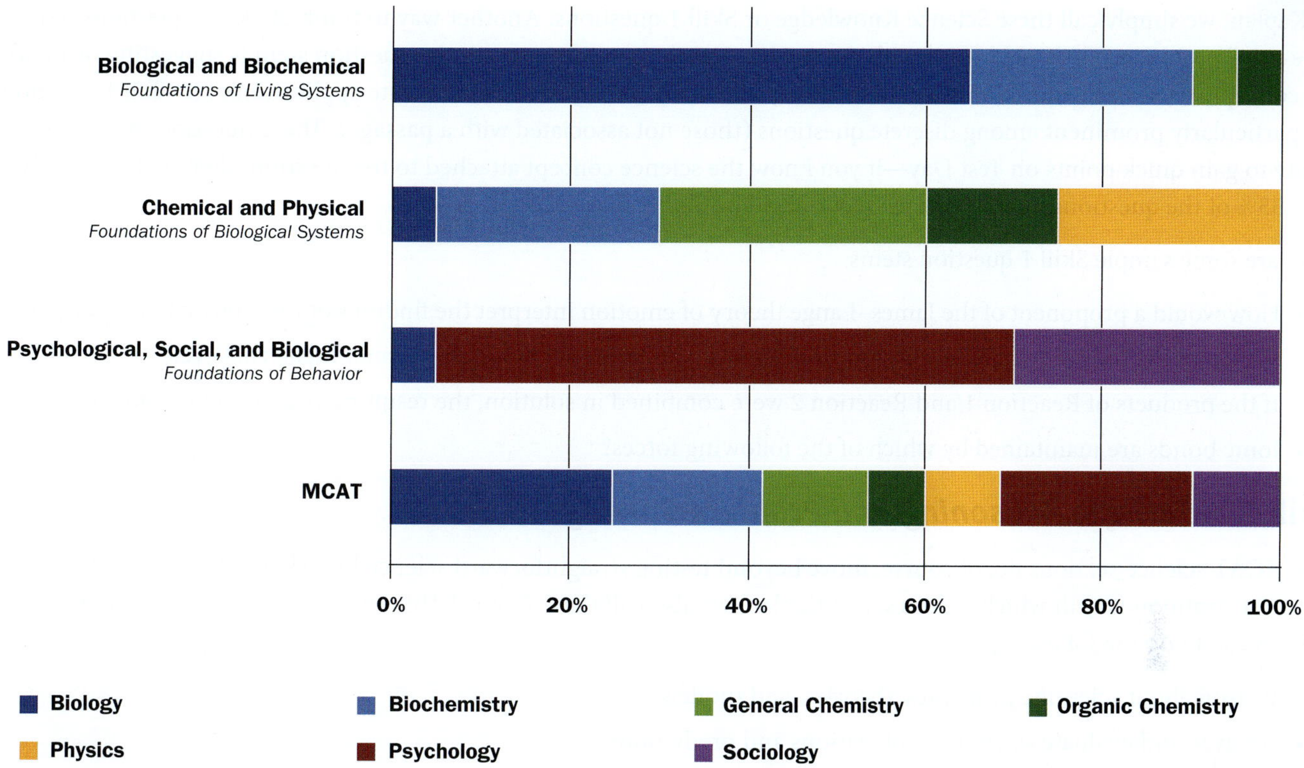

Scientific Inquiry and Reasoning Skills (SIRS)

The AAMC has defined four *Scientific Inquiry and Reasoning Skills* (SIRS) that will be tested in the three science sections of the MCAT:

1. *Knowledge of Scientific Concepts and Principles* (35% of questions)
2. *Scientific Reasoning and Problem-Solving* (45% of questions)
3. *Reasoning About the Design and Execution of Research* (10% of questions)
4. *Data-Based and Statistical Reasoning* (10% of questions)

Let's see how each one breaks down into more specific Test Day behaviors. Note that the bullet points of specific objectives for each of the SIRS are taken directly from the *Official Guide to the MCAT Exam*; the descriptions of what these behaviors mean and sample question stems, however, are written by Kaplan.

Skill 1: *Knowledge of Scientific Concepts and Principles*

This is probably the least surprising of the four SIRS; the testing of science knowledge is, after all, one of the signature qualities of the MCAT. Skill 1 questions will require you to do the following:

- Recognize correct scientific principles
- Identify the relationships among closely related concepts
- Identify the relationships between different representations of concepts (verbal, symbolic, graphic)
- Identify examples of observations that illustrate scientific principles
- Use mathematical equations to solve problems

At Kaplan, we simply call these Science Knowledge or Skill 1 questions. Another way to think of Skill 1 questions is as "one-step" problems. The single step is either to realize which scientific concept the question stem is suggesting or to take the concept stated in the question stem and identify which answer choice is an accurate application of it. Skill 1 questions are particularly prominent among discrete questions (those not associated with a passage). These questions are an opportunity to gain quick points on Test Day—if you know the science concept attached to the question, then that's it! On Test Day, 35% of the questions in each science section will be Skill 1 questions.

Here are some sample Skill 1 question stems:

- How would a proponent of the James–Lange theory of emotion interpret the findings of the study cited in the passage?
- Which of the following most accurately describes the function of FSH in the human menstrual cycle?
- If the products of Reaction 1 and Reaction 2 were combined in solution, the resulting reaction would form:
- Ionic bonds are maintained by which of the following forces?

Skill 2: *Scientific Reasoning and Problem-Solving*

The MCAT science sections do, of course, move beyond testing straightforward science knowledge; Skill 2 questions are the most common way in which it does so. At Kaplan, we also call these Critical Thinking questions. Skill 2 questions will require you to do the following:

- Reason about scientific principles, theories, and models
- Analyze and evaluate scientific explanations and predictions
- Evaluate arguments about causes and consequences
- Bring together theory, observations, and evidence to draw conclusions
- Recognize scientific findings that challenge or invalidate a scientific theory or model
- Determine and use scientific formulas to solve problems

Just as Skill 1 questions can be thought of as "one-step" problems, many Skill 2 questions are "two-step" problems, and more difficult Skill 2 questions may require three or more steps. These questions can require a wide spectrum of reasoning skills, including integration of multiple facts from a passage, combination of multiple science content areas, and prediction of an experiment's results. Skill 2 questions also tend to ask about science content without actually mentioning it by name. For example, a question might describe the results of one experiment and ask you to predict the results of a second experiment without actually telling you what underlying scientific principles are at work—part of the question's difficulty will be figuring out which principles to apply in order to get the correct answer. On Test Day, 45% of the questions in each science section will be Skill 2 questions.

Here are some sample Skill 2 question stems:

- Which of the following experimental conditions would most likely yield results similar to those in Figure 2?
- All of the following conclusions are supported by the information in the passage EXCEPT:
- The most likely cause of the anomalous results found by the experimenter is:
- An impact to a person's chest quickly reduces the volume of one of the lungs to 70% of its initial value while not allowing any air to escape from the mouth. By what percentage is the force of outward air pressure increased on a 2 cm^2 portion of the inner surface of the compressed lung?

Skill 3: *Reasoning About the Design and Execution of Research*

The MCAT is interested in your ability to critically appraise and analyze research, as this is an important day-to-day task of a physician. We call these questions Skill 3 or Experimental and Research Design questions for short. Skill 3 questions will require you to do the following:

- Identify the role of theory, past findings, and observations in scientific questioning
- Identify testable research questions and hypotheses
- Distinguish between samples and populations and distinguish results that support generalizations about populations
- Identify independent and dependent variables
- Reason about the features of research studies that suggest associations between variables or causal relationships between them (such as temporality and random assignment)
- Identify conclusions that are supported by research results
- Determine the implications of results for real-world situations
- Reason about ethical issues in scientific research

Over the years, the AAMC has received input from medical schools to require more practical research skills of MCAT test takers, and Skill 3 questions are the response to these demands. This skill is unique in that the outside knowledge you need to answer Skill 3 questions is not taught in any one undergraduate course; instead, the research design principles needed to answer these questions are learned gradually throughout your science classes and especially through any laboratory work you have completed. It should be noted that Skill 3 comprises 10% of the questions in each science section on Test Day.

Here are some sample Skill 3 question stems:

- What is the dependent variable in the study described in the passage?
- The major flaw in the method used to measure disease susceptibility in Experiment 1 is:
- Which of the following procedures is most important for the experimenters to follow in order for their study to maintain a proper, randomized sample of research subjects?
- A researcher would like to test the hypothesis that individuals who move to an urban area during adulthood are more likely to own a car than are those who have lived in an urban area since birth. Which of the following studies would best test this hypothesis?

Skill 4: *Data-Based and Statistical Reasoning*

Lastly, the science sections of the MCAT test your ability to analyze the visual and numerical results of experiments and studies. We call these Data and Statistical Analysis questions. Skill 4 questions will require you to do the following:

- Use, analyze, and interpret data in figures, graphs, and tables
- Evaluate whether representations make sense for particular scientific observations and data
- Use measures of central tendency (mean, median, and mode) and measures of dispersion (range, interquartile range, and standard deviation) to describe data
- Reason about random and systematic error

- Reason about statistical significance and uncertainty (interpreting statistical significance levels and interpreting a confidence interval)
- Use data to explain relationships between variables or make predictions
- Use data to answer research questions and draw conclusions

Skill 4 is included in the MCAT because physicians and researchers spend much of their time examining the results of their own studies and the studies of others, and it's very important for them to make legitimate conclusions and sound judgments based on that data. The MCAT tests Skill 4 on all three science sections with graphical representations of data (charts and bar graphs), as well as numerical ones (tables, lists, and results summarized in sentence or paragraph form). On Test Day, 10% of the questions in each science section will be Skill 4 questions.

Here are some sample Skill 4 question stems:

- According to the information in the passage, there is an inverse correlation between:
- What conclusion is best supported by the findings displayed in Figure 2?
- A medical test for a rare type of heavy metal poisoning returns a positive result for 98% of affected individuals and 13% of unaffected individuals. Which of the following types of error is most prevalent in this test?
- If a fourth trial of Experiment 1 was run and yielded a result of 54% compliance, which of the following would be true?

SIRS Summary

Discussing the SIRS tested on the MCAT is a daunting prospect given that the very nature of the skills tends to make the conversation rather abstract. Nevertheless, with enough practice, you'll be able to identify each of the four skills quickly, and you'll also be able to apply the proper strategies to solve those problems on Test Day. If you need a quick reference to remind you of the four SIRS, these guidelines may help:

Skill 1 (**Science Knowledge**) questions ask:

- Do you remember this science content?

Skill 2 (**Critical Thinking**) questions ask:

- Do you remember this science content? And if you do, could you please apply it to this novel situation?
- Could you answer this question that cleverly combines multiple content areas at the same time?

Skill 3 (**Experimental and Research Design**) questions ask:

- Let's forget about the science content for a while. Could you give some insight into the experimental or research methods involved in this situation?

Skill 4 (**Data and Statistical Analysis**) questions ask:

- Let's forget about the science content for a while. Could you accurately read some graphs and tables for a moment? Could you make some conclusions or extrapolations based on the information presented?

Critical Analysis and Reasoning Skills (CARS)

The *Critical Analysis and Reasoning Skills* (CARS) section of the MCAT tests three discrete families of textual reasoning skills; each of these families requires a higher level of reasoning than the last. Those three skills are as follows:

1. *Foundations of Comprehension* (30% of questions)
2. *Reasoning Within the Text* (30% of questions)
3. *Reasoning Beyond the Text* (40% of questions)

These three categories of skills are tested through nine humanities- and social sciences–themed passages, with approximately 5 to 7 questions per passage. Let's take a more in-depth look into these three types. Again, the bullet points of specific objectives for each of the CARS are taken directly from the *Official Guide to the MCAT Exam*; the descriptions of what these behaviors mean and sample question stems, however, are written by Kaplan.

Foundations of Comprehension

Questions in this category will ask for basic facts and simple inferences about the passage; the questions themselves will be similar to those seen on reading comprehension sections of other standardized exams like the SAT® and ACT®. *Foundations of Comprehension* questions will require you to do the following:

- Understand the basic components of the text
- Infer meaning from rhetorical devices, word choice, and text structure

This covers a wide range of question skills (Summarize Text, Recognize Opinion, Paraphrase Detail, and Interpret Meaning), but finding the correct answer to all *Foundations of Comprehension* questions will follow from a basic understanding of the passage and the point of view of its author (and occasionally that of other voices in the passage). Because these questions tend to avoid digging too deeply into the passage, Kaplan calls these *surface* questions.

Here are some sample *Foundations of Comprehension* question stems:

- **Summarize Text**—The author's primary thesis in this passage is:
- **Recognize Opinion**—Based on the information in the second paragraph, which of the following is the most accurate summary of the opinion held by Schubert's critics?
- **Paraphrase Detail**—According to the passage, which of the following is FALSE about literary reviews in the 1920s?
- **Interpret Meaning**—The word "obscure" (paragraph 3), when used in reference to the historian's actions, most nearly means:

Reasoning Within the Text

While *Foundations of Comprehension* questions will usually depend on interpreting a single piece of information in the passage or understanding the passage as a whole, *Reasoning Within the Text* questions require more thought because they will ask you to identify the purpose of a particular piece of information in the context of the passage, or ask how one piece of information relates to another. *Reasoning Within the Text* questions will require you to:

- Integrate different components of the text to draw relevant conclusions

In other words, questions in this type often ask either *How do these two details relate to one another?* or *What else must be true that the author didn't say?* The CARS section will also ask you to judge certain parts of the passage or even judge the author. These questions, which fall under the *Reasoning Within the Text* skill, can ask you to identify authorial bias, evaluate the credibility of cited sources, determine the logical soundness of an argument, identify the importance of a particular fact or statement in the context of the passage, or search for relevant evidence in the passage to support a given conclusion. This category, which Kaplan refers to as *deep* questions because of their tendency to venture into the deep reasoning of the passage, encompasses the following skills: Describe Purpose, Evaluate Reasoning, and Make Deduction.

Here are some sample *Reasoning Within the Text* question stems:

- **Describe Purpose**—The author's discussion of the effect of socioeconomic status on social mobility primarily serves which of the following functions?
- **Evaluate Reasoning**—Which of the following facts is used in the passage as the most prominent piece of evidence in favor of the author's conclusions?
- **Make Deduction**—In putting together the argument in the passage, the author most likely assumes:

Reasoning Beyond the Text

The distinguishing factor of *Reasoning Beyond the Text* questions is in the title of the category: the word *Beyond*. Questions of this type, which make up a larger share of the CARS section than questions from either of the other two types, will always introduce a completely new situation that was not present in the passage itself; these questions will ask you to determine how one influences the other. *Reasoning Beyond the Text* questions will require you to:

- Apply or extrapolate ideas from the passage to new contexts
- Assess the impact of introducing new factors, information, or conditions to ideas from the passage

Because they always introduce ideas not discussed in the passage, Kaplan refers to these as *new info* questions. They test the following skills: Anticipate Response, Predict Outcome/Explanation, Imagine Example/Analogy, and Strengthen/Weaken Argument.

Here are some sample *Reasoning Beyond the Text* question stems:

- **Anticipate Response**—If a document were located that demonstrated Berlioz intended to include a chorus of at least 700 in his *Grande Messe des Morts*, how would the author likely respond?
- **Imagine Example/Analogy**—Which of the following is the best example of a "virtuous rebellion," as it is defined in the passage?
- **Predict Outcome/Explanation**—Extending the author's discussion of ancient Greek history, a conflict between a democracy and an oligarchy would most likely result in:
- **Strengthen/Weaken Argument**—Which of the following sentences, if added to the end of the passage, would most WEAKEN the author's conclusions in the last paragraph?

CARS Summary

Through the *Foundations of Comprehension* category of skills, the CARS section tests many of the reading skills you have been building on since grade school, albeit in the context of very challenging doctorate-level passages. But through the two other categories (*Reasoning Within the Text* and *Reasoning Beyond the Text*), the MCAT demands that you understand the deep structure of passages and the arguments within them at an advanced level. And, of course, all of this is tested under very tight timing restrictions: only 102 seconds per question—and that doesn't even include the time spent reading the passages.

Here's a quick reference guide to the three categories and 11 skills tested in CARS:

Foundations of Comprehension skills:

- Interpret Meaning: Use context to determine what a word/phrase from the passage is intended to communicate.
- Recognize Opinion: Identify what the author or someone else feels about a passage idea based on word choice or other context clues.
- Paraphrase Detail: Recognize a specific piece of information that is stated or strongly implied at one location in the passage.
- Summarize Text: Articulate the main idea of the passage or of a part of it.

Reasoning Within the Text skills:

- Describe Purpose: Identify why the author wrote the passage or a part of it.
- Evaluate Reasoning: Characterize logical connections between ideas in the passage.
- Make Deduction: Infer a claim that follows from multiple parts of the passage, such as an assumption in an argument.

Reasoning Beyond the Text skills:

- Anticipate Response: Identify what the author or someone else would feel/say/do about a new situation based on its similarities to passage ideas.
- Predict Outcome/Explanation: Apply causal reasoning or another connection from the passage to a new situation.
- Strengthen/Weaken Argument: Characterize the logical relationship between a new claim and arguments from the passage.
- Imagine Example/Analogy: Identify new examples of categories defined in the passage or analogies of passage concepts.

Scoring

Each of the four sections of the MCAT is scored between 118 and 132, with the median at approximately 125. This means the total score ranges from 472 to 528, with the median at about 500. Why such peculiar numbers? The AAMC stresses that this scale emphasizes the importance of the central portion of the score distribution, where most students score (around 125 per section, or 500 total), rather than putting undue focus on the high end of the scale.

Note that there is no wrong answer penalty on the MCAT, so you should select an answer for every question—even if it is only a guess.

The AAMC has released the 2022–2024 correlation between scaled score and percentile, as shown on the following page. It should be noted that the percentile scale is adjusted and renormalized over time and thus can shift slightly from year to year. Percentile rank updates are released by the AAMC around May 1 of each year.

Total Score	Percentile	Total Score	Percentile
528	100	499	46
527	100	498	42
526	100	497	39
525	100	496	36
524	100	495	34
523	99	494	31
522	99	493	28
521	98	492	25
520	97	491	23
519	96	490	21
518	95	489	18
517	94	488	16
516	92	487	14
515	91	486	12
514	89	485	11
513	87	484	9
512	84	483	8
511	82	482	6
510	79	481	5
509	77	480	4
508	74	479	3
507	71	478	2
506	68	477	2
505	65	476	1
504	62	475	1
503	58	474	<1
502	55	473	<1
501	52	472	<1
500	49		

Source: AAMC. 2025. *Summary of MCAT Total and Section Scores*. Accessed October 2025.
https://students-residents.aamc.org/mcat-research-and-data/percentile-ranks-mcat-exam

Further information on score reporting is included at the end of the next section (see *After Your Test*).

MCAT Policies and Procedures

We strongly encourage you to download the latest copy of *MCAT® Essentials*, available on the AAMC's website, to ensure that you have the latest information about registration and Test Day policies and procedures; this document is updated annually. A brief summary of some of the most important rules is provided here.

MCAT Registration

The only way to register for the MCAT is online. You can access AAMC's registration system at **www.aamc.org/mcat**.

The AAMC posts the schedule of testing, registration, and score release dates in the fall before the MCAT testing year, which runs from January into September. See the AAMC's website for the exact dates that registration opens each year. There is one standard registration fee, but the fee for changing your test date or test center increases the closer you get to your MCAT.

Fees and the Fee Assistance Program (FAP)

Payment for test registration must be made by American Express, Discover, MasterCard, or VISA. As described earlier, the fee for rescheduling your exam or changing your testing center increases as one approaches Test Day. In addition, it is not uncommon for test centers to fill up well in advance of the registration deadline. For these reasons, we recommend identifying your preferred Test Day as soon as possible and registering. There are ancillary benefits to having a set Test Day, as well: when you know the date you're working toward, you'll study harder and are less likely to keep pushing back the exam. The AAMC offers a Fee Assistance Program (FAP) for students with financial hardship to help reduce the cost of taking the MCAT, as well as for the American Medical College Application Service (AMCAS®) application. Further information on the FAP can be found at **www.aamc.org/students/applying/fap**.

Testing Security

On Test Day, you will be required to present a qualifying form of ID. Generally, a current driver's license or United States passport will be sufficient (consult the AAMC website for the full list of qualifying criteria). When registering, take care to spell your first and last names (middle names, suffixes, and prefixes are not required and will not be verified on Test Day) precisely the same as they appear on this ID; failure to provide this ID at the test center or differences in spelling between your registration and ID will be considered a "no-show," and you will not receive a refund for the exam.

During Test Day registration, other identity data collected may include: a digital palm vein scan, a Test Day photo, a digitization of your valid ID, and signatures. Some testing centers may use a metal detection wand to ensure that no prohibited items are brought into the testing room. Prohibited items include all electronic devices, including watches and timers, calculators, cell phones, and any and all forms of recording equipment; food, drinks (including water), and cigarettes or other smoking paraphernalia; hats and scarves (except for religious purposes); and books, notes, or other study materials. If you require a medical device, such as an insulin pump or pacemaker, you must apply for accommodated testing. During breaks, you are allowed access to food and drink, but not to electronic devices, including cell phones.

Testing centers are under video surveillance and the AAMC does not take potential violations of testing security lightly. The bottom line: *know the rules and don't break them.*

Accommodations

Students with disabilities or medical conditions can apply for accommodated testing. Documentation of the disability or condition is required, and requests may take two months—or more—to be approved. For this reason, it is recommended that you begin the process of applying for accommodated testing as early as possible. More information on applying for accommodated testing can be found at **www.aamc.org/students/applying/mcat/accommodations**.

After Your Test

When your MCAT is all over, no matter how you feel you did, be good to yourself when you leave the test center. Celebrate! Take a nap. Watch a movie. Get some exercise. Plan a trip or outing. Call up all of your neglected friends or message them on social media. Go out for snacks or drinks with people you like. Whatever you do, make sure that it has absolutely nothing to do with thinking too hard—you deserve some rest and relaxation.

Perhaps most importantly, do not discuss specific details about the test with anyone. For one, it is important to let go of the stress of Test Day, and reliving your exam only inhibits you from being able to do so. But more significantly, the Examinee Agreement you sign at the beginning of your exam specifically prohibits you from discussing or disclosing exam content. The AAMC is known to seek out individuals who violate this agreement and retains the right to prosecute these individuals at their discretion. This means that you should not, under any circumstances, discuss the exam in person or over the phone with other individuals—including us at Kaplan—or post information or questions about exam content to Facebook, Student Doctor Network, or other online social media. You are permitted to comment on your "general exam experience," including how you felt about the exam overall or an individual section, but this is a fine line. In summary: *if you're not certain whether you can discuss an aspect of the test or not, just don't do it!* Do not let a silly Facebook post stop you from becoming the doctor you deserve to be.

Scores are typically released approximately one month after Test Day. The release is staggered during the afternoon and evening, ending at 5 p.m. Eastern. This means that not all examinees receive their scores at exactly the same time. Your score report will include a scaled score for each section between 118 and 132, as well as your total combined score between 472 and 528. These scores are given as confidence intervals. For each section, the confidence interval is approximately the given score ± 1; for the total score, it is approximately the given score ± 2. You will also be given the corresponding percentile rank for each of these section scores and the total score.

AAMC Contact Information

For further questions, contact the MCAT team at the Association of American Medical Colleges:

MCAT Resource Center
Association of American Medical Colleges
www.aamc.org/mcat
(202) 828-0600
www.aamc.org/contactmcat

HOW THIS BOOK WAS CREATED

The *Kaplan MCAT Review* project began shortly after the release of the *Preview Guide for the MCAT 2015 Exam*, 2nd edition. Through thorough analysis by our staff psychometricians, we were able to analyze the relative yield of the different topics on the MCAT, and we began constructing tables of contents for the books of the *Kaplan MCAT Review* series. A dedicated staff of 30 writers, 7 editors, and 32 proofreaders worked over 5,000 combined hours to produce these books. The format of the books was heavily influenced by weekly meetings with Kaplan's learning science team.

In the years since this book was created, a number of opportunities for expansion and improvement have occurred. This edition is the product of our largest revision since the series' creation more than a decade ago.

To better accommodate students who prefer learning visually, our six science titles have added more than 500 new images and updated more than a hundred existing figures. All of these new images were chosen by an expert team of MCAT faculty members, led by veteran teachers and tutors with advanced science or medical degrees. Our objective with these new images was not to add visual flair but to enhance student learning outcomes. Toward that end, our team of medical illustrators partnered with our MCAT experts to ensure scientific accuracy and relevance for the exam.

On top of this extensive science image expansion, we completely rewrote *Critical Analysis and Reasoning Skills Review* based on what we've learned from more than ten years of helping students improve on the CARS section in our classrooms. In addition to this collective experience, internal data suggests that our new approach is more effective at helping students get higher CARS scores. Our streamlined and simplified CARS strategies accompany an extended focus on the critical thinking skills tested on the exam, best embodied by our new Skillbuilder activities that enable targeted skill practice in a lower pressure setting.

These books were submitted for publication in January 2026. For any updates after this date, please visit www.kaptest.com/retail-book-corrections-and-updates.

If you have any questions about the content presented here, email KaplanMCATfeedback@kaplan.com. For other questions not related to content, email booksupport@kaplan.com.

Each book has been vetted through at least ten rounds of review. To that end, the information presented in these books is true and accurate to the best of our knowledge. Still, your feedback helps us improve our prep materials. Please notify us of any inaccuracies or errors in the books by sending an email to KaplanMCATfeedback@kaplan.com.

USING THIS BOOK

Kaplan MCAT Biochemistry Review, and the other six books in the *Kaplan MCAT Review* series, bring the Kaplan classroom experience to you—right in your home, at your convenience. This book offers the same Kaplan content review, strategies, and practice that make Kaplan the #1 choice for MCAT prep.

This book is designed to help you review the biochemistry topics covered on the MCAT. Please understand that content review—no matter how thorough—is not sufficient preparation for the MCAT! The MCAT tests not only your science knowledge but also your critical reading, reasoning, and problem-solving skills. Do not assume that simply memorizing the contents of this book will earn you high scores on Test Day; to maximize your scores, you must also improve your reading and test-taking skills through MCAT-style questions and practice tests.

Learning Objectives

At the beginning of each section, you'll find a short list of objectives describing the skills and strategies covered within that section. Learning objectives for these texts were developed in conjunction with Kaplan's learning science team, and have been designed specifically to focus your attention on tasks and concepts that are likely to show up on your MCAT. These learning objectives will function as a means to guide your study, and indicate what information and relationships you should be focused on within each section. Before starting each section, read these learning objectives carefully. They will not only allow you to assess your existing familiarity with the content, but also provide a goal-oriented focus for your studying experience of the section.

MCAT Concept Checks

At the end of each section, you'll find a few open-ended questions that you can use to assess your mastery of the material. These MCAT Concept Checks were introduced after numerous conversations with Kaplan's learning science team. Research has demonstrated repeatedly that introspection and self-analysis improve mastery, retention, and recall of material. Complete these MCAT Concept Checks to ensure that you've got the key points from each section before moving on!

Science Mastery Assessments

At the beginning of each chapter, you'll find 15 concept-focused multiple-choice questions. These are designed to help you assess your understanding of the chapter before you begin reading the chapter. Using the guidance provided with the assessment, you can determine the best way to review each chapter based on your personal strengths and weaknesses. Most of the questions in the Science Mastery Assessments focus on the first of the *Scientific Inquiry and Reasoning Skills* (*Knowledge of Scientific Concepts and Principles*), although there are occasional questions that fall into the second or fourth SIRS (*Scientific Reasoning and Problem-Solving* and *Data-Based and Statistical Reasoning*, respectively). You can complete each chapter's assessment in a testing interface in your online resources, where you'll also find a test-like passage set covering the same content you just studied to ensure you can also apply your knowledge the way the MCAT will expect you to!

Guided Examples with Expert Thinking

Embedded in each chapter of this book is a Guided Example with Expert Thinking. Each of these guided examples will be located in the same section as the content used in that example. Each example will feature an MCAT-level scientific article, that simulates an MCAT experiment passage. Read through the passage as you would on the real MCAT, referring to the Expert Thinking material to the right of the passage to clarify the key information you should be gathering from each paragraph. Read and attempt to answer the associated question once you have worked through the passage. There is a full explanation, including the correct answer, following the given question. These passages and questions are designed to help build your critical thinking, experimental reasoning, and data interpretation skills as preparation for the challenges you will face on the MCAT.

Sidebars

The following is a guide to the five types of sidebars you'll find in *Kaplan MCAT Biochemistry Review:*

- **Bridge:** These sidebars create connections between science topics that appear in multiple chapters throughout the *Kaplan MCAT Review* series.
- **Key Concept:** These sidebars draw attention to the most important takeaways in a given topic, and they sometimes offer synopses or overviews of complex information. If you understand nothing else, make sure you grasp the Key Concepts for any given subject.
- **MCAT Expertise:** These sidebars point out how information may be tested on the MCAT or offer key strategy points and test-taking tips that you should apply on Test Day.
- **Mnemonic:** These sidebars present memory devices to help recall certain facts.
- **Real World:** These sidebars illustrate how a concept in the text relates to the practice of medicine or the world at large. While this is not information you need to know for Test Day, many of the topics in Real World sidebars are excellent examples of how a concept may appear in a passage or discrete (stand-alone) question on the MCAT.

What This Book Covers

The information presented in the *Kaplan MCAT Review* series covers everything listed on the official MCAT content lists. Every topic in these lists is covered in the same level of detail as is common to the undergraduate and postbaccalaureate classes that are considered prerequisites for the MCAT. Note that your premedical classes may include topics not discussed in these books, or they may go into more depth than these books do. Additional exposure to science content is never a bad thing, but all of the content knowledge you are expected to have walking in on Test Day is covered in these books.

Chapter profiles, on the first page of each chapter, represent a holistic look at the content within the chapter, and will include a pie chart as well as text information. The pie chart analysis is based directly on data released by the AAMC, and will give a rough estimate of the importance of the chapter in relation to the book as a whole. Further, the text portion of the Chapter Profiles includes which AAMC content categories are covered within the chapter. These are referenced directly from the AAMC MCAT exam content listing, available on the testmaker's website.

You'll also see High-Yield badges scattered throughout the sections of this book:

In This Chapter

1.1 Amino Acids Found in Proteins High Yield

LEARNING OBJECTIVES

After Chapter 1.1, you will be able to:

These badges represent the top 100 topics most tested by the AAMC. In other words, according to the testmaker and all our experience with their resources, a High-Yield badge means more questions on Test Day.

This book also contains a thorough glossary and index for easy navigation of the text.

Additional guidance on how to use the different chapters of this book can be found in Chapter 1. In the end, this is your book, so write in the margins, draw diagrams, highlight the key points—do whatever is necessary to help you get that higher score. We look forward to working with you as you achieve your dreams and become the doctor you deserve to be!

Studying with This Book

In addition to providing you with the best practice questions and test strategies, Kaplan's team of learning scientists are dedicated to researching and testing the best methods for getting the most out of your study time. Here are their top four tips for improving retention:

Review multiple topics in one study session. This may seem counterintuitive—we're used to practicing one skill at a time in order to improve each skill. But research shows that weaving topics together leads to increased learning. Beyond that consideration, the MCAT often includes more than one topic in a single question. Studying in an integrated manner is the most effective way to prepare for this test.

Customize the content. Drawing attention to difficult or critical content can ensure you don't overlook it as you read and re-read sections. The best way to do this is to make it more visual—highlight, make tabs, use stickies, whatever works. We recommend highlighting only the most important or difficult sections of text. Selective highlighting of up to about 10% of text in a given chapter is great for emphasizing parts of the text, but over-highlighting can have the opposite effect.

Repeat topics over time. Many people try to memorize concepts by repeating them over and over again in succession. Our research shows that retention is improved by spacing out the repeats over time and mixing up the order in which you study content. For example, try reading chapters in a different order the second (or third!) time around. Revisit practice questions that you answered incorrectly in a new sequence. Perhaps information you reviewed more recently will help you better understand those questions and solutions you struggled with in the past.

Take a moment to reflect. When you finish reading a section for the first time, stop and think about what you just read. Jot down a few thoughts in the margins or in your notes about why the content is important or what topics came to mind when you read it. Associating learning with a memory is a fantastic way to retain information! This also works when answering questions. After answering a question, take a moment to think through each step you took to arrive at a solution. What led you to the answer you chose? Understanding the steps you took will help you make good decisions when answering future questions.

Online Resources

In addition to the resources located within this text, you also have online resources awaiting you. If you purchased this book as part of a 7-book set, scan the QR code that appears on your slipcase (the illustrated box that originally contained the books) and enter your unique access code, which appears on a sticker on the front of that slipcase. If you purchased this book separately, book-specific resources are available at **www.kaptest.com/booksonline**. Make sure to log on and take advantage of free practice and other resources!

Please note that access to the online resources is limited to the original owner of this book.

STUDYING FOR THE MCAT

The first year of medical school is a frenzied experience for most students. To meet the requirements of a rigorous work schedule, students either learn to prioritize their time or else fall hopelessly behind. It's no surprise, then, that the MCAT, the test specifically designed to predict success in medical school, is a high-speed, time-intensive test. The MCAT demands excellent time-management skills, endurance, and grace under pressure both during the test as well as while preparing for it. Having a solid plan of attack and sticking with it are key to giving you the confidence and structure you need to succeed.

Creating a Study Plan

The best time to create a study plan is at the beginning of your MCAT preparation. If you don't already use a calendar, you will want to start. You can purchase a planner, print out a free calendar from the Internet, use a built-in calendar or app on one of your smart devices, or keep track using an interactive online calendar. Pick the option that is most practical for you and that you are most likely to use consistently. If you purchased this book new as part of a set, your online resources come with a study plan to space out your readings, chapter quizzes, full-length practice tests, and other study materials (see the previous page for how to log on).

Once you have a calendar, you'll be able to start planning your study schedule with the following steps:

1. **Fill in your obligations and choose a day off.**

   Write in all your school, extracurricular, and work obligations first: class sessions, work shifts, and meetings that you must attend. Then add in your personal obligations: appointments, lunch dates, family and social time, etc. Making an appointment in your calendar for hanging out with friends or going to the movies may seem strange at first, but planning social activities in advance will help you achieve a balance between personal and professional obligations even as life gets busy. Having a happy balance allows you to be more focused and productive when it comes time to study, so stay well-rounded and don't neglect anything that is important to you.

   In addition to scheduling your personal and professional obligations, you should also plan your time off. Taking some time off is just as important as studying. Kaplan recommends taking at least one full day off per week, ideally from all your study obligations but at minimum from studying for the MCAT.

2. **Add in study blocks around your obligations.**

   Once you have established your calendar's framework, add in study blocks around your obligations, keeping your study schedule as consistent as possible across days and across weeks. Studying at the same time of day as your official test is ideal for promoting recall, but if that's not possible, then fit in study blocks wherever you can.

   To make your studying as efficient as possible, block out short, frequent periods of study time throughout the week. From a learning perspective, studying one hour per day for six days per week is much more valuable than studying for six hours all at once one day per week. Specifically, Kaplan recommends studying for no longer than three hours in one sitting. Within those three-hour blocks, also plan to take ten-minute breaks every hour. Use these breaks to get up from your seat, do some quick stretches, get a snack and drink, and clear your mind. Although ten minutes of break for every 50 minutes of studying may sound like a lot, these breaks will allow you to deal with distractions and rest your brain so that, during the 50-minute study blocks, you can remain fully engaged and completely focused.

3. **Add in your full-length practice tests.**

   Next, you'll want to add in full-length practice tests. You'll want to take one test very early in your prep and then spread your remaining full-length practice tests evenly between now and your test date. Staggering tests in this way allows you to form a baseline for comparison and to determine which areas to focus on right away, while also providing realistic feedback throughout your prep as to how you will perform on Test Day.

When planning your calendar, aim to finish your full-length practice tests and the majority of your studying by one week before Test Day, which will allow you to spend that final week completing a brief review of what you already know. In your online resources, you'll find a sample study calendar to use as a starting point. This sample calendar may include more focus than you need in some areas, and less in others, and it may not fit your timeline to Test Day. You will need to customize your study calendar to your needs using the steps above.

The total amount of time you spend studying each week will depend on your schedule, your personal prep needs, and your time to Test Day, but it is recommended that you spend somewhere in the range of 300–350 hours preparing before taking the official MCAT. One way you could break this down is to study for three hours per day, six days per week, for four months, but this is just one approach. You might study six days per week for more than three hours per day. You might study over a longer period of time if you don't have much time to study each week. No matter what your plan is, ensure you complete enough practice to feel completely comfortable with the MCAT and its content. A good sign you're ready for Test Day is when you begin to earn your goal score consistently in practice.

How to Study

The MCAT covers a large amount of material, so studying for Test Day can initially seem daunting. To combat this we have some tips for how to take control of your studying and make the most of your time.

Goal Setting

To take control of the amount of content and practice required to do well on the MCAT, break the content down into specific goals for each week instead of attempting to approach the test as a whole. A goal of "I want to increase my overall score by 5 points" is too big, abstract, and difficult to measure on the small scale. More reasonable goals are "I will read two chapters each day this week." Goals like this are much less overwhelming and help break studying into manageable pieces.

Active Reading

As you go through this book, much of the information will be familiar to you. After all, you have probably seen most of the content before. However, be very careful: Familiarity with a subject does not necessarily translate to knowledge or mastery of that subject. Do not assume that if you recognize a concept you actually know it and can apply it quickly at an appropriate level. Don't just passively read this book. Instead, read actively. Highlighting can be an excellent tool, but use it sparingly: highlighting every sentence isn't active reading, it's coloring. Frequently stop and ask yourself questions while you read (e.g., *What is the main point? How does this fit into the overall scheme of things? Could I thoroughly explain this to someone else?*). By making connections and focusing on the grander scheme, not only will you ensure you know the essential content, but you also prepare yourself for the level of critical thinking required by the MCAT.

Focus on Areas of Greatest Opportunity

If you are limited by only having a minimal amount of time to prepare before Test Day, focus on your biggest areas of opportunity first. Areas of opportunity are topic areas that are highly tested and that you have not yet mastered. You likely won't have time to take detailed notes for every page of these books; instead, use your results from practice materials to determine which areas are your biggest opportunities and seek those out. After you've taken a full-length test, make sure you are using your performance report to best identify areas of opportunity. Skim over content matter for which you are already demonstrating proficiency, pausing to read more thoroughly when something looks unfamiliar or particularly difficult. Begin with the Science Mastery Assessment at the beginning of each chapter. If you can get all of those questions correct within a reasonable amount of time, you may be able to quickly skim through that chapter, but if the questions prove to be more difficult, then you may need to spend time reading the chapter or certain subsections of the chapter more thoroughly.

Practice, Review, and Tracking

Leave time to review your practice questions and full-length tests. You may be tempted, after practicing, to push ahead and cover new material as quickly as possible, but failing to schedule ample time for review will actually throw away your greatest opportunity to improve your performance. The brain rarely remembers anything it sees or does only once. When you carefully review the questions you've solved (and the explanations for them), the process of retrieving that information reopens and reinforces the connections you've built in your brain. This builds long-term retention and repeatable skill sets—exactly what you need to beat the MCAT!

One useful tool for making the most of your review is the How I'll Fix It (HIFI) sheet. You can create a HIFI sheet, such as the sample below, to track questions throughout your prep that you miss or have to guess on. For each such question, figure out why you missed it and supply at least one action step for how you can avoid similar mistakes in the future. As you move through your MCAT prep, adjust your study plan based on your available study time and the results of your review. Your strengths and weaknesses are likely to change over the course of your prep. Keep addressing the areas that are most important to your score, shifting your focus as those areas change.

Section	Q #	Topic or skill	Why I missed it	How I'll fix it
Chem/Phys	*42*	*Nuclear chem.*	*Confused electron absorption and emission*	*Reread Physics Chapter 9.2*
Chem/Phys	*47*	K_{eq}	*Didn't know right equation*	*Memorize equation for* K_{eq}
CARS	*2*	*Paraphrase Detail*	*Didn't read "not" in answer choice*	*Slow down when finding match*
CARS	*4*	*Make Deduction*	*Forgot to research answer*	*Reread passage and predict first*

Where to Study

One often-overlooked aspect of studying is the environment where the learning actually occurs. Although studying at home is many students' first choice, several problems can arise in this environment, chief of which are distractions. Studying can be a mentally draining process, so as time passes, these distractions become ever more tempting as escape routes. Although you may have considerable willpower, there's no reason to make staying focused harder than it needs to be. Instead of studying at home, head to a library, quiet coffee shop, or another new location whenever possible. This will eliminate many of the usual distractions and also promote efficient studying; instead of studying off and on at home over the course of an entire day, you can stay at the library for three hours of effective studying and enjoy the rest of the day off from the MCAT.

No matter where you study, make your practice as much like Test Day as possible. Just as is required during the official test, don't have snacks or chew gum during your study blocks. Turn off your music, television, and phone. Practice on the computer with your online resources to simulate the computer-based test environment. When completing practice questions, do your work on scratch paper or noteboard sheets rather than writing directly on any printed materials since you won't have that option on Test Day. Because memory is tied to all of your senses, the more test-like you can make your studying environment, the easier it will be on Test Day to recall the information you're putting in so much work to learn.

CHAPTER 1

AMINO ACIDS, PEPTIDES, AND PROTEINS

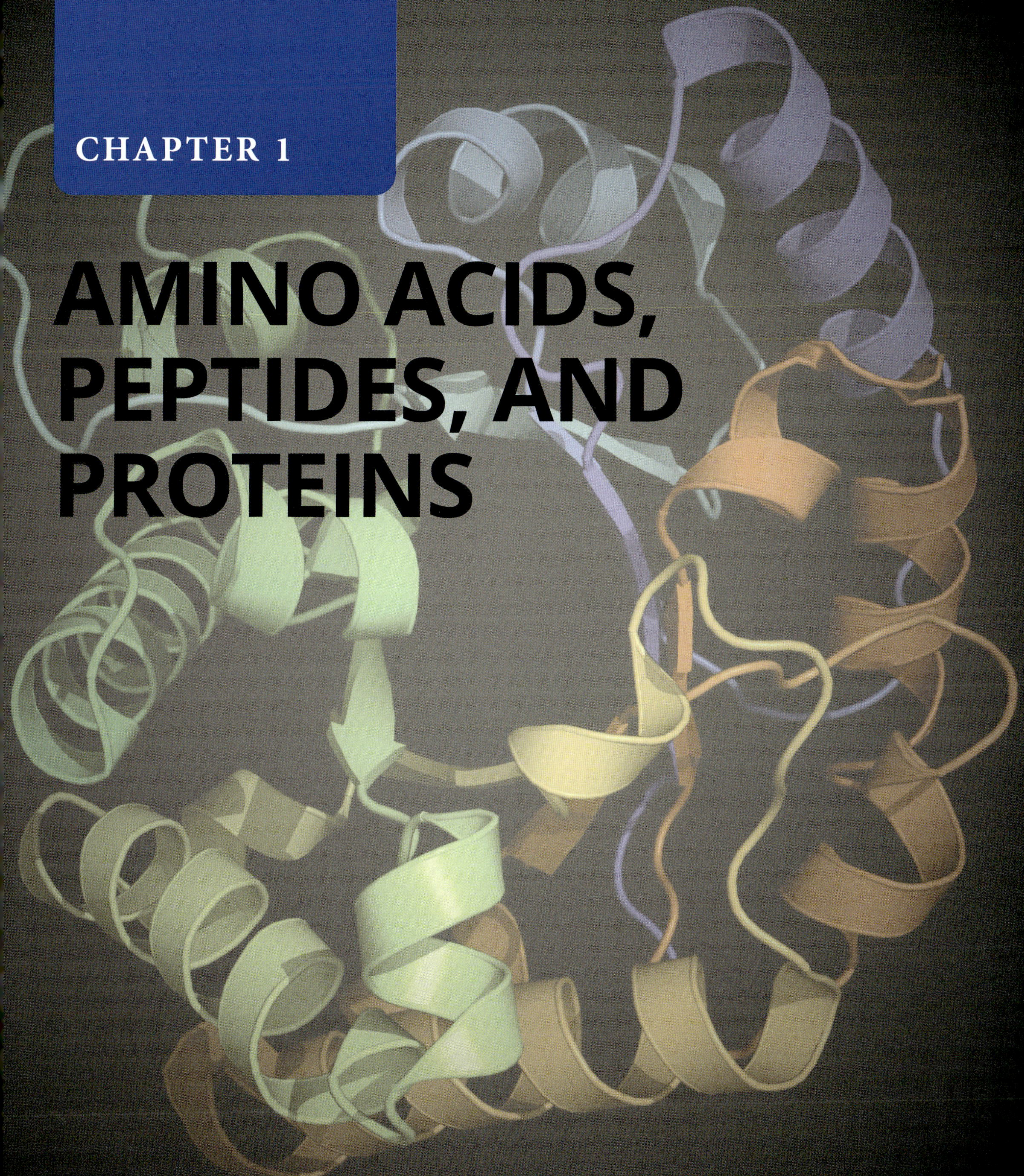

SCIENCE MASTERY ASSESSMENT

Every pre-med knows this feeling: there is so much content I have to know for the MCAT! How do I know what to do first or what's important?

While the high-yield badges throughout this book will help you identify the most important topics, this Science Mastery Assessment is another tool in your MCAT prep arsenal. This quiz (which can also be taken in your online resources) and the guidance below will help ensure that you are spending the appropriate amount of time on this chapter based on your personal strengths and weaknesses. Don't worry though—skipping something now does not mean you'll never study it. Later on in your prep, as you complete full-length tests, you'll uncover specific pieces of content that you need to review and can come back to these chapters as appropriate.

How to Use This Assessment

If you answer 0–7 questions correctly:

Spend about 1 hour to read this chapter in full and take limited notes throughout. Follow up by reviewing **all** quiz questions to ensure that you now understand how to solve each one.

If you answer 8–11 questions correctly:

Spend 20–40 minutes reviewing the quiz questions. Beginning with the questions you missed, read and take notes on the corresponding subchapters. For questions you answered correctly, ensure your thinking matches that of the explanation and you understand why each choice was correct or incorrect.

If you answer 12–15 questions correctly:

Spend less than 20 minutes reviewing all questions from the quiz. If you missed any, then include a quick read-through of the corresponding subchapters, or even just the relevant content within a subchapter, as part of your question review. For questions you got correct, ensure your thinking matches that of the explanation and review the Concept Summary at the end of the chapter.

1. In a neutral solution, most amino acids exist as:
   - **A.** positively charged compounds.
   - **B.** zwitterions.
   - **C.** negatively charged compounds.
   - **D.** hydrophobic molecules.

2. At pH 7, the charge on a glutamic acid molecule is:
   - **A.** -2.
   - **B.** -1.
   - **C.** 0.
   - **D.** $+1$.

3. Which of the following statements is most likely to be true of nonpolar R groups in aqueous solution?
   - **A.** They are hydrophilic and found buried within proteins.
   - **B.** They are hydrophilic and found on protein surfaces.
   - **C.** They are hydrophobic and found buried within proteins.
   - **D.** They are hydrophobic and found on protein surfaces.

4. Scientists discover a cDNA sequence for an uncharacterized protein. In their initial studies, they use a computer program designed to predict protein structure. Which of the following levels of protein structure can be most accurately predicted?
   - **A.** Primary structure
   - **B.** Secondary structure
   - **C.** Tertiary structure
   - **D.** Quaternary structure

5. How many distinct tripeptides can be formed from one valine molecule, one alanine molecule, and one leucine molecule?
   - **A.** 1
   - **B.** 3
   - **C.** 6
   - **D.** 27

6. Which of the following best describes the change in entropy that occurs during protein folding?
   - **A.** Entropy of both the water and the protein increase.
   - **B.** Entropy of the water increases; entropy of the protein decreases.
   - **C.** Entropy of the water decreases; entropy of the protein increases.
   - **D.** Entropy of both the water and the protein decrease.

7. An α-helix is most likely to be held together by:
   - **A.** disulfide bonds.
   - **B.** hydrophobic effects.
   - **C.** hydrogen bonds.
   - **D.** ionic attractions between side chains.

8. Which of the following is least likely to cause denaturation of proteins?
   - **A.** Heating the protein to 100°C
   - **B.** Adding 8 M urea
   - **C.** Moving it to a more hypotonic environment
   - **D.** Adding a detergent such as sodium dodecyl sulfate

9. A particular α-helix is known to cross the cell membrane. Which of these amino acids is most likely to be found in the transmembrane portion of the helix?
   - **A.** Glutamate
   - **B.** Lysine
   - **C.** Phenylalanine
   - **D.** Aspartate

10. Which of these amino acids has a chiral carbon in its side chain?

I. Serine

II. Threonine

III. Isoleucine

A. I only
B. II only
C. II and III only
D. I, II, and III

11. Following translation and folding, many receptor tyrosine kinases exist as monomers in their inactive state on the cell membrane. Upon the binding of a ligand, these proteins dimerize and initiate a signaling cascade. During this process, their highest element of protein structure changes from:

A. secondary to tertiary.
B. tertiary to quaternary.
C. primary to secondary.
D. secondary to quaternary.

12. Which of these amino acids has a side chain that can become ionized in cells?

A. Histidine
B. Leucine
C. Proline
D. Threonine

13. In lysine, the pK_a of the side chain is about 10.5. Assuming that the pK_a of the carboxyl and amino groups are 2 and 9, respectively, the pI of lysine is closest to:

A. 5.5.
B. 6.2.
C. 7.4.
D. 9.8.

14. Which of the following is a reason for conjugating proteins?

I. To direct their delivery to a particular organelle

II. To direct their delivery to the cell membrane

III. To add a cofactor needed for their activity

A. I only
B. II only
C. II and III only
D. I, II, and III

15. Collagen consists of three helices with carbon backbones that are tightly wrapped around one another in a “triple helix.” Which of these amino acids is most likely to be found in the highest concentration in collagen?

A. Proline
B. Glycine
C. Threonine
D. Cysteine

Answer Key

1. **B** (See section 1.1)
2. **B** (See section 1.2)
3. **C** (See section 1.1)
4. **A** (See section 1.4)
5. **C** (See section 1.3)
6. **B** (See section 1.5)
7. **C** (See section 1.4)
8. **C** (See section 1.6)
9. **C** (See section 1.1)
10. **C** (See section 1.1)
11. **B** (See section 1.5)
12. **A** (See section 1.1)
13. **D** (See section 1.2)
14. **D** (See section 1.3)
15. **B** (See section 1.1)

The relevant section of the chapter to review for each question is given in parentheses after the correct answer. Detailed explanations can be found at the end of the chapter.

CHAPTER 1

AMINO ACIDS, PEPTIDES, AND PROTEINS

In This Chapter

Introduction

How important are amino acids? Consider sickle cell disease. People with sickle cell disease have red blood cells that, under certain conditions, can become rigid and sickle-shaped. Those sickle-shaped cells can become stuck in capillaries, blocking them. In severe cases, it can block enough of the blood supply to cause damage to several organs, such as the kidneys, liver, and spleen. This happens because of a mutation in hemoglobin, the protein in red blood cells that transports oxygen. Remarkably, the difference between the normal form of hemoglobin, HbA, and the one that causes sickle cell disease, HbS, is a seemingly minor one. All it takes is a change in a single amino acid on the surface of hemoglobin: the sixth amino acid in two of its four chains is changed from glutamic acid to valine. That minor difference allows the deoxygenated form of HbS to aggregate and precipitate, which leads to the sickled shape—and all the symptoms—of sickle cell disease.

In this chapter, we'll take a look at the basics of proteins by focusing on the amino acids that compose them and how those amino acids contribute to the physical and chemical properties of proteins.

CHAPTER PROFILE

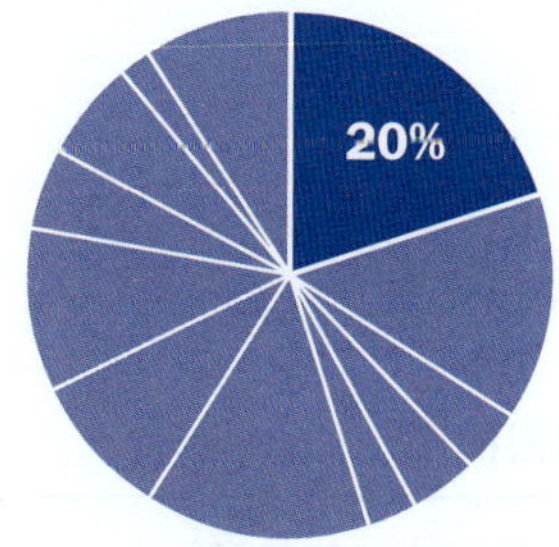

The content in this chapter should be relevant to about 20% of all questions about biochemistry on the MCAT.

This chapter covers material from the following AAMC content categories:

1A: Structure and function of proteins and their constituent amino acids

5D: Structure, function, and reactivity of biologically-relevant molecules

MCAT EXPERTISE

This chapter represents a whopping 20% of all biochemistry questions you will see on Test Day. That makes amino acids one of the highest yield subjects within any of the review books! Make sure to work sufficient study of these materials into your study plan.

1.1 Amino Acids Found in Proteins High Yield

MCAT EXPERTISE

The "High-Yield" badge on this section indicates that the content is frequently tested on the MCAT.

LEARNING OBJECTIVES

After Chapter 1.1, you will be able to:

- Recognize common abbreviations for amino acids, such as Glu and Y
- Distinguish the stereochemistries, typical cellular locations, and reactivities of the 20 major amino acids
- Identify the major amino acids, such as:

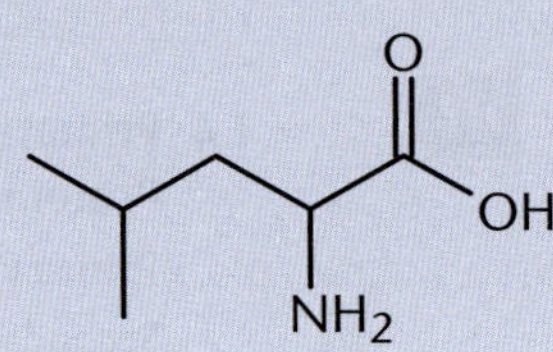

BRIDGE

Remember that for carboxylic acids, the α-carbon is the carbon *adjacent* to the carboxyl carbon. The structure and nomenclature of carboxylic acids are discussed in Chapter 8 of *MCAT Organic Chemistry Review*.

Amino acids are molecules that contain two functional groups: an amino group ($-NH_2$) and a carboxyl group ($-COOH$). In this chapter, we'll focus specifically on the α-amino acids, in which the amino group and the carboxyl group are bonded to the same carbon, the α-carbon of the carboxylic acid. Think of the α-carbon as the central carbon of the amino acid, as shown in Figure 1.1.

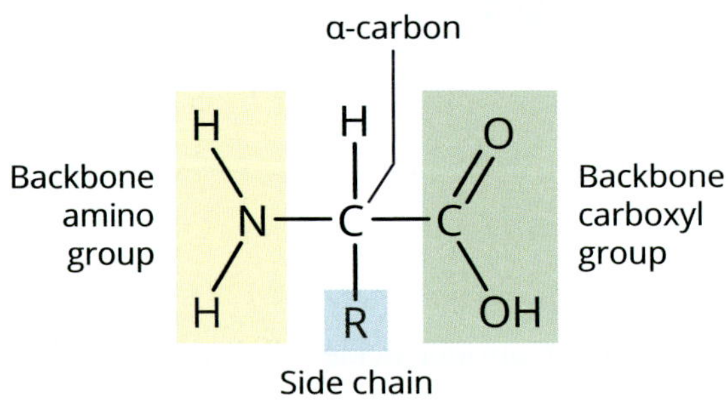

Figure 1.1 Amino Acid Structure

KEY CONCEPT

The side chains (R groups) of amino acids determine their chemical properties.

In addition to the amino and carboxyl groups, the α-carbon has two other groups attached to it: a hydrogen atom and a **side chain**, also called an **R group**, which is specific to each amino acid. The side chains determine the properties of amino acids, and therefore their functions.

A Note on Terminology

MCAT EXPERTISE

While the MCAT *could* include passages on GABA or other nonstandard amino acids, they are *not* part of the background information you're expected to know for Test Day.

Amino acids do not *need* to have both the amino and carboxyl groups bonded to the same carbon. For example, the neurotransmitter γ-*aminobutyric acid* (GABA) has the amino group on the gamma (γ) carbon, *three* carbons away from the carboxyl group, as shown in Figure 1.2. Similarly, not every amino acid found in the human body is specified by a codon in the genetic code or incorporated into proteins. One example is *ornithine*, one of the intermediates in the urea cycle, the metabolic process by which the body excretes excess nitrogen. There are also some amino acids that are specifically modified for specialized roles in the body; for example, lysine is sometimes converted into pyrrolysine.

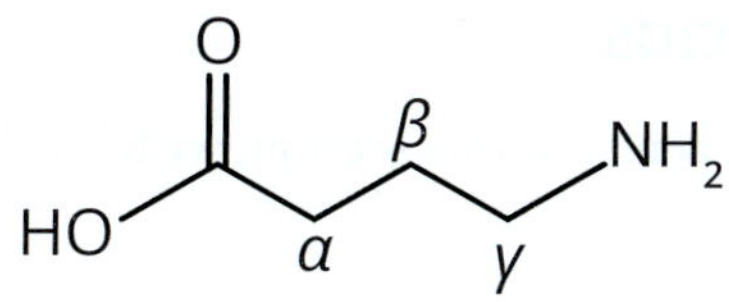

Figure 1.2 GABA

That said, the Association of American Medical Colleges (AAMC) has specifically stated they'll focus on the 20 α-amino acids encoded by the human genetic code, also called **proteinogenic amino acids**. So, for the rest of this chapter, we'll use the term *amino acid* to refer specifically to these compounds.

Stereochemistry of Amino Acids

For most amino acids, the α-carbon is a chiral (or stereogenic) center, as it has four different groups attached to it. Thus, most amino acids are optically active. The one exception is **glycine**, which has a hydrogen atom as its R group, making it achiral, as shown in Figure 1.3.

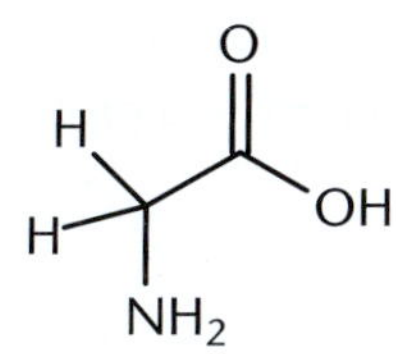

Figure 1.3 Glycine

All chiral amino acids used in eukaryotes are L-amino acids, so the amino group is drawn on the left in a Fischer projection, as demonstrated in Figure 1.4.

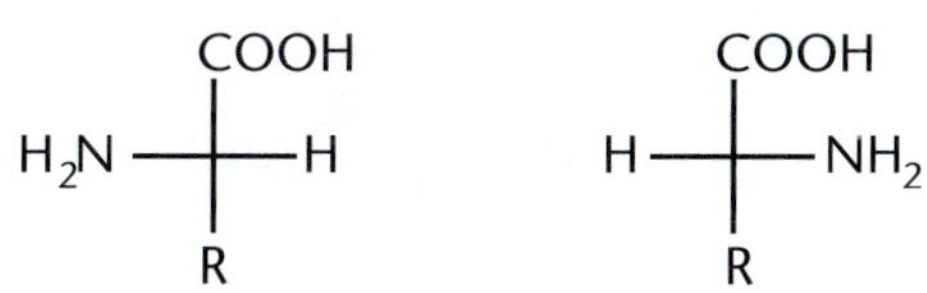

L-amino acid   D-amino acid

Figure 1.4 L- and D-Amino Acids

In the Cahn–Ingold–Prelog system, this translates to an (*S*) absolute configuration for almost all chiral amino acids. The only exception is **cysteine**, which, while still being an L-amino acid, has an (*R*) absolute configuration, as shown in Figure 1.5, because the $-CH_2SH$ group has priority over the $-COOH$ group.

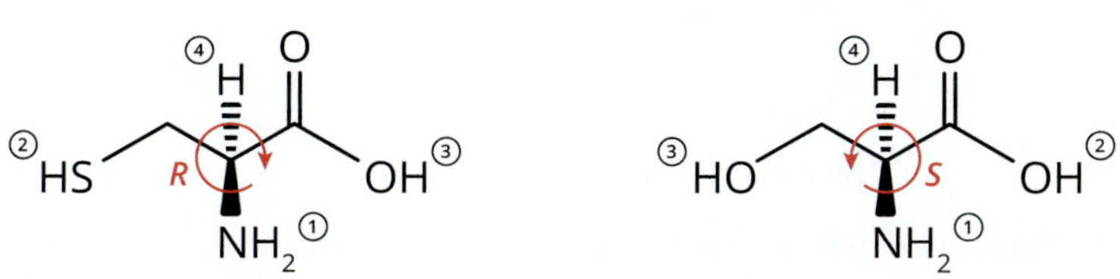

L-(*R*)-cysteine   L-(*S*)-serine

Figure 1.5 Cysteine Has an (*R*) Absolute Configuration

KEY CONCEPT

Except for glycine, all amino acids are chiral—and except for cysteine, all of them have an (*S*) absolute configuration.

REAL WORLD

While L-amino acids are the only ones found in eukaryotic proteins, D-amino acids do exist. One example is *gramicidin*, an antibiotic produced by a soil bacterium called *Bacillus brevis*, in which D- and L-amino acids alternate in the primary structure.

Structures of the Amino Acids

There are several ways to classify amino acids. In this section, we'll break them down by the structures of their side chains.

Nonpolar, Nonaromatic Side Chains

Seven amino acids, shown in Figure 1.6(a), fall into this class. **Glycine**, discussed earlier, has a single hydrogen atom as its side chain and is therefore achiral. It is also the smallest amino acid. Four other amino acids—**alanine**, **valine**, **leucine**, and **isoleucine**—have alkyl side chains containing one to four carbons.

Methionine is one of only two amino acids that contains a sulfur atom in its side chain. Nevertheless, because the sulfur has a methyl group attached, it is considered relatively nonpolar.

Finally, **proline** is unique in that it forms a *cyclic* amino acid. In all the other amino acids, the amino group is attached *only* to the α-carbon. In proline, however, the amino nitrogen becomes a part of the side chain, forming a five-membered ring. That ring places notable constraints on the flexibility of proline, which limits where it can appear in a protein and can have significant effects on proline's role in secondary structure.

MCAT EXPERTISE

The AAMC's practice materials have made it clear that test takers are expected to know the structures, names, and three-letter and one-letter abbreviations for the amino acids.

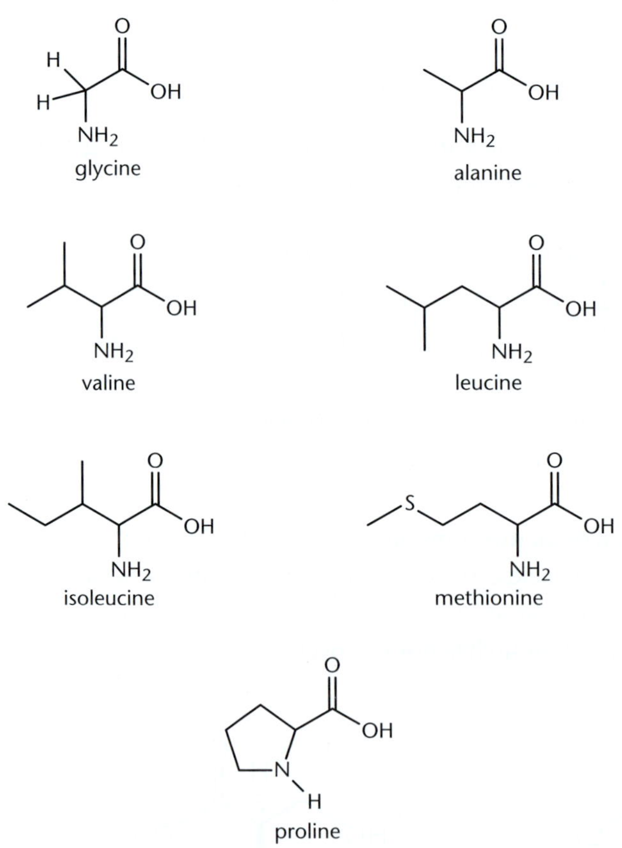

Figure 1.6(a) Amino Acids with Nonpolar, Nonaromatic Side Chains

Aromatic Side Chains

Three amino acids have uncharged aromatic side chains and are depicted in Figure 1.6(b). The largest of these is **tryptophan**, which has a double-ring heterocyclic system called an **indole** that contains a nitrogen atom. The smallest is **phenylalanine**, which has a benzyl side chain (a benzene ring plus a $-CH_2-$ group). Adding an $-OH$ group to phenylalanine gives the third member, **tyrosine**. The $-OH$ group makes tyrosine relatively polar compared to phenylalanine, though still net nonpolar.

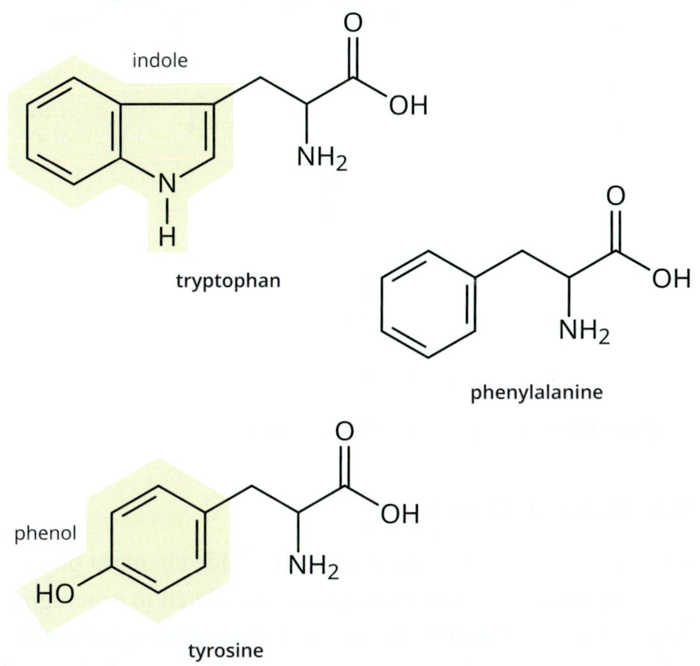

Figure 1.6(b) Amino Acids with Aromatic Side Chains

MCAT EXPERTISE

The MCAT writers strive to avoid misuse of terminology. Some textbooks problematically describe proline as an *imino* acid because the amino nitrogen forms two bonds to carbon. The MCAT won't use this term because an *imine* is specifically a molecule with a carbon–nitrogen double bond.

Polar Side Chains

Five amino acids, shown in Figure 1.6(c), have side chains that are polar but not aromatic. **Serine** and **threonine** both have $-OH$ groups in their side chains, which makes them highly polar and able to participate in hydrogen bonding. **Asparagine** and **glutamine** have amide side chains. Unlike the amino group common to all amino acids, the amide nitrogens do *not* gain or lose protons with changes in pH; they do not become charged.

The last amino acid with a polar side chain is **cysteine**, which has a **thiol** ($-SH$) group in its side chain. Because sulfur is larger than oxygen, the S$-$H bond is longer and weaker than the O$-$H bond. In addition, sulfur is less electronegative than oxygen. This leaves the thiol group in cysteine prone to oxidation, a reaction we'll study later in this chapter.

BRIDGE

Make sure you know your carboxylic acid derivatives for Test Day! They are discussed in Chapter 9 of *MCAT Organic Chemistry Review*.

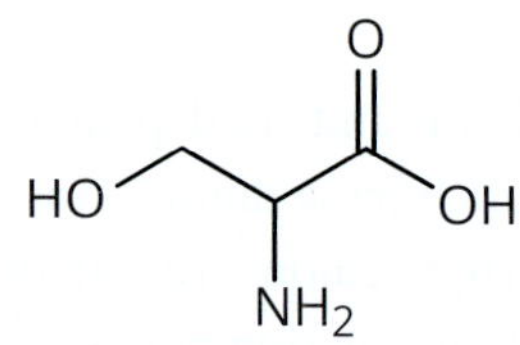

serine

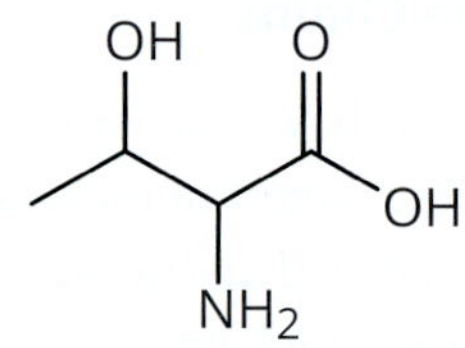

threonine

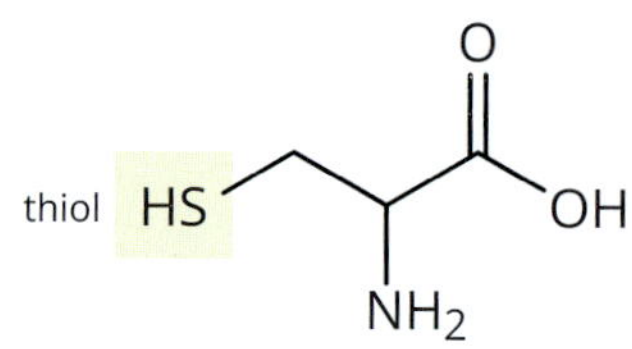

cysteine

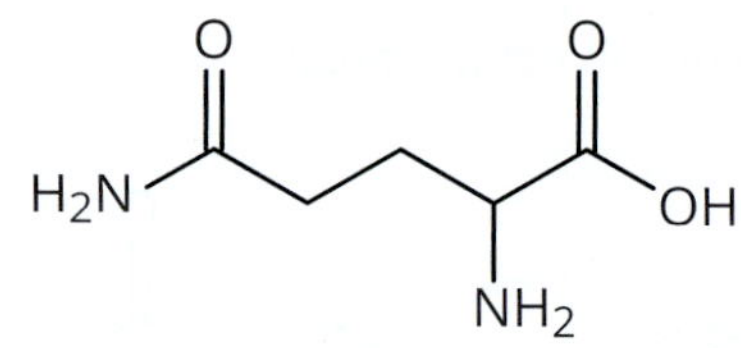

glutamine

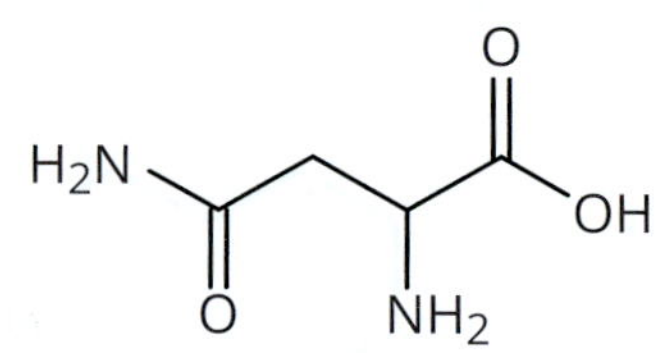

asparagine

Figure 1.6(c) Amino Acids with Polar Side Chains

Negatively Charged (Acidic) Side Chains

Only two of the 20 amino acids have negative charges on their side chains at physiological pH (7.4). Those two are **aspartic acid (aspartate)**, which is related to asparagine, and **glutamic acid (glutamate)**, which is related to glutamine. Unlike asparagine and glutamine, aspartate and glutamate have carboxylate ($-COO^-$) groups in their side chains, rather than amides. Note that aspartate is simply the deprotonated form of aspartic acid, and glutamate is the deprotonated form of glutamic acid. These two amino acids are depicted in Figure 1.6(d).

MCAT EXPERTISE

On the MCAT, you're likely to see anion names (aspartate and glutamate) instead of acid names (aspartic acid and glutamic acid) because most acids in cells exist in the deprotonated form. This also applies to molecules other than amino acids (*malate* instead of *malic acid*).

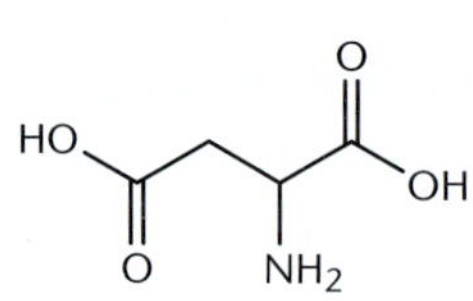

aspartic acid

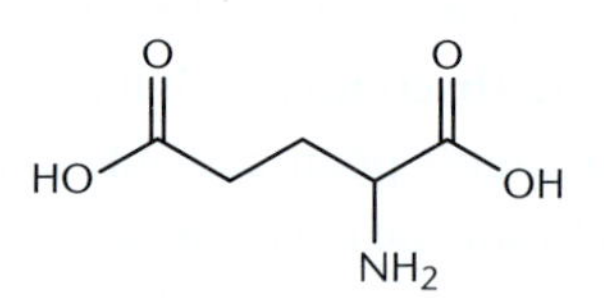

glutamic acid

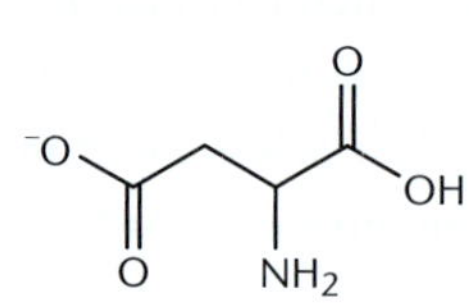

(anion is aspartate)

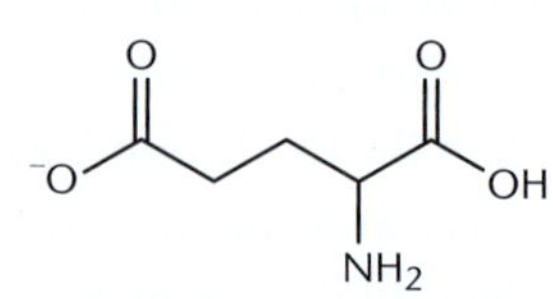

(anion is glutamate)

Figure 1.6(d) Amino Acids with Negatively Charged Side Chains

Positively Charged (Basic) Side Chains

The remaining three amino acids, shown in Figure 1.6(e), have side chains that have positively charged nitrogen atoms. **Lysine** has a terminal primary amino group, while **arginine** has three nitrogen atoms in its side chain, forming a **guanidine**; the positive charge is delocalized over all three nitrogen atoms. The final amino acid, **histidine**, has an aromatic ring with two nitrogen atoms (this ring is called an **imidazole**). You might be wondering how histidine can acquire a positive charge. The pK_a of the side chain is relatively close to 7.4—it's about 6—so, at physiologic pH, one nitrogen atom is protonated and the other isn't. Under more acidic conditions, the second nitrogen atom can become protonated, giving the side chain a positive charge.

BRIDGE

The catalytic triad found in *chymotrypsin* makes use of the histidine side chain's ability to gain a proton. The histidine residue in its active site removes a proton from the –OH group of a serine residue side chain, which facilitates nucleophilic attack by the serine residue on the carbonyl carbon atom of the substrate. Chymotrypsin's role as a digestive enzyme is discussed in Chapter 9 of *MCAT Biology Review*.

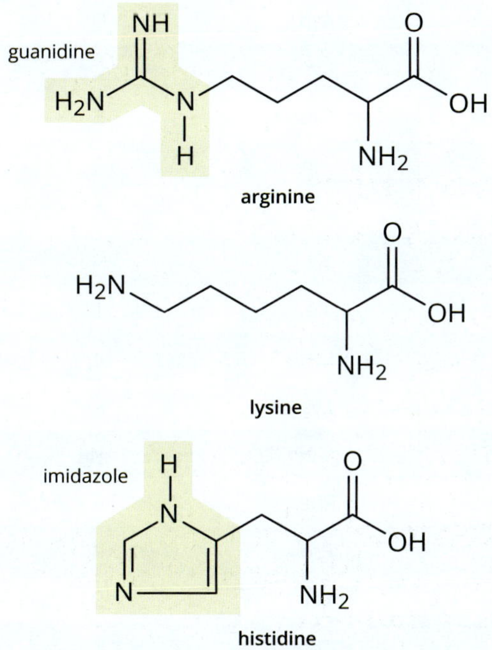

Figure 1.6(e) Amino Acids with Positively Charged Side Chains

Hydrophobic and Hydrophilic Amino Acids

Classifying amino acid side chains as hydrophobic or hydrophilic is actually a very complex matter. For example, tyrosine has both an –OH group and an aromatic ring—so which one "wins"?

A few clear conclusions can be drawn, though. First, the amino acids with long alkyl side chains—alanine, isoleucine, leucine, valine, and phenylalanine—are all strongly hydrophobic and thus more likely to be found in the interior of proteins, away from water on the surface of the protein. Second, all the amino acids with charged side chains—positively charged histidine, arginine, and lysine, plus negatively charged glutamate and aspartate—are hydrophilic, as are the amides asparagine and glutamine. The remaining amino acids lie somewhere in the middle and are neither particularly hydrophilic nor particularly hydrophobic.

KEY CONCEPT

The surface of a protein tends to be rich in amino acids with charged side chains. Strongly hydrophobic amino acids tend to be found in the interior of proteins.

Amino Acid Abbreviations

Now that we have explored the structures of the 20 proteinogenic amino acids, it is worth mentioning that you are expected to be able to identify an amino acid on the MCAT not only by name, but also by its three-letter and one-letter abbreviations. These abbreviations are listed in Table 1.1.

MCAT EXPERTISE

It bears repeating: the structures and abbreviations (both three- and one-letter) have been tested *heavily* on both natural science sections of the MCAT. Make sure you know this page by heart!

AMINO ACID	THREE-LETTER ABBREVIATION	ONE-LETTER ABBREVIATION
Alanine	Ala	A
Arginine	Arg	R
Asparagine	Asn	N
Aspartic acid	Asp	D
Cysteine	Cys	C
Glutamic acid	Glu	E
Glutamine	Gln	Q
Glycine	Gly	G
Histidine	His	H
Isoleucine	Ile	I
Leucine	Leu	L
Lysine	Lys	K
Methionine	Met	M
Phenylalanine	Phe	F
Proline	Pro	P
Serine	Ser	S
Threonine	Thr	T
Tryptophan	Trp	W
Tyrosine	Tyr	Y
Valine	Val	V

Table 1.1 Three- and One-Letter Abbreviations of Amino Acids

Mutagenesis

Mutagenesis describes the process by which mutations are deliberately introduced into a DNA sequence in order to produce a mutant gene or protein. Mutagenesis is commonly used by researchers interested in determining the function of specific amino acids within proteins or of specific nucleotides within DNA or RNA, where the specific sites are mutated to see if the mutation disrupts normal protein or nucleotide function. For instance, a researcher interested in determining if certain amino acids within a protein are phosphorylated may generate mutant proteins that contain alanine mutations (which are not amino acids that undergo phosphorylation) at the putative phosphorylation sites. The researcher can then compare the levels of phosphorylation in the wild-type protein to the mutated proteins. If one of the amino acids that was mutated to an alanine originally was phosphorylated, levels of phosphorylation would be expected to decrease on the mutant protein compared to the wild-type protein. However, if the amino acid that was mutated was never phosphorylated to begin with, there would be no change in the levels of phosphorylation, indicating that amino acid is not a phosphorylation site. Alternatively, to mimic the effects of constitutive phosphorylation, a target amino acid can be mutated to a negatively charged residue like glutamate (E) or aspartate (D), whose side chain imitates the negative charge of the phosphate group.

A mainstay of mutagenesis is **site-directed mutagenesis**, which is a method used to introduce specific mutations into DNA. First, DNA primers are synthesized that contain the mutation of interest. Surrounding the site of mutation are sequences complementary to the template DNA. The primers are then used to introduce the mutation into each newly-synthesized DNA molecule.

As shown in the preceding table, each amino acid has a one-letter code. This one-letter code is commonly used as a shorthand to denote single amino acid mutations: The original amino acid is listed first, which is then followed by a number denoting the position of the mutated amino acid in the primary sequence relative to the N-terminus, before ending with a second letter that denotes the substituted amino acid. For example, S46A indicates that the 46th amino acid, which was originally a serine (S), has been mutated to an alanine (A). This type of shorthand will show up on not just one, but all three, of the science sections of the MCAT on Test Day.

BRIDGE

Solutions to concept checks for a given chapter in *MCAT Biochemistry Review* can be found near the end of the chapter in which the concept check is located, following the Concept Summary for that chapter.

MCAT CONCEPT CHECK 1.1

Before you move on, assess your understanding of the material with these questions.

1. What are the four groups attached to the central (α) carbon of a proteinogenic amino acid?

____

2. What is the stereochemistry of the chiral amino acids that appear in eukaryotic proteins?
   - L or D?
   - (*R*) or (*S*)? (Exception:) _______________

3. Which amino acids fit into each of these categories? (Note: The number in parentheses indicates the number of amino acids in that category.)
   - Nonpolar, nonaromatic (7):

   ____

   - Aromatic (3):

   ____

   - Polar (5):

   ____

   - Negatively charged/acidic (2):

   ____

   - Positively charged/basic (3):

   ____

4. Where do hydrophobic amino acids tend to reside within a protein? What about hydrophilic ones?
   - Hydrophobic:

   ____

   - Hydrophilic:

   ____

5. Identify the amino acids below by their one-letter abbreviation.

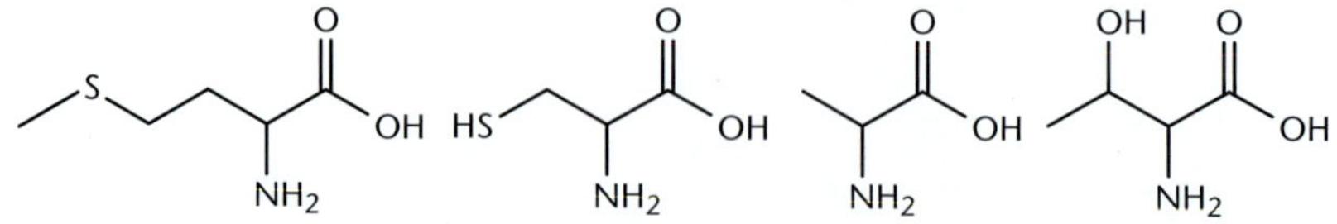

1.2 Acid–Base Chemistry of Amino Acids

LEARNING OBJECTIVES

After Chapter 1.2, you will be able to:

- Identify the predominant ion form of the generic amino acid backbone given a pH value
- Calculate pI values for an amino acid given pK_a values for backbone and side chains
- Predict the general form of the titration curve for an amino acid

The AAMC loves to use amino acids to test your understanding of acid–base chemistry because they have both an acidic carboxylic acid group and a basic amino group. That makes them **amphoteric species**, as they can either accept a proton or donate a proton; how they react depends on the pH of their environment. The key to understanding the behavior of amino acids is to remember two facts:

- Ionizable groups tend to gain protons under acidic conditions and lose them under basic conditions. So, in general, at low pH, ionizable groups tend to be protonated; at high pH, they tend to be deprotonated.
- The pK_a of a group is the pH at which, on average, half of the molecules of that species are deprotonated; that is, [protonated version of the ionizable group] = [deprotonated version of the ionizable group] or [HA] = [A^-]. If the pH is less than the pK_a, a majority of the species will be protonated. If the pH is higher than the pK_a, a majority of the species will be deprotonated. (These relationships are depicted in Figure 1.7.)

MCAT EXPERTISE

You are *not* expected to know exact values for isoelectric points or side chain pK_a values. The MCAT will either provide you with numerical data to use in answering a question or test clear-cut distinctions that can be made without additional information (such as, *Which is more hydrophilic, valine or lysine?* but not *Which is more hydrophobic, valine or alanine?*).

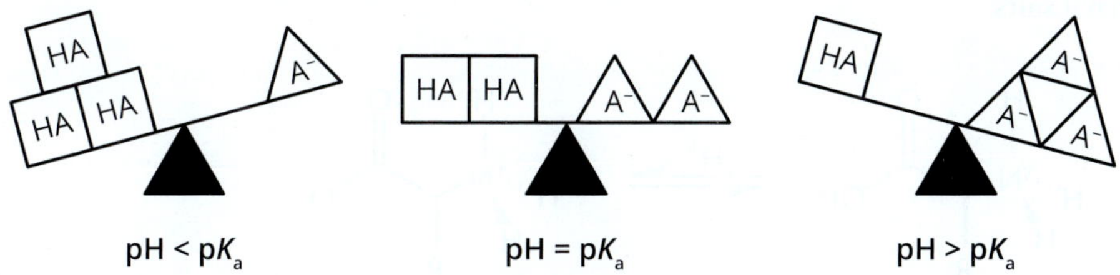

Figure 1.7 Protonation Depends on pH and pK_a

Protonation and Deprotonation

Because all amino acids have at least two groups that can be deprotonated, they all have at least two pK_a values. The first one, pK_{a_1}, is the pK_a for the carboxyl group and is usually around 2. For most amino acids, the second pK_a value, pK_{a_2}, is the pK_a for the amino group, which is usually between 9 and 10. For amino acids with an ionizable side chain, there will be three pK_a values, but we'll come back to that later. As an example, let's take glycine, which doesn't have an ionizable side chain.

KEY CONCEPT

Like all polyprotic acids, each ionizable proton has its own pK_a at which it is "half-deprotonated."§

Positively Charged under Acidic Conditions

At pH 1 (below even the pH of the stomach), there are plenty of protons in solution. Because we're far below the pK_a of the amino group, the amino group will be fully protonated ($-NH_3^+$) and thus positively charged. Because we're also below the pK_a of the carboxylic acid group, it too will be fully protonated ($-COOH$) and thus neutral. Therefore, at very acidic pH values, amino acids tend to be positively charged, as shown in Figure 1.8.

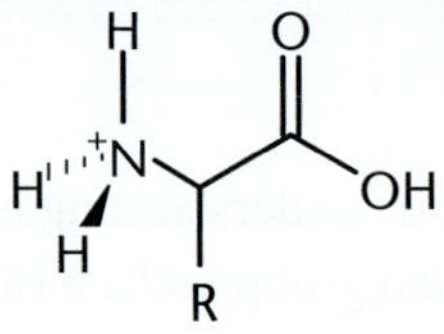

Figure 1.8 Amino Acid Structure at Acidic pH

Zwitterions at Intermediate pH

If we increase the pH of the amino acid solution from pH 1 to pH 7.4, the normal pH of human blood, we've moved far above the pK_a of the carboxylic acid group. At physiological pH, you will not find amino acids with the carboxylate group protonated ($-COOH$) and the amino group unprotonated ($-NH_2$). Under these conditions, the carboxyl group will be in its conjugate base form and be deprotonated, becoming $-COO^-$. Conversely, we're still well below the pK_a of the basic amino group, so it will remain fully protonated and in its conjugate acid form ($-NH_3^+$). Thus, we have a molecule that has both a positive charge and a negative charge, but overall, the molecule is electrically neutral. We call such molecules dipolar ions, or **zwitterions** (from the German *zwitter*, or "hybrid"), as depicted in Figure 1.9. The two charges neutralize one another, and zwitterions exist in water as internal salts.

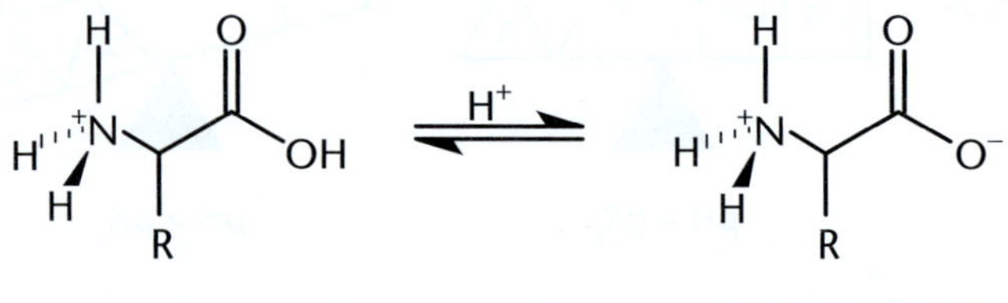

Figure 1.9 Carboxylic Acids Become Deprotonated at Neutral pH, Forming Zwitterions

Negatively Charged under Basic Conditions

Milk of magnesia, which is often used as an antacid, has a pH around 10.5. At that pH, the carboxylate group is already deprotonated and thus remains $-COO^-$. On the other hand, we are now well above the pK_a for the amino group, so it deprotonates too, becoming $-NH_2$. So, at highly basic pH, glycine is now negatively charged, as depicted in Figure 1.10.

KEY CONCEPT

At very acidic pH values, amino acids tend to be positively charged. At very alkaline pH values, amino acids tend to be negatively charged.

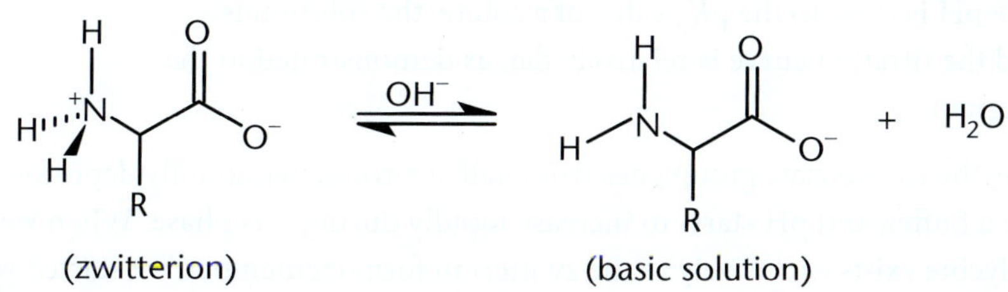

Figure 1.10 Amino Groups Become Deprotonated at Basic pH, Forming an Anion

Titration of Amino Acids

Because of these acid–base properties, amino acids are great candidates for titrations. We assume that the titration of each proton occurs as a distinct step, resembling that of a simple monoprotic acid. Thus, the titration curve looks like a combination of two monoprotic acid titration curves (or three curves, if the side chain is charged). Figure 1.11 shows the titration curve for glycine. After we inspect this curve, we'll look at the differences for the amino acids with charged side chains.

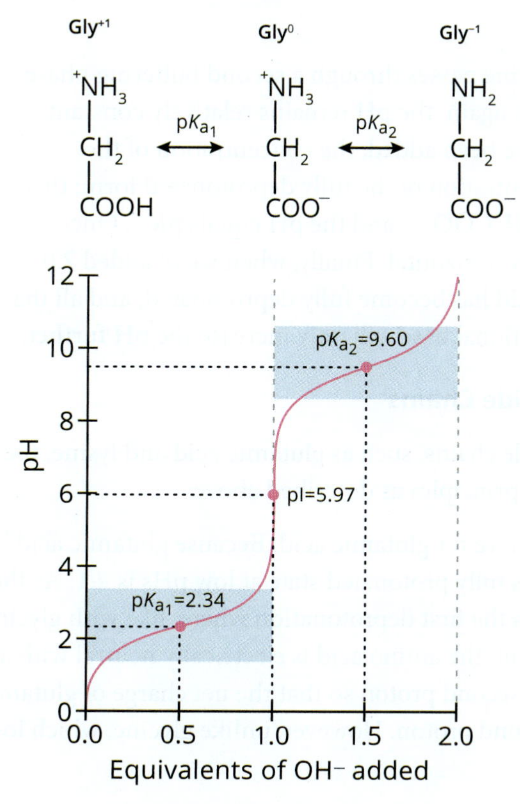

Figure 1.11 Titration Curve for Glycine

Imagine an acidic 1 M glycine solution. At low pH values, glycine exists predominantly as $^{+}NH_3CH_2COOH$; it is fully protonated, with a positive charge. As the solution is titrated with NaOH, the carboxyl group will deprotonate first because it is more acidic than the amino group. When 0.5 equivalents of base have been added to the solution, the concentrations of the fully protonated glycine and its zwitterion, $^{+}NH_3CH_2COO^{-}$, are equal; that is, $[^{+}NH_3CH_2COOH] = [^{+}NH_3CH_2COO^{-}]$. At this point, the pH equals pK_{a_1}. Remember: when the pH is close to the pK_a value of a solute, the solution is acting as a buffer and the titration curve is relatively flat, as demonstrated in the blue boxes in the diagram.

KEY CONCEPT

When the pH of a solution is approximately equal to the pK_a of the solute, the solution acts as a buffer.

As we add more base, the carboxylate group goes from half-deprotonated to fully deprotonated. The amino acid stops acting like a buffer, and pH starts to increase rapidly during this phase. When we've added 1.0 equivalent of base, glycine exists exclusively as the zwitterion form (remember, we started with 1.0 equivalent of glycine). This means that every molecule is now electrically neutral, and thus the pH equals the **isoelectric point (pI)** of glycine. This is true of all amino acids: the isoelectric point is the pH at which the molecule is electrically neutral. For neutral amino acids, it can be calculated by averaging the two pK_a values for the amino and carboxyl groups:

$$pI_{\text{neutral amino acid}} = \frac{pK_{a,NH_3^+\text{ group}} + pK_{a,COOH\text{ group}}}{2}$$

Equation 1.1

For glycine, the pI value is $(2.34 + 9.60) \div 2 = 5.97$. Remember that when the molecule is neutral, it is especially sensitive to pH changes, and the titration curve is nearly vertical.

As we continue adding base, glycine passes through a second buffering phase as the amino group deprotonates; again, the pH remains relatively constant. When 1.5 equivalents of base have been added, the concentration of the zwitterion form equals the concentration of the fully deprotonated form; that is, $[^{+}NH_3CH_2COO^{-}] = [NH_2CH_2COO^{-}]$, and the pH equals pK_{a_2}. Once again, the titration curve is nearly horizontal. Finally, when we've added 2.0 equivalents of base, the amino acid has become fully deprotonated, and all that remains is $NH_2CH_2COO^{-}$; additional base will only increase the pH further.

KEY CONCEPT

When the pH of an amino acid solution equals the isoelectric point (pI) of the amino acid, it exists as electrically neutral molecules. The pI is calculated as the average of the two nearest pK_a values. For amino acids with non-ionizable side chains, the pI is usually around 6.

Amino Acids with Charged Side Chains

For amino acids with charged side chains, such as glutamic acid and lysine, the titration curve has an extra "step," but works along the same principles as described above.

Figure 1.12 shows the titration curve for glutamic acid. Because glutamic acid has two carboxyl groups and one amino group, its charge in its fully protonated state at low pHs is +1. As the glutamic acid solution is titrated with NaOH, it undergoes the first deprotonation where, like with glycine, a proton is lost from the main carboxyl group. At that point, the amino acid is electrically neutral with a net charge of 0. As the pH continues to increase, it loses its second proton so that the net charge of glutamic acid becomes −1, just as it does when glycine loses its second proton. However, unlike glycine, which loses its second proton from the amino group, the second proton that is removed from glutamic acid comes from the side chain carboxyl group! The side chain carboxyl group on glutamic acid is a relatively acidic group, with a pK_a of around 4.2. Therefore, the pI of glutamic acid is around 3.2.

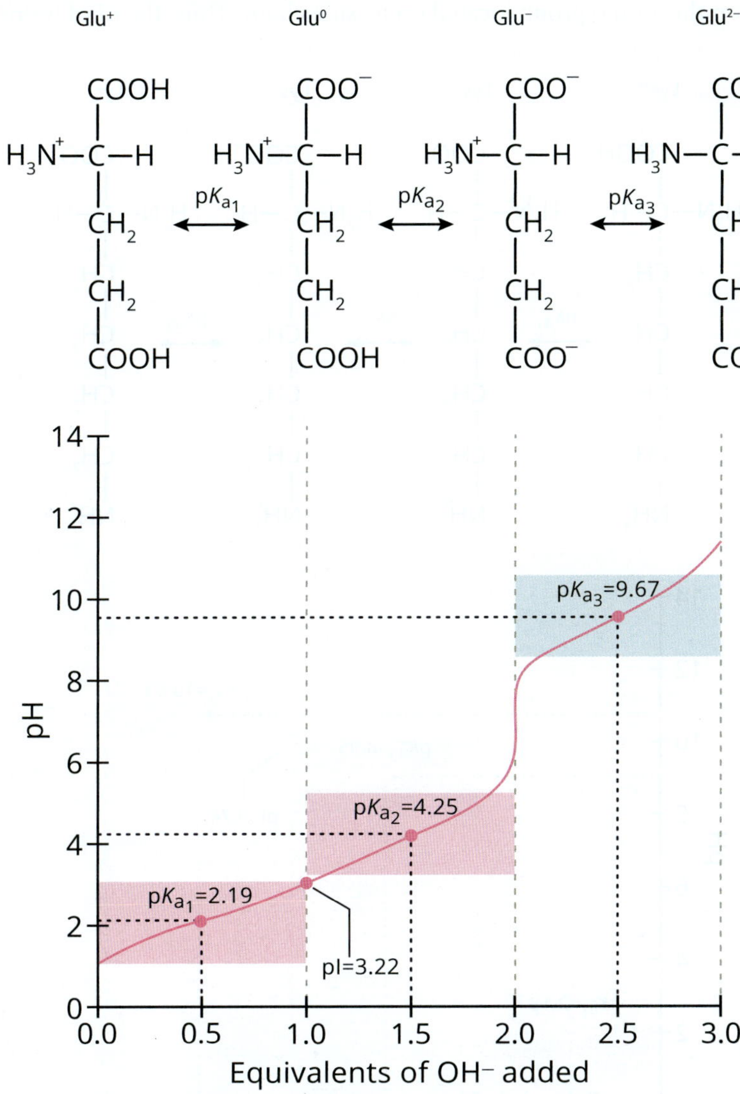

Figure 1.12 Titration Curve for Glutamic Acid

The isoelectric point for an acidic amino acid can be calculated by averaging the pI values of the acidic side chain and carboxylic acid group, as shown below:

$$pI_{\text{acidic amino acid}} = \frac{pK_{\text{a,R group}} + pK_{\text{a,COOH group}}}{2}$$

Equation 1.2

Figure 1.13 shows the titration curve for lysine. Lysine has two amino groups and one carboxyl group. Thus, its charge in its fully protonated state is +2, not +1. Losing the carboxyl proton, which still happens around pH 2, brings the charge down to +1. However, lysine does not become electrically neutral until it loses the proton from its main amino group, which happens around pH 9. It gains a negative charge around pH 10.5, at which point it loses the proton on the amino group located on its side chain. Thus, the pI of lysine is around 9.7.

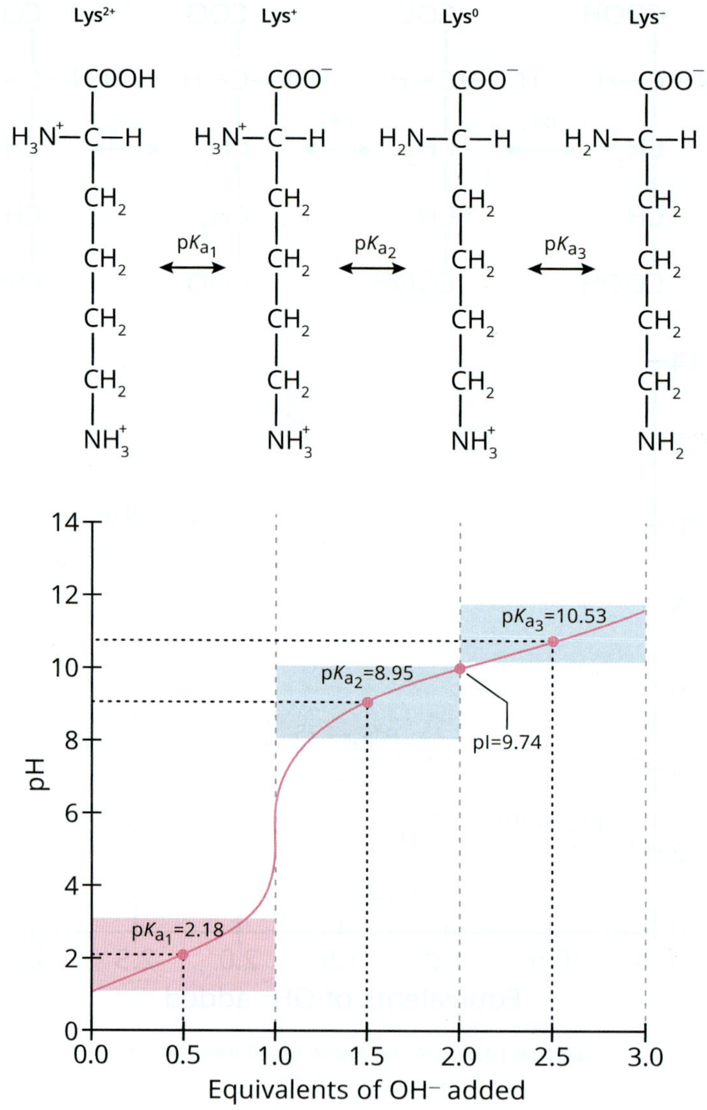

Figure 1.13 Titration Curve for Lysine

The pI for a basic amino acid can be calculated by averaging the pI values of the basic side chain and the amino group, as shown below:

$$pI_{\text{basic amino acid}} = \frac{pK_{a,\text{NH}_3^+ \text{ group}} + pK_{a,\text{R group}}}{2}$$

Equation 1.3

The take-home message: amino acids with acidic side chains have relatively low values for pI while those with basic side chains have relatively high ones.

KEY CONCEPT

Amino acids with acidic side chains have pI values well below 6; amino acids with basic side chains have pI values well above 6.

MCAT CONCEPT CHECK 1.2

Before you move on, assess your understanding of the material with these questions.

1. For a generic amino acid, $NH_2CRHCOOH$, with an uncharged side chain, what would be the predominant form at each of the following pH values?
   - pH = 1:

   ____
   - pH = 7:

   ____
   - pH = 11:

   ____

2. Given the following pK_a values, what is the value of the pI for each of the amino acids listed below?
   - Aspartic acid (pK_{a_1} = 1.88, pK_{a_2} = 3.65, pK_{a_3} = 9.60): pI = __________
   - Arginine (pK_{a_1} = 2.17, pK_{a_2} = 9.04, pK_{a_3} = 12.48): pI = __________
   - Valine (pK_{a_1} = 2.32, pK_{a_2} = 9.62): pI = __________

1.3 Peptide Bond Formation and Hydrolysis

High Yield

LEARNING OBJECTIVES

After Chapter 1.3, you will be able to:

- Recognize the relationship of nomenclature with length, such as predicting the length of a compound called a "tripeptide"
- Apply the hydrolytic mechanisms of trypsin and chymotrypsin to novel peptide chains
- Predict the products of peptide bond formation and cleavage reactions:

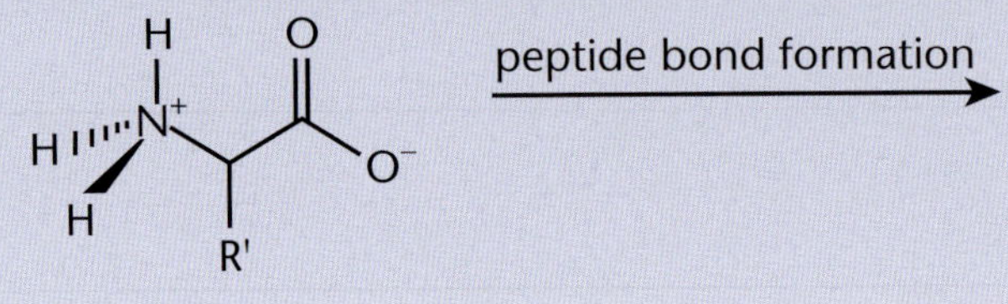

Peptides are composed of amino acid subunits, sometimes called **residues**, as shown in Figure 1.14. **Dipeptides** consist of two amino acid residues; **tripeptides** have three. The term **oligopeptide** is used for relatively small peptides, up to about 20 residues; while longer chains are called **polypeptides**.

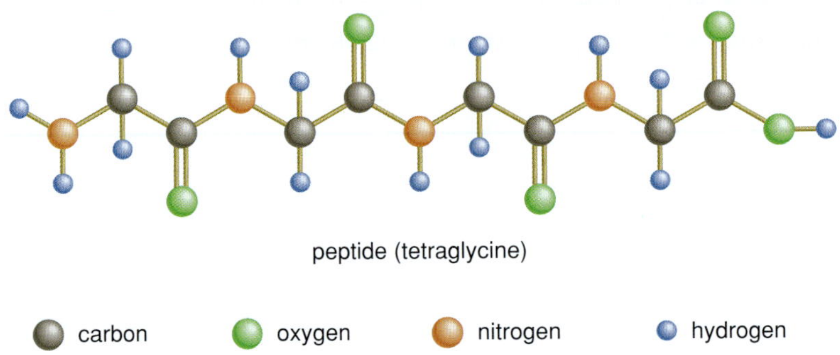

Figure 1.14 Peptide Residues

The residues in peptides are joined together through **peptide bonds**, a specialized form of an amide bond, which form between the $-COO^-$ group of one amino acid and the NH_3^+ group of another amino acid. This forms the functional group $-C(O)NH^-$. In this section, we'll look at the key reactions involved in forming and breaking peptide bonds.

BRIDGE

For Test Day, you also need to know how peptide bonds are formed in the context of ribosomes, which is covered in Chapter 7 of *MCAT Biochemistry Review*.

Peptide Bond Formation

Peptide bond formation is an example of a **condensation** or **dehydration** reaction because it results in the removal of a water molecule (H_2O); it can also be viewed as an acyl substitution reaction, which can occur with all carboxylic acid derivatives. When a peptide bond forms, as shown in Figure 1.15, the electrophilic carbonyl carbon on the first amino acid is attacked by the nucleophilic amino group on the second amino acid. After that attack, the hydroxyl group of the carboxylic acid is kicked off. The result is the formation of a peptide (amide) bond.

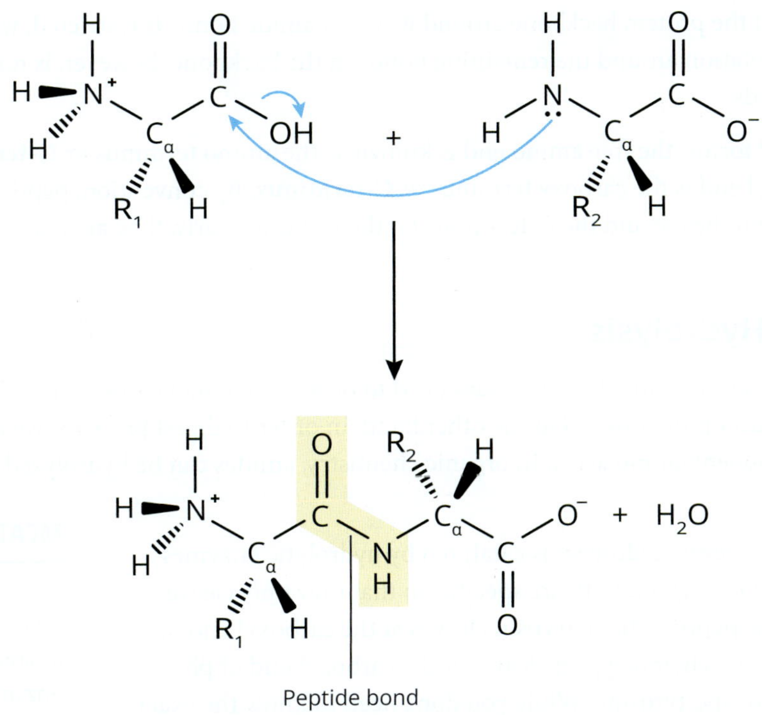

Figure 1.15 Peptide Bond Formation

Because amide groups have delocalizable π electrons in the carbonyl and in the lone pair on the amino nitrogen, they can exhibit resonance; thus, the C—N bond in the amide has partial double bond character, as shown in Figure 1.16.

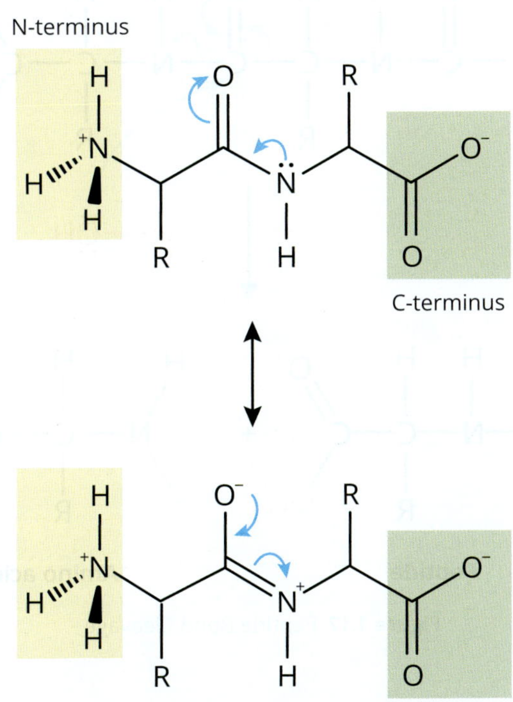

Figure 1.16 Resonance in the Peptide Bond

BRIDGE

The peptide is drawn in the same order that it is synthesized by ribosomes: from the N-terminus to the C-terminus! Translation is covered in Chapter 7 of *MCAT Biochemistry Review*.

As a result, rotation of the protein backbone around its C—N amide bonds is restricted, which makes the protein more rigid. Rotation around the remaining bonds in the backbone, however, is not restricted, as those remain single (σ) bonds.

When a peptide bond forms, the free amino end is known as the amino terminus or **N-terminus**, while the free carboxyl end is the carboxy terminus or **C-terminus**. By convention, peptides are drawn with the N-terminus on the left and the C-terminus on the right; similarly, they are read from N-terminus to C-terminus.

Peptide Bond Hydrolysis

For enzymes to carry out their function, peptides need to be relatively stable in solution. Therefore, they don't normally fall apart on their own. On the other hand, in order to digest proteins, we need to break them down into their component amino acids. In organic chemistry, amides can be hydrolyzed using acid or base catalysis.

In living organisms, however, hydrolysis is catalyzed by hydrolytic enzymes such as *trypsin* and *chymotrypsin*. Both are specific, in that they only cleave at specific points in the peptide chain: trypsin cleaves at the carboxyl end of arginine and lysine, while chymotrypsin cleaves at the carboxyl end of phenylalanine, tryptophan, and tyrosine. While you don't need to know the exact mechanism of how these enzymes catalyze hydrolysis, you do need to understand the main idea: they break apart the amide bond by adding a hydrogen atom to the amide nitrogen and an OH group to the carbonyl carbon as shown in Figure 1.17. This is the reverse reaction shown before in Figure 1.15.

MCAT EXPERTISE

You do *not* need to memorize the specific amino acids that hydrolytic enzymes recognize or the exact mechanisms for those reactions. On the other hand, you could certainly encounter a passage describing them.

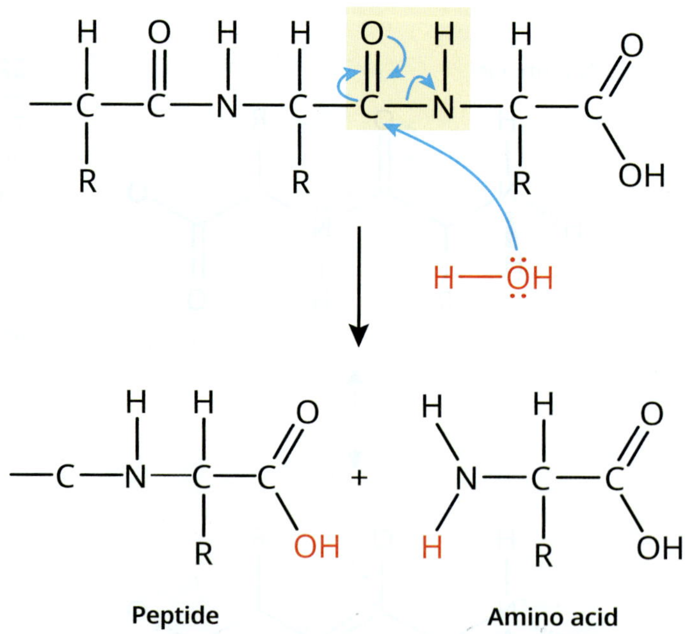

Figure 1.17 Peptide Bond Cleavage

MCAT CONCEPT CHECK 1.3

Before you move on, assess your understanding of the material with these questions.

1. What is the difference between an amino acid, a dipeptide, a tripeptide, an oligopeptide, and a polypeptide?

____

2. What molecule is released during formation of a peptide bond?

____

3. If chymotrypsin cleaves at the carboxyl end of phenylalanine, tryptophan, and tyrosine, how many oligopeptides would be formed in enzymatic cleavage of the following molecule with chymotrypsin?

   Val – Phe – Glu – Lys – Tyr – Phe – Trp – Ile – Met – Tyr – Gly – Ala

1.4 Primary and Secondary Protein Structure High Yield

LEARNING OBJECTIVES

After Chapter 1.4, you will be able to:

- Describe all four levels of protein structure
- Recognize the unique role of proline in secondary protein structure
- Recall the structural features of α-helices and β-pleated sheets

Proteins are polypeptides that range from just a few amino acids in length up to thousands. They serve many functions in biological systems, functioning as enzymes, hormones, membrane pores and receptors, and elements of cell structure. Proteins are the main actors in cells; the genetic code, after all, is simply a recipe for making thousands of proteins.

Proteins have four levels of structure: **primary** (1°), **secondary** (2°), **tertiary** (3°), and **quaternary** (4°). In this section, we'll examine the first two; we'll discuss tertiary and quaternary structure in the next section.

Primary Structure

The primary structure of a protein is the linear arrangement of amino acids coded in an organism's DNA. It's the sequence of amino acids, listed from the N-terminus, or amino end, to the C-terminus, or carboxyl end, as shown in Figure 1.18. So, for example, the first ten amino acids of the β-chain of hemoglobin are normally valine, histidine, leucine, threonine, proline, glutamate, glutamate, lysine, serine, and alanine. Primary structure is stabilized by the formation of covalent peptide bonds between adjacent amino acids.

MCAT EXPERTISE

The MCAT will not expect you to memorize the exact primary sequence of any protein!

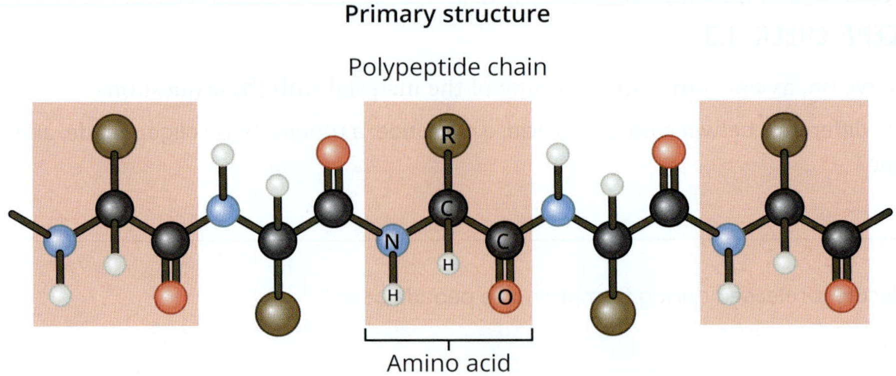

Figure 1.18 Primary Structure

The primary structure alone encodes all the information needed for folding at all of the higher structural levels; the secondary, tertiary, and quaternary structures a protein adopts are the most energetically favorable arrangements of the primary structure in a given environment. The primary structure of a protein can be determined by a laboratory technique called **sequencing**. This is most easily done using the DNA that coded for that protein, although it can also be done from the protein itself.

Secondary Structure

A protein's secondary structure is the local structure of neighboring amino acids. Secondary structures are primarily the result of hydrogen bonding between nearby amino acids. The two most common secondary structures are **α-helices** and **β-pleated sheets**. The key to the stability of both structures is the formation of intramolecular hydrogen bonds between different residues.

KEY CONCEPT

The primary structure of a protein is the order of its amino acids. The two main secondary structures are the α-helix and β-pleated sheet, which both result from hydrogen bonding.

α-Helices

The α-helix, shown in Figure 1.19, is a rodlike structure in which the peptide chain coils clockwise around a central axis. The helix is stabilized by intramolecular hydrogen bonds between a carbonyl oxygen atom and an amide hydrogen atom four residues down the chain. One complete turn of the α-helix has 3.6 amino acids residues.The side chains of the amino acids in the α-helical conformation point away from the helix core. The α-helix is an important component in the structure of **keratin**, a fibrous structural protein found in human skin, hair, and fingernails.

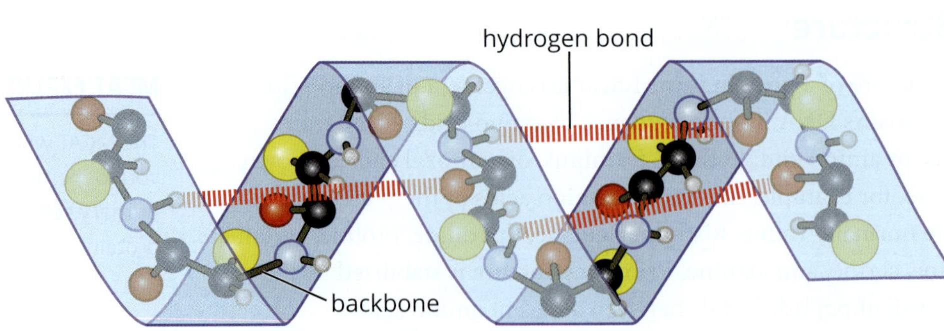

Figure 1.19 Hydrogen Bonding and Spatial Configuration of an α-Helix

β-Pleated Sheets

In β-pleated sheets, which can be parallel or antiparallel, the peptide chains lie alongside one another, forming rows or strands held together by hydrogen bonds between carbonyl oxygen atoms on one chain and amide hydrogen atoms in an adjacent chain, as shown in Figure 1.20.

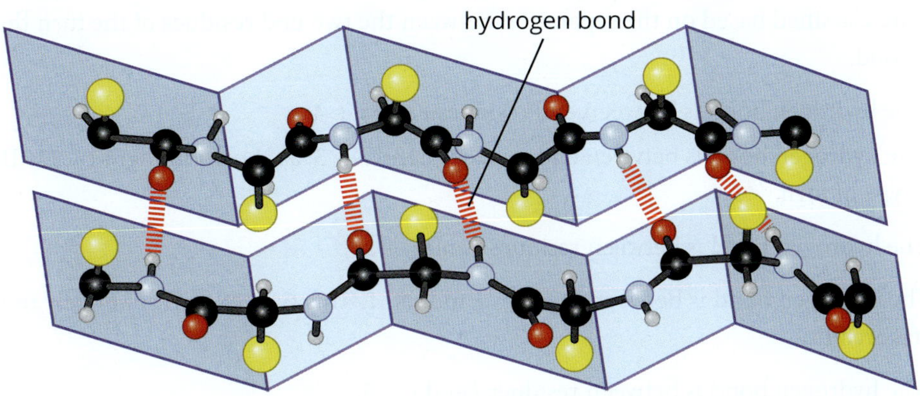

Figure 1.20 Hydrogen Bonding and Spatial Configuration of a β-Pleated Sheet

To accommodate as many hydrogen bonds as possible, the β-pleated sheets assume a pleated, or rippled, shape. The R groups of amino residues point above and below the plane of the β-pleated sheet. The adjacent peptide chains can either form a parallel or antiparallel orientation, as shown in Figure 1.21. *Fibroin*, the primary protein component of silk fibers, is composed of β-pleated sheets.

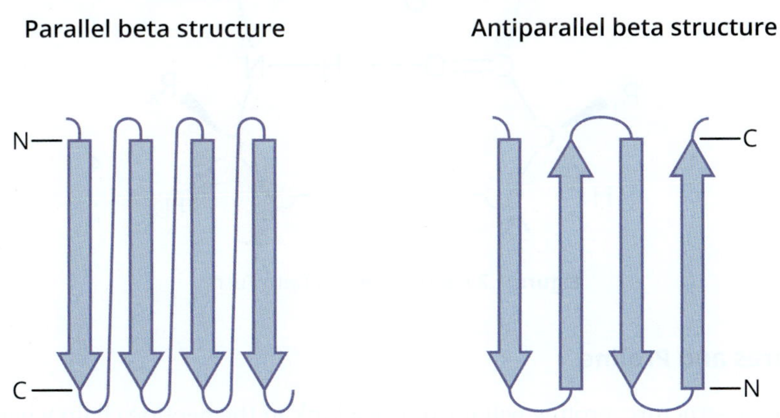

Figure 1.21 Parallel and Antiparallel β-Pleated Sheets

Turns

Turns are secondary structural motifs that lead to a change in the direction of the polypeptide chain. These motifs usually contain between one to five amino acids and join secondary structural elements together, where the first amino acid is labeled i, with subsequent ones labeled $i+1$, $i+2$, $i+3$, and so on. The structure of the turns often allows for the formation of a main chain hydrogen bond between the residues that start and end the turn. They are classified based on the separation between the two end residues of the turn that are joined by a hydrogen bond.

- α-**turn:** The hydrogen bond is between end residues i and $i+4$.
- β-**turn:** The hydrogen bond is between end residues i and $i+3$, as shown in Figure 1.22. This is the most common type of turn.
- γ-**turn:** The hydrogen bond is between residues i and $i+2$.
- δ-**turn:** The hydrogen bond is between residues i and $i+1$. This type of turn is unlikely to form due to steric unfavorability.
- π-**turn:** The hydrogen bond is between residues i and $i+5$.

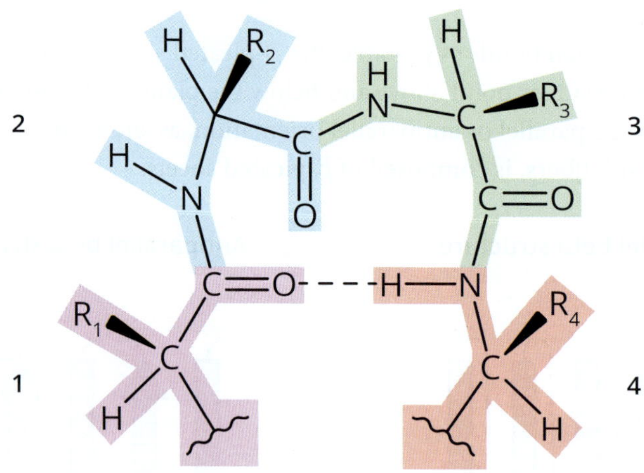

Figure 1.22 Structure of a Beta Turn

Secondary Structures and Proline

Because of its rigid cyclic structure, proline will introduce a kink in the peptide chain when it is found in the middle of an α-helix (see Figure 1.23). Proline residues are thus rarely found in α-helices, except in helices that cross the cell membrane. Similarly, it is rarely found in the middle of pleated sheets. On the other hand, proline is often found in the turns between the chains of a β-pleated sheet, and it is often found as the residue at the start of an α-helix.

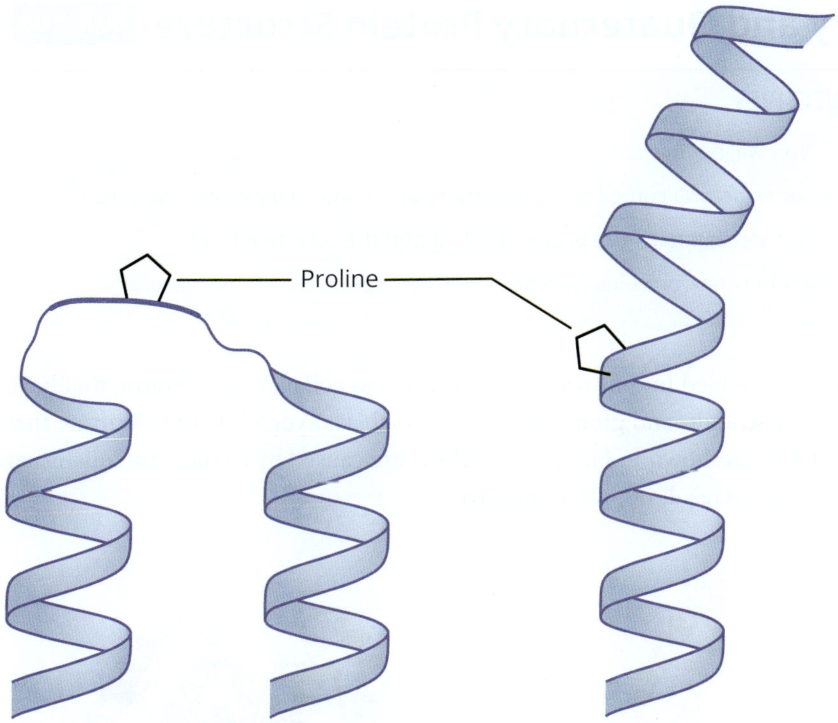

Figure 1.23 Proline in Secondary Structure

MCAT CONCEPT CHECK 1.4

Before you move on, assess your understanding of the material with these questions.

1. What are the definitions of primary and secondary structure, and how do they differ in subtypes and the bonds that stabilize them?

Structural Element	Definition	Subtypes	Stabilizing Bonds
Primary structure (1°)			
Secondary structure (2°)			

2. What role does proline serve in secondary structure?

____

3. Describe the key structural features of the following secondary structures.

   - α-helix:

   ____

   - β-pleated sheet:

   ____

1.5 Tertiary and Quaternary Protein Structure High Yield

LEARNING OBJECTIVES

After Chapter 1.5, you will be able to:

- Identify the major structural components of tertiary and quaternary protein structure
- Recognize the relationship between protein folding and the solvation layer
- Recall the nomenclature of proteins with prosthetic groups, such as nucleoproteins

Proteins can be broadly divided into **fibrous** proteins, such as collagen and keratin, that have structures that resemble sheets or long strands, and **globular** proteins, such as myoglobin and albumin, that tend to be spherical (that is, like a globe), as shown in Figure 1.24. These are caused by tertiary and quaternary protein structures, both of which are the result of protein folding.

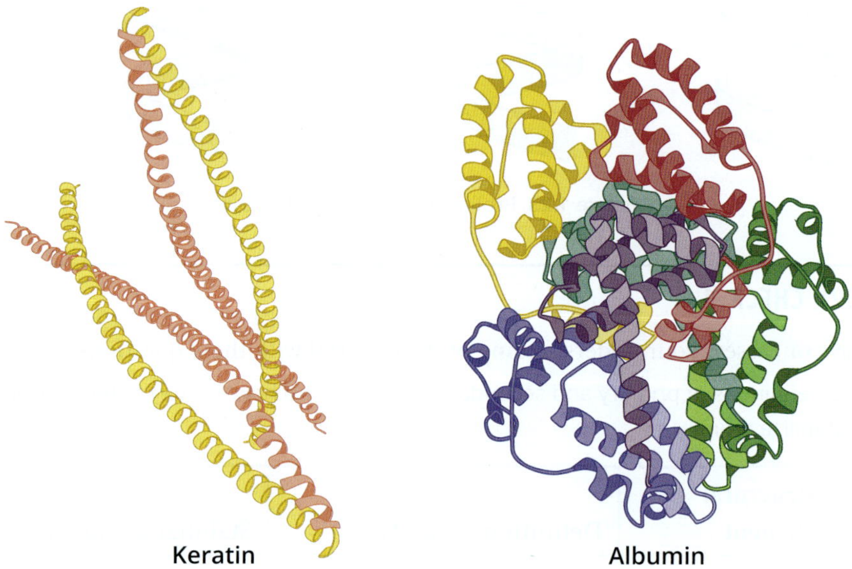

Figure 1.24 Fibrous vs. Globular Proteins

Tertiary Structure

A protein's tertiary structure is its three-dimensional shape. Tertiary structures are mostly determined by hydrophilic and hydrophobic interactions between R groups of amino acids. Hydrophobic residues prefer to be on the interior of proteins, which reduces their proximity to water. Hydrophilic N—H and C=O bonds found in the polypeptide chain get pulled in by these hydrophobic residues. These hydrophilic bonds can then form electrostatic interactions and hydrogen bonds that further stabilize the protein from the inside. As a result of these hydrophobic interactions, most of the amino acids on the surface of proteins have hydrophilic (polar or charged) R groups; highly hydrophobic R groups, such as phenylalanine, are almost never found on the surface of a protein.

KEY CONCEPT

The tertiary structure of a protein is primarily the result of moving hydrophobic amino acid side chains into the interior of the protein.

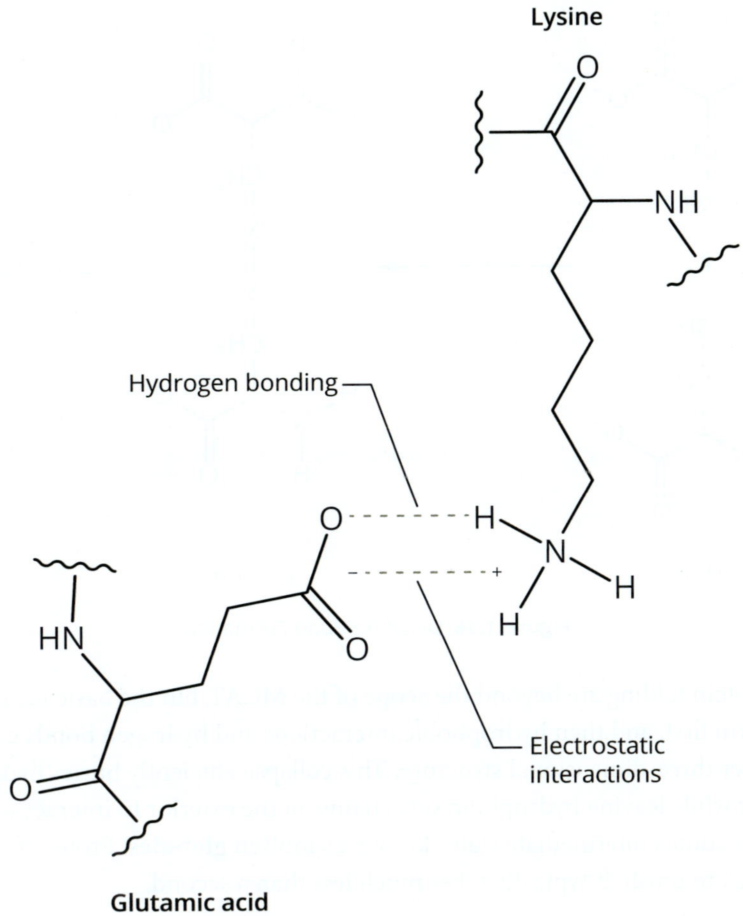

Figure 1.25 Salt Bridge Interaction

The three-dimensional structure can also be determined by hydrogen bonding, as well as acid–base interactions between amino acids with charged R groups. When an interaction consists of both a hydrogen bond and an ionic bond, as shown in Figure 1.25, it is referred to as a **salt bridge**. A particularly important component of tertiary structure is the presence of **disulfide bonds**, the bonds that form when two **cysteine** molecules become oxidized to form **cystine**, as shown in Figure 1.26. Disulfide bonds create loops in the protein chain. In addition, disulfide bonds determine how wavy or curly human hair is: the more disulfide bonds, the curlier it is. Note that forming a disulfide bond requires the loss of two protons and two electrons (oxidation).

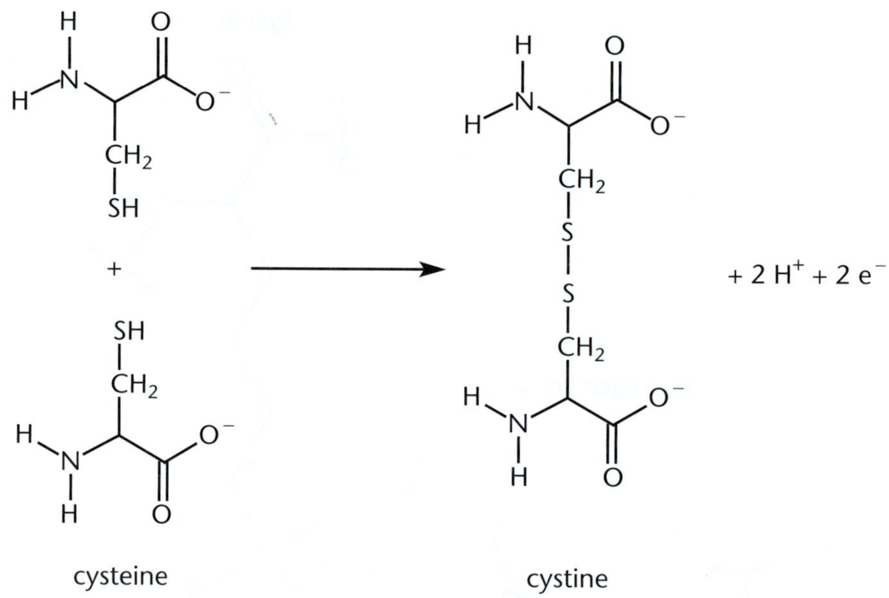

Figure 1.26 Disulfide Bond Formation

The exact details of protein folding are beyond the scope of the MCAT, but the basic idea is that the secondary structures probably form first, and then hydrophobic interactions and hydrogen bonds cause the protein to "collapse" into its proper three-dimensional structure. This collapse efficiently buries hydrophobic side chains in the protein's interior while leaving hydrophilic side chains on the exterior to interact with the surrounding water. Along the way, it adopts intermediate states known as **molten globules**. Protein folding is an extremely rapid process: from start to finish, it typically takes much less than a second.

If a protein loses its tertiary structure, a process commonly called **denaturation**, it loses its function.

Folding and the Solvation Layer

Why do hydrophobic residues tend to occupy the interior of a protein, while hydrophilic residues tend to accumulate on the exterior portions? The answer can be summed up in one word: entropy.

Whenever a solute dissolves in a solvent, the nearby solvent molecules form a **solvation layer** around that solute. From an enthalpy standpoint, the process is surprisingly favorable ($\Delta H < 0$) even for a hydrocarbon—this is not due to the hydrocarbon itself, but because the water molecules in the solvation layer form very stable, energy-releasing hydrogen bonds with each other. However, when a hydrophobic side chain, such as those in phenylalanine and leucine, is placed in aqueous solution, the water molecules in the solvation layer cannot form hydrogen bonds with the side chain. As depicted in Figure 1.27, this forces the nearby water molecules to rearrange themselves into specific arrangements to maximize hydrogen bonding—which means a negative change in entropy, ΔS. Remember that negative changes in entropy represent increasing order (decreasing disorder) and thus are unfavorable. This entropy change makes the overall process nonspontaneous ($\Delta G > 0$).

BRIDGE

Make sure you understand the basic thermodynamic properties of enthalpy, entropy, and Gibbs free energy, discussed in Chapter 7 of *MCAT General Chemistry Review*. On Test Day, they can be tested on both natural sciences sections!

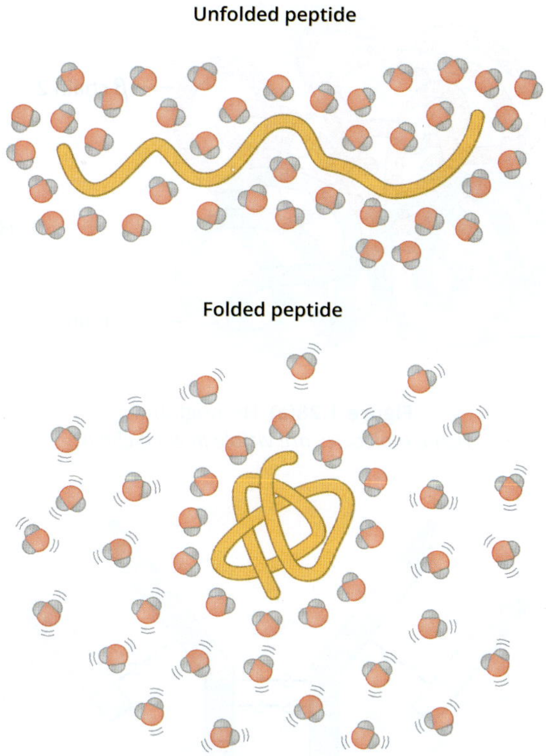

Figure 1.27 Protein Folding and Entropy

On the other hand, putting hydrophilic residues such as serine or lysine on the exterior of the protein allows the nearby water molecules more latitude in their positioning, thus increasing their entropy ($\Delta S > 0$), and making the overall solvation process spontaneous. Thus, by moving hydrophobic residues away from water molecules and hydrophilic residues toward water molecules, a protein achieves maximum stability.

Quaternary Structure

All proteins have elements of primary, secondary, and tertiary structure; not all proteins have quaternary structure. Quaternary structures only exist for proteins that contain more than one polypeptide chain. For these proteins, the quaternary structure is an aggregate of smaller globular peptides, or **subunits**, and represents the functional form of the protein. The classic examples of quaternary structure are hemoglobin and immunoglobulins, shown in Figures 1.28(a) and 1.28(b). Hemoglobin consists of four distinct subunits, each of which can bind one molecule of oxygen. Similarly, immunoglobulin G (IgG) antibodies also contain a total of four subunits each, held together by disulfide bonds.

MNEMONIC

The primary structure of a protein acts like letters. The secondary structure acts like words: only certain orderings of letters make sense (CAT is a word, while CAQ is not). The tertiary structure acts like sentences: words combine to form a functioning whole. The quaternary structure acts like paragraphs: they're not always present, but subunits can combine to make a cohesive whole.

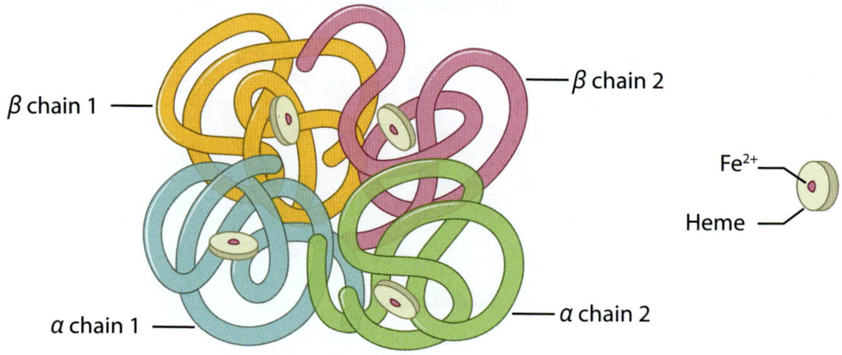

Figure 1.28(a) Hemoglobin
Heme molecules are visible in each chain.

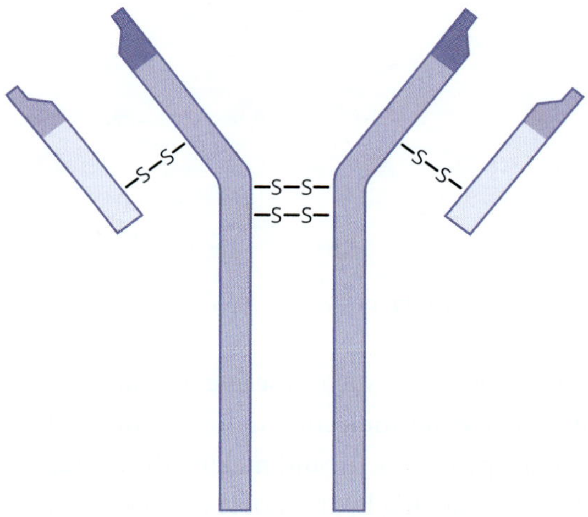

Figure 1.28(b) Immunoglobulin G1

The formation of quaternary structures can serve several roles. First, they can be more stable, by further reducing the surface area of the protein complex. Second, they can reduce the amount of DNA needed to encode the protein complex. Third, they can bring catalytic sites close together, allowing intermediates from one reaction to be directly shuttled to a second reaction. Finally, and most important, they can induce **cooperativity**, or **allosteric effects**. We'll discuss this much further in the next chapter (especially for hemoglobin), but the basic idea is that one subunit can undergo conformational or structural changes, which either enhance or reduce the activity of the other subunits.

BRIDGE

The reduction of genetic material is crucial for viruses. The genome for most viruses is tiny. Thus, their viral coats typically consist of one small protein repeated dozens or even hundreds of times. Viral structure is discussed in Chapter 1 of *MCAT Biology Review*.

Conjugated Proteins

Conjugated proteins derive part of their function from covalently attached molecules called **prosthetic groups**. These prosthetic groups can be organic molecules, such as vitamins, or even metal ions, such as iron. Proteins with lipid, carbohydrate, and nucleic acid prosthetic groups are referred to as **lipoproteins**, **glycoproteins** (see Figure 1.29), and **nucleoproteins**, respectively. These prosthetic groups have major roles in determining the function of their respective proteins. For example, each of hemoglobin's subunits (as well as myoglobin) contains a prosthetic group called **heme**. The heme group is composed of four **pyrrole** rings. Pyrroles are five-membered heterocyclic aromatic compounds, in which the nitrogen of each pyrrole acts to coordinate the central iron ion. The iron atom binds to and carries oxygen; as such, hemoglobin is inactive without the heme group. These groups can also direct the protein to be delivered to a certain location, such as the cell membrane, nucleus, lysosome, or endoplasmic reticulum.

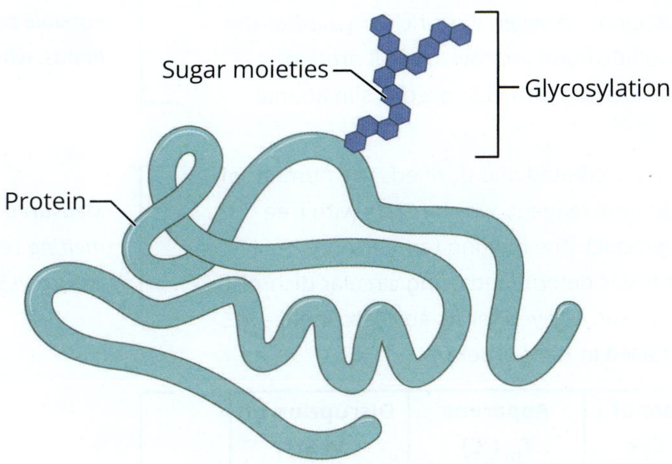

Figure 1.29 Glycosylation

BIOCHEMISTRY GUIDED EXAMPLE WITH EXPERT THINKING

Ricin is a highly toxic ribosome-inactivating protein (RIP) that can be obtained easily from the widely available castor bean, *Ricinus communis*, making it a potential bioterrorist and biowarfare agent. There is no known antidote, but toxoid and recombinant vaccines have been shown to be effective in raising protective immunity and preventing the lethal effects of ricin.

This is just background info on ricin and vaccines

Currently, variants of ricin that do not bind to ribosomes exist, and show promising results as a human immunogen in Phase 1 clinical trials. However, the vaccines suffer from instability and aggregation, and can still cause serious effects like vascular leak syndrome (VLS). Based on previous X-ray crystal structures of RTA1-33/44-198 (an inactive variant), introduction of a disulfide bond stabilizes a disordered loop. However, it is unclear whether the mutations made to introduce the disulfide bond improve overall protein stability and how the mutant proteins interact with VLS receptors in animal models.

Problem statement: issue with current vaccines

Possible solution: introduce disulfide bonds, which may help with stability

A series of RTA1-33/44-198 mutants were created and purified. The number of free cysteines were assayed using Ellman's reagent, which reacts with free sulfhydryl groups to yield a colored product. The melting temperature (apparent T_m) of each purified protein was determined using circular dichroism measurements. Finally, each construct was assayed for its ability to induce VLS in animal models. The results are detailed in Table 1 below.

Measured: free cysteines (via assay), melting temperature, and ability to induce VLS

RTA1-33/44-198 types	Number of free Cys	Apparent T_m (°C)	Disruption of VLS?
wild-type	0.97 ± 0.03	57.9 ± 0.03	No
R48C/T77C	1.00 ± 0.08	62.9 ± 0.22	No
V49C/E99C	0.96 ± 0.05	62.9 ± 0.21	No
R48C/T77C/D75N	1.04 ± 0.02	63.2 ± 0.26	Yes
V49C/E99C/V76I	0.99 ± 0.03	62.6 ± 0.21	Yes
V49C/E99C/D75N	1.10 ± 0.06	62.2 ± 0.13	Yes
R48C/T77C/V76I	1.89 ± 0.03	59.3 ± 0.60	Yes

Table 1

Look for trends and outliers!
The last construct has a different number of free Cys and a T_m similar to WT; the bottom four constructs disrupt VLS

Adapted from Janosi, L., Compton, J. R., Legler, P. M., Steele, K. E., Davis, J. M., Matyas, G. R., & Millard, C. B. (2013). Disruption of the putative vascular leak peptide sequence in the stabilized ricin vaccine candidate RTA1-33/44-198. *Toxins*, 5(2), 224-48. doi:10.3390/toxins5020224.

Is R48C/T77C/V76I a suitable candidate for further testing? Why or why not?

This question is asking us to interpret the study results, but we'll want to start with the purpose of the study to be able to go through the data efficiently. The goal is to develop a vaccine for ricin poisoning. The second paragraph starts with what has already been done, which is the creation of a possible working vaccine. Since it's based on the ricin protein, we can use our background knowledge and critical reasoning to assume that the vaccine is similar enough to the ricin protein to elicit a proper immune response, but does not inhibit ribosome function. Notice the keyword "however" in the second paragraph—this indicates that there is still a problem. In this case, the current vaccine is not stable, which would presumably affect its efficacy. Also, the vaccine seems to have a serious side effect (VLS), which is something the researchers want to eliminate. We're given a hint about a possible solution to the stability issue—creating a disulfide bond. This means that the disulfide is not native to the protein, but created by mutating select amino acids to cysteines.

Following that possible solution in paragraph 2, the researchers generated a series of protein mutations, which are outlined in the first column of Table 1. Notice the notation: letter-number-letter. We know from the passage that these are mutants and, in looking at this code, we can infer that the first letter is the original amino acid, the number is its position in the sequence, and the second letter is the mutated amino acid. This style of notation is common in scientific papers, so we'll likely want to keep this in mind even on Test Day as a possibility when we see similar notation. For instance, R48C is arginine at position 48 mutated to cysteine. Notice that in each mutation, there is a pair of amino acids mutated to cysteine to create the opportunity for a disulfide bond. The second column tells us about the success of creating a disulfide bond. Since the wild-type protein has one free cysteine, and the mutants introduce two more cysteines for the purpose of a creating a disulfide bond, a successful disulfide bond formation will eliminate two sulfhydryls, leaving the original free cysteine. R48C/T77C/V76I has approximately two (1.89 ± 0.03) free cysteines, suggesting an incomplete formation of the disulfide bond. The third column determines the effect of the disulfide bond formation on stability. Melting temperature (T_m) is a great indication for stability—the higher the temperature, the more energy it takes to break all bonds to unfold the protein. Both wild-type and R48C/T77C/V76I have markedly lower T_m compared to the other constructs, which we can conclude means they have reduced stability. Finally, the last column provides information about whether the construct induced VLS. We can see that R48C/T77C/V76I did not induce VLS, making it 'safer' from the perspective of risk for this dangerous syndrome.

Given the data from the passage, while R48C/T77C/V76I does address the issue of not inducing VLS in animal models, the construct is not stable, and therefore would not be suitable for additional testing.

MCAT CONCEPT CHECK 1.5

Before you move on, assess your understanding of the material with these questions.

1. What are the definitions of tertiary and quaternary structure, and how do they differ in subtypes and the bonds that stabilize them?

Structural Element	Definition	Subtypes	Stabilizing Bonds
Tertiary structure (3°)			
Quaternary structure (4°)			

2. What is the primary motivation for hydrophobic residues in a polypeptide to move to the interior of the protein?

___

3. List three different prosthetic groups that can be attached to a protein and name the conjugated protein.

___

1.6 Denaturation

LEARNING OBJECTIVE

After Chapter 1.6, you will be able to:

- Predict the impact of denaturation via heat or solute

BRIDGE

Heat denatures proteins for the same reason that raising a reaction's temperature increases its rate: increased average kinetic energy of molecules means increased molecular motion. The relationship between temperature and kinetic energy is discussed in Chapter 7 of *MCAT General Chemistry Review*.

In the previous section, we discussed protein folding. The reverse of this process is **denaturation**, in which a protein loses its three-dimensional structure. Although it is sometimes reversible, denaturation is often irreversible; whether its denaturation is reversible or not, unfolded proteins cannot catalyze reactions. The two main causes of denaturation are heat and solutes.

As with all molecules, when the temperature of a protein increases, its average kinetic energy increases. When the temperature gets high enough, this extra energy can be enough to overcome the hydrophobic interactions that hold a protein together, causing the protein to unfold. This is what happens when egg whites are cooked: in the uncooked egg whites, albumin is folded, which makes it transparent; cooking them causes the albumin molecules to denature and aggregate, forming a solid, rubbery white mass that will not revert to its transparent form.

On the other hand, solutes such as urea denature proteins by directly interfering with the forces that hold the protein together. They can disrupt tertiary and quaternary structures by interrupting non-covalent interactions like hydrogen bonds and other side chain interactions that hold α-helices and β-pleated sheets intact. Similarly, detergents such as SDS (sodium dodecyl sulfate, also called sodium lauryl sulfate) can solubilize proteins, disrupting noncovalent bonds and promoting denaturation. Note that both urea and SDS do not interfere with any covalent bonds, including disulfide and peptide bonds.

KEY CONCEPT

Denatured proteins lose their three-dimensional structure and are thus inactive.

The stability of proteins to thermal or chemical denaturation can be assessed using denaturation curves, which plot the fraction of unfolded protein against increasing amounts of a denaturant. The denaturation midpoint describes the point at which there are equal amounts of the folded and unfolded proteins. When assessing the effect of temperature on protein unfolding, the midpoint is called the **melting point** (**T_m**), and when using a chemical denaturant to assess protein stability, the midpoint is referred to as a **midpoint concentration** (**C_m**). Changes in the midpoint indicate changes in protein folding stability: For example, Figure 1.30 shows the melting curves of two variants of a protein, Variant A and Variant B. Comparing the two thermal denaturation curves shows that Variant B has a higher T_m, suggesting Variant B requires higher temperatures to denature, while Variant A is less thermally stable and will unfold at lower temperatures.

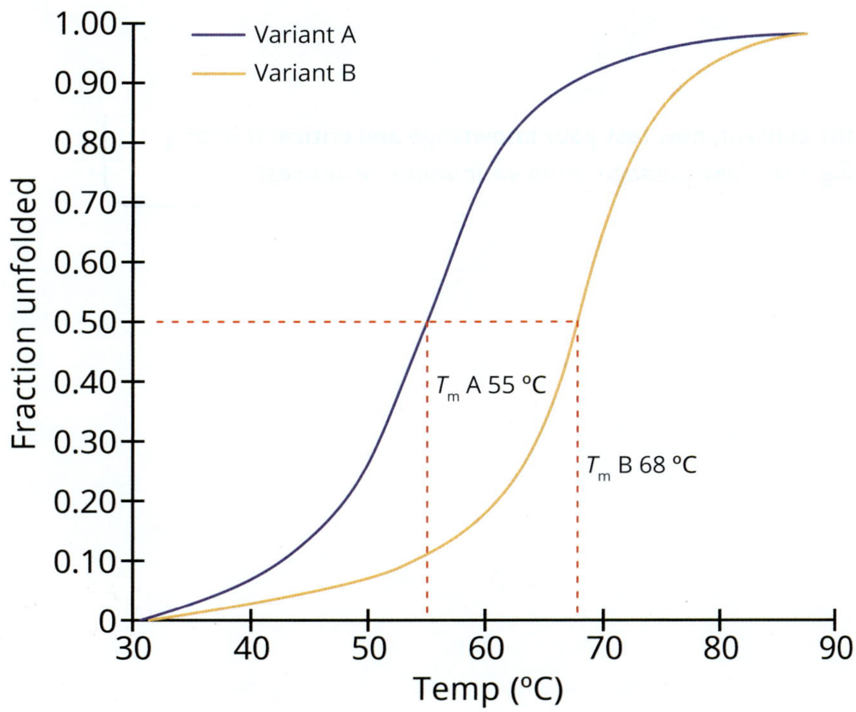

Figure 1.30 Thermal Denaturation Curve
Changes in T_m correlate to protein folding stability.

MCAT CONCEPT CHECK 1.6

Before you move on, assess your understanding of the material with this question.

1. Why are proteins denatured by heat and solutes, respectively?
   - Heat:

   ____

   - Solutes:

   ____

Conclusion

Nearly every part of a cell involves proteins in some way, from the nucleus to the mitochondria to the cell membrane. The MCAT will test your understanding of key concepts regarding amino acids because the amino acids that compose a protein determine its structure. In the next chapter, we'll discuss the best-known function of proteins: their role as enzymes.

GO ONLINE

You've reviewed the content, now test your knowledge and critical thinking skills by completing a test-like passage set in your online resources!

CONCEPT SUMMARY

Amino Acids Found in Proteins

- **Amino acids** have four groups attached to a central (α) carbon: an amino group, a carboxylic acid group, a hydrogen atom, and an **R group**.
  - The R group determines chemistry and function of that amino acid.
  - Twenty amino acids appear in the proteins of eukaryotic organisms.
- The stereochemistry of the α-carbon is L for all chiral amino acids in eukaryotes.
  - D-amino acids can exist in prokaryotes.
  - All chiral amino acids except **cysteine** have an (*S*) configuration.
  - All amino acids are chiral except **glycine**, which has a hydrogen atom as its R group.
- Side chains can be polar or nonpolar, aromatic or nonaromatic, charged or uncharged.
  - **Nonpolar, nonaromatic:** glycine, alanine, valine, leucine, isoleucine, methionine, proline
  - **Aromatic:** tryptophan, phenylalanine, tyrosine
  - **Polar:** serine, threonine, asparagine, glutamine, cysteine
  - **Negatively charged (acidic):** aspartate, glutamate
  - **Positively charged (basic):** lysine, arginine, histidine
- Amino acids with long alkyl chains are hydrophobic, and those with charges are hydrophilic; many others fall somewhere in between.

Acid–Base Chemistry of Amino Acids

- Amino acids are **amphoteric**; that is, they can accept or donate protons.
- The **pK_a** of a group is the pH at which half of the species are deprotonated; $[HA] = [A^-]$.
- Amino acids exist in different forms at different pH values.
  - At low (acidic) pH, the amino acid is fully protonated.
  - At pH near the pI of the amino acid, the amino acid is a neutral **zwitterion**.
  - At high (alkaline) pH, the amino acid is fully deprotonated.
- The **isoelectric point (pI)** of an amino acid without a charged side chain can be calculated by averaging the two pK_a values.
- Amino acids can be titrated.
  - The titration curve is nearly flat at the pK_a values of the amino acid.
  - The titration curve is nearly vertical at the pI of the amino acid.

- Amino acids with charged side chains have an additional pK_a value, and their pI is calculated by averaging the two pK_a values that correspond to protonation and deprotonation of the zwitterion.
  - Amino acids without charged side chains have a pI around 6.
  - Acidic amino acids have a pI well below 6.
  - Basic amino acids have a pI well above 6.

Peptide Bond Formation and Hydrolysis

- Dipeptides have two amino acid residues; tripeptides have three. Oligopeptides have a "few" amino acid residues (<20); polypeptides have "many" (>20).
- Forming a peptide bond is a **condensation** or **dehydration** reaction (releasing one molecule of water).
  - The nucleophilic amino group of one amino acid attacks the electrophilic carbonyl group of another amino acid.
  - Amide bonds are rigid because of resonance.
- Breaking a peptide bond is a **hydrolysis** reaction.

Primary and Secondary Protein Structure

- **Primary structure** is the linear sequence of amino acids in a peptide and is stabilized by peptide bonds.
- **Secondary structure** is the local structure of neighboring amino acids, and is stabilized by hydrogen bonding between amino groups and nonadjacent carboxyl groups.
  - **α-helices** are clockwise coils around a central axis.
  - **β-pleated sheets** are rippled strands that can be parallel or antiparallel.
  - **Proline** can interrupt secondary structure because of its rigid cyclic structure.

Tertiary and Quaternary Protein Structure

- **Tertiary structure** is the three-dimensional shape of a single polypeptide chain, and is stabilized by hydrophobic interactions, acid–base interactions (salt bridges), hydrogen bonding, and disulfide bonds.
  - **Hydrophobic interactions** push hydrophobic R groups to the interior of a protein, which increases entropy of the surrounding water molecules and creates a negative Gibbs free energy.
  - **Disulfide bonds** occur when two **cysteine** molecules are oxidized and create a covalent bond to form **cystine**.
- **Quaternary structure** is the interaction between peptides in proteins that contain multiple subunits.
- Proteins with covalently attached molecules are termed **conjugated proteins**. The attached molecule is a **prosthetic group**, and may be a metal ion, vitamin, lipid, carbohydrate, or nucleic acid.

Denaturation

- Both heat and increasing solute concentration can lead to loss of three-dimensional protein structure, which is termed **denaturation**.

ANSWERS TO CONCEPT CHECKS

1.1

1. The four groups are an amino group ($-NH_2$), a carboxylic acid group ($-COOH$), a hydrogen atom, and an R group.
2. All chiral eukaryotic amino acids are L. All chiral eukaryotic amino acids are (*S*), with the exception of cysteine (because cysteine is the only amino acid with an R group that has a higher priority than a carboxylic acid according to Cahn–Ingold–Prelog rules).
3. Nonpolar, nonaromatic: glycine, alanine, valine, leucine, isoleucine, methionine, proline

   Aromatic: tryptophan, phenylalanine, tyrosine

   Polar: serine, threonine, asparagine, glutamine, cysteine

   Negatively charged/acidic: aspartate, glutamate

   Positively charged/basic: lysine, arginine, histidine
4. Hydrophobic amino acids tend to reside in the interior of a protein, away from water. Hydrophilic amino acids tend to remain on the surface of the protein, in contact with water.
5. From left to right the amino acids are methionine (M), cysteine (C), alanine (A), and threonine (T): MCAT.

1.2

1. pH = 1: $^{+}NH_3CRHCOOH$; pH = 7: $^{+}NH_3CRHCOO^{-}$; pH = 11: $NH_2CRHCOO^{-}$
2. Aspartic acid: $pI = (1.88 + 3.65) \div 2 = 2.77$

   Arginine: $pI = (9.04 + 12.48) \div 2 = 10.76$

   Valine: $pI = (2.32 + 9.62) \div 2 = 5.97$

1.3

1. These species differ by the number of amino acids that make them up: amino acid = 1, dipeptide = 2, tripeptide = 3, oligopeptide = "few" (< 20), polypeptide = "many" (> 20)
2. Water (H_2O)
3. 4: Val – Phe; Glu – Lys – Tyr; Ile – Met – Tyr; Gly–Ala. A single amino acid on its own is not considered an oligopeptide.

1.4

1.

Structural Element	Definition	Subtypes	Stabilizing Bonds
Primary structure (1°)	Linear sequence of amino acids in chain	(none)	Peptide (amide) bond
Secondary structure (2°)	Local structure determined by nearby amino acids	• α-helix • β-pleated sheet	Hydrogen bonds

2. Proline's rigid structure causes it to introduce kinks in α-helices or create turns in β-pleated sheets.
3. The α-helix is a rod-like structure in which the peptide chain coils clockwise around a central axis. In β-pleated sheets the peptide chains lie alongside one another, forming rows or strands held together by intramolecular hydrogen bonds between carbonyl oxygen atoms on one chain and amide hydrogen atoms in an adjacent chain.

1.5

1.

Structural Element	Definition	Subtypes	Stabilizing Bonds
Tertiary structure (3°)	Three-dimensional shape of protein	• Hydrophobic interactions • Acid–base/salt bridges • Disulfide links	• van der Waals forces • Hydrogen bonds • Ionic bonds • Covalent bonds
Quaternary structure (4°)	Interaction between separate subunits of a multisubunit protein	(none)	Same as tertiary structure

2. Moving hydrophobic residues to the interior of a protein increases entropy by allowing water molecules on the surface of the protein to have more possible positions and configurations. This positive ΔS makes $\Delta G < 0$, stabilizing the protein.
3. Examples of common prosthetic groups include lipids, carbohydrates, and nucleic acids; they are known as lipoproteins, glycoproteins, and nucleoproteins, respectively.

1.6

1. Heat denatures proteins by increasing their average kinetic energy, thus disrupting hydrophobic interactions. Solutes denature proteins by disrupting elements of secondary, tertiary, and quaternary structure.

SCIENCE MASTERY ASSESSMENT EXPLANATIONS

1. **B**

Most amino acids (except the acidic and basic amino acids) have two sites for protonation: the carboxylic acid and the amine. At neutral pH, the carboxylic acid will be deprotonated ($-COO^-$) and the amine will remain protonated ($-NH_3^+$).This dipolar ion is a zwitterion, so **(B)** is the correct answer.

2. **B**

Glutamic acid is an acidic amino acid because it has an extra carboxyl group. At neutral pH, both carboxyl groups are deprotonated and thus negatively charged. The amino group has a positive charge because it remains protonated at pH 7. Overall, therefore, glutamic acid has a net charge of -1, and **(B)** is correct. Notice that you do not even need to know the pI values to solve this question; as an acidic amino acid, glutamic acid must have a pI below 7.

3. **C**

Nonpolar groups are not capable of forming dipoles or hydrogen bonds; this makes them hydrophobic. Burying hydrophobic R groups inside proteins means they don't have to interact with water, which is polar. This makes **(C)** correct. **(A)** and **(B)** are incorrect because nonpolar molecules are hydrophobic, not hydrophilic; **(D)** is incorrect because they are not generally found on protein surfaces.

4. **A**

The cDNA sequence is a DNA copy of the mRNA used to generate a protein. A computer program can quickly identify the amino acid that corresponds to each codon and generate a list of these amino acids. This amino acid sequence is the primary structure of the protein. These observations support **(A)** as the correct answer. By contrast, the secondary, tertiary, and quaternary structures involve higher level interactions between the backbone and R groups and are increasingly difficult to predict.

5. **C**

There are three choices for the first amino acid, leaving two choices for the second, and one choice for the third. Multiplying those numbers gives us a total of $3 \times 2 \times 1 = 6$ distinct tripeptides. (Using the one-letter codes for valine (V), alanine (A), and leucine (L), those six tripeptides are VAL, VLA, ALV, AVL, LVA, and LAV.)

6. **B**

As the protein folds, it takes on an organized structure and thus its entropy decreases. However, the opposite trend is true for the water surrounding the protein. Prior to protein folding, hydrophobic amino acid residues are exposed and the water molecules must form structured hydration shells around these hydrophobic residues. During folding, these hydrophobic residues are generally buried in the interior of the protein so that the surrounding water molecules gain more latitude in their interactions. Thus, the entropy of the surrounding water increases, making the correct answer **(B)**.

7. **C**

The α-helix is held together primarily by hydrogen bonds between the carboxyl groups and amino groups of amino acids. Disulfide bridges, **(A)**, and hydrophobic effects, **(B)**, are primarily involved in tertiary structures, not secondary. Even if they were charged, the side chains of amino acids are too far apart to participate in strong interactions in secondary structure.

8. **C**

High salt concentrations and detergents can denature a protein, as can high temperatures. But moving a protein to a hypotonic environment—that is, a lower solute concentration—should not lead to denaturation.

9. **C**

An amino acid likely to be found in a transmembrane portion of an α-helix will be exposed to a hydrophobic environment, so we need an amino acid with a hydrophobic side chain. The only choice that has a hydrophobic side chain is **(C)**, phenylalanine. The other choices are all polar or charged.

10. **C**

Every amino acid except glycine has a chiral α-carbon, but only two of the 20 amino acids—threonine and isoleucine—also have a chiral carbon in their side chains as well. Thus, the correct answer is **(C)**. Just as only one configuration is normally seen at the α carbon, only one configuration is seen in the side chain chiral carbon.

11. **B**

In their inactive state, the receptor tyrosine kinases are fully folded single polypeptide chains and thus have tertiary structure. When these monomers dimerize, they become a protein complex and thus have elements of quaternary structure. This change from tertiary to quaternary structure justifies **(B)**.

12. **A**

Histidine has an ionizable side chain: its imidazole ring has a nitrogen atom that can be protonated. None of the remaining answers have ionizable atoms in their side chains.

13. **D**

Because lysine has a basic side chain, we ignore the pK_a of the carboxyl group, and average the pK_a of the side chain and the amino group; the average of 9 and 10.5 is 9.75, which is closest to **(D)**.

14. **D**

Conjugated proteins can have lipid or carbohydrate "tags" added to them. These tags can indicate that these proteins should be directed to the cell membrane (especially lipid tags) or to specific organelles (such as the lysosome). They can also provide the activity of the protein; for example, the heme group in hemoglobin is needed for it to bind oxygen. Thus, **(D)** is the correct answer.

15. **B**

Because collagen has a triple helix, the carbon backbones are very close together. Thus, steric hindrance is a potential problem. To reduce that hindrance, we need small side chains; glycine has the smallest side chain of all: a hydrogen atom.

GO ONLINE

Consult your online resources for additional practice.

EQUATIONS TO REMEMBER

(1.1) **Isoelectric point of a neutral amino acid:**

$$pI_{\text{neutral amino acid}} = \frac{pK_{a,NH_3^+\text{ group}} + pK_{a,COOH\text{ group}}}{2}$$

(1.2) **Isoelectric point of an acidic amino acid:**

$$pI_{\text{acidic amino acid}} = \frac{pK_{a,R\text{ group}} + pK_{a,COOH\text{ group}}}{2}$$

(1.3) **Isoelectric point of a basic amino acid:**

$$pI_{\text{basic amino acid}} = \frac{pK_{a,NH_3^+\text{ group}} + pK_{a,R\text{ group}}}{2}$$

SHARED CONCEPTS

Biochemistry Chapter 2
Enzymes

Biochemistry Chapter 3
Nonenzymatic Protein Function and Protein Analysis

Biochemistry Chapter 7
RNA and the Genetic Code

Biology Chapter 1
The Cell

Biology Chapter 9
The Digestive System

General Chemistry Chapter 7
Thermochemistry

Organic Chemistry Chapter 8
Carboxylic Acids

Organic Chemistry Chapter 9
Carboxylic Acid Derivatives

CHAPTER 2

ENZYMES

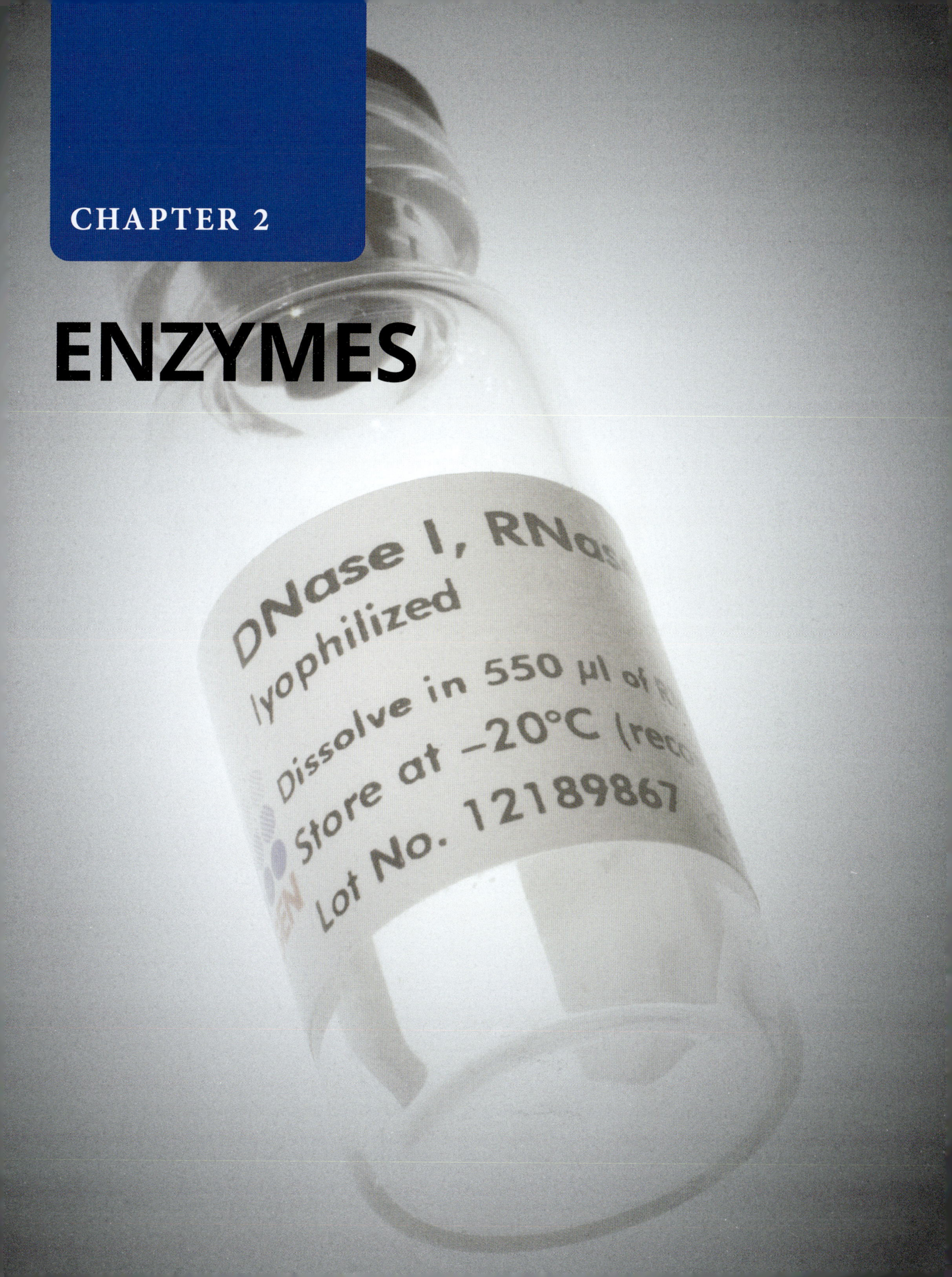

SCIENCE MASTERY ASSESSMENT

Every pre-med knows this feeling: there is so much content I have to know for the MCAT! How do I know what to do first or what's important?

While the high-yield badges throughout this book will help you identify the most important topics, this Science Mastery Assessment is another tool in your MCAT prep arsenal. This quiz (which can also be taken in your online resources) and the guidance below will help ensure that you are spending the appropriate amount of time on this chapter based on your personal strengths and weaknesses. Don't worry though—skipping something now does not mean you'll never study it. Later on in your prep, as you complete full-length tests, you'll uncover specific pieces of content that you need to review and can come back to these chapters as appropriate.

How to Use This Assessment

If you answer 0–7 questions correctly:

Spend about 1 hour to read this chapter in full and take limited notes throughout. Follow up by reviewing **all** quiz questions to ensure that you now understand how to solve each one.

If you answer 8–11 questions correctly:

Spend 20–40 minutes reviewing the quiz questions. Beginning with the questions you missed, read and take notes on the corresponding subchapters. For questions you answered correctly, ensure your thinking matches that of the explanation and you understand why each choice was correct or incorrect.

If you answer 12–15 questions correctly:

Spend less than 20 minutes reviewing all questions from the quiz. If you missed any, then include a quick read-through of the corresponding subchapters, or even just the relevant content within a subchapter, as part of your question review. For questions you got correct, ensure your thinking matches that of the explanation and review the Concept Summary at the end of the chapter.

CHAPTER 2
ENZYMES

1. Consider a biochemical reaction A → B, which is catalyzed by *A–B dehydrogenase*. Which of the following statements is true?
   - **A.** The reaction will proceed until the enzyme concentration decreases.
   - **B.** The reaction will be most favorable at 0°C.
   - **C.** A component of the enzyme is transferred from A to B.
   - **D.** The free energy change (ΔG) of the catalyzed reaction is the same as for the uncatalyzed reaction.

2. Which of the following statements about enzyme kinetics is FALSE?
   - **A.** An increase in the substrate concentration (at constant enzyme concentration) leads to proportional increases in the rate of the reaction.
   - **B.** Most enzymes operating in the human body work best at a temperature of 37°C.
   - **C.** An enzyme–substrate complex can either form a product or dissociate back into the enzyme and substrate.
   - **D.** Maximal activity of many human enzymes occurs around pH 7.4.

3. Some enzymes require the presence of a nonprotein molecule to behave catalytically. An enzyme devoid of this molecule is called a(n):
   - **A.** holoenzyme.
   - **B.** apoenzyme.
   - **C.** coenzyme.
   - **D.** zymoenzyme.

4. Which of the following factors determine an enzyme's specificity?
   - **A.** The three-dimensional shape of the active site
   - **B.** The Michaelis constant
   - **C.** The type of cofactor required for the enzyme to be active
   - **D.** The prosthetic group on the enzyme

5. Human DNA polymerase is removed from the freezer and placed in a 60°C water bath. Which of the following best describes the change in enzyme activity as the polymerase sample comes to thermal equilibrium with the water bath?
   - **A.** Increases then decreases
   - **B.** Decreases then plateaus
   - **C.** Increases then plateaus
   - **D.** Decreases then increases

6. In the equation below, substrate C is an allosteric inhibitor to enzyme 1. Which of the following is another mechanism necessarily caused by substrate C?

$$A \xrightarrow[\text{enzyme 1}]{} B \xrightarrow[\text{enzyme 2}]{} C$$

   - **A.** Competitive inhibition
   - **B.** Irreversible inhibition
   - **C.** Feedback enhancement
   - **D.** Negative feedback

7. The activity of an enzyme is measured at several different substrate concentrations, and the data are shown in the table below.

[S] (mM)	$v\left(\frac{\text{mmol}}{\text{sec}}\right)$
0.01	1
0.05	9.1
0.1	17
0.5	50
1	67
5	91
10	95
50	99
100	100

K_m for this enzyme is approximately:
   - **A.** 0.5
   - **B.** 1.0
   - **C.** 10.0
   - **D.** 50.0

Questions 8 and 9 refer to the following statement:

Consider a reaction catalyzed by enzyme A with a K_m value of 5×10^{-6} M and V_{max} of 20 $\frac{\text{mmol}}{\text{min}}$.

8. At a concentration of 5×10^{-6} M substrate, the rate of the reaction will be:
   - **A.** 10 $\frac{\text{mmol}}{\text{min}}$.
   - **B.** 20 $\frac{\text{mmol}}{\text{min}}$.
   - **C.** 30 $\frac{\text{mmol}}{\text{min}}$.
   - **D.** 40 $\frac{\text{mmol}}{\text{min}}$.

9. At a concentration of 5×10^{-4} M substrate, the rate of the reaction will be:
   - **A.** 10 $\frac{\text{mmol}}{\text{min}}$.
   - **B.** 15 $\frac{\text{mmol}}{\text{min}}$.
   - **C.** 20 $\frac{\text{mmol}}{\text{min}}$.
   - **D.** 30 $\frac{\text{mmol}}{\text{min}}$.

10. The graph below shows kinetic data obtained for flu virus enzyme activity as a function of substrate concentration in the presence and absence of two antiviral drugs.

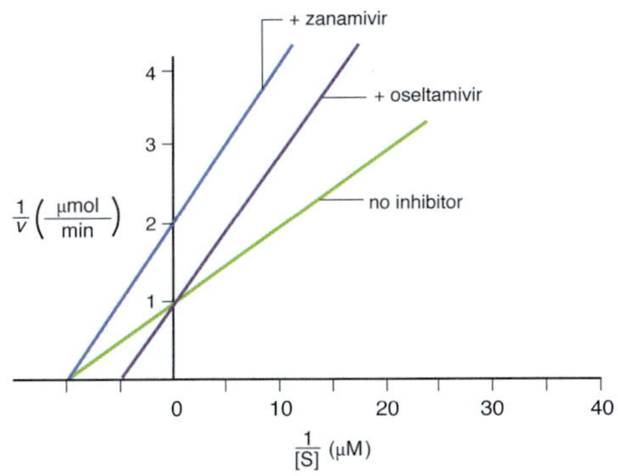

Based on the graph, which of the following statements is correct?
   - **A.** Both drugs are noncompetitive inhibitors of the viral enzyme.
   - **B.** Oseltamivir increases the K_m value for the substrate compared to Relenza.
   - **C.** Zanamivir increases the V_{max} value for the substrate compared to Tamiflu.
   - **D.** Both drugs are competitive inhibitors of the viral enzyme.

11. The conversion of ATP to cyclic AMP and inorganic phosphate is most likely catalyzed by which class of enzyme?
   - **A.** Ligase
   - **B.** Hydrolase
   - **C.** Lyase
   - **D.** Transferase

12. Which of the following is NOT a method by which enzymes decrease the activation energy for biological reactions?
   - **A.** Modifying the local charge environment
   - **B.** Forming transient covalent bonds
   - **C.** Acting as electron donors or receptors
   - **D.** Breaking bonds in the enzyme irreversibly to provide energy

13. A certain enzyme that displays positive cooperativity has four subunits, two of which are bound to substrate. Which of the following statements must be true?
   - **A.** The affinity of the enzyme for the substrate has just increased.
   - **B.** The affinity of the enzyme for the substrate has just decreased.
   - **C.** The affinity of the enzyme for the substrate is half of what it would be if four sites had substrate bound.
   - **D.** The affinity of the enzyme for the substrate is greater than with one substrate bound.

14. Which of the following is LEAST likely to be required for a series of metabolic reactions?
   - **A.** Triacylglycerol acting as a coenzyme
   - **B.** Oxidoreductase enzymes
   - **C.** Magnesium acting as a cofactor
   - **D.** Transferase enzymes

15. How does the ideal temperature for a reaction change with and without an enzyme catalyst?
   - **A.** The ideal temperature is generally higher with a catalyst than without.
   - **B.** The ideal temperature is generally lower with a catalyst than without.
   - **C.** The ideal temperature is characteristic of the reaction, not the enzyme.
   - **D.** No conclusion can be made without knowing the enzyme type.

Answer Key

1. **D** (See section 2.1)
2. **A** (See section 2.3)
3. **B** (See section 2.5)
4. **A** (See section 2.5)
5. **A** (See section 2.4)
6. **D** (See section 2.5)
7. **A** (See section 2.3)
8. **A** (See section 2.3)
9. **C** (See section 2.3)
10. **B** (See section 2.3)
11. **C** (See section 2.1)
12. **D** (See section 2.2)
13. **D** (See section 2.5)
14. **A** (See section 2.1)
15. **B** (See section 2.4)

The relevant section of the chapter to review for each question is given in parentheses after the correct answer. Detailed explanations can be found at the end of the chapter.

CHAPTER 2

ENZYMES

In This Chapter

CHAPTER PROFILE

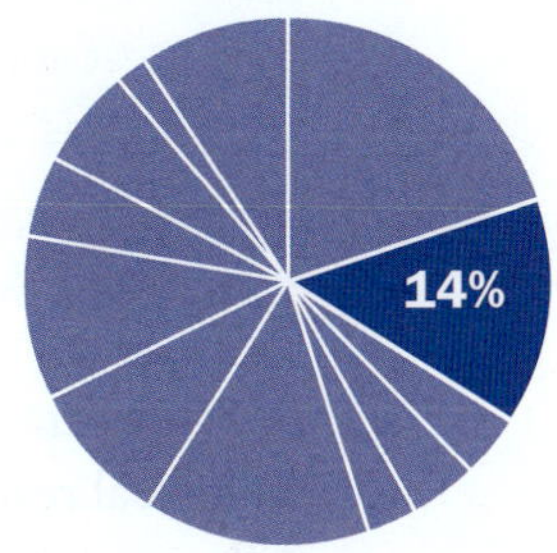

The content in this chapter should be relevant to about 14% of all questions about biochemistry on the MCAT.

This chapter covers material from the following AAMC content categories:

1A: Structure and function of proteins and their constituent amino acids

5E: Principles of chemical thermodynamics and kinetics

Introduction

Obesity is increasingly common in the United States and is paralleled by an increase in high blood pressure, or hypertension. This is extremely relevant to medical students because hypertension increases the risk of stroke, heart failure, and kidney failure.

Each year, physicians encourage millions of Americans to improve their diets, add exercise to their daily regimens, or even take prescription drugs to control their hypertension. Many of these anti-hypertensive medications are called ACE (*angiotensin-converting enzyme*) inhibitors. In healthy patients, ACE catalyzes a reaction that converts a peptide called angiotensin I to angiotensin II. The angiotensin II peptide then not only directly causes constriction of the blood vessels to raise blood pressure, but also stimulates the release of the hormone aldosterone, which activates the kidneys to reabsorb more water back into the bloodstream. The increase in blood volume also increases blood pressure. Physicians take advantage of this complicated pathway with a straightforward solution: stop the pathway early by inhibiting ACE and blood pressure will decrease.

Enzymes are crucial proteins that dramatically increase the rate of biological reactions. They're used to regulate homeostatic mechanisms in every organ system and are highly regulated themselves by environmental conditions, activators, and inhibitors. These regulators may be naturally occurring or may be given as a drug, such as the ACE inhibitors used to treat hypertension. Some enzymes are kept in an inactivated form called a zymogen and are only activated as needed. In this chapter, we'll learn about how enzymes work and how different conditions influence their activity. We'll also see how enzymes are regulated, which will help us tie together concepts about every organ system and metabolic process we learn about for the MCAT.

2.1 Enzymes as Biological Catalysts High Yield

LEARNING OBJECTIVES

After Chapter 2.1, you will be able to:

- Explain the major features of enzyme function, including specificity and catalysis
- Describe all seven classes of enzymes: oxidoreductases, transferases, hydrolases, lyases, isomerases, ligases, and translocases
- Recognize how enzymes affect thermodynamics and kinetics of a reaction

Enzymes are incredibly important as biological catalysts. **Catalysts** do not impact the thermodynamics of a biological reaction; that is, the ΔH_{rxn} and equilibrium position do not change. Instead, they help the reaction proceed at a much faster rate. As a catalyst, the enzyme is not changed during the course of the reaction. Enzymes increase the reaction rate of a process by a factor of 100, 1000, or even 1,000,000,000,000 (10^{12}) times when compared to the uncatalyzed reaction. Without this increase, we wouldn't be alive. Table 2.1 summarizes the key points to remember about enzymes.

Lower the activation energy
Increase the rate of the reaction
Do not alter the equilibrium constant
Are not changed or consumed in the reaction (which means that they will appear in both the reactants and products)
Are pH- and temperature-sensitive, with optimal activity at specific pH ranges and temperatures
Do not affect the overall ΔG of the reaction
Are specific for a particular reaction or class of reactions

Table 2.1 Key Features of Enzymes

Enzyme Classifications

Enzymes are picky. The molecules upon which an enzyme acts are called substrates; a given enzyme will only catalyze a single reaction or class of reactions with these substrates, a property known as **enzyme specificity**. For example, *urease* only catalyzes the breakdown of urea. *Chymotrypsin*, on the other hand, can cleave peptide bonds around the amino acids phenylalanine, tryptophan, and tyrosine in a variety of polypeptides. Although those amino acids aren't identical, they all contain an aromatic ring, which makes chymotrypsin specific for a class of molecules.

Enzymes can be classified into seven categories, based on their function or mechanism. We'll review each type of enzyme and give examples of those that you are most likely to see on Test Day. If you encounter an unfamiliar enzyme on the MCAT, keep in mind that most enzymes have descriptive names ending in the suffix *–ase*: *lactase*, for example, breaks down lactose.

BRIDGE

The convention for naming reductants and oxidants of oxidoreductases is the same as the convention for naming reducing agents and oxidizing agents in general and organic chemistry. This is a good time to brush up on oxidation–reduction reactions if you haven't seen them in a while—they're covered in Chapter 11 of *MCAT General Chemistry Review* and Chapter 4 of *MCAT Organic Chemistry Review*.

Oxidoreductases

Oxidoreductases catalyze oxidation–reduction reactions; that is, the transfer of electrons between biological molecules. They often have a cofactor that acts as an electron carrier, such as NAD^+ or $NADP^+$. In reactions catalyzed by oxidoreductases, the electron donor is known as the **reductant**, and the electron acceptor is known as the **oxidant**. Enzymes with *dehydrogenase* or *reductase* in their names are usually oxidoreductases. Enzymes in which oxygen is the final electron acceptor often include *oxidase* in their names. Malate dehydrogenase is an example of an oxidoreductase; it oxidizes malate to oxaloacetate or reduces oxaloacetate to malate, as seen in Figure 2.1.

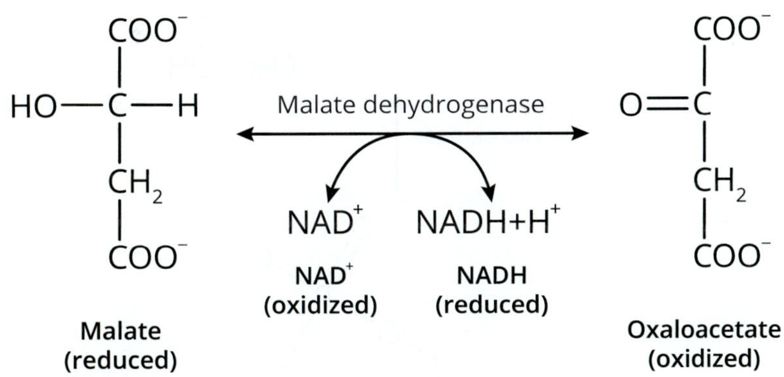

Figure 2.1 Oxidoreductases Catalyze Oxidation-Reduction Reactions

Transferases

Transferases catalyze the movement of a functional group from one molecule to another. For example, in protein metabolism, an *aminotransferase* can convert aspartate and α-ketoglutarate, as a pair, to glutamate and oxaloacetate by moving the amino group from aspartate to α-ketoglutarate. Most transferases will be straightforwardly named, but remember that *kinases* are also a member of this class. **Kinases** catalyze the transfer of a phosphate group, generally from ATP, to another molecule. Figure 2.2 shows an example of the transferase (and kinase) hexokinase transferring ATP onto a glucose molecule.

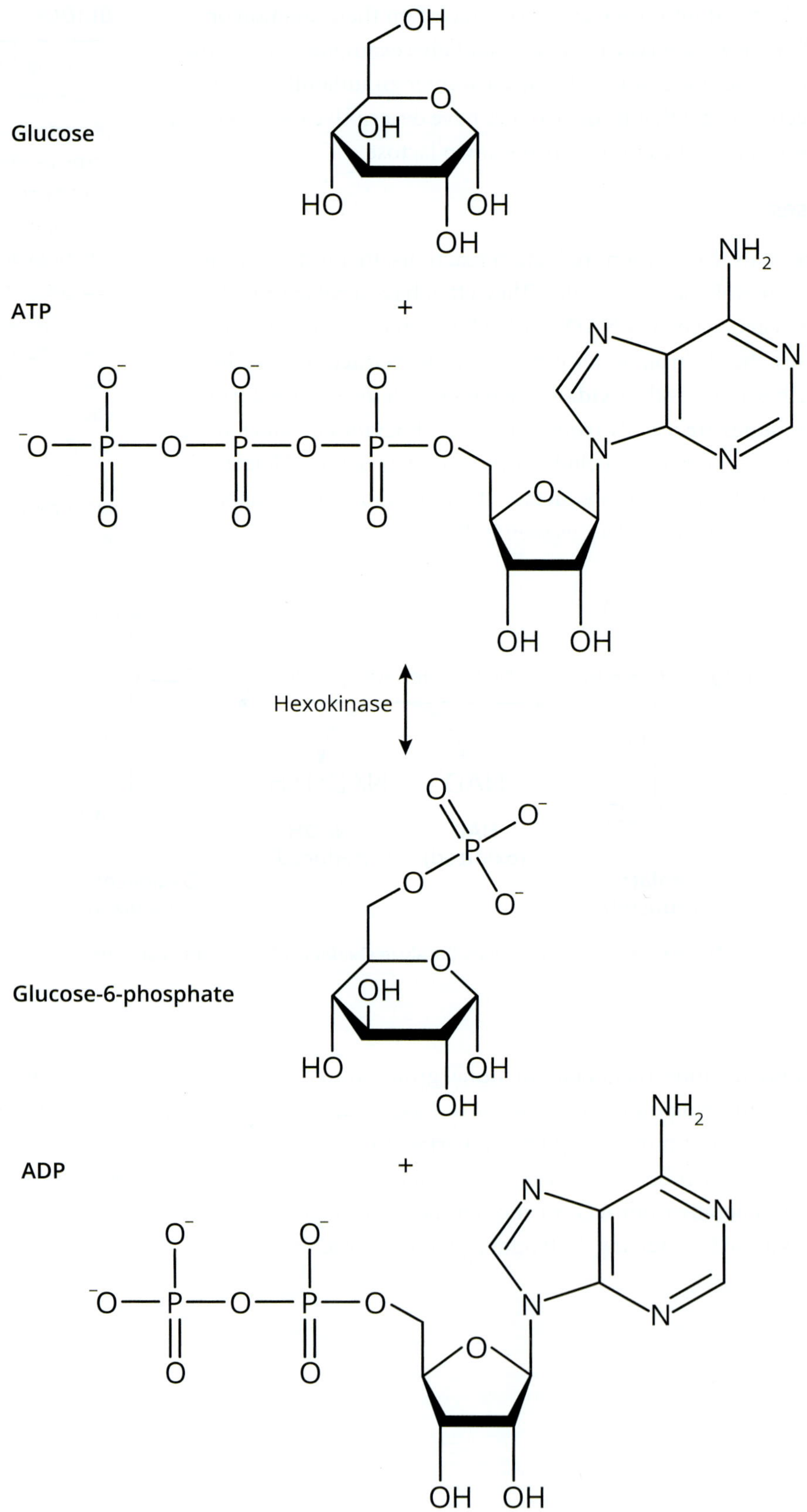

Figure 2.2 Transferases Move Functional Groups between Molecules

Hydrolases

Hydrolases catalyze the breaking of a compound into two molecules using the addition of water, as seen in Figure 2.3. In common usage, many hydrolases are named only for their substrate. For example, one of the most common hydrolases you will encounter on the MCAT is a *phosphatase*, which cleaves a phosphate group from another molecule. Other hydrolases include *peptidases*, *nucleases*, and *lipases,* which break down proteins, nucleic acids, and lipids, respectively.

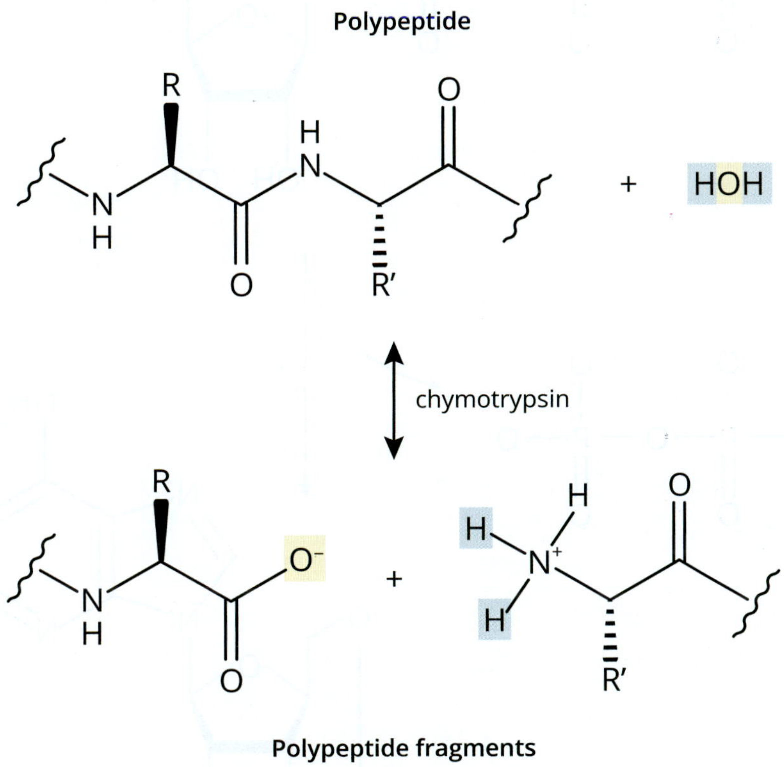

Figure 2.3 Hydrolases Use Water to Cleave Bonds

Lyases

Lyases catalyze the cleavage of a single molecule into two products without the use of water and without acting as oxidoreductases. Adenylyl cyclase (AC), shown converting ATP into cyclic AMP in Figure 2.4, is one example of a lyase. Because most enzymes can also catalyze the reverse of their specific reactions, the synthesis of two molecules into a single molecule may also be catalyzed by a lyase. When fulfilling this function, it is common for them to be referred to as *synthases*.

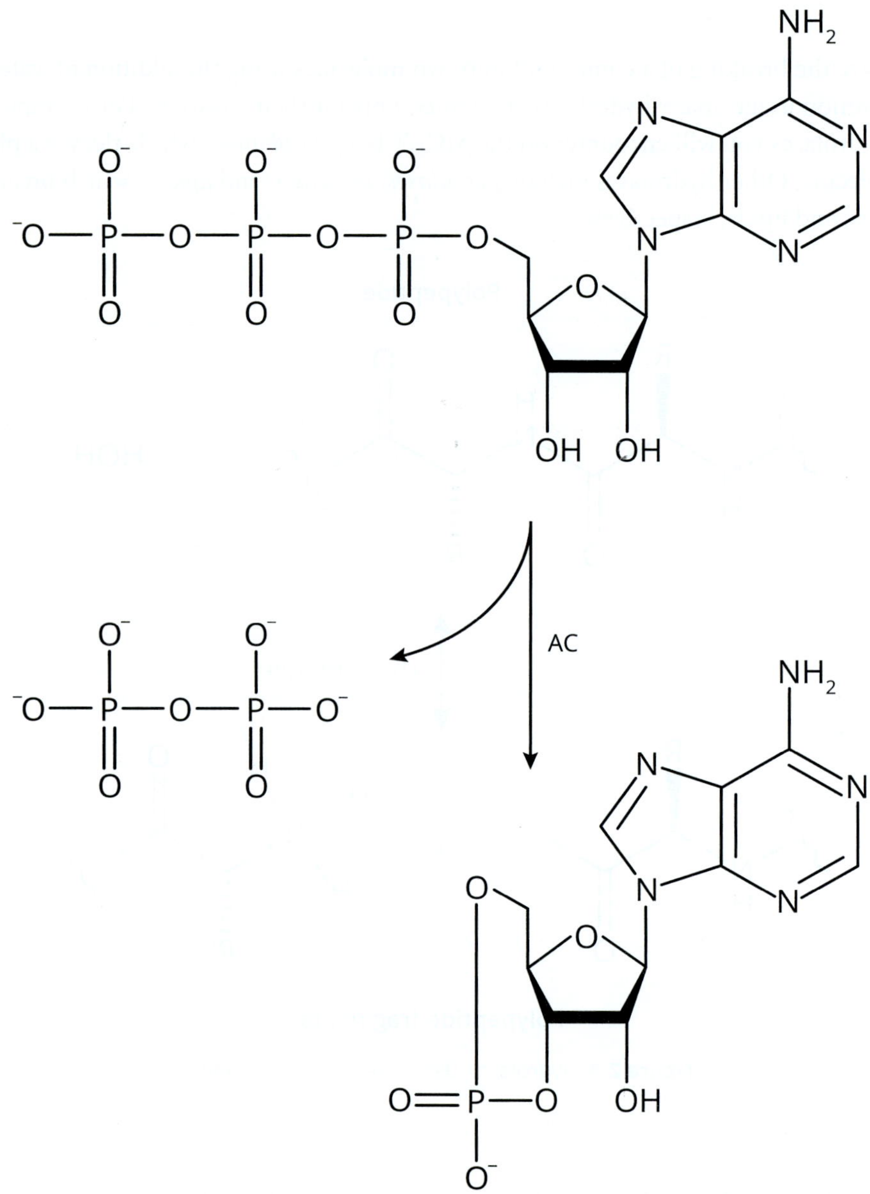

Figure 2.4 Lyases Like Adenylyl Cyclase (AC) Cleave Bonds without Using Water

Isomerases

Isomerases catalyze the rearrangement of bonds within a molecule. Some isomerases can also be classified as oxidoreductases, transferases, or lyases, depending on the mechanism of the enzyme. Keep in mind that isomerases catalyze reactions between stereoisomers as well as constitutional isomers. Figure 2.5 shows the conversion between the isomers citrate and isocitrate, which is catalyzed by the isomerase aconitase.

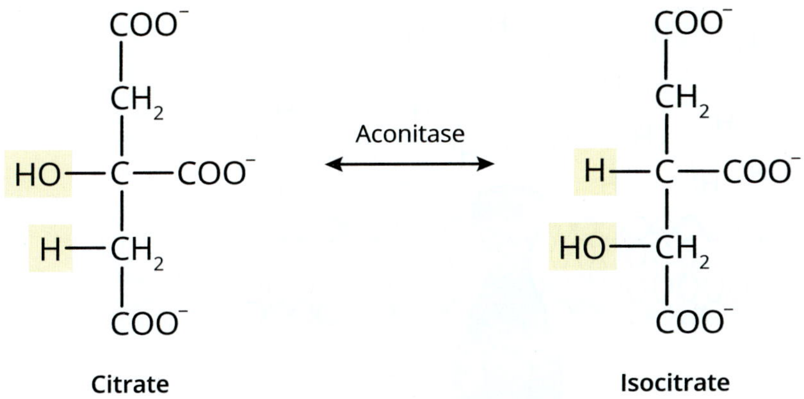

Figure 2.5 Isomerases Rearrange Bonds within Molecules

Ligases

Ligases catalyze addition or synthesis reactions, generally between large, similar molecules, and often require ATP. Synthesis reactions with smaller molecules are generally accomplished by lyases. Ligases are most likely to be encountered in nucleic acid synthesis and repair on Test Day. An example of a ligase is the enzyme acetyl-CoA carboxylase, shown in Figure 2.6, which adds a molecule of CO_2 onto acetyl-CoA to create malonyl-CoA.

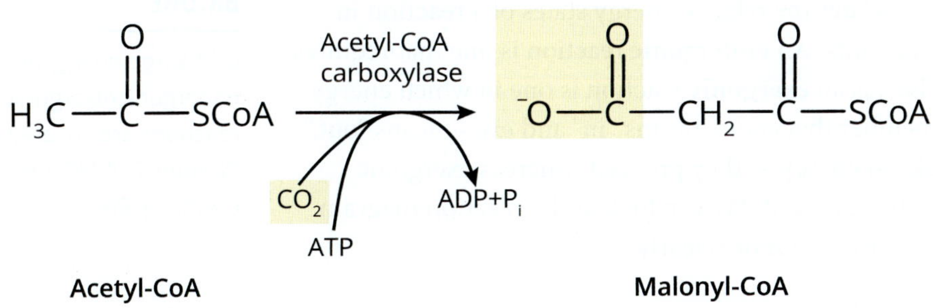

Figure 2.6 Ligases Join Large Molecules Together

Translocases

Enzymes originally were classified into six groups: oxidoreductases, transferases, hydrolases, lyases, isomerases, and ligases, which are described in more detail above. However, certain important enzymes did not properly fit into any of those six classes, so as of 2018, a seventh type was recognized: ***translocases***. Translocases are proteins that help catalyze the transport of molecules across a cell membrane. ATP synthase, shown in Figure 2.7, is an important enzyme that falls under this class. To create ATP, the F_O subunit of ATP synthase translocates protons across the inner mitochondrial membrane, where the energy from the electrochemical proton gradient is used by the F_1 subunit of ATP synthase to create ATP.

MNEMONIC

Major Enzyme Classifications: **LI'L HOTT**

- **L**igase
- **I**somerase
- **L**yase
- **H**ydrolase
- **O**xidoreductase
- **T**ransferase
- **T**ranslocase

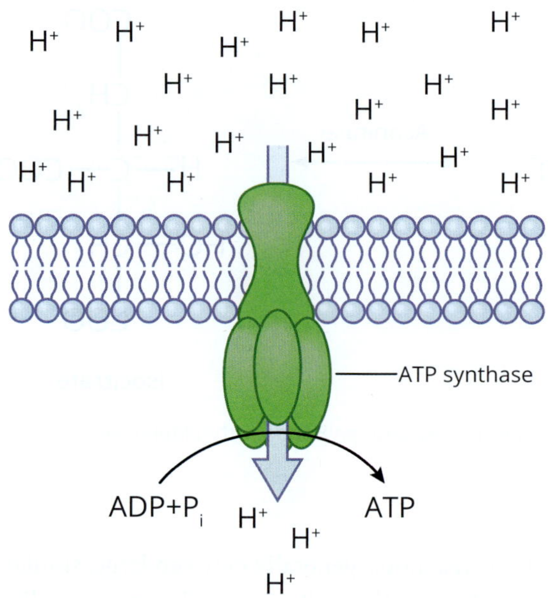

Figure 2.7 Translocases Move Molecules across Membranes

Impact on Activation Energy

Recall that thermodynamics relates the relative energy states of a reaction in terms of its products and reactants. An **endergonic** reaction is one that requires energy input ($\Delta G > 0$), whereas an **exergonic** reaction is one in which energy is given off ($\Delta G < 0$). Remember that *endo–* means "in" and *exo–* means "out," so endergonic reactions take in energy as they proceed, whereas exergonic reactions release energy as they proceed. We can look at the reaction diagram in Figure 2.8 to see this demonstrated more clearly.

BRIDGE

Gibbs free energy and endergonic/exergonic reactions are covered in Chapter 7 of *MCAT General Chemistry Review.*

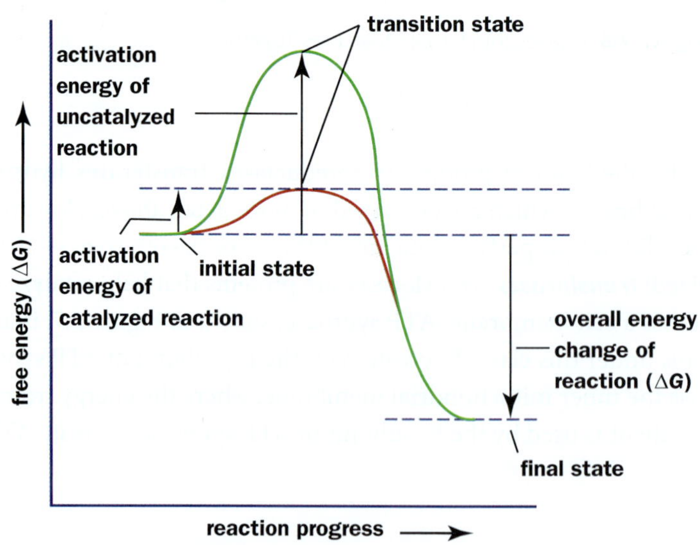

Figure 2.8 Exergonic Reaction Diagram
The activation energy required for a catalyzed reaction is lower than that of an uncatalyzed reaction while the ΔG (and ΔH) remains the same.

The reaction shown in Figure 2.8 is spontaneous. Note that the ΔG for this reaction is negative. A very important characteristic of enzymes is that they do not alter the overall free energy change for a reaction, nor do they change the equilibrium of a reaction. Rather, they affect the rate (kinetics) at which a reaction occurs; thus, they can affect how quickly a reaction gets to equilibrium but not the actual equilibrium state itself. For example, a reaction could take years to approach equilibrium without an enzyme. In comparison, with the enzyme, equilibrium might be attained within seconds. Enzymes ensure that many important reactions can occur in a reasonable amount of time in biological systems. Recall that enzymes, as catalysts, are unchanged by the reaction. What is the functional consequence of this? Far fewer copies of the enzyme are required relative to the overall amount of substrate because one enzyme can act on many, many molecules of substrate over time.

Catalysts exert their effect by lowering the **activation energy** of a reaction; in other words, they make it easier for the substrate to reach the transition state. Imagine having to walk to the other side of a tall hill. The only way to get there is to climb to the top of the hill and then walk down the other side—but wouldn't it be easier if the top of the hill was cut off so one wouldn't have to climb so high? That's exactly what catalysts do for chemical reactions when they make it easier for substrates to achieve their transition state. Most reactions catalyzed by enzymes are technically reversible, although that reversal may be extremely energetically unfavorable and therefore essentially nonexistent. Figure 2.9 summarizes the seven types of enzymes: oxidoreductase, transferase, hydrolase, lyase, ligase, transferase, and translocase.

Ligase	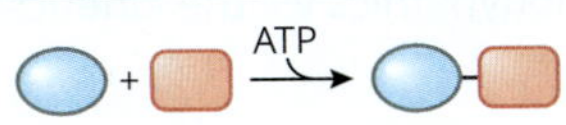	Joins molecules together
Isomerase	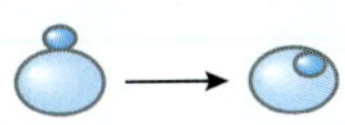	Rearranges atoms to form isomers
Lyase	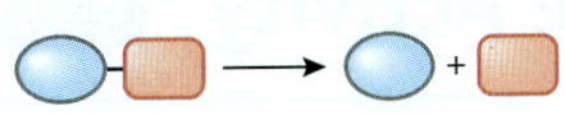	Breaks bonds without hydrolysis or oxidation
Hydrolase	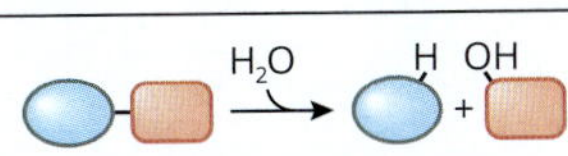	Breaks bonds with water
Oxidoreductase	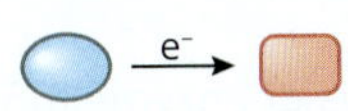	Transfers electrons
Transferase	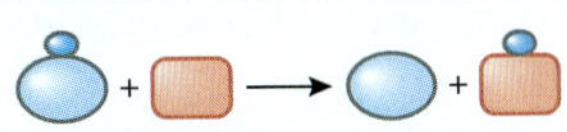	Transfers functional groups
Translocase	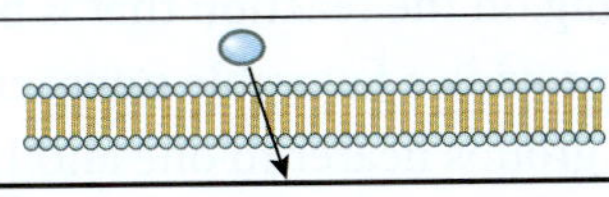	Moves molecules across membranes

Figure 2.9 The Seven Major Classes of Enzymes

MCAT CONCEPT CHECK 2.1

Before you move on, assess your understanding of the material with these questions.

1. How do enzymes function as biological catalysts?

___

2. What is enzyme specificity?

___

3. What are the names and main functions of the seven different classes of enzymes?

Name	Function

4. In what ways do enzymes affect the thermodynamics vs. the kinetics of a reaction?

___

2.2 Mechanisms of Enzyme Activity High Yield

LEARNING OBJECTIVES

After Chapter 2.2, you will be able to:

- Differentiate between coenzymes and cofactors
- Compare the induced fit and lock and key models of enzyme function

While enzyme mechanisms will vary depending on the reaction that is being catalyzed, they tend to share some common features. Enzymes may act to provide a favorable microenvironment in terms of charge or pH, stabilize the transition state, or bring reactive groups nearer to one another in the active site. The formation of the enzyme–substrate complex in the active site of an enzyme is the key catalytic activity of the enzyme, which reduces the activation energy of the reaction as described above. This interaction between a substrate and the active site of an enzyme also accounts for the selectivity and some regulatory mechanisms of enzymes.

Enzyme–Substrate Binding

The molecule upon which an enzyme acts is known as its **substrate**. The physical interaction between these two is referred to as the **enzyme–substrate complex**. The **active site** is the location within the enzyme where the substrate is held during the chemical reaction, as shown in Figure 2.10.

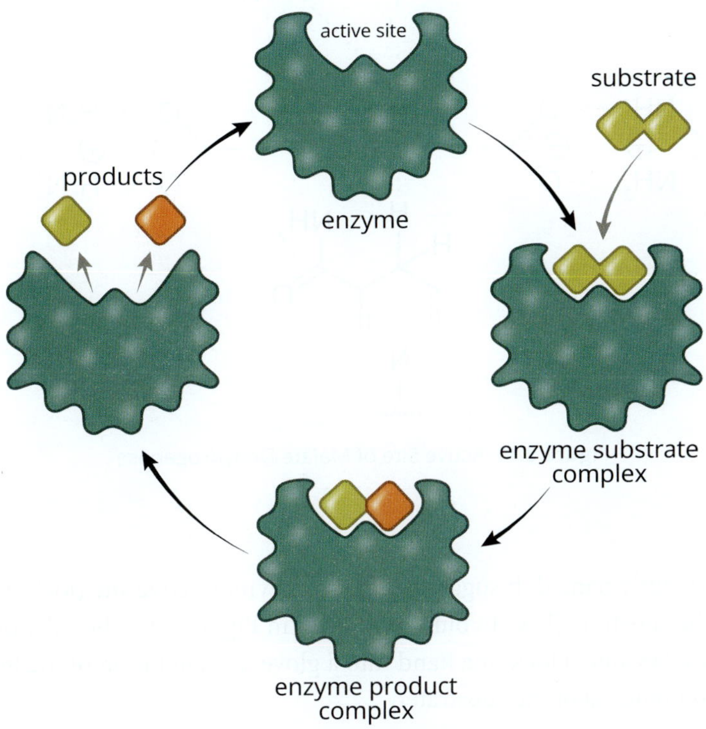

Figure 2.10 Reaction Catalysis in the Active Site of an Enzyme

The active site assumes a defined spatial arrangement in the enzyme–substrate complex, which dictates the specificity of that enzyme for a molecule or group of molecules. Hydrogen bonding, ionic interactions, and transient covalent bonds within the active site all stabilize this spatial arrangement and contribute to the efficiency of the enzyme, as shown in Figure 2.11. Two competing theories explain how enzymes and substrates interact, but one of the two is better supported than the other.

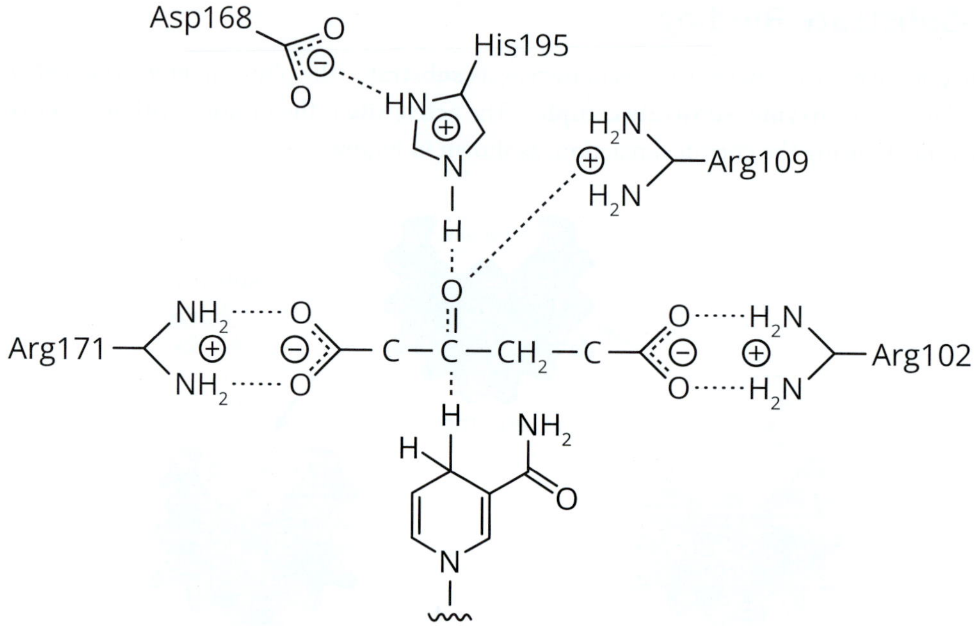

Figure 2.11 Active Site of Malate Dehydrogenase

Lock and Key Theory

The **lock and key theory** is aptly named. It suggests that the enzyme's active site (lock) is already in the appropriate conformation for the substrate (key) to bind. As shown in Figure 2.12, the substrate can then easily fit into the active site, like a key into a lock or a hand into a glove. No alteration of the tertiary or quaternary structure is necessary upon binding of the substrate.

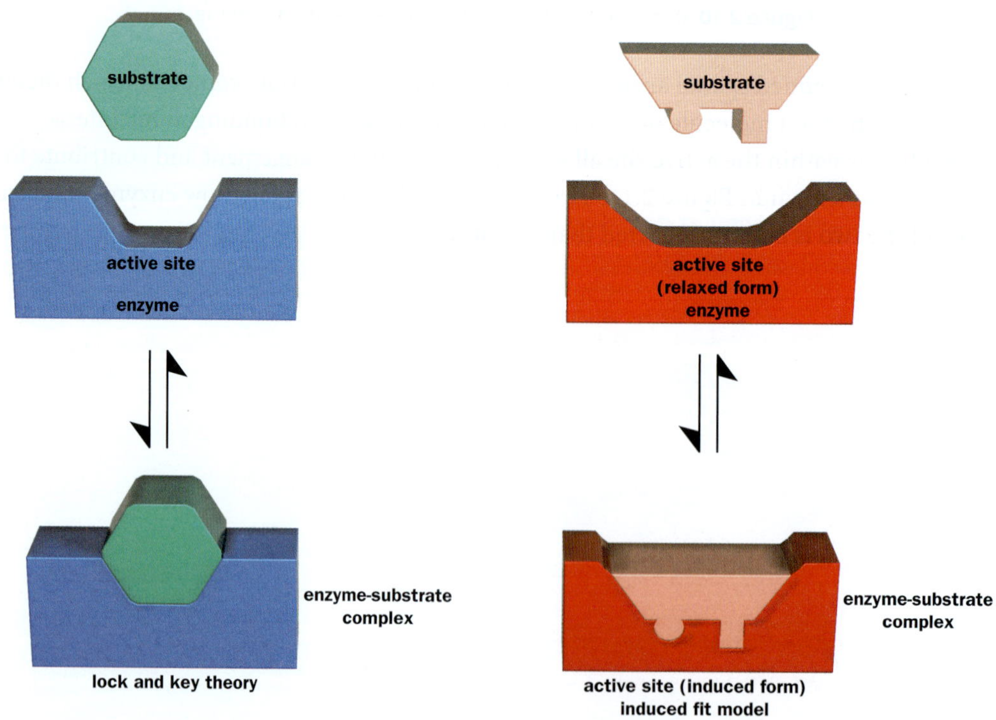

Figure 2.12 Lock and Key Theory vs. Induced Fit Model for Enzyme Catalysis

Induced Fit Model

The more scientifically accepted theory is the induced fit model; this is the one you are more likely to see referenced on Test Day. Imagine that the enzyme is a foam stress ball and the substrate is a frustrated MCAT student's hand. What's the desired interaction? The student wants to release some stress and relax. As the student's hand squeezes the ball, both change conformation. The ball is no longer spherical and the hand is no longer flat because they adjust to fit each other well. In this case, the substrate (the student) has induced a change in the shape of the enzyme (the stress ball). This interaction requires energy, and therefore, this part of the reaction is endergonic. Once the student lets go of the stress ball, we have our desired product: a relaxed, more confident test taker. Letting go of the stress ball is pretty easy and doesn't require extra energy; so, this part of the reaction is exergonic. Just like enzymes, foam stress balls return to their original shape once their crushers (substrates) let go of them. On a molecular level, demonstrated in Figure 2.12, the induced fit model starts with a substrate and an enzyme active site that don't seem to fit together. However, once the substrate is present and ready to interact with the active site, the molecules find that the induced form, or transition state, is more comfortable for both of them. Thus, the shape of the active site becomes truly complementary only after the substrate begins binding to the enzyme. Similarly, a substrate of the wrong type will not cause the appropriate conformational shift in the enzyme. Thus, the active site will not be adequately exposed, the transition state is not preferred, and no reaction occurs.

REAL WORLD

Deficiencies in vitamin cofactors can result in devastating disease. Thiamine is an essential cofactor for several enzymes involved in cellular metabolism and nerve conduction. Thiamine deficiency, often a result of excess alcohol consumption and poor diet, results in diseases including Wernicke–Korsakoff syndrome. In this disorder, patients suffer from a variety of neurologic deficits, including delirium, balance problems, and, in severe cases, the inability to form new memories.

Cofactors and Coenzymes

Many enzymes require nonprotein molecules called **cofactors** or **coenzymes** to be effective. These cofactors and coenzymes tend to be small in size so they can bind to the active site of the enzyme and participate in the catalysis of the reaction, usually by carrying charge through ionization, protonation, or deprotonation. Cofactors and coenzymes are usually kept at low concentrations in cells, so they can be recruited only when needed. Enzymes without their cofactors are called **apoenzymes**, whereas those containing them are **holoenzymes**, as depicted in Figure 2.13. Cofactors are attached in a variety of ways, ranging from weak noncovalent interactions to strong covalent ones. Tightly bound cofactors or coenzymes that are necessary for enzyme function are known as **prosthetic groups**.

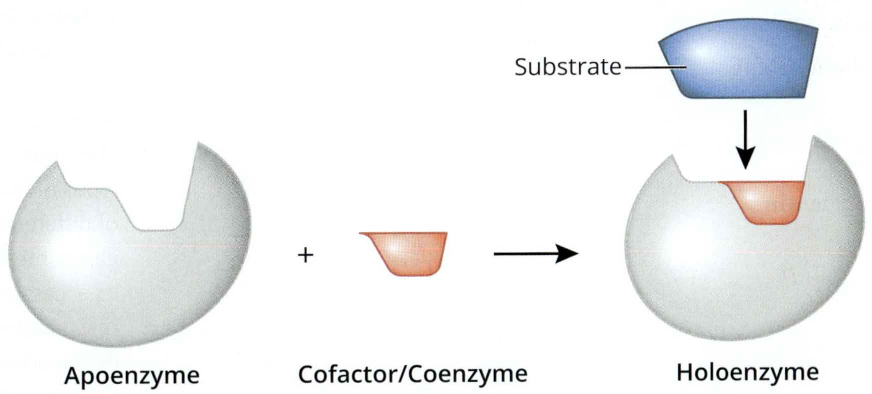

Figure 2.13 Apoenzyme vs. Holoenzyme

Cofactors and coenzymes are topics that we are likely to see on Test Day, so they are important to know. Cofactors are generally inorganic molecules or metal ions, and are often ingested as dietary minerals. In addition to inorganic ions, cofactors can also be large organic molecules, like the heme group shown in Figure 2.14. Coenzymes are small organic groups, the vast majority of which are vitamins or derivatives of vitamins such as NAD^+, FAD, and coenzyme A. The water-soluble vitamins include the B complex vitamins and ascorbic acid (vitamin C), and are important coenzymes that must be replenished regularly because they are easily excreted. The fat-soluble vitamins—A, D, E, and K—are better regulated by partition coefficients, which quantify the ability of a molecule to dissolve in a polar vs. nonpolar environment. Enzymatic reactions are not restricted to a single cofactor or coenzyme. For example, metabolic reactions often require magnesium, NAD^+ (derived from vitamin B_3), and biotin (vitamin B_7) simultaneously.

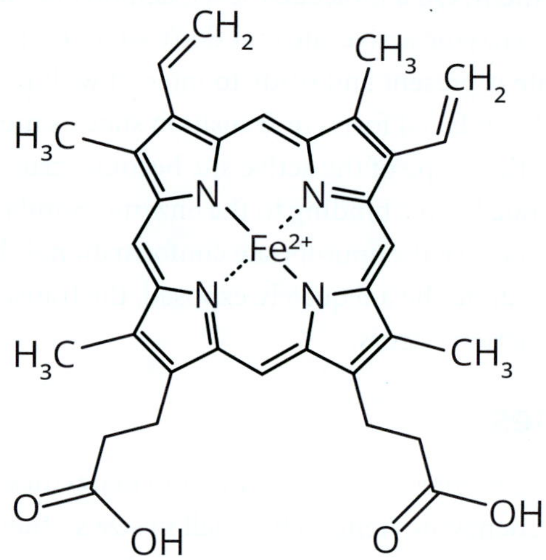

Figure 2.14 Organic Cofactor (Heme)

BRIDGE

Vitamins come in two major classes: fat- and water-soluble. This is important to consider in digestive diseases, where different parts of the gastrointestinal tract may be affected by different disease processes. Because different parts of the gastrointestinal tract specialize in the absorption of different types of biomolecules, loss of different parts of the gastrointestinal tract or its accessory organs may result in different vitamin deficiencies. The digestive system is discussed in Chapter 9 of *MCAT Biology Review*.

Memorization of the B vitamins is low yield for the MCAT, though testable; however, familiarity with their names may make biochemistry passages easier on Test Day:

- B_1: thiamine
- B_2: riboflavin
- B_3: niacin
- B_5: pantothenic acid
- B_6: pyridoxal phosphate
- B_7: biotin
- B_9: folic acid
- B_{12}: cyanocobalamin

MCAT CONCEPT CHECK 2.2

Before you move on, assess your understanding of the material with these questions.

1. How do the lock and key theory and induced fit model differ?

Lock and Key	Induced Fit

2. What do cofactors and coenzymes do? How do they differ?

____

2.3 Enzyme Kinetics High Yield

LEARNING OBJECTIVES

After Chapter 2.3, you will be able to:

- Predict how changes in enzyme and solute concentration will affect enzyme kinetics
- Define enzyme cooperativity
- Compare Lineweaver–Burk and Michaelis–Menten plots
- Explain key points on a Lineweaver–Burk or Michaelis–Menten plot:

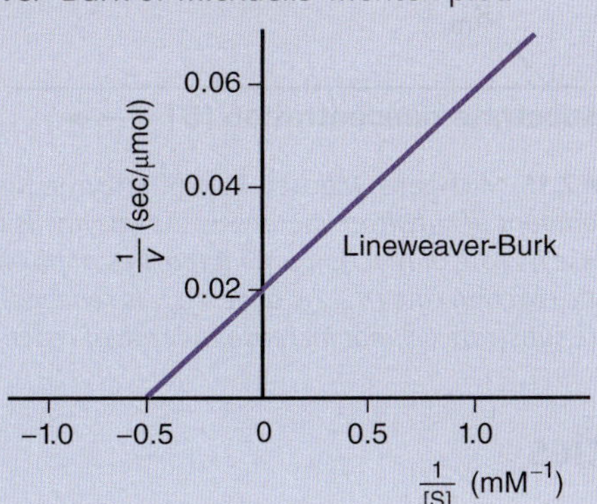

Kinetics of Monomeric Enzymes

Enzyme kinetics is a high-yield topic that can score us several points on Test Day. Just as the relief our student derives from squeezing a stress ball depends on a number of factors, such as size and shape of the ball and the student's baseline level of stress, enzyme kinetics are dependent on factors like environmental conditions and concentrations of substrate and enzyme.

The concentrations of the substrate, [S], and enzyme, [E], greatly affect how quickly a reaction will occur. Let's say that we have 100 stress balls (enzymes) and only 10 frustrated students (substrates) to derive stress relief from them. This represents a high enzyme concentration relative to substrate. Because there are many active sites available, we will quickly form products (students letting go and feeling relaxed); in a chemical sense, we would reach equilibrium quickly. As we slowly add more substrate (students), the rate of the reaction will increase; that is, more people will relax in the same amount of time because we have plenty of available stress balls for them to squeeze. However, as we add more and more people (and start approaching 100 students), we begin to level off and reach a maximal rate of relaxation. There are fewer and fewer available stress balls until finally all active sites are occupied. Unlike before, inviting more students into the room will not change the rate of the reaction. It cannot go any faster once it has reached **saturation**. At this rate, the enzyme is working at maximum velocity, denoted by $\mathbf{V_{max}}$. The only way to increase V_{max} is by increasing the enzyme concentration. In the cell, this can be accomplished by inducing the expression of the gene encoding the enzyme. These concepts are represented graphically in Figure 2.15.

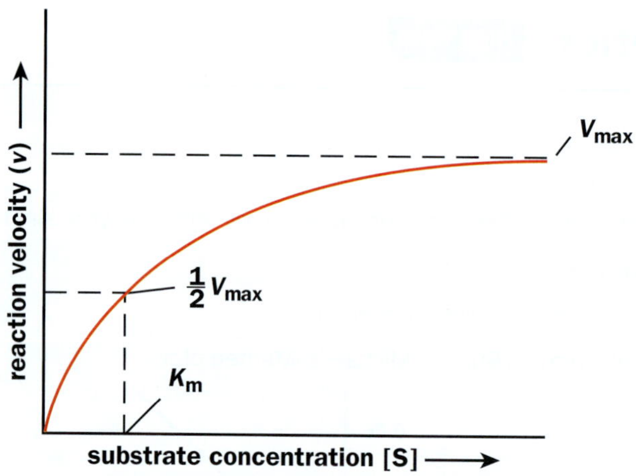

Figure 2.15 Michaelis–Menten Plot of Enzyme Kinetics
As the amount of substrate increases, the enzyme is able to increase its rate of reaction until it reaches a maximum enzymatic reaction rate (V_{max}); once V_{max} is reached, adding more substrate will not increase the rate of reaction.

Michaelis–Menten Kinetics

For most enzymes with one substrate, the Michaelis–Menten equation describes how the rate of the reaction, v, depends on the concentration of both the enzyme, [E], and the substrate, [S], to form the product, [P]. The equation presumes a simple two-step reaction: enzyme–substrate complexes form at a rate k_1; then the ES complex can either dissociate at a rate k_{-1} or turn into E + P at a rate k_{cat}:

$$E + S \underset{k_{-1}}{\overset{k_1}{\rightleftharpoons}} ES \xrightarrow{k_{cat}} E + P$$

Equation 2.1

Note that in either case, the enzyme is regenerated. Michaelis–Menten kinetics presumes a set of assumptions and conditions:

1. Measurements of the initial enzyme velocity (v_o) must be at early time points, where [P] = 0.
2. The concentration of substrate must be in excess of the concentration of enzyme ([S] >> [E]) so that [S] is effectively constant at early time points.
3. The binding of E to S ($E + S \rightleftharpoons ES$) is fast, allowing for [E], [S], and [ES] to reach steady state and therefore equilibrium ratios. The catalytic step ($ES \longrightarrow P$) is slow and rate-limiting.
4. There are only two forms of the enzyme: E and ES. The total concentration of enzyme [E_T] is the sum of the free enzyme and enzyme-substrate complex ([E_T] = [E] + [ES]).

On Test Day, the concentration of enzyme will be kept constant unless otherwise stated. Under these conditions, we can relate the velocity of the enzyme to substrate concentration using the Michaelis–Menten equation:

$$v = \frac{V_{max}\,[S]}{K_m + [S]}$$

Equation 2.2

Some important and Test Day–relevant math can be derived from this equation. When the reaction rate is equal to half of V_{max}, K_m = [S]:

$$\frac{V_{max}}{2} = \frac{V_{max}\,[S]}{K_m + [S]}$$

$$V_{max}(K_m + [S]) = 2(V_{max}[S])$$

$$K_m + [S] = 2[S]$$

$$K_m = [S]$$

K_m can, therefore, be understood to be the substrate concentration at which half of the enzyme's active sites are full (half the stress balls are in use). $\boldsymbol{K_m}$ is the **Michaelis constant** and is often used to compare enzymes. Under certain conditions, K_m is a measure of the affinity of the enzyme for its substrate. When comparing two enzymes, the one with the higher K_m has the lower affinity for its substrate because it requires a higher substrate concentration to be half-saturated. The K_m value is an intrinsic property of the enzyme–substrate system and cannot be altered by changing the concentration of substrate or enzyme.

KEY CONCEPT

We can assess an enzyme's affinity for a substrate by noting the K_m. A low K_m reflects a high affinity for the substrate (low [S] required for 50% enzyme saturation). Conversely, a high K_m reflects a low affinity of the enzyme for the substrate.

For a given concentration of enzyme, the Michaelis–Menten relationship generally graphs as a hyperbola, as seen in the Michaelis–Menten plot in Figure 2.15. When substrate concentration is less than K_m, changes in substrate concentration will greatly affect the reaction rate. At high substrate concentrations exceeding K_m, the reaction rate increases much more slowly as it approaches V_{max}, where it becomes independent of substrate concentration.

The variable V_{max} represents maximum enzyme velocity and is measured in moles of enzyme per second. Also, V_{max} can be mathematically related to $\boldsymbol{k_{cat}}$, which has units of s^{-1}:

$$V_{max} = [E]\,k_{cat}$$

Equation 2.3

Qualitatively speaking, k_{cat} measures the number of substrate molecules "turned over," or converted to product, per enzyme molecule per second. Most enzymes have k_{cat} values between 10^1 and 10^3. The Michaelis–Menton equation above can be restated using k_{cat}:

$$v = \frac{k_{cat}[E][S]}{K_m + [S]}$$

At very low substrate concentrations, where $K_m >> [S]$, this derived equation can be further simplified as:

$$v = \frac{k_{cat}}{K_m}[E][S]$$

The ratio of k_{cat}/K_m is referred to as the **catalytic efficiency** of the enzyme. A large k_{cat} (high turnover) or a small K_m (high substrate affinity) will result in a higher catalytic efficiency, which indicates a more efficient enzyme.

Lineweaver–Burk Plots

The Lineweaver–Burk plot is a double reciprocal graph of the Michaelis–Menten equation. The same data graphed in this way yield a straight line as shown in Figure 2.16. The actual data are represented by the portion of the graph to the right of the y-axis, but the line is extrapolated into the upper left quadrant to determine its intercept with the x-axis. The intercept of the line with the x-axis gives the value of $-\frac{1}{K_m}$. The intercept of the line with the y-axis gives the value of $\frac{1}{V_{max}}$. The Lineweaver–Burk plot is especially useful when determining the type of inhibition that an enzyme is experiencing because V_{max} and K_m can be compared without estimation.

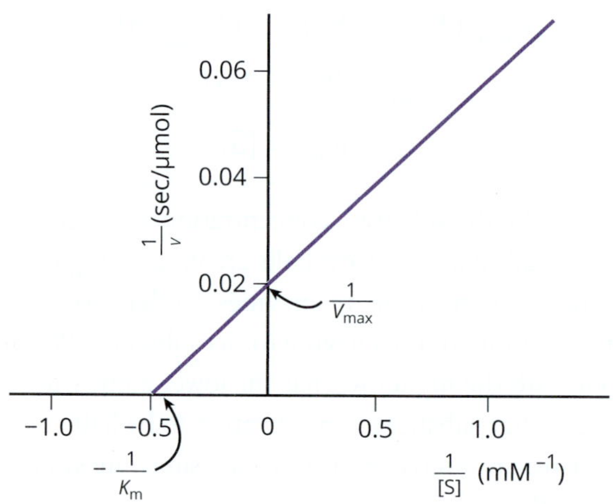

Figure 2.16 Experimentally Determined Lineweaver–Burk (Double Reciprocal) Plot Used to Calculate the Values of K_m and V_{max}

Cooperativity

Certain enzymes do not show the normal hyperbola when graphed on a Michaelis–Menten plot (v vs. [S]), but rather show sigmoidal (S-shaped) kinetics owing to cooperativity among substrate binding sites, as shown in Figure 2.18. Cooperative enzymes have multiple subunits and multiple active sites. Subunits and enzymes may exist in one of two states: a low-affinity tense state (T) or a high-affinity relaxed state (R), as shown in Figure 2.17. Binding of the substrate encourages the transition of other subunits from the T state to the R state, which increases the likelihood of substrate binding by these other subunits. Conversely, loss of substrate can encourage the transition from the R state to the T state, and promote dissociation of substrate from the remaining subunits. Think of cooperative enzyme kinetics like a party. As more people start arriving, the atmosphere becomes more relaxed and the party seems more appealing, but as people start going home the party dies down and more people are encouraged to leave so the tense hosts can clean up. Enzymes showing cooperative kinetics are often regulatory enzymes in pathways, like *phosphofructokinase-1* in glycolysis. Cooperative enzymes are also subject to activation and inhibition, both competitively and through allosteric sites.

MCAT EXPERTISE

The cooperative binding of hemoglobin, which acts as a transport protein rather than an enzyme, results in a characteristic sigmoidal binding curve that is an MCAT favorite.

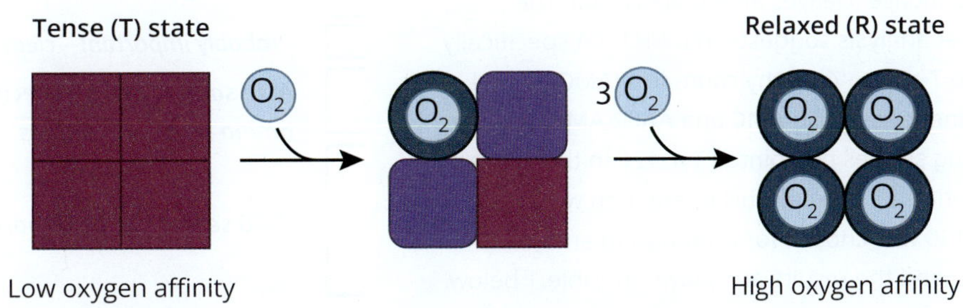

Figure 2.17 Low-affinity Tense State (T) vs. High-affinity Relaxed State (R)

Cooperativity can also be quantified using a numerical value called **Hill's coefficient**. The value of Hill's coefficient indicates the nature of binding by the molecule:

- If Hill's coefficient > 1, positively cooperative binding is occurring, such that after one ligand is bound the affinity of the enzyme for further ligand(s) increases.
- If Hill's coefficient < 1, negatively cooperative binding is occurring, such that after one ligand is bound the affinity of the enzyme for further ligand(s) decreases.
- If Hill's coefficient $= 1$, the enzyme does not exhibit cooperative binding.

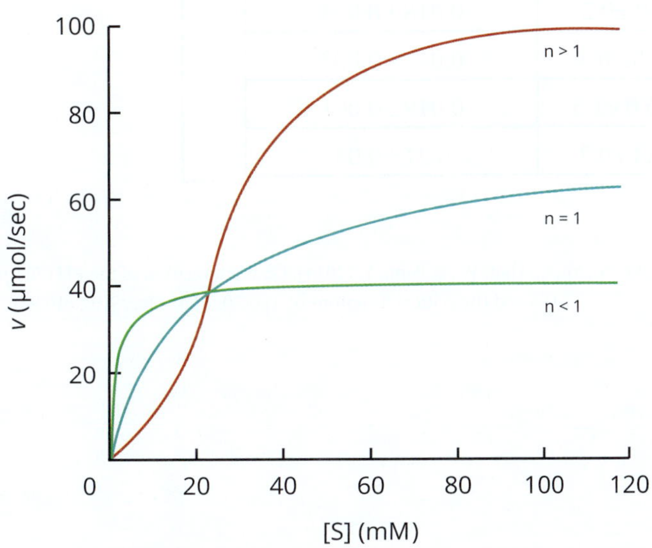

Figure 2.18 Cooperativity in Enzyme Kinetics

BIOCHEMISTRY GUIDED EXAMPLE WITH EXPERT THINKING

The PH1704 protease from *Pyrococcus horikoshii* OT3 is a hyperthermophilic enzyme that belongs to the DJ-1/ThiJ/PfpI superfamily. One of its members, the human protein DJ-1, has recently been reported to cause certain types of early-onset Parkinsonism. Thus, an increasing number of studies on this superfamily are being conducted. Despite this growing interest, few members of this superfamily have been biochemically characterized.

This is just a lot of context; the useful info is that PH1704 is a protease, which means it is an enzyme that cleaves peptide bonds

PH1704 has both endopeptidase (cleaves nonterminal amino acids) and aminopeptidase (cleaves amino acids from the N-terminus) activity.

2 kinds of protease activity for this enzyme

Further analysis suggests that PH1704 specifically cleaves after arginine.

Probably important—cleaves after arginine!

Two 7-amino-4-methylcoumarin (AMC)-linked substrates were used in kinetic assays: R-AMC and AAFR-AMC.

AMC sounds like a molecule attached to amino acids or peptides

Predictive substrate docking studies pinpointed Tyr-120 in the active site, possibly involved in aromatic and hydrophobic interaction with the substrate. Therefore, Tyr-120 was chosen for mutation to analyze the effects on PH1704 kinetics, and the results are shown in Table 1 below.

Y120 seems like an important residue

Enzyme	Aminopeptidase (R-AMC)		
	K_{cat} (min^{-1})	K_m (μM)	K_{cat}/K_m (min^{-1} μM^{-1})
WT	0.646±0.05	12±0.65	0.052±0.008
Y120S	0.147±0.01	9.0±0.43	0.024±0.004
Y120W	1.2±0.07	20.6±0.77	0.066±0.005
Y120P	4.37±0.12	11.3±0.59	0.398±0.025
Enzyme	**Endopeptidase (AAFR-AMC)**		
	K_{cat} (min^{-1})	K_m (μM)	K_{cat}/K_m (min^{-1} μM^{-1})
WT	0.11±0.02	10±0.2	0.018±0.004
Y120S	0.084±0.01	6.5±0.4	0.017±0.003
Y120W	0.12±0.01	16.0±1.5	0.019±0.001
Y120P	1.13±0.07	5.4±0.3	0.21±0.03

Table 1

Trends: catalytic efficiency (k_{cat}/K_m) seems much higher for Y120P, Y120S is much slower at producing product in both cases (lower k_{cat}), and, in general, efficiency is higher for aminopeptidase than for endopeptidase activity

Adapted from Zhan, D., Bai, A., Yu, L., Han, W., & Feng, Y. (2014). Characterization of the PH1704 protease from *Pyrococcus horikoshii* OT3 and the critical functions of Tyr120. *PLoS One*, 9(9), e103902. doi:10.1371/journal.pone.010390.

According to the data, does PH1704 have equivalent aminopeptidase and endopeptidase activity? Why or why not?

The question asks us for data analysis, so we know we should start by making sure we understand what the given material is telling us. A quick scan of the passage reveals unfamiliar enzymes, terminology, and a data-packed table, so a careful read of the passage for the big picture will be important in order to relate what the table is trying to prove. We are also definitely going to need to bring in some of our outside knowledge about enzymes. The passage describes an enzyme called PH1704, which has several characteristics outlined in the first half of the paragraph. We're told it's a protease, which means it breaks peptide bonds, and it's hyperthermophilic. Breaking down the term hyperthermophilic, we get *hyper-* (higher) *-thermo-* (heat) *-philic* (love), and we can thus deduce that the enzyme is from a bacterial species that lives in high temperatures. Next, we're told it's an endopeptidase (*endo-* meaning between) and an aminopeptidase with a strong preference for arginine. There are two substrates described in the study. Notice how only R-AMC can be used to discern the aminopeptidase activity, and AAFR-AMC can be used to test endopeptidase activity. Finally, we're told that Tyr-120 can be important for activity, so researchers created mutations of this residue and the kinetic information of the resulting mutants is described in Table 1.

The question asks us to determine whether PH1704 acts equally as an aminopeptidase and an endopeptidase. In order to answer this question, first note that the mutation data for Y120 is not needed since we are only being asked about the wild-type PH1704 enzyme.

All we really need is a comparison between the WT enzyme with R-AMC as a substrate, and WT enzyme with AAFR-AMC as a substrate. Also, we need to determine whether k_{cat}, k_m, or k_{cat}/k_m will be most useful. Recall that k_{cat} provides information about how much product is produced per unit time, and k_m is a measure of substrate affinity. To have an enzyme that is maximally efficient, you want both a high catalytic turnover (high k_{cat}) and a high substrate affinity (low k_m), so the best comparison would be the k_{cat}/k_m data, which is equal to the catalytic efficiency of an enzyme. The catalytic efficiency for PH1704 as an aminopeptidase is 0.052 $min^{-1}/\mu M$, and for PH1704 as an endopeptidase efficiency is 0.018 $min^{-1}/\mu M$.

Since these values of catalytic efficiency are different when measuring aminopeptidase and endopeptidase activity, we can conclude that PH1704 functions more effectively as an aminopeptidase than as an endopeptidase.

Multi-Substrate Reactions

The Michaelis–Menten model of enzyme kinetics deals with single substrate reactions, but the majority of known enzymatic reactions involve more than one substrate. Some of the multi-substrate reactions are detailed in Figure 2.19.

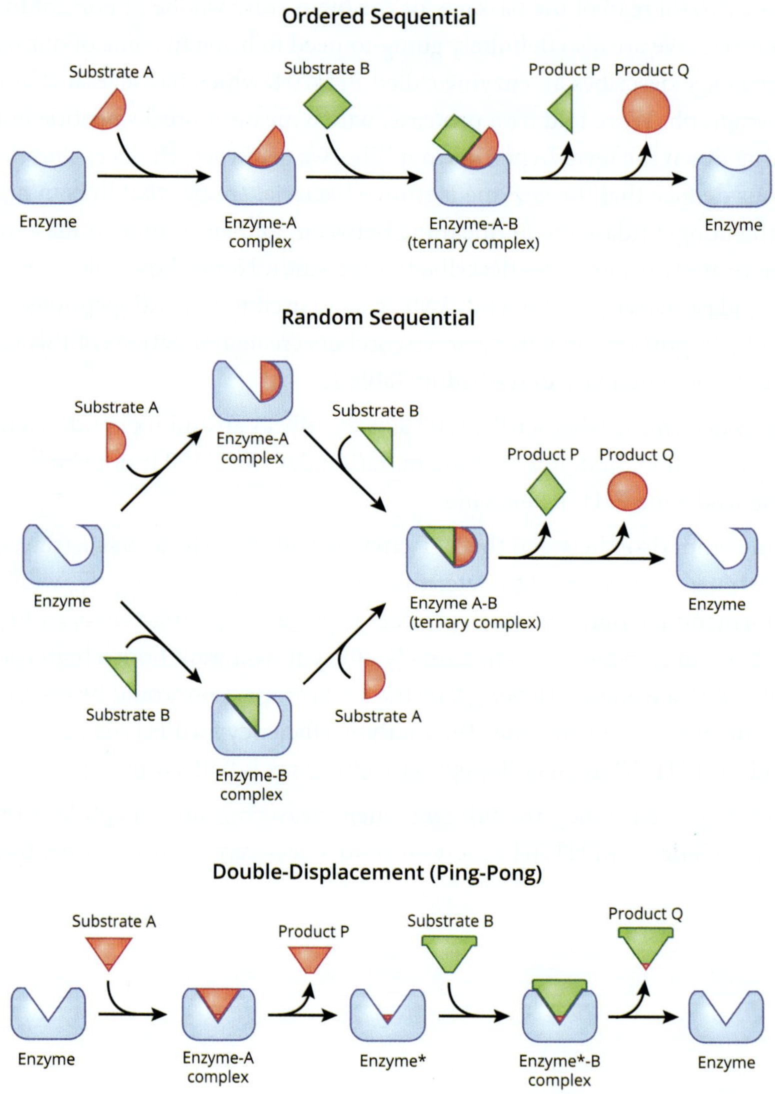

Figure 2.19 Multi-Substrate Reaction Mechanisms

In an **ordered sequential reaction**, substrates bind to the enzyme in a specific sequence. The conversion of pyruvate into lactate by lactate dehydrogenase demonstrates this type of reaction mechanism: Coenzyme NADH binds to lactate dehydrogenase first, and only then can pyruvate bind for the catalyzation of NADH into NAD^+ and pyruvate into lactate.

In contrast to an ordered sequential reaction, a **random sequential reaction** is unordered, meaning that the substrates and products can bind and release without a preference in order. The enzyme creatinine kinase follows this mechanism, where either ATP or creatinine can first bind the active site to make ADP and phosphocreatine.

In a **double-displacement (ping-pong)** reaction, one substrate binds first to the enzyme and is turned into product, leaving behind an intermediate form of the enzyme. The modified enzyme can then bind a second substrate and turn it into product. The formation of phosphocholine from choline by choline kinase occurs by this mechanism, where ATP binds to choline kinase, resulting in the formation of ADP and phosphorylation of choline kinase. This modified enzyme then binds to choline after ADP ejection, leading to phosphorylation of choline to create phosphocholine and dephosphorylation of the enzyme to revert it back to its original form.

MCAT CONCEPT CHECK 2.3

Before you move on, assess your understanding of the material with these questions.

1. What are the effects of increasing [S] on enzyme kinetics? What about increasing [E]?
   - Increasing [S]:

   ____

   - Increasing [E]:

   ____

2. How are the Michaelis–Menten and Lineweaver–Burk plots similar? How are they different?
   - Similarities:

   ____

   - Differences:

   ____

3. What does K_m represent? What would an increase in K_m signify?

   ____

   ____

4. What do the *x*- and *y*-intercepts in a Lineweaver–Burk plot represent?
   - *x*-intercept:

   ____

   - *y*-intercept:

   ____

5. What is enzyme cooperativity?

   ____

2.4 Effects of Local Conditions on Enzyme Activity High Yield

LEARNING OBJECTIVES

After Chapter 2.4, you will be able to:

- Predict how changes to the environment will alter enzyme behavior
- Estimate the ideal pH and temperature for enzymes found in the human body

The activity of an enzyme is heavily influenced by its environment; in particular, temperature, acidity or alkalinity (pH), and high salinity have significant effects on the ability of an enzyme to carry out its function. Note that the terms **enzyme activity**, **enzyme velocity**, and **enzyme rate** are all used synonymously on the MCAT.

Temperature

Enzyme-catalyzed reactions tend to double in velocity for every 10°C increase in temperature until the optimum temperature is reached; for the human body, this is 37°C (98.6°F or 310 K). After this, activity falls off sharply, as the enzyme will denature at higher temperatures, as shown in Figure 2.20. Some enzymes that are overheated may regain their function if cooled. A real-life example of temperature dependence occurs in Siamese cats. Siamese cats are dark on their faces, ears, tails, and feet but white elsewhere. Why? The enzyme responsible for pigmentation, *tyrosinase*, is mutated in Siamese cats. It is ineffective at body temperature but at cooler temperatures becomes active. Thus, only the tail, feet, ears, and face (cooled by air passing through the nose and mouth) have an active form of the enzyme and are dark.

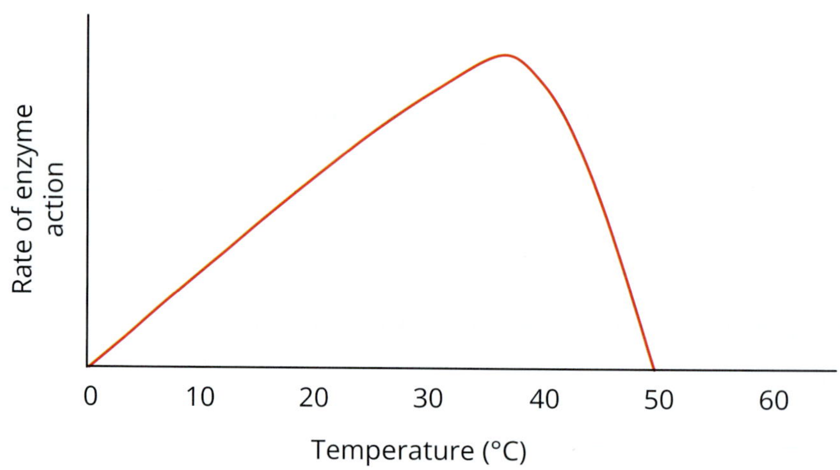

Figure 2.20 Effect of Temperature on the Rate of Enzyme Action

pH

Most enzymes also depend on pH in order to function properly, not only because pH affects the ionization of the active site, but also because changes in pH can lead to denaturation of the enzyme. For enzymes that circulate and function in human blood, this optimal pH is 7.4. A pH < 7.35 in human blood is termed acidemia. Even though it's more basic than *chemically* neutral 7.0, it is more acidic than *physiologically* neutral 7.4. Where might exceptions to this pH 7.4 occur? Both are in our digestive tract. Pepsin, which works in the stomach, has maximal activity around pH 2, whereas pancreatic enzymes, which work in the small intestine, work best around pH 8.5. The graph in Figure 2.21 shows the different optimal pH ranges for the enzymes pepsin, salivary amylase, and trypsin.

BRIDGE

The pH levels in the stomach and intestine, and their effects on these gastric and pancreatic enzymes, are covered in Chapter 9 of *MCAT Biology Review*.

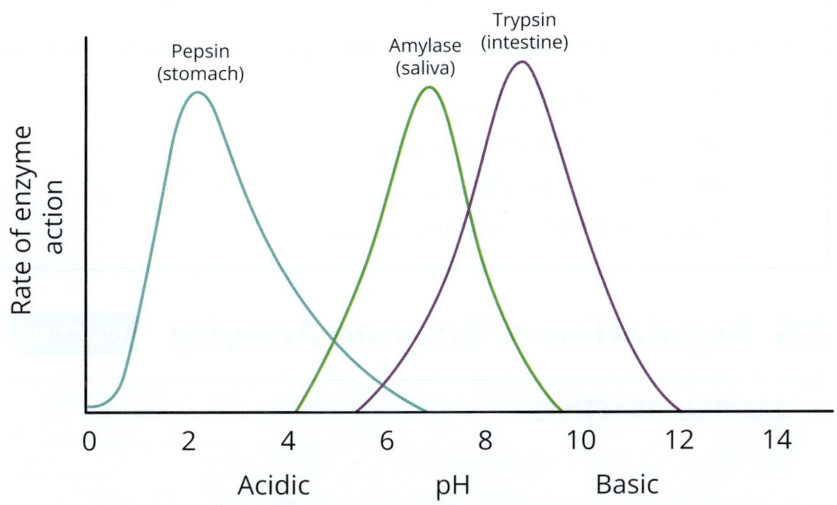

Figure 2.21 Different Enzymes Have Different Optimal pH Ranges

Salinity

While the effect of salinity or osmolarity is not generally of physiologic significance, altering the concentration of salt can change enzyme activity *in vitro*. Increasing levels of salt can disrupt hydrogen and ionic bonds, causing a partial change in the conformation of the enzyme, and in some cases causing denaturation.

MCAT CONCEPT CHECK 2.4

Before you move on, assess your understanding of the material with these questions.

1. What are the effects of temperature, pH, and salinity on the function of enzymes?
   - Temperature:

   ____

   - pH:

   ____

   - Salinity:

   ____

2. What is the ideal temperature for most enzymes in the body? The ideal pH?
   - Ideal temperature: _______ °C = _______ °F = _______ K
   - Ideal pH (most enzymes): _______
   - Ideal pH (gastric enzymes): _______
   - Ideal pH (pancreatic enzymes): _______

2.5 Regulation of Enzyme Activity High Yield

LEARNING OBJECTIVES

After Chapter 2.5, you will be able to:

- Explain feedback inhibition and irreversible inhibition
- Differentiate between the four types of reversible inhibition
- Differentiate between transient and covalent enzyme modifications
- Recall the traits of zymogens

BRIDGE

Negative feedback is an important topic in both enzymology and the endocrine system. Remember that most hormonal feedback loops are also inhibited by negative feedback. The endocrine system is discussed in Chapter 5 of *MCAT Biology Review*.

Although enzymes are useful, the body must be able to control when they work; for example, enzymes involved in mitosis should be shut off when cells are no longer dividing (in the G_0 phase). This may be accomplished in a variety of ways, as described below.

Feedback Regulation

Enzymes are often subject to regulation by products further down a given metabolic pathway, a process called **feedback regulation**. Less often, enzymes may be regulated by intermediates that precede the enzyme in the pathway, also called **feed-forward regulation**. This is clearly evident in the study of metabolism, as discussed in Chapters 9 through 12 of *MCAT Biochemistry Review*. While there are some examples of feedback activation, feedback inhibition is far more common. Feedback inhibition, or **negative feedback**, helps maintain homeostasis: once we have enough of a given product, we want to turn off the pathway that creates that product, rather than creating more. In feedback inhibition, the product may bind to the active site of an enzyme or multiple enzymes that acted earlier in its biosynthetic pathway, thereby competitively inhibiting these enzymes and making them unavailable for use. This is schematically represented in Figure 2.22, as we see product D feeding back to inhibit the first enzyme in the pathway.

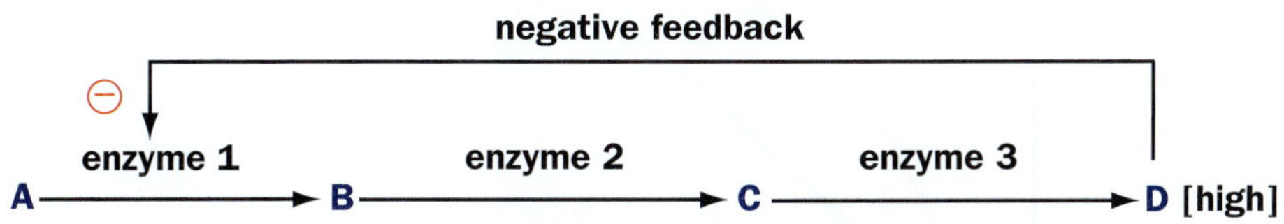

Figure 2.22 Feedback Inhibition by the Product of a Metabolic Pathway
A high concentration of the product, D, inhibits enzyme 1, slowing the entire pathway.

Reversible Inhibition

There are four types of reversible inhibition: competitive, noncompetitive, uncompetitive, and mixed. The MCAT typically tests the first three types of inhibition directly, while mixed inhibition is tested through exclusion by way of presenting an inhibitor that does not fall under the three prior categories. Table 2.2 at the end of this section summarizes the features of each type of reversible inhibition.

Competitive Inhibition

Competitive inhibition simply involves occupancy of the active site, as shown in Figure 2.23. Substrates cannot access enzymatic binding sites if there is an inhibitor in the way.

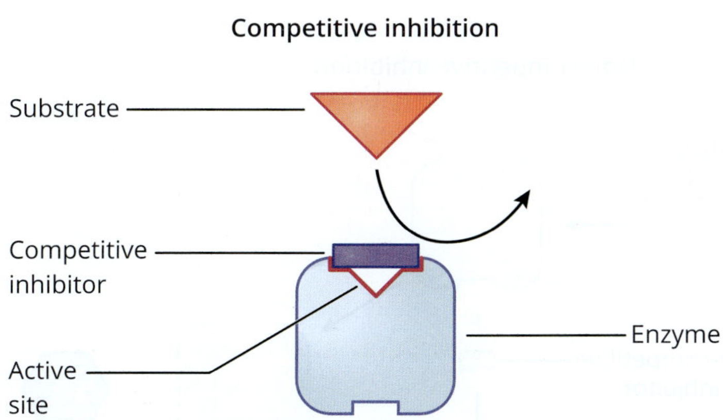

Figure 2.23 Competitive Inhibition

REAL WORLD

The concept of competitive inhibition has relevance in the clinical setting. For example, methanol (wood alcohol), if ingested, is enzymatically converted to toxic metabolites, which can cause blindness and even death. Administration of intravenous ethanol is the treatment of choice for a patient suffering from methanol poisoning. Ethanol works by competing with methanol for the active sites of the enzymes involved.

Competitive inhibition can be overcome by adding more substrate so that the substrate-to-inhibitor ratio is higher. If more molecules of substrate are available than molecules of inhibitor, then the enzyme will be more likely to bind substrate than inhibitor (assuming the enzyme has equal affinity for both molecules). Adding a competitive inhibitor does not alter the value of V_{max} because if enough substrate is added, it will outcompete the inhibitor and be able to run the reaction at maximum velocity. A competitive inhibitor does increase the measured value of K_m. This is because the substrate concentration has to be higher to reach half the maximum velocity in the presence of the inhibitor. A Lineweaver–Burk plot comparing an enzyme with and without a competitive inhibitor is shown in Figure 2.24.

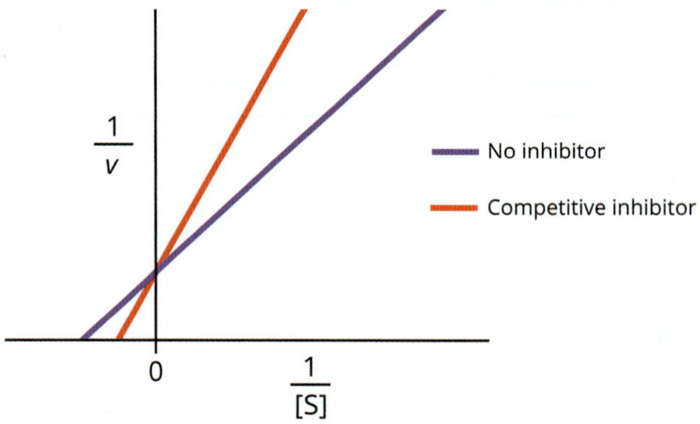

Figure 2.24 Lineweaver–Burk Plot of Competitive Inhibition

Noncompetitive Inhibition

Noncompetitive inhibitors bind to an allosteric site instead of the active site, which induces a change in enzyme conformation. Allosteric sites are non-catalytic regions of the enzyme that bind regulators. Because the two molecules do not compete for the same site, inhibition is considered noncompetitive and cannot be overcome by adding more substrate. Noncompetitive inhibitors bind equally well to the enzyme and the enzyme–substrate complex, unlike mixed inhibitors. As shown in Figure 2.25, once the enzyme's conformation is altered by the binding of the inhibitor, no amount of extra substrate will be conducive to forming an enzyme–substrate complex.

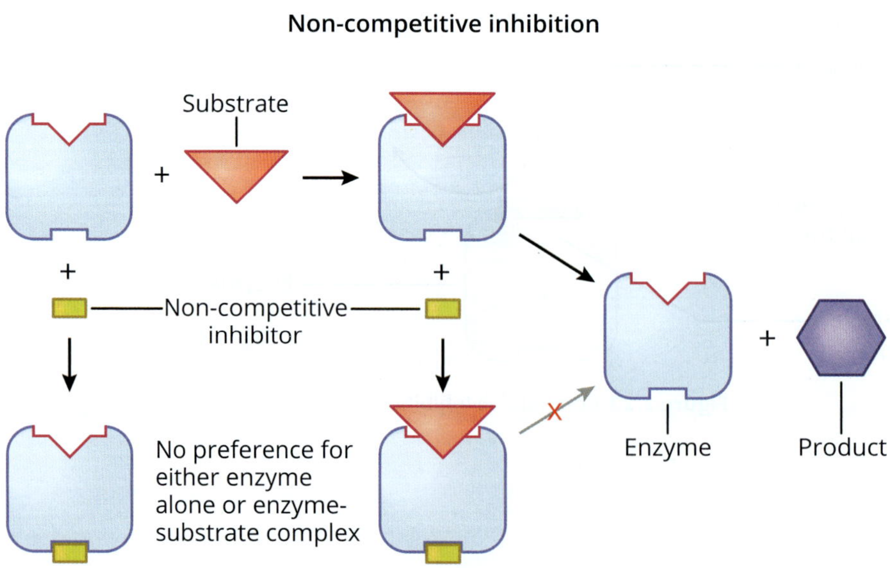

Figure 2.25 Noncompetitive Inhibition

Adding a noncompetitive inhibitor decreases the measured value of V_{max} because there is less enzyme available to react; it does not, however, alter the value of K_m because any copies of the enzyme that are still active maintain the same affinity for their substrate. A Lineweaver–Burk plot of an enzyme with and without a noncompetitive inhibitor is shown in Figure 2.26.

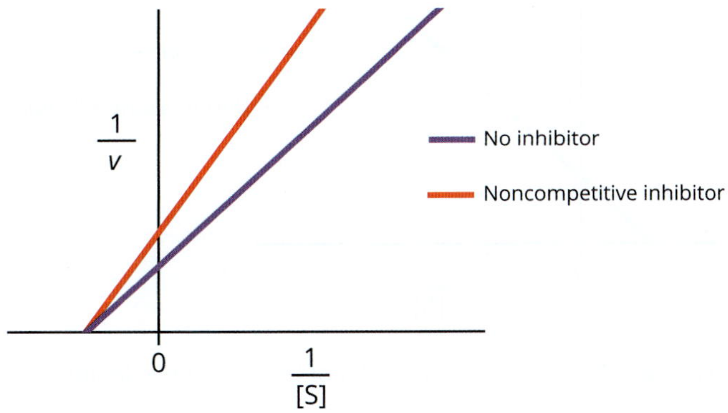

Figure 2.26 Lineweaver–Burk Plot of Noncompetitive Inhibition

Uncompetitive Inhibition

Uncompetitive inhibitors bind only to the enzyme–substrate complex and essentially lock the substrate in the enzyme, preventing its release and inhibiting substrate conversion into product, as shown in Figure 2.27. This can be interpreted as increasing affinity between the enzyme and substrate. Because the enzyme–substrate complex has already formed upon binding, uncompetitive inhibitors must bind at an allosteric site; in fact, it is the formation of the enzyme–substrate complex that creates a conformational change that allows the uncompetitive inhibitor to bind.

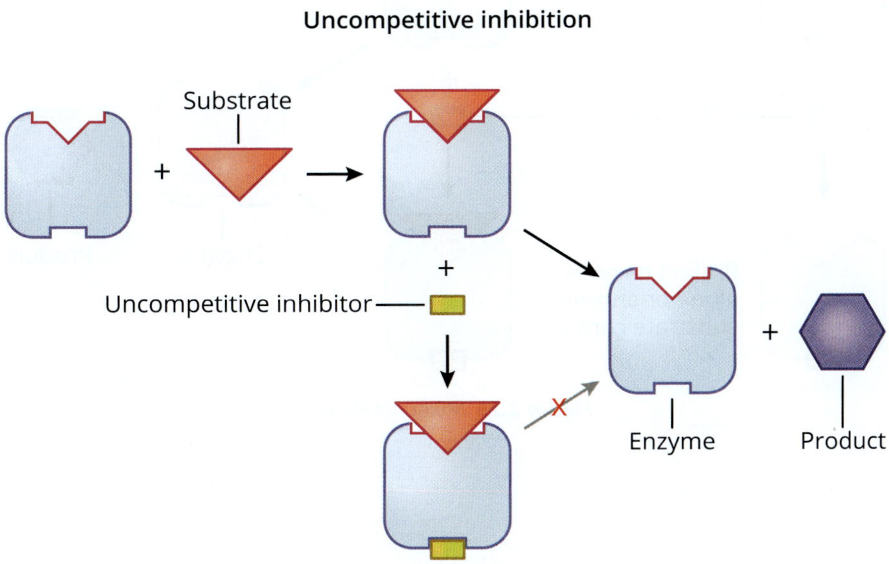

Figure 2.27 Uncompetitive Inhibition

Thus, uncompetitive inhibitors lower K_m and V_{max}. On a Lineweaver–Burk plot, as shown in Figure 2.28, the curves for activity with and without an uncompetitive inhibitor are parallel.

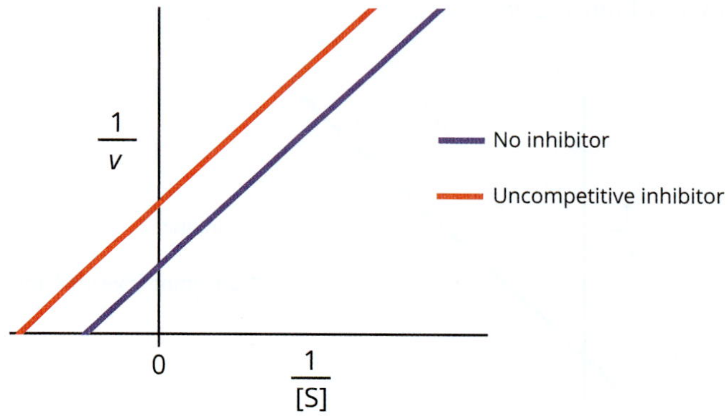

Figure 2.28 Lineweaver-Burk Plot of Uncompetitive Inhibition

Mixed Inhibition

Mixed inhibition results when an inhibitor can bind to either the enzyme or the enzyme–substrate complex, but has different affinity for each. If the inhibitor had the same affinity for both, it would be a noncompetitive inhibitor. As shown in Figure 2.29, mixed inhibitors do not bind at the active site, but at an allosteric site.

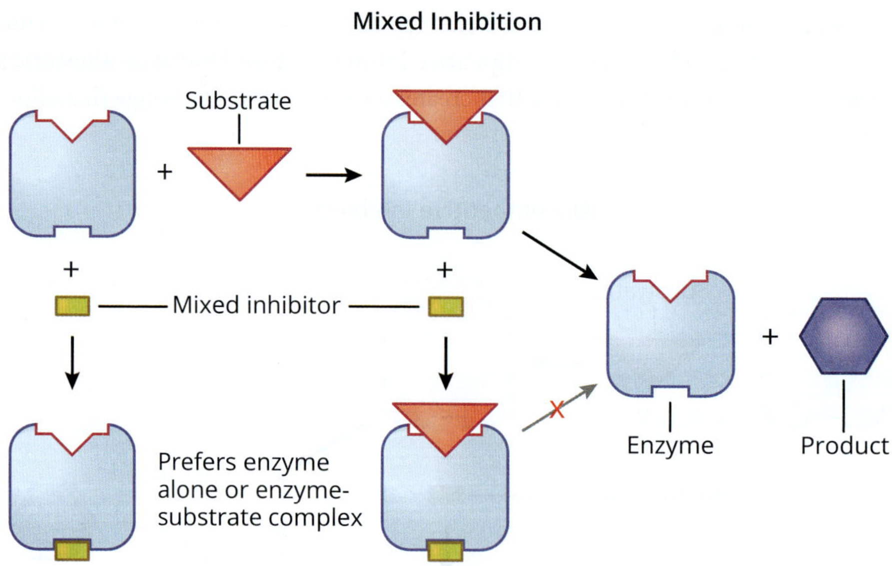

Figure 2.29 Mixed Inhibition

Mixed inhibition alters the experimental value of K_m depending on the preference of the inhibitor for the enzyme vs. the enzyme–substrate complex. If the inhibitor preferentially binds to the enzyme, it increases the K_m value (lowers affinity); if the inhibitor binds to the enzyme–substrate complex, it lowers the K_m value (increases affinity). In either case, V_{max} is decreased. On a Lineweaver–Burk plot, as shown in Figure 2.30, the curves for the activity with and without the inhibitor intersect at a point that is not on either axis.

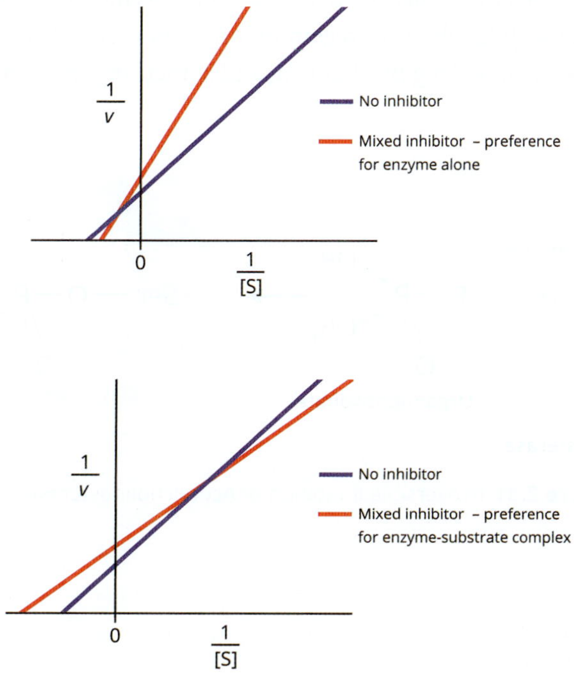

Figure 2.30 Lineweaver-Burk Plots of Mixed Inhibition

Inhibitor type	Binds to	Effect on K_m	Effect on affinity	Effect on V_{max}	Lineweaver-Burk plot
Competitive	Enzyme active site	↑ K_m	↓ affinity	Unchanged	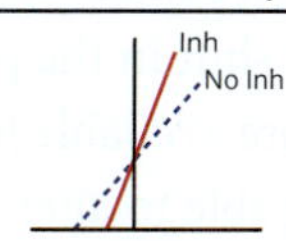
Noncompetitive	Either enzyme or ES complex equally, allosteric	Unchanged	Unchanged	↓ V_{max}	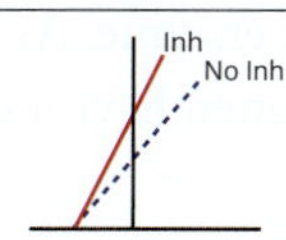
Uncompetitive	Only ES complex, allosteric	↓ K_m	↑ affinity	↓ V_{max}	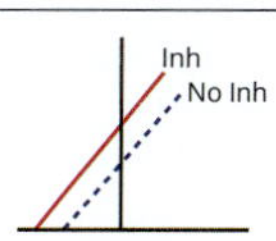
Mixed (preference ES complex)	Either enzyme or ES complex but prefer ES, allosteric	↓ K_m	↑ affinity	↓ V_{max}	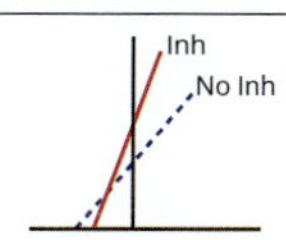
Mixed (preference enzyme)	Either enzyme or ES complex but prefer enzyme, allosteric	↑ K_m	↓ affinity	↓ V_{max}	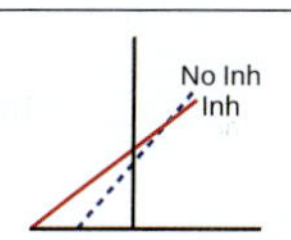

Table 2.2 Comparison of Reversible Inhibitors

Irreversible Inhibition

In this type of inhibition, the active site is made unavailable for a prolonged period of time, or the enzyme is permanently altered. In other words, this type of inhibition is not easily overcome or reversed. A real-world example is the inhibition of acetylcholinesterase (AChE) by organophosphates (found in many pesticides and nerve agents). As shown in Figure 2.31, the organophosphate forms a covalent bond with a critical serine residue in the active site of AChE. This permanently inactivates the enzyme, preventing it from breaking down its substrate, the neurotransmitter acetylcholine. To regain function, new acetylcholinesterase must be synthesized. Irreversible inhibition is a prime drug mechanism, and something that you will come across often in medical school.

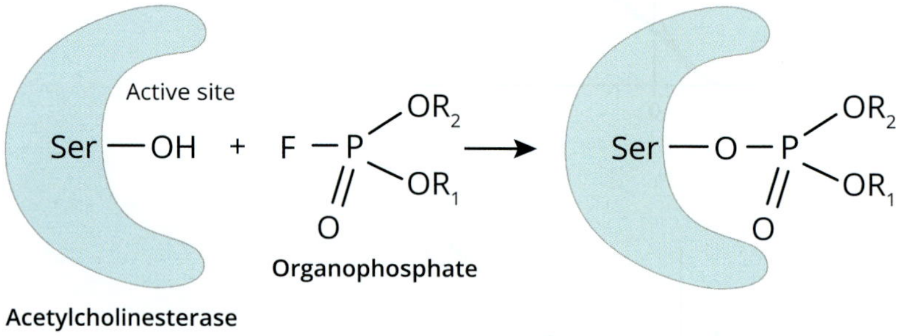

Figure 2.31 Irreversible Inhibition of Acetylcholinesterase

Regulated Enzymes

Allosteric Enzymes

Enzymes that are allosteric have multiple binding sites. The active site is present, as well as at least one other regulatory site known as an **allosteric site**, as illustrated in Figure 2.32. **Allosteric enzymes** alternate between an active and an inactive form. The inactive form cannot carry out the enzymatic reaction. Molecules that bind to the allosteric site may be either **allosteric activators** or **allosteric inhibitors**. Binding of either causes a conformational shift in the protein; however, the effect differs. An activator will result in a shift that makes the active site more available for binding to the substrate, whereas an inhibitor will make it less available. In addition to being able to alter the conformation of the protein, binding of activators or inhibitors may alter the activity of the enzyme. As shown in Figure 2.18 above, Michaelis–Menten plots of cooperative allosteric enzyme kinetics often have a sigmoidal (S-shaped) curve.

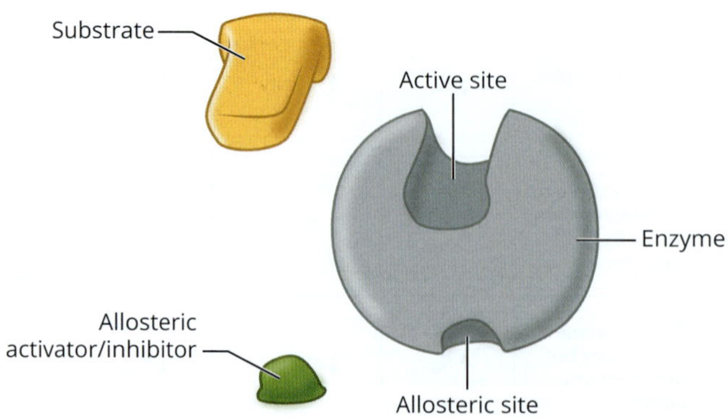

Figure 2.32 Allosteric vs. Active Sites

Covalently Modified Enzymes

In addition to transient interactions, enzymes are often subject to covalent modification. For example, enzymes can be activated or deactivated by **phosphorylation** or **dephosphorylation**. One cannot predict whether phosphorylation or dephosphorylation will activate an enzyme without experimental determination. **Glycosylation**, the covalent attachment of sugar moieties, is another covalent enzyme modification. Glycosylation can tag an enzyme for transport within the cell, or can modify protein activity and selectivity. Figure 2.33 shows a protein that has been phosphorylated and glycosylated. There are many other types of covalently-linked modifications, some of which are further detailed in Chapter 7 of *MCAT Biochemistry Review*, but specific mechanisms for the modifications of enzymes are still being studied and are beyond the scope of the MCAT.

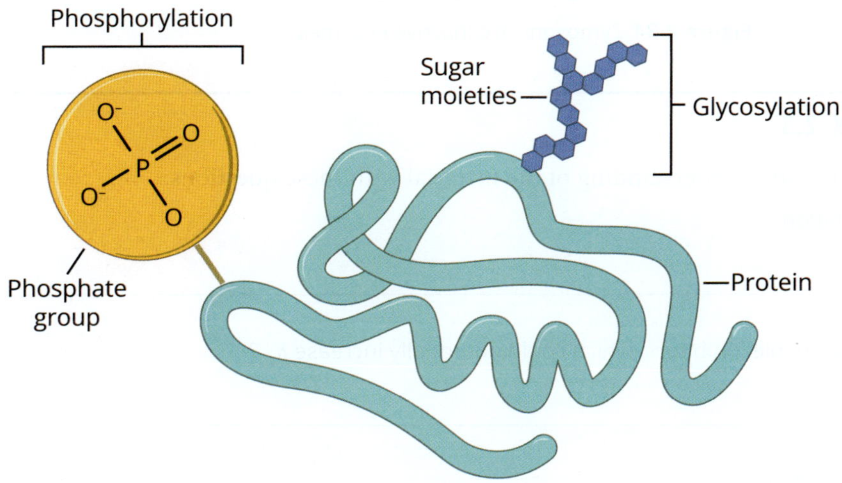

Figure 2.33 Examples of Covalent Protein Modifications

Zymogens

Certain enzymes are particularly dangerous if they are not tightly controlled. These include the digestive enzymes like *trypsin*, which, if released from the pancreas in an uncontrolled manner, would digest the organ itself. To avoid this danger, these enzymes and many others are secreted as inactive **zymogens** like *trypsinogen*. Zymogens contain a catalytic (active) domain and regulatory domain. The regulatory domain must be either removed or altered to expose the active site (see Figure 2.34 for an example). Apoptotic enzymes (*caspases*) exhibit similar regulation. Most zymogens have the suffix ***–ogen***.

BRIDGE

Consider that digestive enzymes, discussed in Chapter 9 of *MCAT Biology Review*, chew up fats, proteins, and carbohydrates—the very same compounds of which our body is made. How do these enzymes know to digest your food but not your body? Simply put, they don't! So, we regulate their activity in a coordinated manner using feedback mechanisms and other substances.

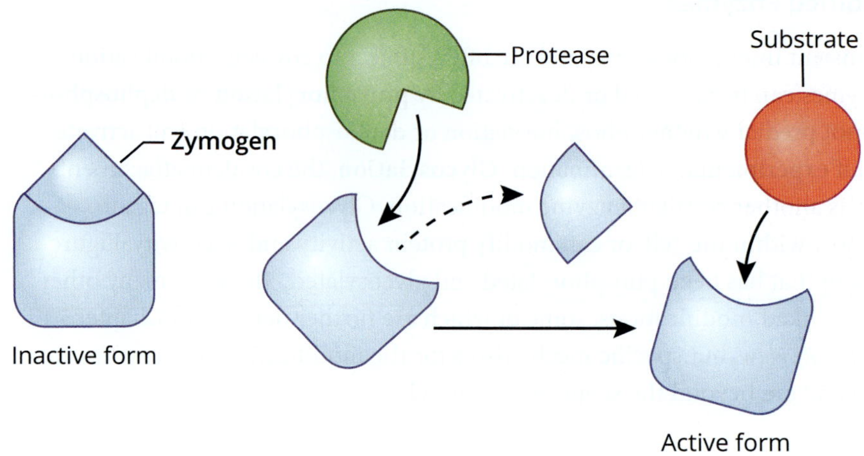

Figure 2.34 Zymogens Are Inactive Enzymes

MCAT CONCEPT CHECK 2.5

Before you move on, assess your understanding of the material with these questions.

1. What is feedback inhibition?

____

2. Of the four types of reversible inhibitors, which could potentially increase K_m?

____

3. What is irreversible inhibition?

____

4. What are some examples of transient and covalent enzyme modifications?
    - Transient:

____

    - Covalent:

____

5. Why are some enzymes released as zymogens?

____

Conclusion

Our current chapter focused on the way in which cells are able to carry out the reactions necessary for life. We began with a discussion of the types of enzymes that you are likely to encounter on Test Day before reviewing thermodynamics and kinetics in relation to enzymes, which are biological catalysts. We went on to discuss the analysis of kinetic data with two different types of graphs, and talked about cooperativity. Because catalysts are generally most active in their native environment, we considered the impact of temperature, pH, and salinity on their activity. All of these are likely to appear on Test Day.

Enzymes need to be regulated; we analyzed the basics of feedback mechanisms. We talked about inhibitors of enzymes, which may be reversible or irreversible. The difference between the types of reversible inhibition is a key Test Day concept. Finally, we discussed changes in enzyme activity that may include allosteric activation, covalent modification, or cleavage of inactive zymogens. Let's move on now to discuss the nonenzymatic functions of proteins. You will notice many parallels between the new material and the concepts described in this chapter, like binding affinity. By the end of the next chapter, you'll be ready to face any protein question the MCAT can throw at you!

GO ONLINE

You've reviewed the content, now test your knowledge and critical thinking skills by completing a test-like passage set in your online resources!

CONCEPT SUMMARY

Enzymes as Biological Catalysts

- **Enzymes** are biological catalysts that are unchanged by the reactions they catalyze and are reusable.
- Each enzyme catalyzes a single reaction or type of reaction with high specificity.
  - **Oxidoreductases** catalyze oxidation–reduction reactions that involve the transfer of electrons.
  - **Transferases** move a functional group from one molecule to another molecule.
  - **Hydrolases** catalyze cleavage with the addition of water.
  - **Lyases** catalyze cleavage without the addition of water and without the transfer of electrons. The reverse reaction (synthesis) is often more important biologically.
  - **Isomerases** catalyze the interconversion of isomers, including both constitutional isomers and stereoisomers.
  - **Ligases** are responsible for joining two large biomolecules, often of the same type.
  - **Translocases** are responsible for transporting molecules across membranes.
- **Exergonic reactions** release energy; ΔG is negative.
- Enzymes lower the activation energy necessary for biological reactions.
- Enzymes do not alter the free energy (ΔG) or enthalpy (ΔH) change that accompanies the reaction nor the final equilibrium position; rather, they change the rate (kinetics) at which equilibrium is reached.

Mechanisms of Enzyme Activity

- Enzymes act by stabilizing the transition state, providing a favorable microenvironment, or bonding with the substrate molecules.
- Enzymes have an **active site**, which is the site of catalysis.
- Binding to the active site is explained by the **lock and key theory** or the **induced fit model**.
  - The lock and key theory hypothesizes that the enzyme and substrate are exactly complementary.
  - The induced fit model hypothesizes that the enzyme and substrate undergo conformational changes to interact fully.
- Some enzymes require metal cation **cofactors** or small organic **coenzymes** to be active.

Enzyme Kinetics

- Enzymes experience **saturation kinetics**: as substrate concentration increases, the reaction rate does as well until a maximum value is reached.
- **Michaelis–Menten** and **Lineweaver–Burk** plots represent this relationship as a hyperbola and line, respectively.
- Enzymes can be compared on the basis of their K_m and V_{max} values.
- **Cooperative enzymes** display a sigmoidal curve because of the change in activity with substrate binding.

Effects of Local Conditions on Enzyme Activity

- Temperature and pH affect an enzyme's activity *in vivo*; changes in temperature and pH can result in denaturing of the enzyme and loss of activity due to loss of secondary, tertiary, or, if present, quaternary structure.
- *In vitro*, salinity can impact the action of enzymes.

Regulation of Enzyme Activity

- Enzyme pathways are highly regulated and subject to inhibition and activation.
- **Feedback inhibition** is a regulatory mechanism whereby the catalytic activity of an enzyme is inhibited by the presence of high levels of a product later in the same pathway.
- **Reversible inhibition** is characterized by the ability to replace the inhibitor with a compound of greater affinity or to remove it using mild laboratory treatment.
  - **Competitive inhibition** results when the inhibitor is similar to the substrate and binds at the active site. Competitive inhibition can be overcome by adding more substrate. V_{max} is unchanged, K_m increases.
  - **Noncompetitive inhibition** results when the inhibitor binds with equal affinity to the enzyme and the enzyme–substrate complex. V_{max} is decreased, K_m is unchanged.
  - **Uncompetitive inhibition** results when the inhibitor binds only with the enzyme–substrate complex. K_m and V_{max} both decrease.
  - **Mixed inhibition** results when the inhibitor binds with unequal affinity to the enzyme and the enzyme–substrate complex. V_{max} is decreased, K_m is increased or decreased depending on if the inhibitor has higher affinity for the enzyme or enzyme–substrate complex.
- **Irreversible inhibition** alters the enzyme in such a way that the active site is unavailable for a prolonged duration or permanently; new enzyme molecules must be synthesized for the reaction to occur again.
- Regulatory enzymes can experience activation as well as inhibition.
  - **Allosteric** sites can be occupied by activators, which increase either affinity or enzymatic turnover.
  - **Phosphorylation** (covalent modification with phosphate) or **glycosylation** (covalent modification with carbohydrate) can alter the activity or selectivity of enzymes.
  - **Zymogens** are secreted in an inactive form and are activated by cleavage.

ANSWERS TO CONCEPT CHECKS

2.1

1. Catalysts are characterized by two main properties: they reduce the activation energy of a reaction, thus speeding up the reaction, and they are not used up in the course of the reaction. Enzymes improve the environment in which a particular reaction takes place, which lowers its activation energy. They are also regenerated at the end of the reaction to their original form.
2. Enzyme specificity refers to the idea that a given enzyme will only catalyze a given reaction or type of reaction. For example, *serine/threonine-specific protein kinases* will only place a phosphate group onto the hydroxyl group of a serine or threonine residue.
3.

Name	Function
Ligase	Addition or synthesis reactions, generally between large molecules, often require ATP
Isomerase	Rearrangement of bonds within a compound
Lyase	Cleavage of a single molecule into two products, or synthesis of small organic molecules
Hydrolase	Breaking of a compound into two molecules using the addition of water
Oxidoreductase	Oxidation–reduction reactions (transferring electrons)
Transferase	Movement of a functional group from one molecule to another
Translocase	Transport of molecules across membranes

4. Enzymes have no effect on the overall thermodynamics of the reaction; they have no effect on the ΔG or ΔH of the reaction, although they do lower the energy of the transition state, thus lowering the activation energy. However, enzymes have a profound effect on the kinetics of a reaction. By lowering activation energy, equilibrium can be achieved faster (although the equilibrium position does not change).

2.2

1.

Lock and Key	Induced Fit
• Active site of enzyme fits exactly around substrate • No alterations to tertiary or quaternary structure of enzyme • Less accurate model	• Active site of enzyme molds itself around substrate only when substrate is present • Tertiary and quaternary structure is modified for enzyme to function • More accurate model

2. Cofactors and coenzymes both act as activators of enzymes. Cofactors tend to be inorganic (minerals), while coenzymes tend to be small organic compounds (vitamins). In both cases, these regulators induce a conformational change in the enzyme that promotes its activity. Tightly bound cofactors or coenzymes that are necessary for enzyme function are termed prosthetic groups.

2.3

1. Increasing [S] has different effects, depending on how much substrate is present to begin with. When the substrate concentration is low, an increase in [S] causes a proportional increase in enzyme activity. At high [S], however, when the enzyme is saturated, increasing [S] has no effect on activity because V_{max} has already been attained.

   Increasing [E] will always increase V_{max}, regardless of the starting concentration of enzyme.
2. Both the Michaelis–Menten and Lineweaver–Burk relationships account for the values of K_m and V_{max} under various conditions. They both provide simple graphical interpretations of these two variables and are derived from the Michaelis–Menten equation. However, the axes of these graphs and visual representation of this information is different between the two. The Michaelis–Menten plot is v vs. [S], which creates a hyperbolic curve for monomeric enzymes. The Lineweaver–Burk plot, on the other hand, is $\frac{1}{v}$ vs. $\frac{1}{[S]}$, which creates a straight line.
3. K_m is a measure of an enzyme's affinity for its substrate, and is defined as the substrate concentration at which an enzyme is functioning at half of its maximal velocity. As K_m increases, an enzyme's affinity for its substrate decreases.
4. The x-intercept represents $-\frac{1}{K_m}$; the y-intercept represents $\frac{1}{V_{max}}$.
5. Cooperativity refers to the interactions between subunits in a multisubunit enzyme or protein. The binding of substrate to one subunit induces a change in the other subunits from the T (tense) state to the R (relaxed) state, which encourages binding of substrate to the other subunits. In the reverse direction, the unbinding of substrate from one subunit induces a change from R to T in the remaining subunits, promoting unbinding of substrate from the remaining subunits.

2.4

1. As temperature increases, enzyme activity generally increases (doubling approximately every 10°C). Above body temperature, however, enzyme activity quickly drops off as the enzyme denatures. Enzymes are maximally active within a small pH range; outside of this range, activity drops quickly with changes in pH as the ionization of the active site changes and the protein is denatured. Changes in salinity can disrupt bonds within an enzyme, causing disruption of tertiary and quaternary structure, which leads to loss of enzyme function.
2. Ideal temperature: 37°C = 98.6°F = 310 K

   Ideal pH for most enzymes is 7.4; for gastric enzymes, around 2; for pancreatic enzymes, around 8.5.

2.5

1. Feedback inhibition refers to the product of an enzymatic pathway turning off enzymes further back in that same pathway. This helps maintain homeostasis: as product levels rise, the pathway creating that product is appropriately downregulated.

2. A competitive inhibitor increases K_m because the substrate concentration has to be higher to reach half the maximum velocity in the presence of the inhibitor. A mixed inhibitor will increase K_m only if the inhibitor preferentially binds to the enzyme over the enzyme–substrate complex.
3. Irreversible inhibition refers to the prolonged or permanent inactivation of an enzyme, such that it cannot be easily renatured to gain function.
4. Examples of transient modifications include allosteric activation or inhibition. Examples of covalent modifications include phosphorylation and glycosylation.
5. Zymogens are precursors of active enzymes. It is critical that certain enzymes (like the digestive enzymes of the pancreas) remain inactive until arriving at their target site.

SCIENCE MASTERY ASSESSMENT EXPLANATIONS

1. **D**

Enzymes catalyze reactions by lowering their activation energy, and are not changed or consumed during the course of the reaction. While the activation energy is lowered, the free energy of the reaction, ΔG, remains unchanged in the presence of an enzyme. A reaction will continue to occur in the presence or absence of an enzyme; it simply runs slower without the enzyme, eliminating **(A)**. Most physiological reactions are optimized at body temperature, 37°C, eliminating **(B)**. Finally, dehydrogenases catalyze oxidation–reduction reactions, not transfer reactions, eliminating **(C)**.

2. **A**

Most enzymes in the human body operate at maximal activity around a temperature of 37°C and a pH of 7.4, which is the pH of most body fluids. In addition, as characterized by the Michaelis–Menten equation, enzymes form an enzyme–substrate complex, which can either dissociate back into the enzyme and substrate or proceed to form a product. So far, we can eliminate **(B)**, **(C)**, and **(D)**, so let's check **(A)**. An increase in the substrate concentration, while maintaining a constant enzyme concentration, leads to a proportional increase in the rate of the reaction only initially. However, once most of the active sites are occupied, the reaction rate levels off, regardless of further increases in substrate concentration. At high concentrations of substrate, the reaction rate approaches its maximal velocity and is no longer changed by further increases in substrate concentration.

3. **B**

An enzyme devoid of its necessary cofactor is called an apoenzyme and is catalytically inactive.

4. **A**

An enzyme's specificity is determined by the three-dimensional shape of its active site. Regardless of which explanation for enzyme specificity we are discussing (lock and key or induced fit), the active site determines which substrate the enzyme will react with.

5. **A**

As the temperature of the DNA polymerase sample increases from 0°C to the usual physiological temperature, i.e. 37°C, the enzyme's activity will increase. However, at temperatures above 37°C, the enzyme's activity will rapidly decline due to denaturation.

6. **D**

By limiting the activity of enzyme 1, the rest of the pathway is slowed, which is the definition of negative feedback. **(A)** is incorrect because there is no competition for the active site with allosteric interactions. While many products do indeed competitively inhibit an enzyme in the pathway that creates them, this is an example of an allosterically inhibited enzyme. There is not enough information for **(B)** to be correct because we aren't told whether the inhibition is reversible. In general, allosteric interactions are temporary. **(C)** is incorrect because it is the opposite of what occurs when enzyme 1 activity is reduced.

7. **A**

While the equations given in the text are useful, recognizing relationships is even more important. You can see that as substrate concentration increases significantly, there is only a small change in the rate. This occurs as we approach V_{max}. Because the V_{max} is near 100 $\frac{\text{mmol}}{\text{min}}$, $\frac{V_{max}}{2}$ equals 50 $\frac{\text{mmol}}{\text{min}}$. The substrate concentration giving this rate is 0.5 mM and corresponds to K_m; therefore, **(A)** is correct.

8. **A**

As with the last question, relationships are important. At a concentration of 5×10^{-6} M, enzyme A is working at one-half of its V_{max} because the concentration is equal to the K_m of the enzyme. Therefore, one-half of 20 $\frac{\text{mmol}}{\text{min}}$ is 10 $\frac{\text{mmol}}{\text{min}}$, which corresponds to **(A)**.

9. **C**

At a concentration of 5×10^{-4} M, there is 100 times more substrate than present at half maximal velocity. At high values (significantly larger than the value of K_m), the enzyme is at or near its V_{max}, which is 20 $\frac{\text{mmol}}{\text{min}}$.

10. **B**

Based on the graph, when the substrate is present, oseltamivir results in the same V_{max} and a higher K_m compared to when no inhibitor is added. These are hallmarks of competitive inhibitors. Noncompetitive inhibitors result in decreased V_{max} and the same K_m as the uninhibited reaction, which is shown by the zanamivir line in the graph. Because the question is only comparing the values between the two inhibitors, and not the enzyme without inhibitor, the mechanism of inhibition is less important to determine than the values of K_m and V_{max}. This is a great example of why previewing the answer choices works well in the sciences.

11. **C**

Lyases are responsible for the breakdown of a single molecule into two molecules without the addition of water or the transfer of electrons. Lyases often form cyclic compounds or double bonds in the products to accommodate this. Water was not a reactant, and no cofactor was mentioned; thus lyase, **(C)**, remains the best answer choice.

12. **D**

Enzymes are not altered by the process of catalysis. A molecule that breaks intramolecular bonds to provide activation energy would not be able to be reused.

13. **D**

Cooperative enzymes demonstrate a change in affinity for the substrate depending on how many substrate molecules are bound and whether the last change was accomplished because a substrate molecule was bound or left the active site of the enzyme. Because we cannot determine whether the most recent reaction was binding or dissociation, **(A)** and **(B)** are eliminated. We can make absolute comparisons though. For enzymes expressing positive cooperativity, the unbound enzyme has the lowest affinity for substrate, and the enzyme with all but one subunit bound has the highest. The increase in affinity is not necessarily linear. Furthermore, if all four sites have substrate bound, the enzyme cannot bind to any more substrate. Therefore, **(C)** is not true. An enzyme with two subunits occupied must have a higher affinity for the substrate than the same enzyme with only one subunit occupied; thus, **(D)** is correct.

14. **A**

Triglycerides are unlikely to act as coenzymes for a few reasons, including their large size, neutral charge, and ubiquity in cells. Cofactors and coenzymes tend to be small in size, such as metal ions like **(C)** or small organic molecules. They can usually carry a charge by ionization, protonation, or deprotonation. Finally, they are usually in low, tightly regulated concentrations within cells. Metabolic pathways would be expected to include both oxidation–reduction reactions and movement of functional groups, thus eliminating **(B)** and **(D)**.

15. **B**

The rate of reaction increases with temperature because of the increased kinetic energy of the reactants, but reaches a peak temperature because the enzyme denatures with the disruption of hydrogen bonds at excessively high temperatures. In the absence of enzyme, this peak temperature is generally much hotter. Heating a reaction provides molecules with an increased chance of achieving the activation energy, but the enzyme catalyst would typically reduce activation energy. Keep in mind that thermodynamics and kinetics are not interchangeable, so we are not considering the impact of heat on the equilibrium position.

▶ GO ONLINE

Consult your online resources for additional practice.

EQUATIONS TO REMEMBER

(2.1) **Michaelis–Menten rates:** $E + S \underset{k_{-1}}{\overset{k_1}{\rightleftharpoons}} ES \xrightarrow{k_{cat}} E + P$

(2.2) **Michaelis–Menten equation:** $v = \frac{V_{max}\,[S]}{K_m + [S]}$

(2.3) **Turnover number (k_{cat}):** $V_{max} = [E]\,k_{cat}$

SHARED CONCEPTS

Biochemistry Chapter 1
Amino Acids, Peptides, and Proteins

Biochemistry Chapter 12
Bioenergetics and Regulation of Metabolism

Biology Chapter 5
The Endocrine System

Biology Chapter 9
The Digestive System

General Chemistry Chapter 5
Chemical Kinetics

General Chemistry Chapter 7
Thermochemistry

General Chemistry Chapter 11
Oxidation–Reduction Reactions

CHAPTER 3

NONENZYMATIC PROTEIN FUNCTION AND PROTEIN ANALYSIS

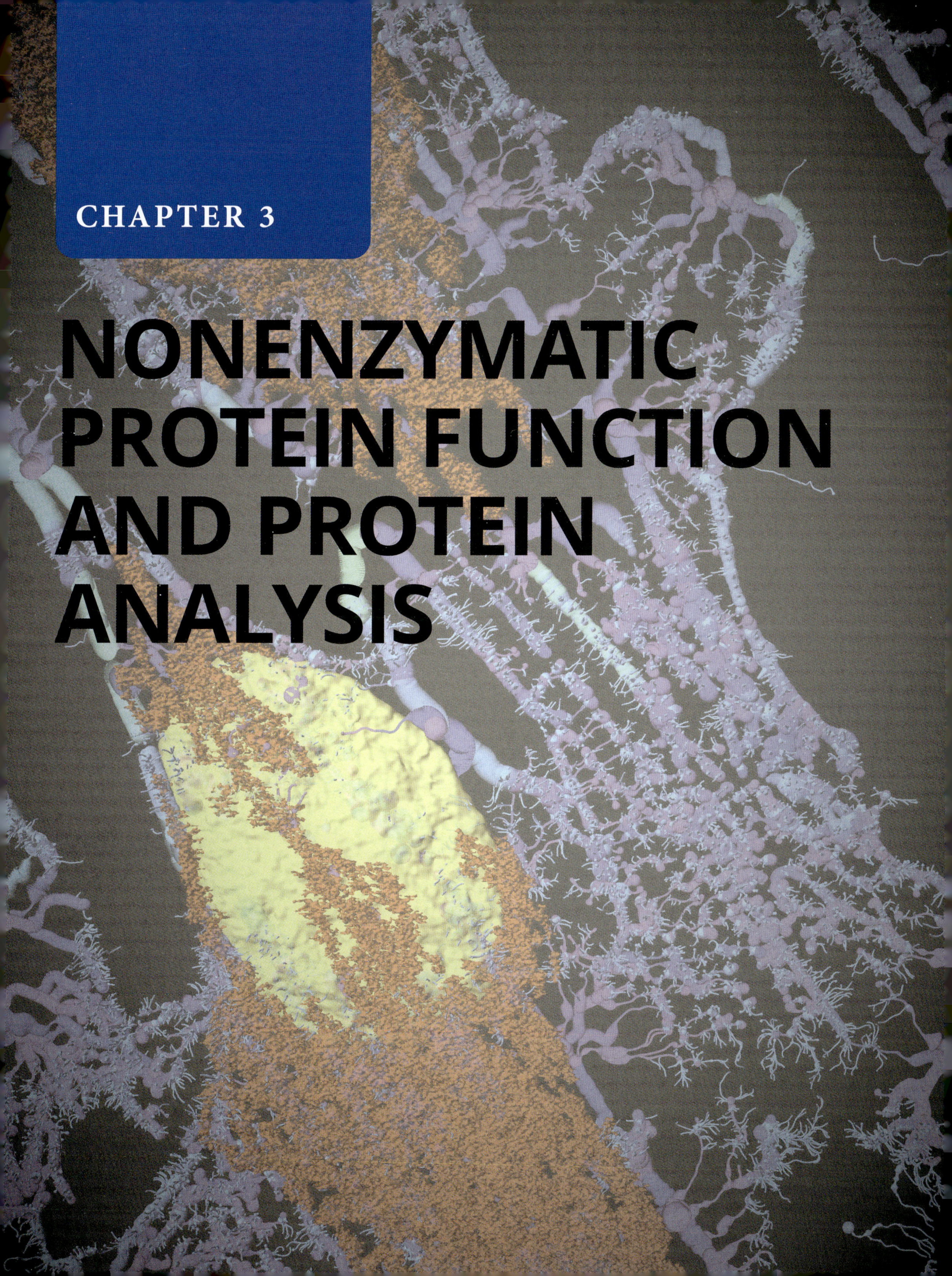

SCIENCE MASTERY ASSESSMENT

Every pre-med knows this feeling: there is so much content I have to know for the MCAT! How do I know what to do first or what's important?

While the high-yield badges throughout this book will help you identify the most important topics, this Science Mastery Assessment is another tool in your MCAT prep arsenal. This quiz (which can also be taken in your online resources) and the guidance below will help ensure that you are spending the appropriate amount of time on this chapter based on your personal strengths and weaknesses. Don't worry though—skipping something now does not mean you'll never study it. Later on in your prep, as you complete full-length tests, you'll uncover specific pieces of content that you need to review and can come back to these chapters as appropriate.

How to Use This Assessment

If you answer 0–7 questions correctly:

Spend about 1 hour to read this chapter in full and take limited notes throughout. Follow up by reviewing **all** quiz questions to ensure that you now understand how to solve each one.

If you answer 8–11 questions correctly:

Spend 20–40 minutes reviewing the quiz questions. Beginning with the questions you missed, read and take notes on the corresponding subchapters. For questions you answered correctly, ensure your thinking matches that of the explanation and you understand why each choice was correct or incorrect.

If you answer 12–15 questions correctly:

Spend less than 20 minutes reviewing all questions from the quiz. If you missed any, then include a quick read-through of the corresponding subchapters, or even just the relevant content within a subchapter, as part of your question review. For questions you got correct, ensure your thinking matches that of the explanation and review the Concept Summary at the end of the chapter.

1. At what pH can protein A best be obtained through electrophoresis? (Note: MM = molar mass)

Protein	pI	MM
Protein A	4.5	25,000
Protein B	6.0	10,000
Protein C	9.5	12,000

   A. 2.5
   B. 3.5
   C. 4.5
   D. 5.5

2. What is the function of sodium dodecyl sulfate (SDS) in SDS-PAGE?
   A. SDS stabilizes the gel matrix, improving resolution during electrophoresis.
   B. SDS solubilizes proteins to give them uniformly negative charges, so the separation is based purely on size.
   C. SDS raises the pH of the gel, separating multiunit proteins into individual subunits.
   D. SDS solubilizes proteins to give them uniformly positive charges, so separation is based purely on pH.

3. Which of the following is NOT involved in cell migration?
   A. Dynein
   B. Flagella
   C. Actin
   D. Centrioles

4. Which of the following proteins is most likely to be found extracellularly?
   A. Tubulin
   B. Myosin
   C. Collagen
   D. Actin

5. Hormones are found in the body in very low concentrations, but tend to have a strong effect. What type of receptor are hormones most likely to act on?
   I. Ligand-gated ion channels
   II. Enzyme-linked receptors
   III. G protein-coupled receptors
   A. I only
   B. III only
   C. II and III only
   D. I, II, and III

6. Which of the following is most likely to be found bound to a protein in the body?
   A. Sodium
   B. Potassium
   C. Chloride
   D. Calcium

7. Which of the following characteristics is NOT attributed to antibodies?
   A. Antibodies bind to more than one distinct antigen.
   B. Antibodies label antigens for targeting by other immune cells.
   C. Antibodies can cause agglutination by interaction with antigen.
   D. Antibodies have two heavy chains and two light chains.

8. Which ion channels are responsible for maintaining the resting membrane potential?
   - **A.** Ungated channels
   - **B.** Voltage-gated channels
   - **C.** Ligand-gated channels
   - **D.** No ion channels are involved in maintenance of the resting membrane potential.

9. Which of the following is NOT a component of all trimeric G proteins?
   - **A.** G_α
   - **B.** G_β
   - **C.** G_γ
   - **D.** G_i

10. Which of the following methods would be best to separate large quantities of the following proteins? (Note: MM = molar mass)

Protein	pI	MM
Protein A	6.5	28,000
Protein B	6.3	70,000
Protein C	6.6	200,000

   - **A.** Ion-exchange chromatography
   - **B.** Size-exclusion chromatography
   - **C.** Isoelectric focusing
   - **D.** Native PAGE

11. Which amino acids contribute most significantly to the pI of a protein?
   - **I.** Lysine
   - **II.** Glycine
   - **III.** Arginine
   - **A.** I only
   - **B.** I and II only
   - **C.** I and III only
   - **D.** II and III only

12. How does the gel for isoelectric focusing differ from the gel for traditional electrophoresis?
   - **A.** Isoelectric focusing uses a gel with much larger pore sizes to allow for complete migration.
   - **B.** Isoelectric focusing uses a gel with SDS added to encourage a uniform negative charge.
   - **C.** Isoelectric focusing uses a gel with a pH gradient that encourages a variable charge.
   - **D.** The gel is unchanged in isoelectric focusing; the protein mixture is treated before loading.

13. Which protein properties allow UV spectroscopy to be used as a method of determining concentration?
   - **A.** Proteins have partially planar characteristics in peptide bonds.
   - **B.** Globular proteins cause scattering of light.
   - **C.** Proteins contain aromatic groups in certain amino acids.
   - **D.** All organic macromolecules can be assessed with UV spectroscopy.

14. A protein collected through affinity chromatography displays no activity even though it is found to have a high concentration using the Bradford protein assay. What best explains these findings?
   - **A.** The Bradford reagent was prepared incorrectly.
   - **B.** The active site is occupied by free ligand.
   - **C.** The protein is bound to the column.
   - **D.** The protein does not catalyze the reaction of interest.

15. What property of protein-digesting enzymes allows for a sequence to be determined without fully degrading the protein?
   - **A.** Selectivity
   - **B.** Sensitivity
   - **C.** Turnover
   - **D.** Inhibition

Answer Key

1. **D** (See section 3.3)
2. **B** (See section 3.3)
3. **D** (See section 3.1)
4. **C** (See section 3.1)
5. **C** (See section 3.2)
6. **D** (See section 3.2)
7. **A** (See section 3.1)
8. **A** (See section 3.2)
9. **D** (See section 3.2)
10. **B** (See section 3.3)
11. **C** (See section 3.3)
12. **C** (See section 3.3)
13. **C** (See section 3.4)
14. **B** (See section 3.3)
15. **A** (See section 3.4)

The relevant section of the chapter to review for each question is given in parentheses after the correct answer. Detailed explanations can be found at the end of the chapter.

CHAPTER 3

NONENZYMATIC PROTEIN FUNCTION AND PROTEIN ANALYSIS

In This Chapter

CHAPTER PROFILE

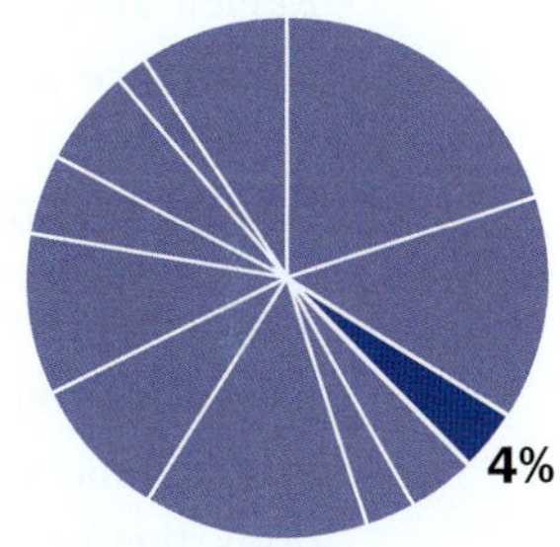

The content in this chapter should be relevant to about 4% of all questions about biochemistry on the MCAT.

This chapter covers material from the following AAMC content categories:

1A: Structure and function of proteins and their constituent amino acids

3A: Structure and functions of the nervous and endocrine systems, and ways in which these systems coordinate the organ systems

5C: Separation and purification methods

5D: Structure, function, and reactivity of biologically relevant molecules

Introduction

Did you ever wonder why some athletes eat raw eggs when training? It doesn't help with digestion or increase enzymatic activity throughout the body; rather, all that protein is used for muscle building. While muscle building does increase cytoplasm and all of the enzymes found therein, the biggest increase is seen in structural and motor proteins like actin and myosin. Valid concerns about bacteria in and on eggs have stopped most athletes from drinking raw eggs, but protein shakes and massive containers of whey protein have replaced them on the shelves of health-food stores, pharmacies, and supermarkets.

In this chapter, we will examine some of the structural and motor proteins that athletes love to build, as well as more complex protein functions in humans, including biosignaling. Finally, we'll learn how to determine which proteins—and their concentrations—are in those eggs through separation and quantitative analysis.

3.1 Cellular Functions

LEARNING OBJECTIVES

After Chapter 3.1, you will be able to:

- Compare and contrast cytoskeletal proteins and motor proteins
- Associate collagen, elastin, keratins, actin, and tubulin with their major functions
- Describe the adhesive properties of cadherins, integrins, and selectins
- Predict the possible outcomes of an antibody binding to its antigen

Typical functions provided by proteins within the cell include supporting cellular shape and organization and acting as enzymes. The enzymatic functions of proteins were detailed in Chapter 2 of *MCAT Biochemistry Review* and we are now ready to look at other protein functions. Structural and motor proteins are found in abundance within individual cells and are also found in the extracellular matrix.

Structural Proteins

The cytoskeleton can be thought of as a three-dimensional web or scaffolding system for the cell. It is comprised of proteins that are anchored to the cell membrane by embedded protein complexes. In addition to intracellular support, extracellular matrices composed of proteins also support the tissues of the body. Tendons, ligaments, cartilage, and basement membranes are all proteinaceous. The primary structural proteins in the body are collagen, elastin, keratin, actin, and tubulin. Structural proteins generally have highly repetitive secondary structure and a supersecondary structure—a repetitive organization of secondary structural elements together sometimes referred to as a **motif**. This regularity gives many structural proteins a fibrous nature.

Collagen

Collagen has a characteristic trihelical fiber (three left-handed helices woven together to form a secondary right-handed helix) and makes up most of the extracellular matrix of connective tissue. It is found throughout the body and is important in providing strength and flexibility.

Elastin

Elastin is another important component of the extracellular matrix of connective tissue. Its primary role is to stretch and then recoil like a spring, which restores the original shape of the tissue.

Keratins

Keratins are intermediate filament proteins found in epithelial cells. Keratins contribute to the mechanical integrity of the cell and also function as regulatory proteins. Keratin is the primary protein that makes up hair and nails.

REAL WORLD

The importance of the structure of collagen is highlighted in the disorder *osteogenesis imperfecta*, also referred to as brittle bone disease. Collagen—a major component of bone—forms a unique and specific secondary helical structure based on the abundance of the amino acid glycine. The replacement of glycine with other amino acids can cause improper folding of the collagen protein and cell death, leading to bone fragility.

Actin

Actin is a protein that makes up microfilaments and the thin filaments in myofibrils. It exists in two forms: a globular monomer known as G-actin and a filamentous polymer known as F-actin, which is formed by the polymerization of G-actin monomers (see Figure 3.1). It is the most abundant protein in eukaryotic cells. Actin proteins have a positive side and a negative side; this polarity allows motor proteins to travel unidirectionally along an actin filament, like a one-way street.

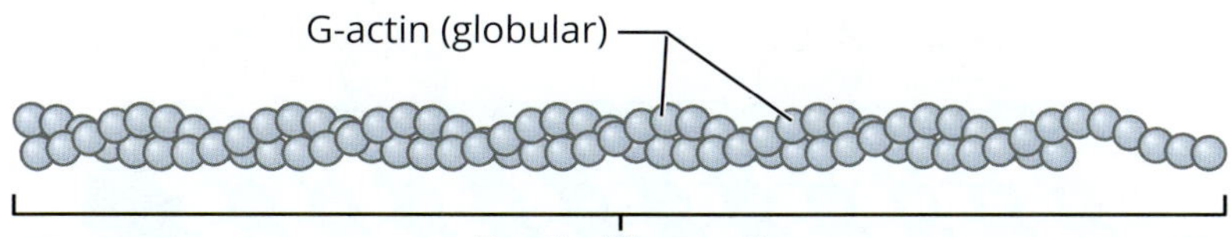

Figure 3.1 G-Actin and F-Actin

Tubulin

Tubulin is the protein that makes up microtubules. Microtubules are important for providing structure, chromosome separation in mitosis and meiosis, and intracellular transport with kinesin and dynein, described in the next section. Like actin, tubulin has polarity: the negative end of a microtubule is usually located adjacent to the nucleus, whereas the positive end is usually in the periphery of a cell.

Motor Proteins

Some structural proteins also have motor functions in the presence of motor proteins. The motile cilia and flagella of bacteria and sperm are prime examples, as is the contraction of the sarcomere in muscle. **Motor proteins** also display enzymatic activity, acting as **ATPases** that power the conformational change necessary for motor function. Motor proteins have transient interactions with either actin or microtubules.

Myosin is the primary motor protein that interacts with actin. In addition to its role as the thick filament in a myofibril, myosin can be involved in cellular transport. Each myosin subunit has a single head and neck; movement at the neck is responsible for the power stroke of sarcomere contraction.

Kinesins and **dyneins** are the motor proteins associated with microtubules. They have two heads, at least one of which remains attached to tubulin at all times. Kinesins play key roles in aligning chromosomes during metaphase and depolymerizing microtubules during anaphase of mitosis. Dyneins are involved in the sliding movement of cilia and flagella. Both proteins are important for vesicle transport in the cell, but have opposite polarities: kinesins bring vesicles toward the positive end of the microtubule, and dyneins bring vesicles toward the negative end, as shown in Figure 3.2.

BRIDGE

Motor proteins are responsible for muscle contraction and cellular movement. Take a moment to review sarcomere structure in Chapter 11 of *MCAT Biology Review* as another example of the interaction between motor proteins and the cytoskeleton.

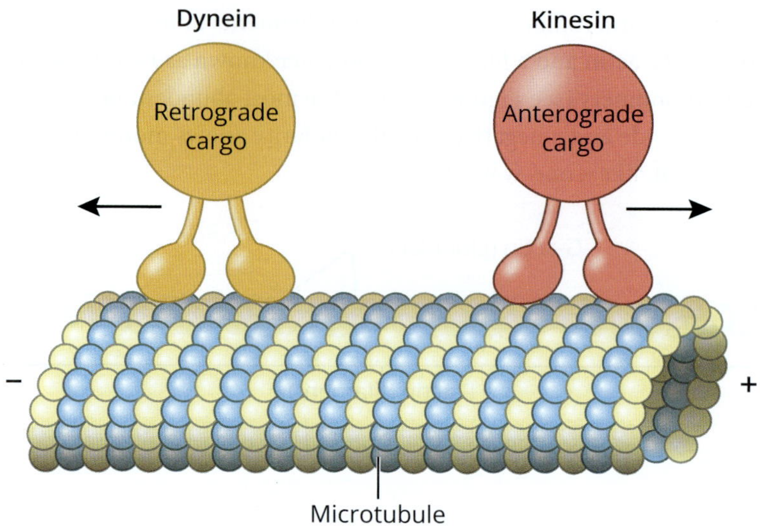

Figure 3.2 Kinesin vs. Dynein

In neurons, we see a classic example of these motor proteins' polarities. Kinesins bring vesicles of neurotransmitter to the positive end of the axonal microtubules (toward the synaptic terminal). In contrast, dyneins bring vesicles of waste or recycled neurotransmitter back toward the negative end of the microtubule (toward the soma) through retrograde transport. The activity of kinesins is illustrated in Figure 3.3 below.

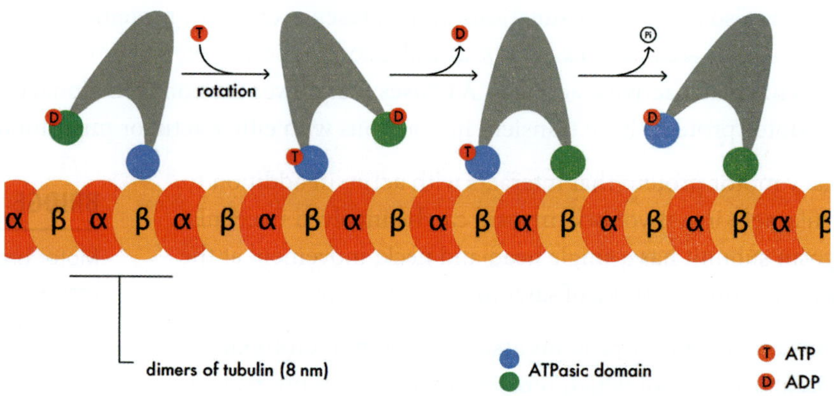

Figure 3.3 Stepwise Activity of Kinesins
Kinesins move along microtubules in a stepping motion such that one or both heads remain attached at all times.

Binding Proteins

While proteins primarily exert enzymatic or structural functions within the cell, they also can have stabilizing functions in individual cells and the body. Proteins that act in this way transport or sequester molecules by binding to them. **Binding proteins** include hemoglobin, calcium-binding proteins, DNA-binding proteins (often transcription factors), and others. Each binding protein has an affinity curve for its molecule of interest; the oxyhemoglobin dissociation curve is one well-known example. This curve differs depending on the goal of the binding protein. When sequestration of a molecule is the goal, the binding protein usually has high affinity for its target across a large range of concentrations so it can keep it bound at nearly 100 percent. A transport protein, which must be able to bind or unbind its target to maintain steady-state concentrations, is likely to have varying affinity depending on the environmental conditions.

Cell Adhesion Molecules

Cell adhesion molecules (**CAMs**) are proteins found on the surface of most cells and aid in binding the cell to the extracellular matrix or other cells. While there are a number of different types of CAMs, they are all integral membrane proteins. Adhesion molecules can be classified into three major families: cadherins, integrins, and selectins.

Cadherins

Cadherins are a group of glycoproteins that mediate calcium-dependent cell adhesion. Cadherins often hold similar cell types together, such as epithelial cells. Different cells usually have type-specific cadherins; for example, epithelial cells use E-cadherin while nerve cells use N-cadherin.

Integrins

Integrins are a group of proteins that all have two membrane-spanning chains called α and β. These chains are very important in binding to and communicating with the extracellular matrix. Integrins also play a very important role in cellular signaling and can greatly impact cellular function by promoting cell division, apoptosis, or other processes. For example, integrin $\alpha_{IIb}\beta_3$ allows platelets to stick to fibrinogen, a clotting factor, which causes activation of platelets to stabilize the clot. Other integrins are used for white blood cell migration, stabilization of epithelium on its basement membrane, and other processes.

Selectins

Selectins are unique because they bind to carbohydrate molecules that project from other cell surfaces. These bonds are the weakest formed by the CAMs discussed here. Selectins are expressed on white blood cells and the endothelial cells that line blood vessels. Like integrins, they play an important role in host defense, including inflammation and white blood cell migration, as shown in Figure 3.4.

REAL WORLD

Many medications target selectins and integrins. For example, research has shown that the ability of cancer cells to metastasize (break away from a tumor and invade other distant tissues) is associated with unique expression patterns of CAMs. By targeting these CAMs, metastasis may be avoided. To stop the clotting process during heart attacks, other medications target CAMs used by platelets.

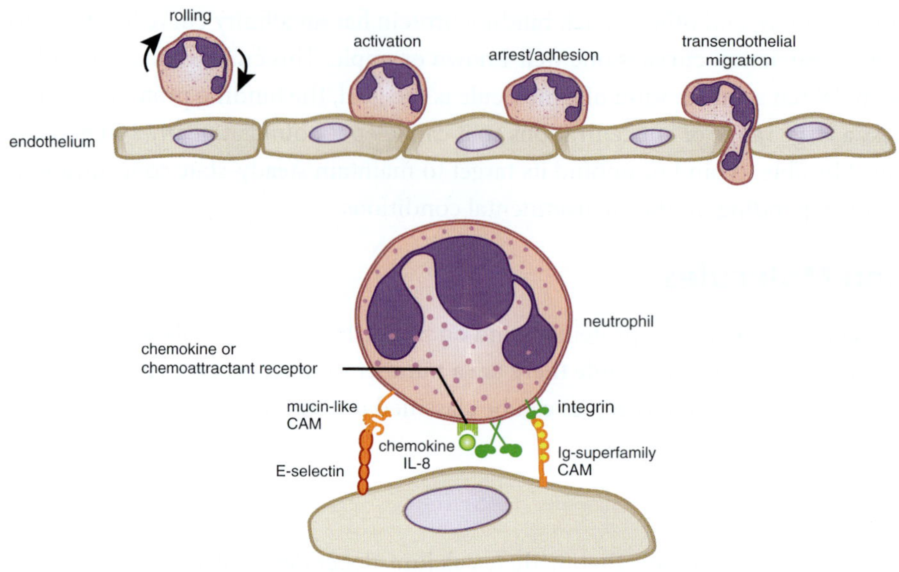

Figure 3.4 White Blood Cell Migration Using Selectins and Integrins
Many other proteins are involved in white blood cell migration, but are outside the scope of the MCAT.

Immunoglobulins

The immune system is very complex and is made up of many different types of cells and proteins. These cells and proteins have a common purpose: to rid the body of foreign invaders. The most prominent type of protein found in the immune system is the antibody. **Antibodies**, also called **immunoglobulins** (**Ig**) are proteins produced by B-cells that function to neutralize targets in the body, such as toxins and bacteria, and then recruit other cells to help eliminate the threat. Antibodies are Y-shaped proteins that are made up of two identical heavy chains and two identical light chains, as shown in Figure 3.5. Disulfide linkages and noncovalent interactions hold the heavy and light chains together. Each antibody has an **antigen-binding region** at the tips of the "Y." Within this region, there are specific polypeptide sequences that will bind one, and only one, specific antigenic sequence. The remaining part of the antibody molecule is known as the constant region, which is involved in recruitment and binding of other cells of the immune system, such as macrophages. Thus, when antibodies bind to their targets, called **antigens**, they can cause one of three outcomes:

- Neutralizing the antigen, making the pathogen or toxin unable to exert its effect on the body
- Marking the pathogen for destruction by other white blood cells immediately; this marking function is also called **opsonization**
- Clumping together (**agglutinating**) the antigen and antibody into large insoluble protein complexes that can be phagocytized and digested by macrophages

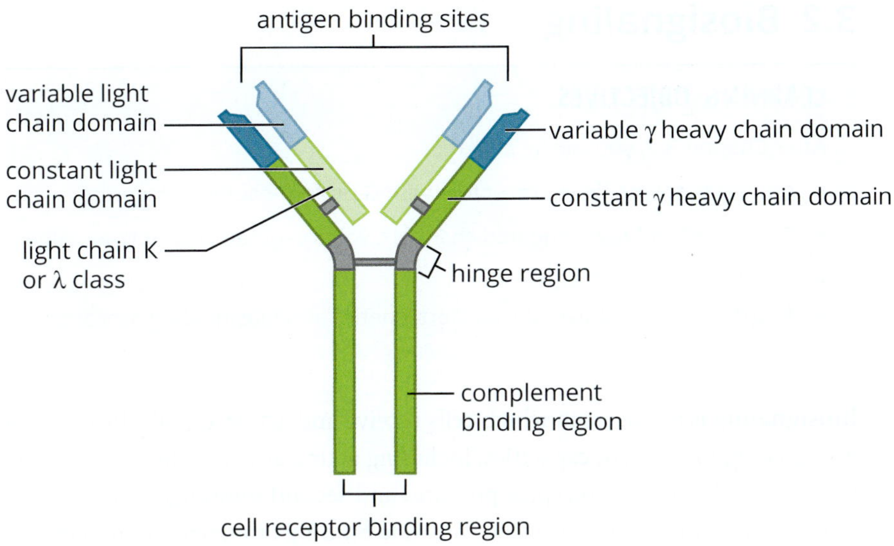

Figure 3.5 Structure of an Antibody Molecule

MCAT CONCEPT CHECK 3.1

Before you move on, assess your understanding of the material with these questions.

1. How do cytoskeletal proteins differ from motor proteins?

____

2. True or False: Motor proteins are not enzymes.

3. What could permit a binding protein involved in sequestration to have a low affinity for its substrate and still have a high percentage of substrate bound?

____

4. What are the three main classes of cell adhesion molecules? What type of adhesion does each class form?

Cell Adhesion Molecule	Type of Adhesion

5. When an antibody binds to its antigen, what are the three possible outcomes of this interaction?

   1. _______________
   2. _______________
   3. _______________

3.2 Biosignaling

LEARNING OBJECTIVES

After Chapter 3.2, you will be able to:

- Contrast enzyme-linked receptors with G protein-coupled receptors
- Distinguish between ungated channels, voltage-gated channels, and ligand-gated channels
- Recognize key features of transport kinetics and biosignaling processes

Biosignaling is a process in which cells receive and act on signals. Proteins participate in biosignaling in different capacities, including acting as extracellular ligands, transporters for facilitated diffusion, receptor proteins, and second messengers. The proteins involved in biosignaling can have functions in substrate binding or enzymatic activity.

REAL WORLD

Hundreds of ion channels have been identified that function in cell signaling and cell excitability. In addition, ion channels are drug targets in the treatment of everything from heart disease (calcium channel blockers) to seizures (sodium channel blockers) to irritable bowel syndrome (acetylcholine receptor/cation channel blockers).

Ion Channels

Ion channels are proteins that create specific pathways for charged molecules. They are classified into three main groups that have different mechanisms of opening, but that all permit facilitated diffusion of charged particles. **Facilitated diffusion**, a type of passive transport, is the diffusion of molecules down a concentration gradient through a pore in the membrane created by this transmembrane protein. It is used for molecules that are impermeable to the membrane (large, polar, or charged). Facilitated diffusion allows integral membrane proteins to serve as channels for these substrates to avoid the hydrophobic fatty acid tails of the phospholipid bilayer. Figure 3.6 shows the three main types of ion channels: ungated, voltage-gated, and ligand-gated.

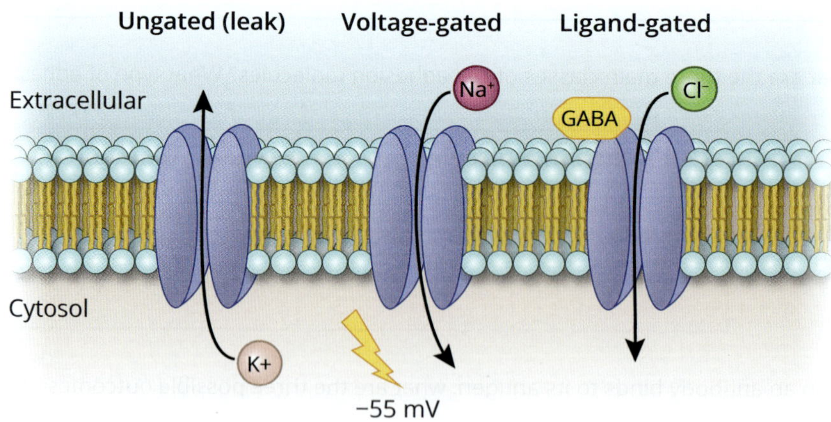

Figure 3.6 Ion Channels

Ungated Channels

As their name suggests, **ungated channels** have no gates and are therefore unregulated. For example, all cells possess ungated potassium channels. This means there will be a net efflux of potassium ions through these channels unless potassium is at equilibrium.

Voltage-Gated Channels

In **voltage-gated channels**, the gate is regulated by the membrane potential change near the channel. For example, many excitable cells such as neurons possess voltage-gated sodium channels. The channels are closed under resting conditions, but membrane depolarization causes a protein conformation change that allows them to quickly open and then quickly close as the voltage increases. Voltage-gated nonspecific sodium–potassium channels are found in cells of the sinoatrial node of the heart. Here, they serve as the pacemaker current; as the voltage drops, these channels open to bring the cell back to threshold and fire another action potential, as shown in Figure 3.7.

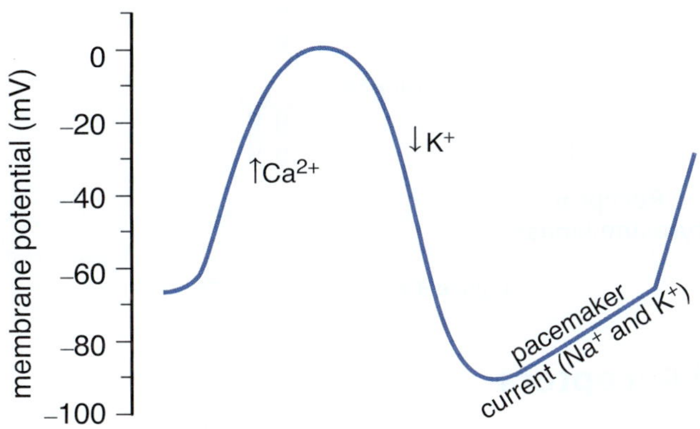

Figure 3.7 Action Potential of the Sinoatrial Node

Ligand-Gated Channels

For **ligand-gated channels**, the binding of a specific substance or ligand to the channel causes it to open or close. For example, neurotransmitters act at ligand-gated channels at the postsynaptic membrane: the inhibitory neurotransmitter γ-aminobutyric acid (GABA) binds to a chloride channel and opens it.

The K_m and V_{max} parameters that apply to enzymes are also applicable to transporters such as ion channels in membranes. The kinetics of transport can be derived from the Michaelis–Menten and Lineweaver–Burk equations, where K_m refers to the solute concentration at which the transporter is functioning at half of its maximum activity.

BRIDGE

The activity at the neuromuscular junction and most chemical synapses relies on ligand-gated ion channels. The nervous system especially makes use of this type of gating, as well as voltage-gated ion channels, as discussed in Chapter 4 of *MCAT Biology Review.*

Enzyme-Linked Receptors

Membrane receptors may also display catalytic activity in response to ligand binding. These **enzyme-linked receptors** have three primary protein domains: a membrane-spanning domain, a ligand-binding domain, and a catalytic domain. The **membrane-spanning domain** anchors the receptor in the cell membrane. The **ligand-binding domain** is stimulated by the appropriate ligand

KEY CONCEPT

Biosignaling can take advantage of either existing gradients (ion channels) or second messenger cascades (enzyme-linked receptors and G protein-coupled receptors).

and induces a conformational change that activates the **catalytic domain**. This often results in the initiation of a **second messenger cascade**. **Receptor tyrosine kinases** (**RTKs**) are classic examples. RTKs are composed of a monomer that dimerizes upon ligand binding. The dimer is the active form that phosphorylates additional cellular enzymes, including the receptor itself (autophosphorylation), as illustrated in Figure 3.8. Other classes of enzyme-linked receptors include *serine/threonine-specific protein kinases* and *receptor tyrosine phosphatases*.

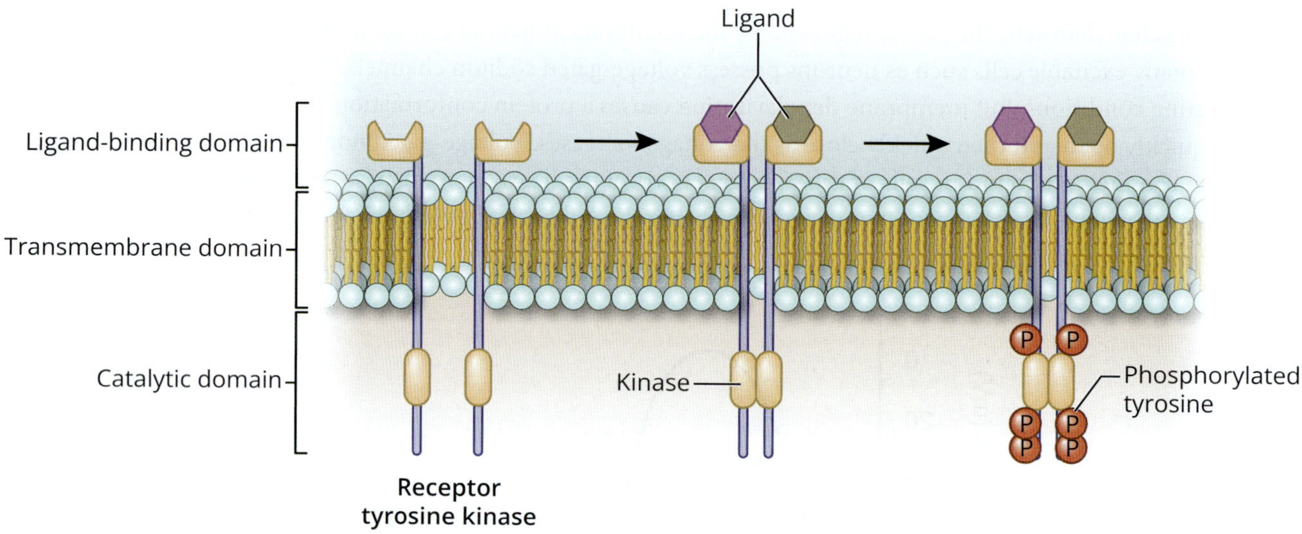

Figure 3.8 Activation of RTK

G Protein-Coupled Receptors

G protein-coupled receptors (**GPCR**) are a large family of integral membrane proteins involved in signal transduction. They are characterized by their seven membrane-spanning α-helices, as shown in Figure 3.9. The receptors differ in specificity of the ligand-binding area found on the extracellular surface of the cell.

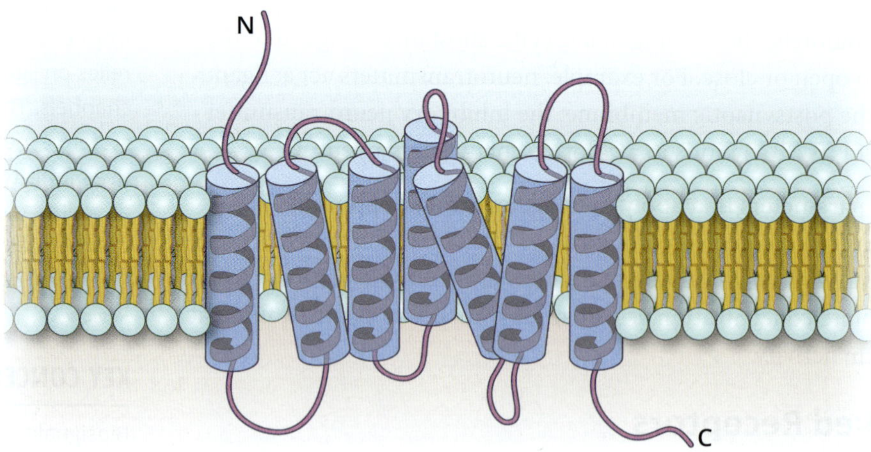

Figure 3.9 Structure of GPCR

In order for GPCRs to transmit signals to an effector in the cell, they utilize a **heterotrimeric G protein**. G proteins are named for their intracellular link to guanine nucleotides (GDP and GTP). The binding of a ligand increases the affinity of the receptor for the G protein. The binding of the G protein represents a switch to the active state and affects the intracellular signaling pathway. There are several different G proteins that can result in either stimulation or inhibition of the signaling pathway. There are three main types of G proteins:

- G_s stimulates adenylate cyclase, which increases levels of cAMP in the cell ($ATP \rightarrow cAMP + PP_i$).
- G_i inhibits adenylate cyclase, which decreases levels of cAMP in the cell.
- G_q activates *phospholipase C*, which cleaves a phospholipid from the membrane to form PIP_2. PIP_2 is then cleaved into DAG and IP_3; IP_3 can open calcium channels in the endoplasmic reticulum, increasing calcium levels in the cell.

MNEMONIC

Functions of heterotrimeric G proteins:

- G_s **s**timulates.
- G_i **i**nhibits.
- "Mind your **p**'s and **q**'s": G_q activates **p**hospholipase C.

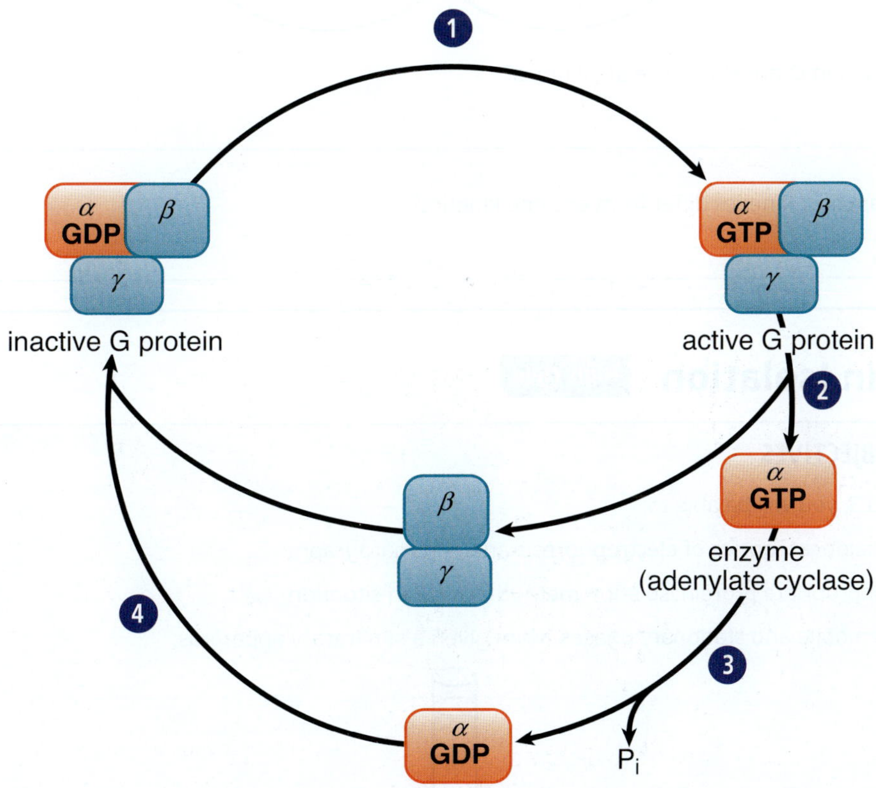

Figure 3.10 Trimeric G Protein Cycle (G_s or G_i)

The three subunits that comprise the G protein are α, β, and γ. In its inactive form, the **α subunit** binds GDP and is in a complex with the **β and γ subunits**. When a ligand binds to the GPCR, the receptor becomes activated and, in turn, engages the corresponding G protein, as shown in Step 1 of Figure 3.10. Once GDP is replaced with GTP, the α subunit is able to dissociate from the β and γ subunits (Step 2). The activated α subunit alters the activity of ***adenylate cyclase***. If the α subunit is α_s, then the enzyme is activated; if the α subunit is α_i, then the enzyme is inhibited. Once GTP on the activated α subunit is dephosphorylated to GDP (Step 3), the α subunit will rebind to the β and γ subunits (Step 4), rendering the G protein inactive.

MCAT CONCEPT CHECK 3.2

Before you move on, assess your understanding of the material with these questions.

1. Contrast enzyme-linked receptors with G protein-coupled receptors:

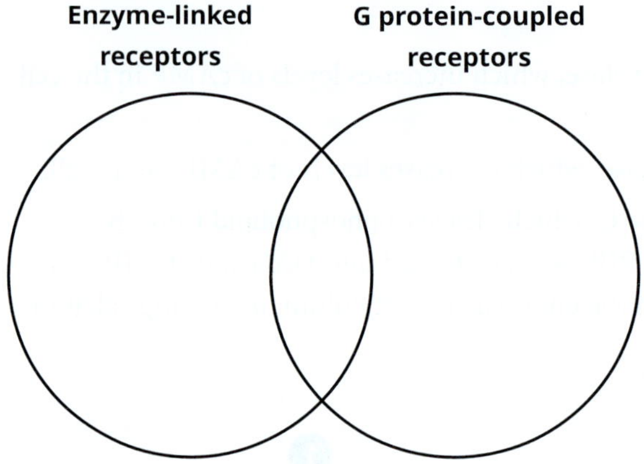

2. What type of ion channel is active at all times?

____

3. How do transport kinetics differ from enzyme kinetics?

____

3.3 Protein Isolation High Yield

LEARNING OBJECTIVES

After Chapter 3.3, you will be able to:

- Recall the major categories of electrophoresis and chromatography
- Select the appropriate protein isolation method in a given situation
- Identify the mobile and stationary phases when given a separatory apparatus:

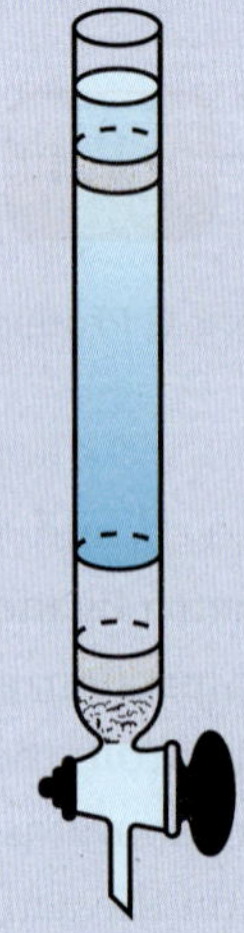

In order to better understand a specific protein, it is important to be able to isolate the protein for study. The purification of proteins can be considered an art form when one considers the difficulty of isolating just one protein from a cell containing hundreds to thousands of proteins. Luckily, as Chapter 1 of *MCAT Biochemistry Review* highlighted, there is a great amount of variation in the physical and chemical properties of proteins and these differences can be exploited in order to purify the protein of interest. Proteins and other biomolecules are isolated from body tissues or cell cultures by cell lysis and **homogenization**—crushing, grinding, or blending the tissue of interest into an evenly mixed solution. **Centrifugation** can then isolate proteins from much smaller molecules before other isolation techniques must be employed. The most common isolation techniques are electrophoresis and chromatography, either of which can be used for native or denatured proteins.

Electrophoresis

One method of separating proteins is with **electrophoresis**. In molecular biology, this is one of the most important analytical techniques. Electrophoresis works by subjecting compounds to an electric field, which moves them according to their net charge and size. Negatively charged compounds will migrate toward the positively charged anode, and positively charged compounds will migrate toward the negatively charged cathode. The velocity of this migration, known as the **migration velocity** of a molecule, **v**, is directly proportional to the electric field strength, **E**, and to the net charge on the molecule, *z*, and is inversely proportional to a frictional coefficient, *f*, which depends on the mass and shape of the migrating molecules:

$$\mathrm{v} = \frac{\mathrm{E}z}{f}$$

Equation 3.1

Polyacrylamide gel is the standard medium for protein electrophoresis. The gel is a slightly porous matrix mixture, which solidifies at room temperature. Proteins travel through this matrix in relation to their size and charge. The gel acts like a sieve, allowing smaller particles to pass through easily while retaining large particles. Therefore, a molecule will move faster through the medium if it is small, highly charged, or placed in a large electric field. Conversely, molecules will migrate slower (or not at all) when they are bigger and more convoluted, electrically neutral, or placed in a small electric field. The size of a standard polyacrylamide gel allows multiple samples to be run simultaneously, as shown in Figure 3.11.

BRIDGE

Electrophoresis uses an electrolytic cell ($\Delta G > 0$, $E_{\text{cell}} < 0$), as described in Chapter 12 of *MCAT General Chemistry Review*. Remember that anions always move toward the anode and cations always move toward the cathode.

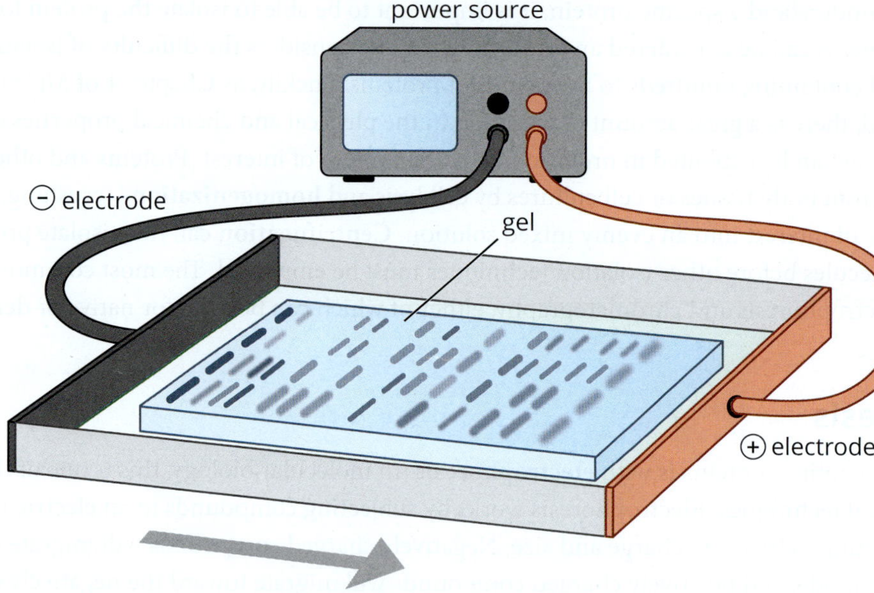

Figure 3.11 Electrophoresis
As an electrolytic (nonspontaneous) cell, electrophoresis moves charged particles toward their respective oppositely charged electrodes; the larger the particle, the more slowly it migrates.

Native PAGE

Polyacrylamide gel electrophoresis (**PAGE**) is a method for analyzing proteins in their native states. Unfortunately, PAGE is limited by the varying mass-to-charge and mass-to-size ratios of cellular proteins because multiple different proteins may experience the same level of migration. In PAGE, the functional native protein can be recovered from the gel after electrophoresis, but only if the gel has not been stained because most stains denature proteins. PAGE is most useful to compare the molecular size or the charge of proteins known to be similar in size from other analytic methods like SDS-PAGE (described below) or size-exclusion chromatography.

SDS-PAGE

Sodium dodecyl sulfate (SDS)–polyacrylamide gel electrophoresis is a useful tool because it separates proteins on the basis of relative molecular mass alone. The **SDS-PAGE** technique starts with the premise of PAGE but adds SDS, a detergent that disrupts all noncovalent interactions. It binds to proteins and creates large chains with net negative charges, thereby neutralizing the protein's original charge and denaturing the protein, as shown in Figure 3.12. As the proteins move through the gel, the only variables affecting their velocity are **E**, the electric field strength, and *f*, the frictional coefficient, which depends on mass. After separation, the gel can be stained so the protein bands can be visualized and the results recorded.

MCAT EXPERTISE

For analytic purposes, protein atomic mass is typically expressed in **daltons (Da)**. A dalton is an alternative term for molar mass $\left(\frac{g}{mol}\right)$. The average molar mass of one amino acid is ~110 daltons, or $110\,\frac{g}{mol}$.

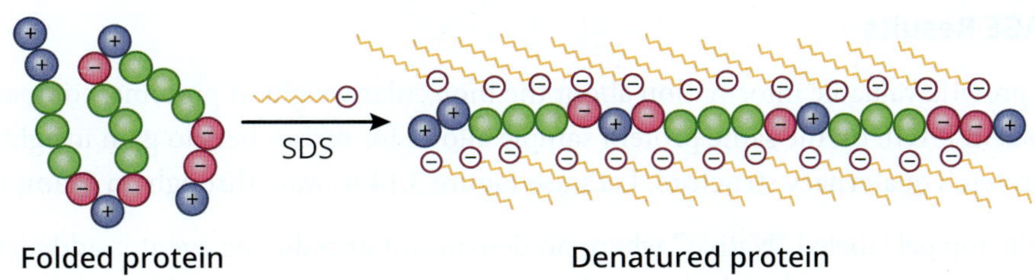

Figure 3.12 Protein Denaturation by SDS

Reducing PAGE

Reducing PAGE works on the same general principle as native PAGE in that all non-covalent interactions are preserved, but the reducing agent will break any disulfide links in the tertiary and quaternary structure by reducing them to cysteines. As seen in Figure 3.13, if disulfide bonds link two polypeptide chains together, in native PAGE or even SDS-PAGE, those two proteins would migrate together as one unit. However, in the presence of a reducing agent like **dithiothreitol (DTT)** or **β-mercaptoethanol (βME)**, the disulfide bond would be broken and the two proteins would migrate separately. Comparing native and reducing PAGE together allows researchers to quickly gain insight into how the quaternary structure of a protein is organized.

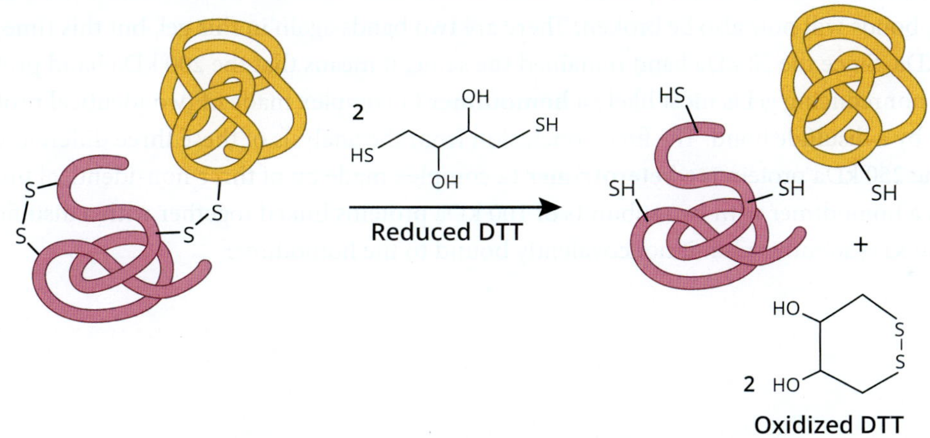

Figure 3.13 Effect of Reducing Agents on Disulfide Bonds

Interpreting PAGE Results

While PAGE can provide valuable information about the molecular weight of proteins, comparing between different conditions in PAGE on the same protein sample allows for researchers to gain insight into the composition of that protein's quaternary structure. Let's use Figure 3.14 to walk through an example analysis.

1. Examining the top gel labeled "Native," where no denaturant or reducing agent is added, the molecular weight markers in the first lane indicate the protein has a molecular weight of approximately 250 kDa (in the real world, native PAGE does not always provide an accurate molecular weight; however, the MCAT will always assume it does). A native gel by itself does not allow for any conclusions on quaternary structure, as protein quaternary structures and protein complexes are not affected in native PAGE.
2. The second gel labeled "SDS nonreducing" has the detergent SDS added, which denatures proteins by breaking any noncovalent interaction and coating the proteins in a uniform negative charge. SDS, however, cannot break disulfide bonds. In this gel, there are two bands: one band at 200 kDa, and another at 50 kDa. When compared to the native gel, this SDS nonreducing gel indicates the protein in the sample has two polypeptides noncovalently linked together that the SDS interrupted.
3. Finally, in the bottom gel labeled SDS reducing, both SDS and a reducing agent were added to the protein sample. As before, SDS breaks any noncovalent interactions, but with the addition of a reducing agent, disulfide bonds will now also be broken. There are two bands again in this gel, but this time at 100 kDa and 50 kDa. Since the 50 kDa band remained the same, it means that the 200 kDa band protein seen on the SDS nonreducing gel is most likely a **homodimer** (a complex made of two identical proteins) linked together by a disulfide bond. The final conclusion from the analysis of these three different types of PAGE is that the 250 kDa protein is a **heterotrimer** (a complex made up of three non-identical proteins) that contains a homodimer with two subunits of 100 kDa proteins linked together with a disulfide bond, and a third 50 kDa subunit subunit noncovalently bound to the homodimer.

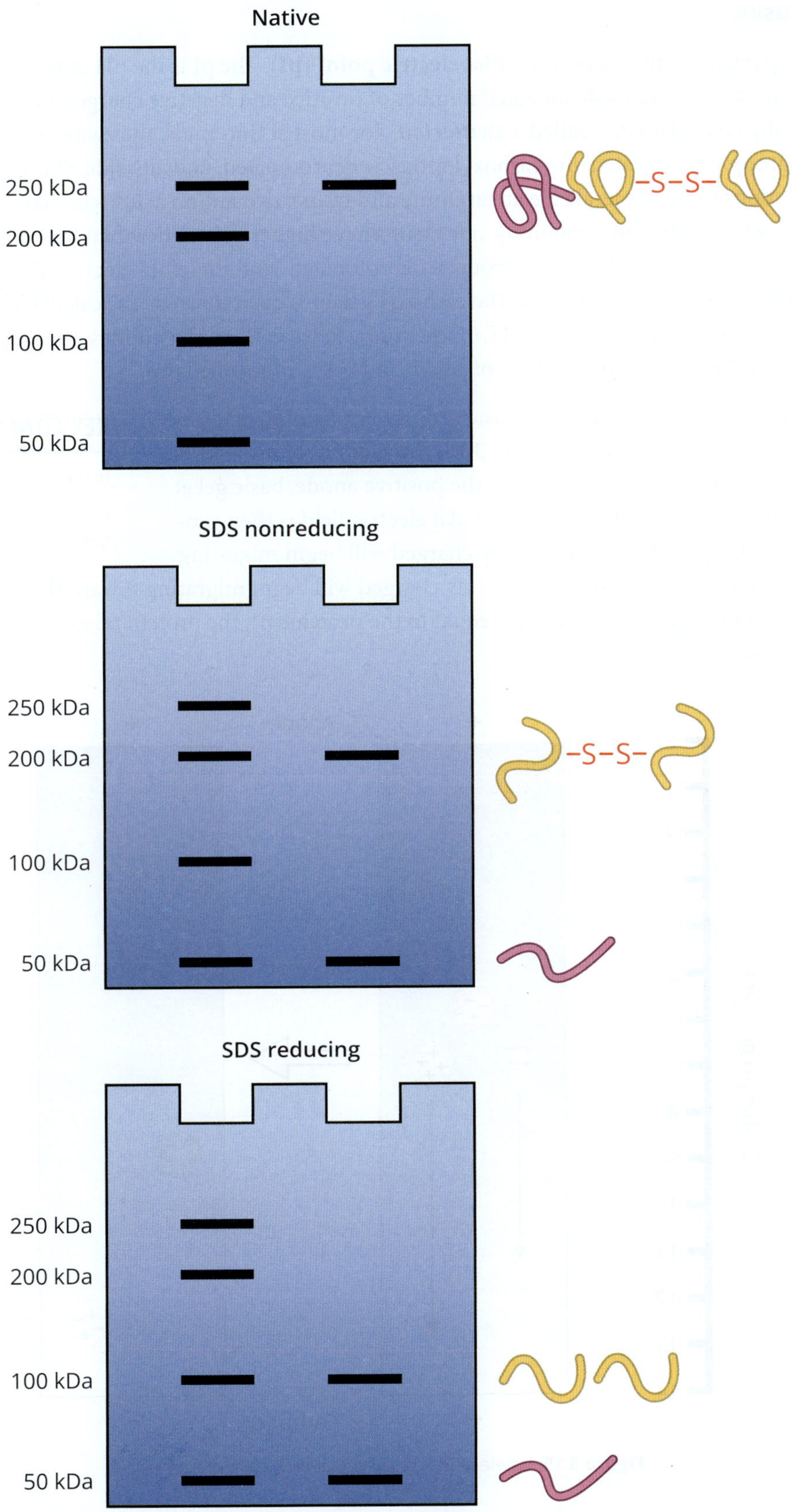

Figure 3.14 Native, SDS Nonreducing, and SDS Reducing PAGE on Example Protein

Isoelectric Focusing

Proteins can be separated on the basis of their **isoelectric point (pI)**. The pI is the pH at which the protein or amino acid is electrically neutral, with an equal number of positive and negative charges. For individual amino acids this electrically neutral form is called a ***zwitterion***. For most amino acids, the zwitterion form occurs when the amino group is protonated, the carboxyl group is deprotonated, and any side chain is electrically neutral. The exceptions to this general rule are arginine and lysine, two amino acids with basic side chains. For these amino acids, whose nitrogen-containing side chains have higher pK_a values than their amino groups, the zwitterion form occurs when the amino group is deprotonated (and therefore electrically neutral), while the nitrogenous side chain is protonated and the carboxyl group is deprotonated. The calculation of the pI for an amino acid was discussed in Chapter 1 of *MCAT Biochemistry Review*. For polypeptides, the isoelectric point is primarily determined by the relative numbers of acidic and basic amino acids.

Isoelectric focusing exploits the acidic and basic properties of amino acids by separating on the basis of pI. As seen in Figure 3.15, the mixture of proteins is placed in a gel with a pH gradient (acidic gel at the positive anode, basic gel at the negative cathode, and neutral in the middle). An electric field is then generated across the gel. Proteins that are positively charged will begin migrating toward the cathode and proteins that are negatively charged will begin migrating toward the anode. As a protein reaches the portion of gel where the pH is equal to the protein's pI, the protein takes on a neutral charge and will stop moving.

KEY CONCEPT

In isoelectric focusing, a protein stops moving when pH = pI.

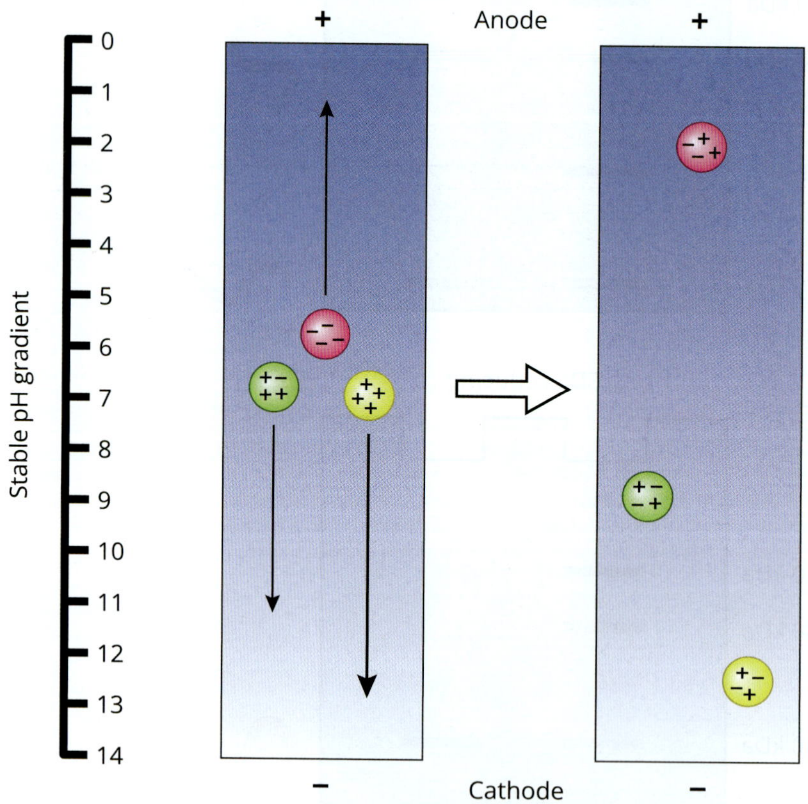

Figure 3.15 Isoelectric Focusing Gel Electrophoresis

Let's take a deeper look. We'll start with a protein that has a pI of 9. When the protein is in an environment with a pH of 9, it will carry no net charge. If we place this protein onto the gel at a pH of 7, there will be more protons around the protein. These protons will attach to the available basic sites on the protein, creating a net positive charge on the molecule, as occurs with the far left green protein in Figure 3.15. This charge will then cause the protein to be attracted to the negatively charged cathode, which is located on the basic side of the gradient. As the protein moves closer to the cathode, the pH of the gel slowly increases. Eventually, as the protein nears a pH of 9, the protons creating the positive charge will dissociate, and the protein will become neutral again. Remember, cations (positively charged species) will always migrate to the cathode, and anions (negatively charged species) will always migrate to the anode.

MNEMONIC

Cations go to the **Cat**hode
Anions go to the **An**ode

Chromatography

Chromatography is another tool that uses physical and chemical properties to separate and identify compounds from a complex mixture. Chromatography refers to a variety of techniques that require the homogenized protein mixture to be fractionated through a porous matrix. One of the reasons chromatography is a valuable tool is that the isolated proteins are immediately available for identification and quantification. In all forms of chromatography discussed here, the concept is identical: the more similar the compound is to its surroundings (by polarity, charge, and so on), the more it will stick to and move slowly through its surroundings. Chromatography is preferred over electrophoresis when large amounts of protein are being separated.

The process begins by placing the sample onto a solid medium called the **stationary phase** or **adsorbent**. The next step is to run the mobile phase through the stationary phase. This will allow the sample to run through the stationary phase, or **elute**. Depending on the relative affinity of the sample for the stationary and mobile phases, different substances will migrate through at different speeds. That is, components that have a high affinity for the stationary phase will barely migrate at all; components with a high affinity for the mobile phase will migrate much more quickly. The amount of time a compound spends in the stationary phase is referred to as the **retention time**. Varying retention times of each compound in the solution results in separation of the components within the stationary phase, or **partitioning**, as demonstrated in Figure 3.16. Each component can then be isolated individually for study.

BRIDGE

Chromatography and other separatory methods are also discussed in Chapter 12 of *MCAT Organic Chemistry Review*.

KEY CONCEPT

All chromatography is about the affinity of a substance for the mobile and stationary phases, except for size-exclusion chromatography.

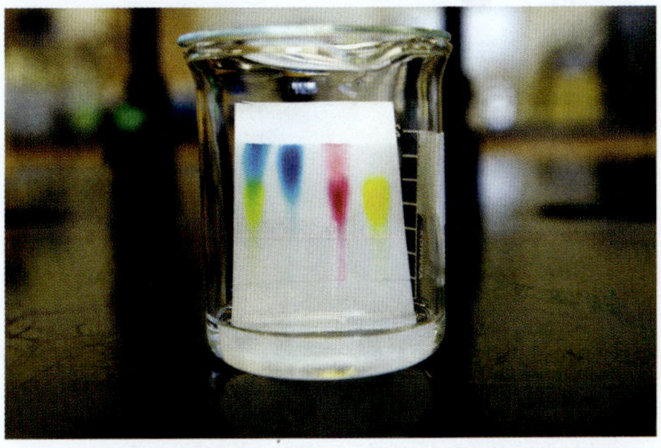

Figure 3.16 Partitioning of Black Ink
Thin-layer chromatography; original spot placed on the bottom of the card. Components with high retention times remain near the bottom of the card; components with low retention times have migrated toward the top of the card.

We can use myriad different media as our stationary phase, each one exploiting different properties that allow us to separate out our compound. In chromatography for protein separation, common properties include charge, pore size, and specific affinities.

Column Chromatography

In **column chromatography**, a column is filled with silica or alumina beads as an adsorbent, and gravity moves the solvent and compounds down the column, shown in Figure 3.17. As the solution flows through the column, both size and polarity have a role in determining how quickly a compound moves through the polar silica or alumina beads: the less polar the compound, the faster it can elute through the column (short retention time). In column chromatography, the solvent polarity, pH, or salinity can easily be changed to help elute the protein of interest.

Eventually, the solvent drips out of the end of the column, and different fractions that leave the column are collected over time. Each fraction contains bands that correspond to different compounds. After collection, the solvent can be evaporated and the compounds of interest kept. Column chromatography is particularly useful in biochemistry because it can be used to separate and collect other macromolecules besides proteins, such as nucleic acids.

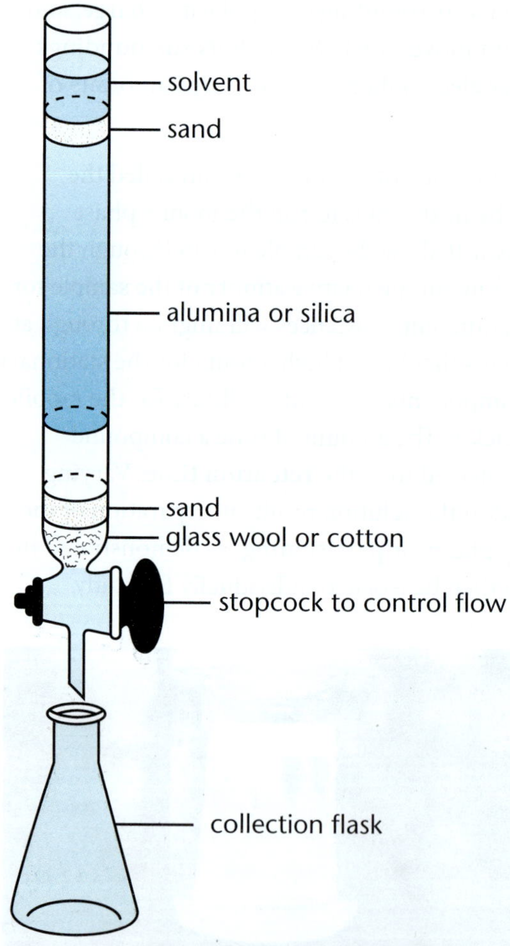

Figure 3.17 Column Chromatography
The sample is added at the top of the column and a solvent is poured over it. The more similar the sample is to the solvent (mobile phase), the more quickly it will elute; the more similar it is to the alumina or silica (stationary phase), the more slowly it will elute—if at all.

Ion-Exchange Chromatography

In this method, the beads in the column are coated with charged substances, so they attract or bind compounds that have an opposite charge, as can be seen in Figure 3.18. For instance, a positively charged column will attract and hold a negatively charged protein as it passes through the column, either increasing its retention time or retaining it completely. After all other compounds have moved through the column, a salt gradient is used to elute the charged molecules that have stuck to the column.

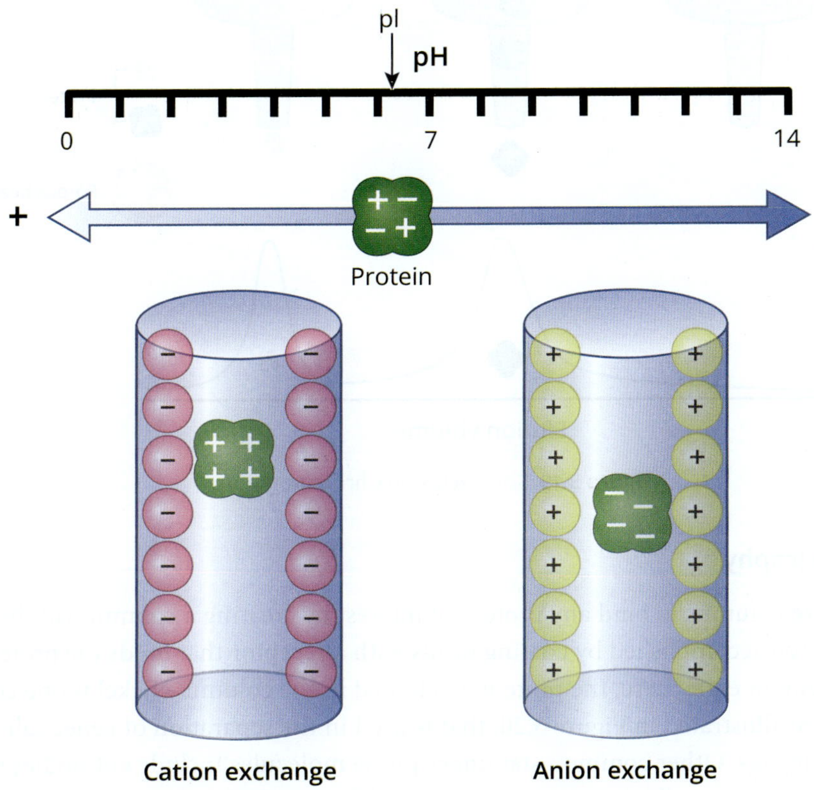

Figure 3.18 Ion-Exchange Chromatography

Size-Exclusion Chromatography

In this method, the beads used in the column contain tiny pores of varying sizes. As demonstrated in Figure 3.19, these tiny pores allow small compounds to enter the beads, thus slowing them down. Large compounds can't fit into the pores, so they will move around them and travel through the column faster. It is important to remember that in this type of chromatography, the small compounds are slowed down and retained longer—which may be counterintuitive. The size of the pores may be varied so that molecules of different molecular weights can be fractionated. A common approach in protein purification is to use an ion-exchange column followed by a size-exclusion column.

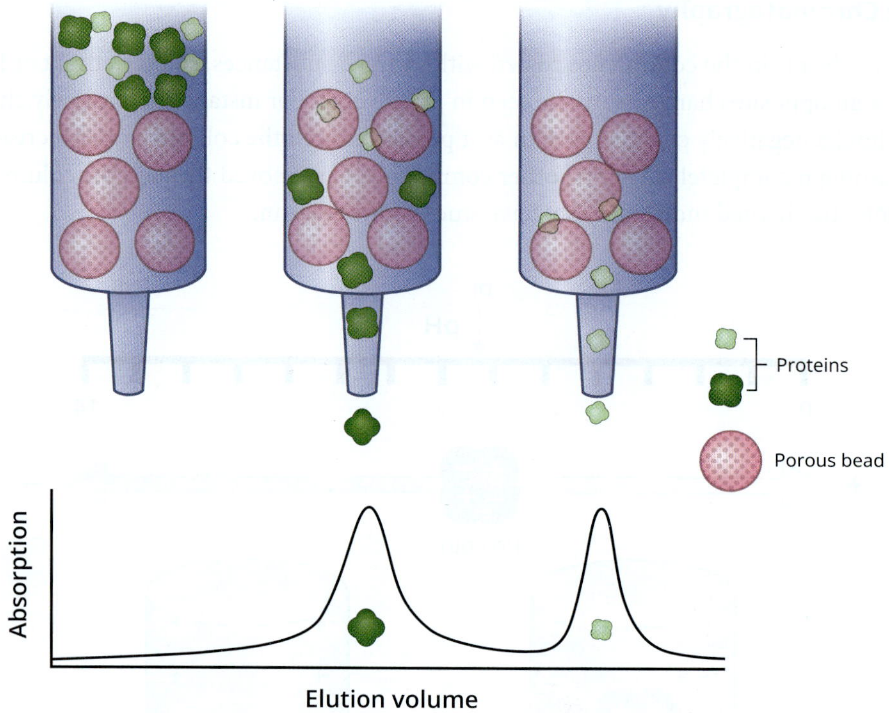

Figure 3.19 Size-Exclusion Chromatography

Affinity Chromatography

We can also customize columns to bind any protein of interest by creating a column with high affinity for that protein. This can be accomplished by coating beads with a receptor that binds the protein or a specific antibody to the protein; in either case, the protein is retained in the column. Nickel is one common choice for stationary phase, as illustrated in Figure 3.20, that is used in the separation of genetically engineered proteins with histidine tags. Other common stationary phase molecules include antibodies (also depicted in Figure 3.20) or antigens, as well as enzyme substrate analogues, which mimic the natural substrate for an enzyme of interest. Once the protein is retained in the column, it can be eluted by washing the column with a free receptor (or target or antibody), which will compete with the bead-bound receptor and ultimately free the protein from the column. Eluents can also be created with a specific pH or salinity level that disrupts the bonds between the ligand and the protein of interest. The only drawback of the elution step is that the recovered substance can be bound to the eluent. If, for example, the eluent was an inhibitor of an enzyme, it could be difficult to remove.

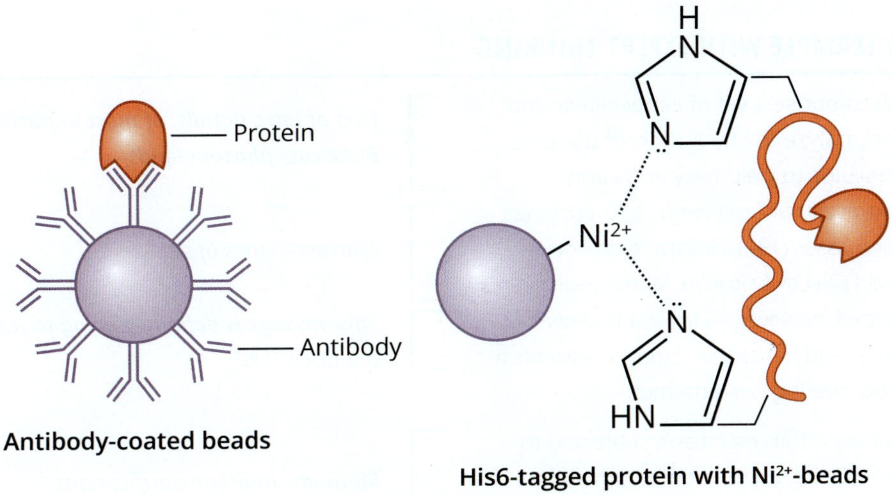

Figure 3.20 Affinity Chromatography

BIOCHEMISTRY GUIDED EXAMPLE WITH EXPERT THINKING

Phospholipases A2 (PLA2) comprise a set of extracellular and intracellular enzymes that catalyze the hydrolysis of the sn-2 fatty acyl bond of phospholipids to yield fatty acids and lysophospholipids. The extracellular (secreted) PLA2 enzymes (sPLA2) have low molecular masses (13–18 kDa) and do not manifest significant fatty acid selectivity *in vitro*. Mammalian sPLA2 enzymes are well characterized; however, much less is known about aquatic sPLA2 enzymes and hence their study represents a great potential source for discovering new enzymes.

Lots of intro details; of most importance is that PLA2 cuts phospholipids

Characteristics of sPLA2

This passage is definitely going to focus on aquatic sPLA2

Pancreases from stingrays were harvested and subjected to multiple purification protocols, including ammonium sulfate precipitation and purification columns while monitoring sPLA2 activity. The final purification step involved a reverse phase high-performance liquid chromatography (RP-HPLC) C8 (nonpolar octylsilane) column, using a dynamic gradient composed of water and acetonitrile. As time increases, the proportion of water decreases and concentration of acetonitrile increases up to 80%. As seen below in Figure 1(a), the eluate was monitored at 280 nm, and the fraction at 23 min was analyzed by 15% SDS-PAGE under reducing conditions and stained with Coomassie blue in Figure 1(b).

Methods: multiple purifications

Final purification: stationary phase (nonpolar) and mobile phase (water and acetonitrile)

Figure shows two things: chromatogram and SDS-PAGE gel

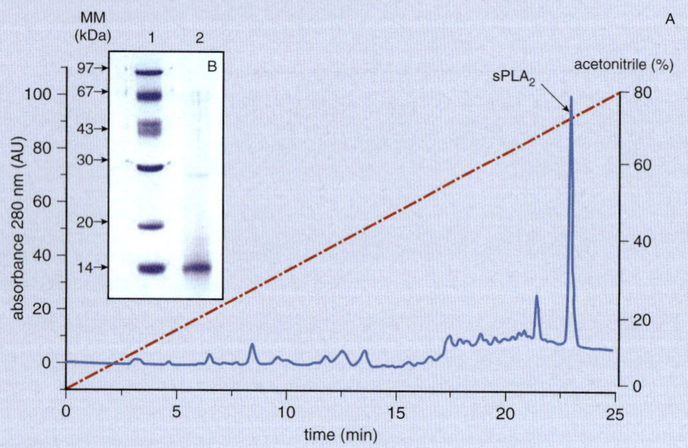

Figure 1(a) (graph) and Figure 1(b) (blot)

Trends: Fig 1(a): big peak at ~23 min at high ACN concentration; Fig 1(b): single band at ~14 kDa

Adapted from Bacha, A. B., Karray, A., Bouchaala, E., Gargouri, Y., & Ali, Y. B. (2011). Purification and biochemical characterization of pancreatic phospholipase A2 from the common stingray *Dasyatis pastinaca*. *Lipids in Health and Disease*, 10, 32. doi:10.1186/1476-511X-10-32

According to the data, what is the approximate monomeric molecular weight of sPLA2? Why is it biologically relevant that sPLA2 required a high acetonitrile concentration to elute o\ff the column?

With "according to the data", this question stem is letting us know we'll need to use one or both parts of the figure to answer. So, let's start with a quick scan of the passage to see the topic and the kind of information presented to better understand the context of the data. The text is focused on a protein called phospholipase A2 (PLA2), and Figure 1 shows peaks with a gel picture inset. The bulk of the passage seems method-heavy (as indicated by the usage of column names and Figure references). We have two questions to answer: the first is asking for the size of the protein, while the second asks for a connection between the biology behind PLA2 and the way PLA2 interacts with the column.

To determine the monomeric molecular weight of sPLA2, we'll need information from the SDS-PAGE data in Figure 1(b). We know from our background content knowledge that an SDS-PAGE gel under reducing conditions will denature proteins and sever any disulfide bonds. Therefore, the bands that appear should only correspond to monomers, and monomers are what this question asked about. The first lane is a series of molecular weight standards measured in kilodaltons (kDa), which are used to estimate the molecular weight of unknown proteins. We're told that the fraction at 23 minutes, which corresponds to the sPLA2 peak on the chromatogram, is analyzed in lane 2 of the gel. The band in lane 2 corresponding to sPLA2 is right next to the 14 kDa standard in lane 1, implying that the sPLA2 protein has a weight of approximately 14 kDa as well. As an extra measure of verification, paragraph 1 stated that sPLA2s have a molecular weight between 13–18 kDa.

Paragraph 2 discusses the method of the experiment, which will help us answer the second part of the question stem. For all the detail in paragraph 2, RP-HPLC is just a type of a column chromatography. Like all types of column chromatography, RP-HPLC has a stationary phase (the column) and a mobile phase (the solvent). We're told that the column is nonpolar, which means nonpolar molecules will stick inside the column. We're also told that the solvent changes composition over time—starting as mostly water, but ending as mostly acetonitrile. Why is this change in composition significant? We recall that water is a polar solvent, while acetonitrile is closer to nonpolar. Therefore, early on, when the solvent is mostly water, polar molecules will flush out of the column because like dissolves like. But near the end of the experiment, when the solvent is mostly acetonitrile, the now nonpolar solvent will dislodge nonpolar molecules. So, nonpolar molecules will elute off the column near the end of the experiment. Finally, we observe that the sPLA2 protein elutes off the column near the end, when the solvent is mostly acetonitrile. This observation implies that the sPLA2 protein is net nonpolar; the nonpolar protein had initially stuck to the nonpolar column, but the protein eventually eluted out of the column once the solvent became nonpolar enough to solvate the protein.

We can thus conclude that sPLA2 monomers have a molecular weight of around 14 kDa and, from the experimental procedure, we can conclude that sPLA2 proteins have a high affinity for nonpolar substances—first for the walls of the nonpolar column, and later for the nonpolar acetonitrile solvent. This behavior makes biological sense because the biological substrates of the sPLA2 protein are phospholipids!

MCAT CONCEPT CHECK 3.3

Before you move on, assess your understanding of the material with these questions.

1. What separation methods can be used to isolate a protein on the basis of isoelectric point?

____

2. What are the relative benefits of native PAGE compared to SDS-PAGE?

____

3. What are two potential drawbacks of affinity chromatography?

    1. _______________
    2. _______________

4. True or False: In size-exclusion chromatography, the largest molecules elute first.

3.4 Protein Analysis

LEARNING OBJECTIVES

After Chapter 3.4, you will be able to:

- Recall the traits that are typically analyzed in proteins
- Describe the Edman degradation and the Bradford assay
- Recognize the limitations of protein separation and analysis techniques

Separating proteins from one another is generally only the first step in analysis. The next step is to study the isolated protein. Protein structure, function, or quantity is often of interest for a researcher or a commercial laboratory. Even after protein identification, protein analysis tools may be used. For example, in the case of protein synthesis for commercial use, purity of the product must be periodically assessed. The protein can be studied as a whole or broken down so that its parts can be examined.

Protein Structure

Protein structure can be determined through **X-ray crystallography** and **nuclear magnetic resonance (NMR) spectroscopy**. Before crystallographic analysis, the protein must be isolated and crystallized. X-ray crystallography is the most reliable and common method; 75 percent of the protein structures known today were analyzed through this method. Crystallography measures electron density on an extremely high-resolution scale and can also be used for nucleic acids. An X-ray diffraction pattern is generated in this method, as shown in Figure 3.21. The small dots in the diffraction pattern can then be interpreted to determine the protein's structure.

BRIDGE

NMR and other forms of spectroscopy are also discussed in Chapter 11 of *MCAT Organic Chemistry Review*.

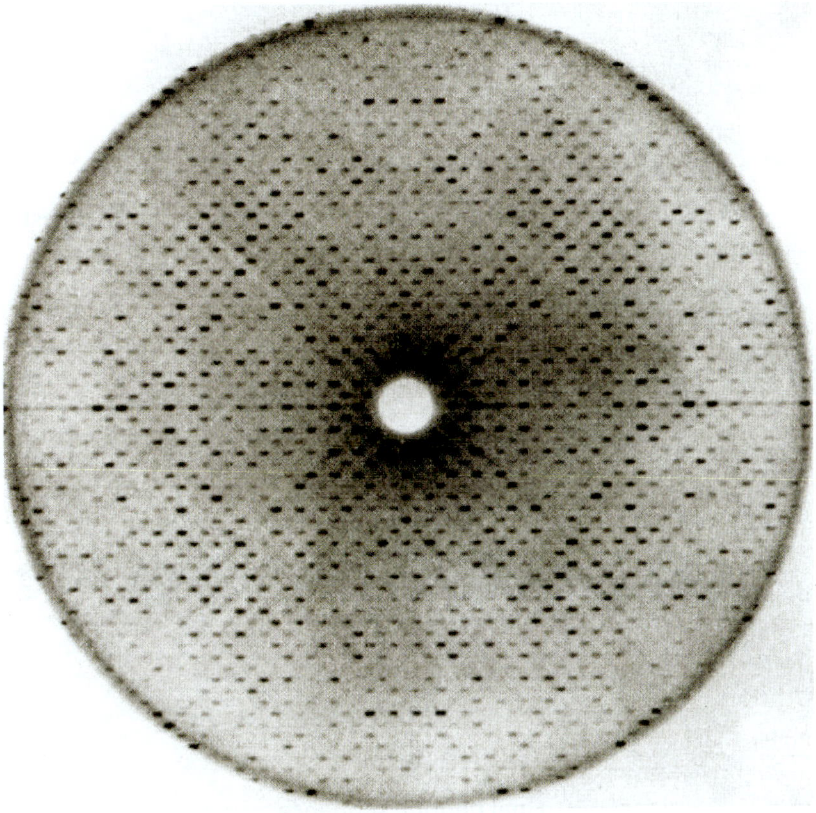

Figure 3.21 Diffraction Pattern in X-Ray Crystallography

The minority of protein structure determination (25 percent) has been accomplished through NMR, as discussed in Chapter 11 of *MCAT Organic Chemistry Review*.

Amino Acid Composition

The amino acids that compose a protein can be determined by complete protein hydrolysis and subsequent chromatographic analysis. However, the random nature of hydrolysis prevents amino acid sequencing. To determine the primary structure of a protein, sequential digestion of the protein with specific cleavage enzymes is used. Small proteins are best analyzed with the **Edman degradation**, which uses cleavage to sequence proteins of up to 50 to 70 amino acids. The Edman degradation selectively and sequentially removes the N-terminal amino acid of the protein, which can be analyzed via mass spectroscopy.

REAL WORLD

Like PCR gene sequencing, protein amino acid sequencing can be automated in a stepwise manner. By combining the information from both techniques, researchers can determine where on a chromosome the gene coding a particular protein resides.

For larger proteins, digestion with *chymotrypsin*, *trypsin*, and *cyanogen bromide*, a synthetic reagent, may be used. This digestion selectively cleaves proteins at specific amino acid residues, creating smaller fragments that can then be analyzed by electrophoresis or the Edman degradation. To determine the full sequence of the original protein, multiple enzymatic digests are performed, and the resulting fragments are sequenced and then aligned by identifying overlapping regions, as illustrated in Figure 3.22. Because disulfide links and salt bridges are broken to reduce the protein to its primary structure, their positions cannot be determined by these methods.

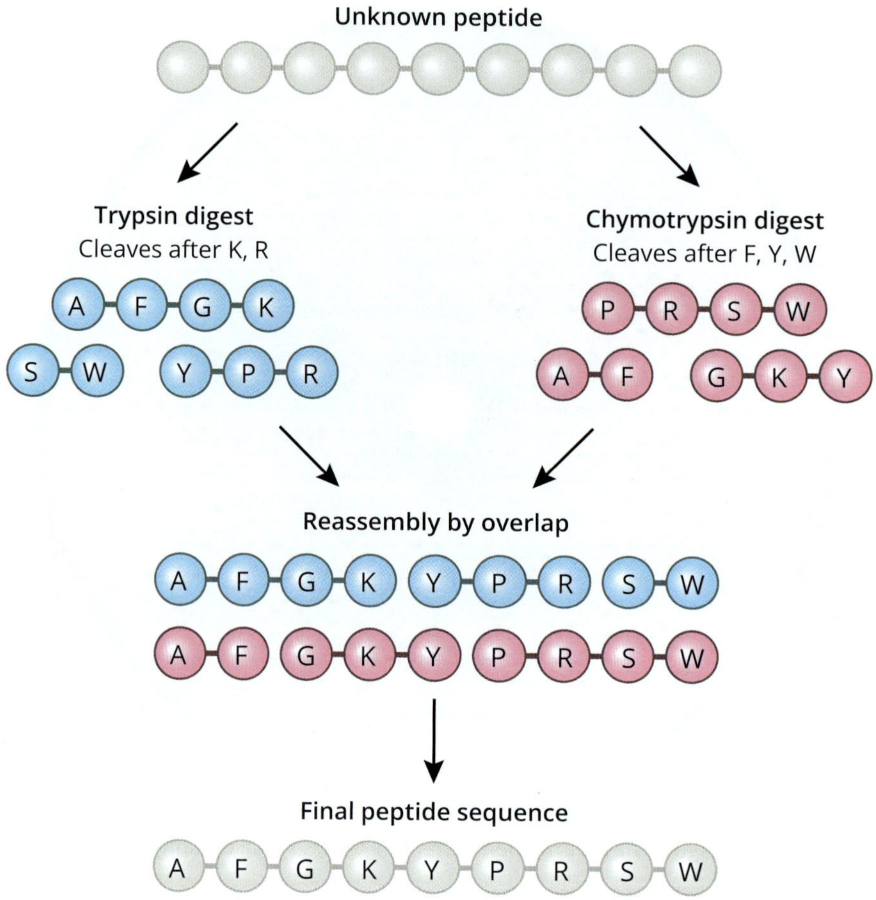

Figure 3.22 Enzymatic Digestion for Peptide Sequencing

Activity Analysis

Protein activity is generally determined by monitoring a known reaction with a given concentration of substrate and comparing it to a standard. Activity is correlated with substrate concentration, but it is also affected by the methods used to purify the enzyme and the specific conditions of the assay. Reactions that lead to a color change have particular applicability because samples with color changes can be rapidly detected using chromatographic analysis. **Enzyme activity** is measured as moles of substrate converted by the enzyme into product per unit of time, with an SI unit of katal, though it is much more commonly measured in units of U. **Specific activity**, however, measures the activity of the enzyme per mass of total protein, and is often used to track the purity of an enzyme within a mixture, like during purification. Comparing the total number of units of activity at the end of the purification to the total units at the beginning of purification can provide an estimate of the **purification yield**.

Concentration Determination

Concentration is determined almost exclusively through spectroscopy. Because proteins contain aromatic side chains, they can be analyzed with **UV spectroscopy** without any treatment; however, this type of analysis is particularly sensitive to sample contaminants. Proteins also cause colorimetric changes with specific reactions, particularly the **bicinchoninic acid (BCA) assay**, **Lowry reagent assay**, and **Bradford protein assay**. The Bradford method is most common because of its reliability and simplicity in basic analyses.

Bradford Protein Assay

The Bradford protein assay mixes a protein in solution with Coomassie Brilliant Blue dye. The dye is protonated and green-brown in color prior to mixing with proteins, as depicted in Figure 3.23. The dye gives up protons upon binding to amino acid groups, turning blue in the process. Ionic attractions between the dye and the protein then stabilize this blue form of the dye; thus, increased protein concentrations correspond to a larger concentration of blue dye in solution. Samples of known protein concentrations are reacted with the Bradford reagent and then absorbance is measured to create a standard curve. The unknown sample is then exposed to the same conditions, and the concentration is determined based on the standard curve. This is a very accurate method when only one type of protein is present in solution, but because of variable binding of the Coomassie dye with different amino acids, it is less accurate when more than one protein is present. The Bradford protein assay is limited by the presence of detergent in the sample or by excessive buffer.

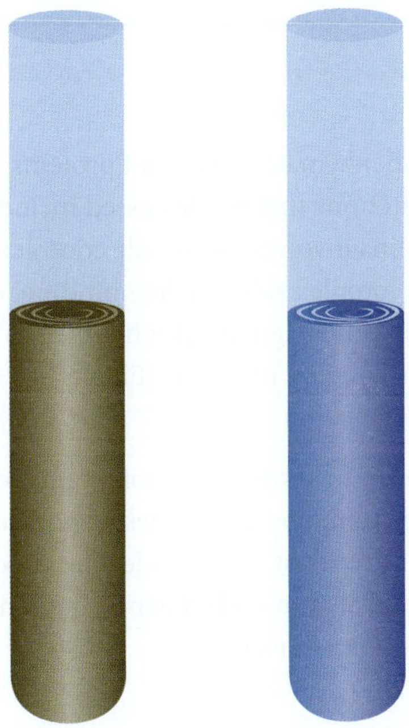

Figure 3.23 Bradford Protein Assay
The acidic form (left) has a brown-green hue; the basic form (right), which is created by interactions with proteins in solution, has a brilliant blue hue.

MCAT CONCEPT CHECK 3.4

Before you move on, assess your understanding of the material with these questions.

1. Why are proteins analyzed after isolation?

 ____

2. What factors would cause an activity assay to display lower activity than expected after concentration determination?

 ____

3. True or False: The Edman degradation proceeds from the carboxy (C-) terminus.

Conclusion

In this chapter, we have explored the nonenzymatic aspects of proteins as well as the ways proteins can be analyzed. The cellular proteins and their functions that we discussed included structural proteins that play a role in cytoskeletal architecture, motor proteins involved in muscle contraction and movement along the cytoskeleton, and other proteins that play more complex roles such as binding, immunologic function, and biosignaling. The more complex proteins involved in biosignaling highlighted in this chapter included ion channels, enzyme-linked receptors, and G protein-coupled receptors. Finally, we determined how to isolate and identify a protein and its relevant properties.

In the next chapter, we'll turn our attention to another class of biomolecules: carbohydrates. As we transition from amino acids, peptides, and proteins to monosaccharides, oligosaccharides, and polysaccharides, look for key connections between the different types of macromolecules used by the body for structure and as fuel sources. In the end, all biomolecules are related to each other through metabolism, which we'll explore in Chapters 9 through 12 of *MCAT Biochemistry Review*.

GO ONLINE

You've reviewed the content, now test your knowledge and critical thinking skills by completing a test-like passage set in your online resources!

CONCEPT SUMMARY

Cellular Functions

- **Structural proteins** compose the cytoskeleton, anchoring proteins, and much of the extracellular matrix.
  - The most common structural proteins are **collagen**, **elastin**, **keratin**, **actin**, and **tubulin**.
  - They are generally fibrous in nature.
- **Motor proteins** have one or more heads capable of force generation through a conformational change.
  - They have catalytic activity, acting as ATPases to power movement.
  - Muscle contraction, vesicle movement within cells, and cell motility are the most common applications of motor proteins.
  - Common examples include **myosin**, **kinesin**, and **dynein**.
- **Binding proteins** bind a specific substrate, either to sequester it in the body or hold its concentration at steady state.
- **Cell adhesion molecules** (**CAM**) allow cells to bind to other cells or surfaces.
  - **Cadherins** are calcium-dependent glycoproteins that hold similar cells together.
  - **Integrins** have two membrane-spanning chains and permit cells to adhere to proteins in the extracellular matrix. Some also have signaling capabilities.
  - **Selectins** allow cells to adhere to carbohydrates on the surfaces of other cells and are most commonly used in the immune system.
- **Antibodies** (or **immunoglobulins**, **Ig**) are used by the immune system to target a specific **antigen**, which may be a protein on the surface of a pathogen (invading organism) or a toxin.
  - Immunoglobulins contain a constant region and a variable region; the variable region is responsible for antigen binding.
  - Two identical heavy chains and two identical light chains form a single antibody; they are held together by disulfide linkages and noncovalent interactions.

Biosignaling

- **Ion channels** can be used for regulating ion flow into or out of a cell. There are three main types of ion channels.
  - **Ungated channels** are always open.
  - **Voltage-gated channels** are open within a range of membrane potentials.
  - **Ligand-gated channels** open in the presence of a specific binding substance, usually a hormone or neurotransmitter.
- **Enzyme-linked receptors** participate in cell signaling through extracellular ligand binding and initiation of second messenger cascades.

- **G protein-coupled receptors** have a membrane-bound protein associated with a trimeric **G protein**. They also initiate second messenger systems.
  - Ligand binding engages the G protein.
  - GDP is replaced with GTP; the α subunit dissociates from the β and γ subunits.
  - The activated α subunit alters the activity of **adenylate cyclase** or **phospholipase C**.
  - GTP is dephosphorylated to GDP; the α subunit rebinds to the β and γ subunits.

Protein Isolation

- **Electrophoresis** uses a gel matrix to observe the migration of proteins in response to an electric field.
  - **Native PAGE** maintains the protein's shape, but results are difficult to compare because the mass-to-charge ratio differs for each protein.
  - **SDS-PAGE** denatures the proteins and masks the native charge so that comparison of size is more accurate, but the functional protein cannot be recaptured from the gel.
  - **Isoelectric focusing** separates proteins by their **isoelectric point** (**pI**); the protein migrates toward an electrode until it reaches a region of the gel where pH = pI of the protein.
- **Chromatography** separates protein mixtures on the basis of their affinity for a **stationary phase** or a **mobile phase**.
  - **Column chromatography** uses beads of a polar compound, like silica or alumina (stationary phase), with a nonpolar solvent (mobile phase).
  - **Ion-exchange chromatography** uses a charged column and a variably saline eluent.
  - **Size-exclusion chromatography** relies on porous beads. Larger molecules elute first because they are not trapped in the small pores.
  - **Affinity chromatography** uses a bound receptor or ligand and an eluent with free ligand or a receptor for the protein of interest.

Protein Analysis

- Protein structure is primarily determined through **X-ray crystallography** after the protein is isolated, although NMR can also be used.
- Amino acid composition can be determined by simple hydrolysis, but amino acid sequencing requires sequential degradation, such as the **Edman degradation**.
- Activity levels for enzymatic samples are determined by following the process of a known reaction, often accompanied by a color change.
- Protein concentration is also determined colorimetrically, either by UV spectroscopy or through a color change reaction.
  - **BCA assay**, **Lowry reagent assay**, and **Bradford protein assay** each test for protein and have different advantages and disadvantages.
  - The Bradford protein assay, which uses a color change from brown-green to blue, is most common.

ANSWERS TO CONCEPT CHECKS

3.1

1. Cytoskeletal proteins tend to be fibrous with repeating domains, while motor proteins tend to have ATPase activity and binding heads. Both types of protein function in cellular motility.
2. False. An enzyme is a protein or RNA molecule with catalytic activity, which motor proteins do have. Motor function is generally considered nonenzymatic, but the ATPase functionality of motor proteins indicates that these molecules do have catalytic activity.
3. If the binding protein is present in sufficiently high quantities relative to the substrate, nearly all substrate will be bound despite a low affinity.
4.

Cell Adhesion Molecule	Type of Adhesion
Cadherin	Two cells of the same or similar type using calcium
Integrin	One cell to proteins in the extracellular matrix
Selectin	One cell to carbohydrates, usually on the surface of other cells

5. Antigen–antibody interactions can result in neutralization of the pathogen or toxin, opsonization (marking) of the antigen for destruction, or creation of insoluble antigen–antibody complexes that can be phagocytized and digested by macrophages (agglutination).

3.2

1.

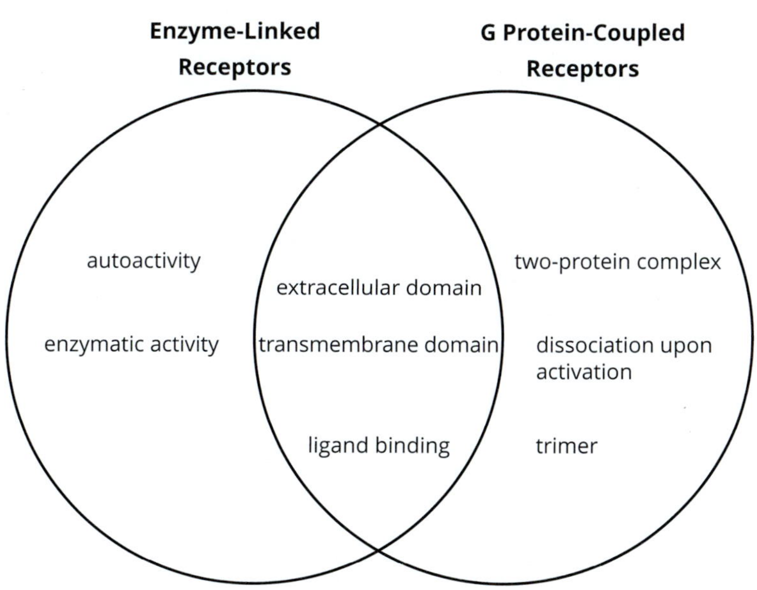

2. Ungated channels are always open.
3. Transport kinetics display both K_m and V_{max} values. They also can be cooperative, like some binding proteins. However, transporters do not have analogous K_{eq} values for reactions because there is no catalysis.

3.3

1. Isoelectric focusing and ion-exchange chromatography both separate proteins based on charge; the charge of a protein in any given environment is determined by its isoelectric point (pI).
2. Native PAGE allows a complete protein to be recovered after analysis; it also more accurately determines the relative globular size of proteins. SDS-PAGE can be used to eliminate conflation from mass-to-charge ratios.
3. The protein of interest may not elute from the column because its affinity is too high or it may be permanently bound to the free receptor in the eluent.
4. True. The small pores in size-exclusion chromatography trap smaller particles, retaining them in the column.

3.4

1. Protein isolation is generally only the first step in an analysis. The protein identity must be confirmed by amino acid analysis or activity. With unknown proteins, classification of their features is generally desired.
2. Contamination of the sample with detergent or SDS could yield an artificially increased protein level, leading to lower activity than expected (because the protein concentration was calculated as higher than its actual value). Alternatively, the enzyme could have been denatured during isolation and analysis.
3. False. The Edman degradation proceeds from the amino (N-) terminus.

SCIENCE MASTERY ASSESSMENT EXPLANATIONS

1. **D**

In most electrophoresis experiments, we attempt to separate out one component from the others. Because we are attempting to isolate protein A only, a pH that causes protein A to be negative while proteins B and C are neutral or positive will be best. pH 5.5 accomplishes this goal; proteins B and C will be positively charged. A pH of 4.5, **(C)**, would make protein A neutral, and it would thus not migrate across the gel. Any neutral impurities would also remain in the well with protein A, making this pH not the best choice.

2. **B**

Sodium dodecyl sulfate is a detergent and will digest proteins to form micelles with uniform negative charges. Because the protein is sequestered within the micelle, other factors such as charge of the protein and shape have minimal roles during separation. In essence, the protein micelles can be modeled as being spheres, dependent only on size.

3. **D**

From the given choices, all of them are involved in cell movement with the exception of **(D)**. Centrioles are composed of microtubules, but are involved in mitosis, not cell migration.

4. **C**

The most prevalent extracellular proteins are keratin, elastin, and collagen. Tubulin and actin are the primary cytoskeletal proteins, while myosin is a motor protein.

5. **C**

For a ligand present in low quantities to have a strong action, we expect it to initiate a second messenger cascade system. Second messenger systems amplify signals because enzymes can catalyze a reaction more than once while they are active, and often activate other enzymes. Both enzyme-linked receptors and G protein-coupled receptors use second messenger systems, while ion channels do not.

6. **D**

Ions that are not readily accessible in the cytoplasm or extracellular space are likely to be bound to a binding protein. Classically, calcium and magnesium are protein-bound. Without this background knowledge, the question can still be answered. Sodium, **(A)**, and potassium, **(B)**, must exist in their free states to participate in action potentials. Chloride, **(C)**, is readily excreted by the kidney, which would not be true if it were protein-bound. Calcium must be sequestered in both the bloodstream and intracellularly because calcium is used for muscle contraction, exocytosis (of neurotransmitters and other signals), and many other cellular processes that must be tightly regulated.

7. **A**

Antibodies are specific to a single antigen. Each B-cell produces a single type of antibody with a constant region that is specific to the host and a variable region that is specific to an antigen.

8. **A**

The resting membrane potential is displayed by cells that are not actively involved in signal transduction. Ungated or "leak" channels permit limited free flow of ions, while the sodium–potassium pump is also active and corrects for this leakage. Ligand-gated and voltage-gated channels are involved in cell signaling and in the pacemaker potentials of certain cells, but cause deviation from—not maintenance of—the resting membrane potential.

9. **D**

All trimeric G proteins have α, β, and γ subunits—**(A)**, **(B)**, and **(C)**, respectively. G_s, G_i, and G_q are subtypes of the G_α subunit of the trimeric G protein and differ depending on the G protein-coupled receptor's function.

10. **B**

The proteins described in the question differ primarily in their molecular weights. Their pI values are very close, so ion-exchange chromatography, **(A)**, is not a good choice. The question specifies a large quantity, which is better processed through chromatography than through electrophoresis—**(C)** and **(D)**—because the gel can only handle a small volume of protein.

11. **C**

The overall pI of a protein is determined by the relative number of acidic and basic amino acids. The basic amino acids are arginine, lysine, and histidine, and the acidic amino acids are aspartic acid and glutamic acid. Glycine's side chain is a hydrogen atom, so it will have the least contribution of all the amino acids.

12. **C**

The gel in isoelectric focusing uses a pH gradient. When a protein is in a region with a pH above its pI, it is negatively charged and moves toward the anode. When it is in a pH region below its pI, it is positively charged and moves toward the cathode. When the pH equals the pI, the migration of the protein is halted.

13. **C**

UV spectroscopy is best used with conjugated systems of double bonds. While the double bond in the peptide bond does display resonance, this is not adequate for UV absorption. However, aromatic systems are conjugated, and phenylalanine, tyrosine, and tryptophan all contain aromatic ring structures.

14. **B**

Protein activity and concentration are generally correlated. Because we have a high concentration of protein, we expect a high activity unless the protein has been damaged or inactivated in some way. The protein could have been inactivated by experimental conditions like detergents, heat, or pH; however, these are not answer choices. Rather, we must consider how the experimental procedure works. Protein elutes off of an affinity column by binding free ligand. In this situation, the binding may not have been reversed and thus the free ligand competes for the active site of the enzyme, lowering its activity.

15. **A**

The selective cleavage of proteins by digestive enzymes allows fragments of different lengths with known amino acid endpoints to be created. By cleaving the protein with several different enzymes, a basic outline of the amino acid sequence can be created.

GO ONLINE

Consult your online resources for additional practice.

EQUATIONS TO REMEMBER

(3.1) **Migration velocity:** $v = \frac{Ez}{f}$

SHARED CONCEPTS

Biochemistry Chapter 1
Amino Acids, Peptides, and Proteins

Biology Chapter 1
The Cell

Biology Chapter 8
The Immune System

Biology Chapter 11
The Musculoskeletal System

General Chemistry Chapter 12
Electrochemistry

Organic Chemistry Chapter 12
Separations and Purifications

CHAPTER 4

CARBOHYDRATE STRUCTURE AND FUNCTION

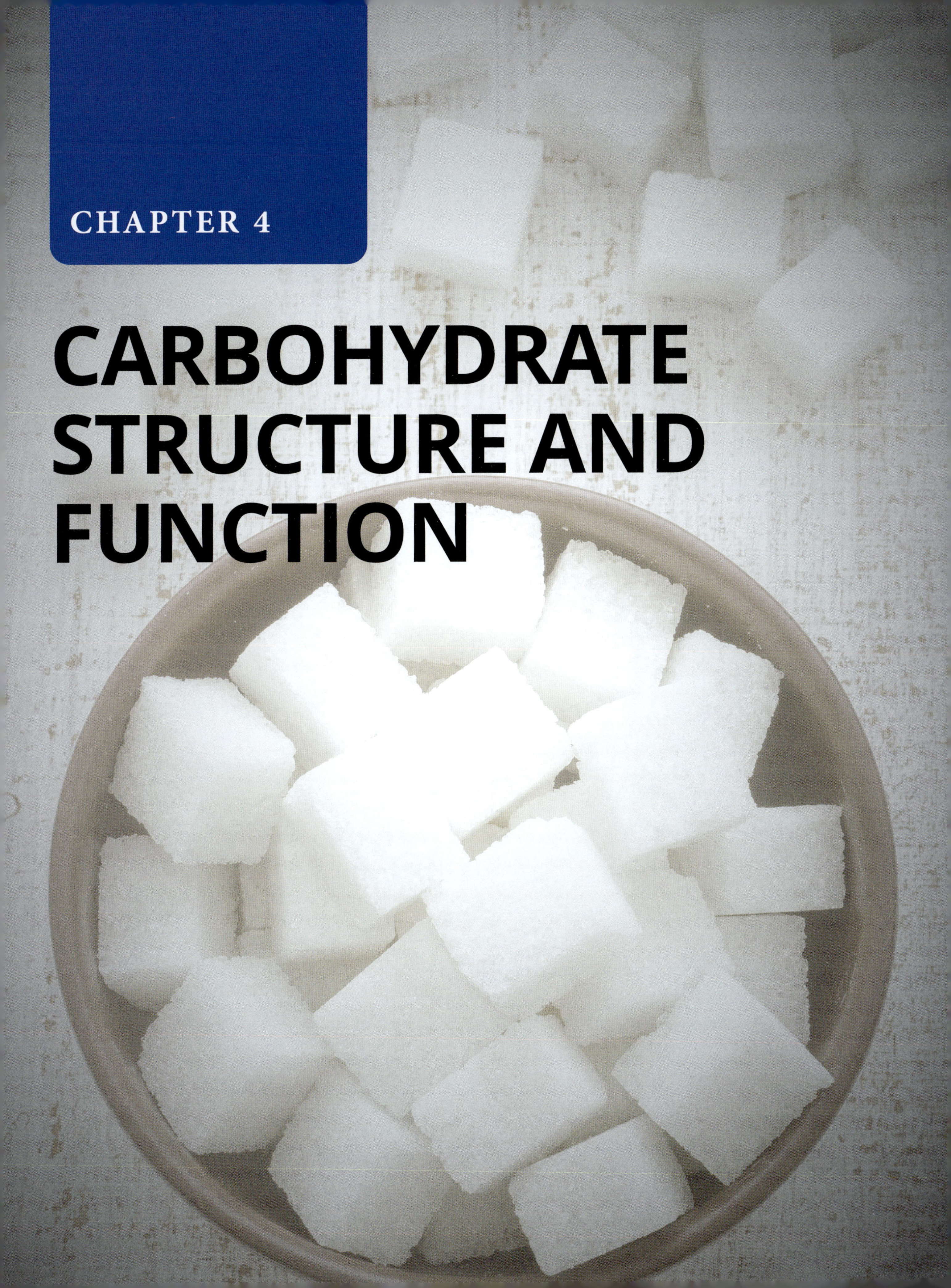

SCIENCE MASTERY ASSESSMENT

Every pre-med knows this feeling: there is so much content I have to know for the MCAT! How do I know what to do first or what's important?

While the high-yield badges throughout this book will help you identify the most important topics, this Science Mastery Assessment is another tool in your MCAT prep arsenal. This quiz (which can also be taken in your online resources) and the guidance below will help ensure that you are spending the appropriate amount of time on this chapter based on your personal strengths and weaknesses. Don't worry though—skipping something now does not mean you'll never study it. Later on in your prep, as you complete full-length tests, you'll uncover specific pieces of content that you need to review and can come back to these chapters as appropriate.

How to Use This Assessment

If you answer 0–7 questions correctly:

Spend about 1 hour to read this chapter in full and take limited notes throughout. Follow up by reviewing **all** quiz questions to ensure that you now understand how to solve each one.

If you answer 8–11 questions correctly:

Spend 20–40 minutes reviewing the quiz questions. Beginning with the questions you missed, read and take notes on the corresponding subchapters. For questions you answered correctly, ensure your thinking matches that of the explanation and you understand why each choice was correct or incorrect.

If you answer 12–15 questions correctly:

Spend less than 20 minutes reviewing all questions from the quiz. If you missed any, then include a quick read-through of the corresponding subchapters, or even just the relevant content within a subchapter, as part of your question review. For questions you got correct, ensure your thinking matches that of the explanation and review the Concept Summary at the end of the chapter.

1. When glucose is in a straight-chain formation, it:
   - **A.** is an aldoketose.
   - **B.** is a pentose.
   - **C.** has five chiral carbons.
   - **D.** is one of a group of 16 stereoisomers.

2. All of the following are true of epimers EXCEPT:
   - **A.** they differ in configuration about only one carbon.
   - **B.** they usually have slightly different chemical and physical properties.
   - **C.** they are diastereomers (with the exception of glyceraldehyde).
   - **D.** they have equal but opposite optical activities.

3. Aldonic acids are compounds that:
   - **A.** can be oxidized, and therefore act as reducing agents.
   - **B.** can be reduced, and therefore act as reducing agents.
   - **C.** have been oxidized, and have acted as reducing agents.
   - **D.** have been oxidized, and have acted as oxidizing agents.

4. The formation of α-D-glucopyranose from β-D-glucopyranose is called:
   - **A.** glycosidation.
   - **B.** mutarotation.
   - **C.** enantiomerization.
   - **D.** racemization.

5. Ketose sugars may have the ability to act as reducing sugars. Which process explains this?
   - **A.** Ketose sugars undergo tautomerization.
   - **B.** The ketone group is oxidized directly.
   - **C.** Ketose sugars undergo anomerization.
   - **D.** The ketone group is reduced directly.

6. What is the product of the following reaction?

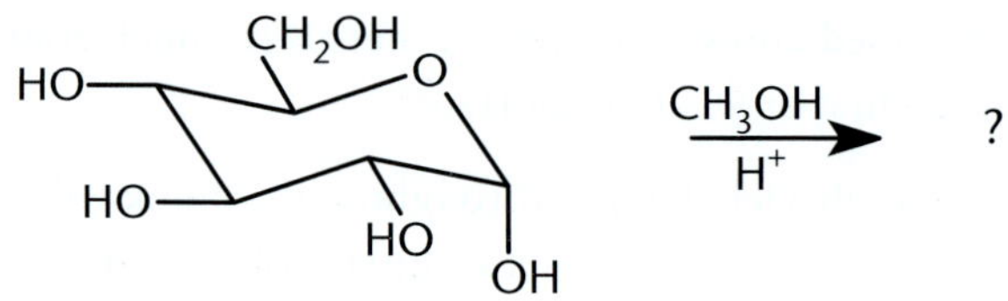

A.

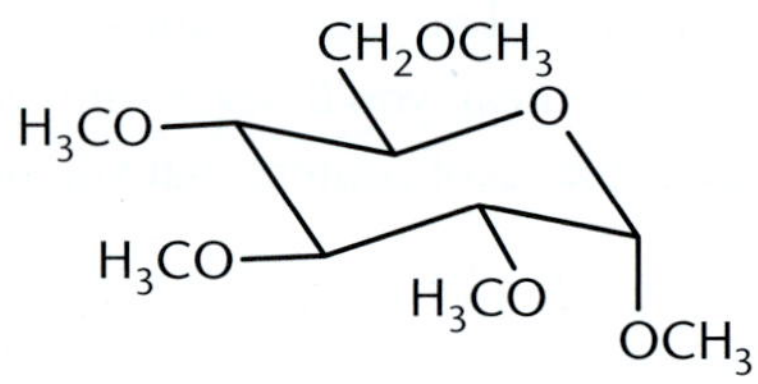

B.

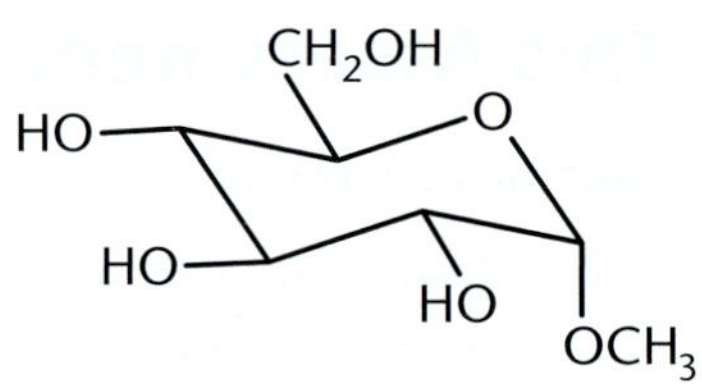

C.

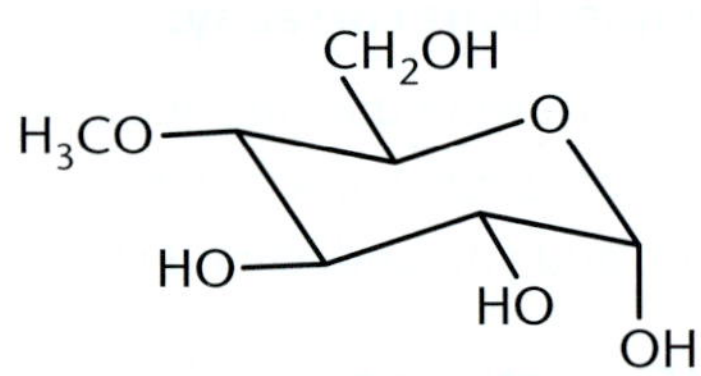

D.

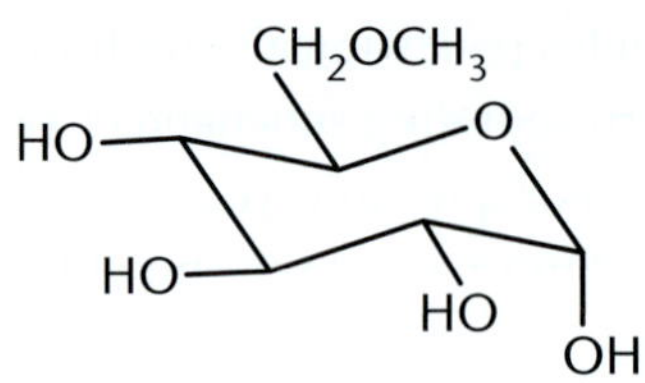

7. Which of the following enzymes cleaves polysaccharide chains and yields maltose exclusively?
   - **A.** α-Amylase
   - **B.** β-Amylase
   - **C.** Debranching enzyme
   - **D.** Glycogen phosphorylase

8. When the following straight-chain Fischer projection is converted to a chair or ring conformation, its structure will be:

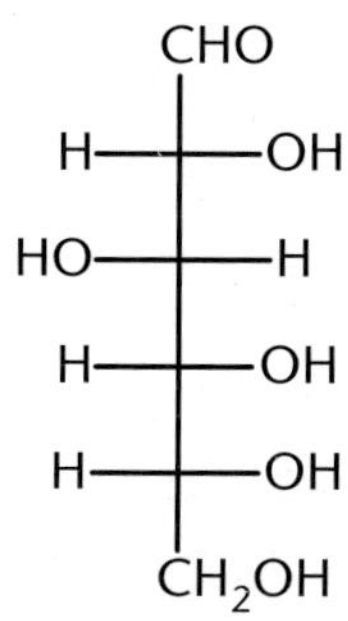

A.

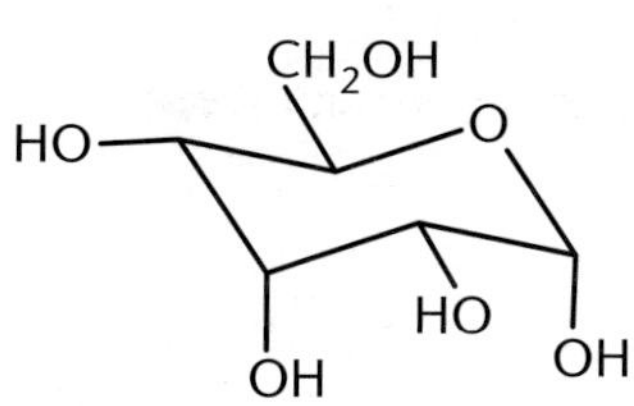

B.

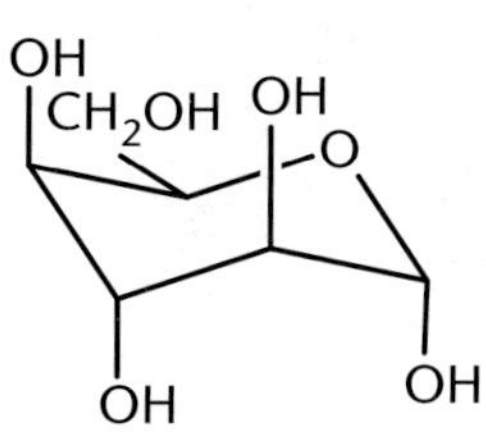

C.

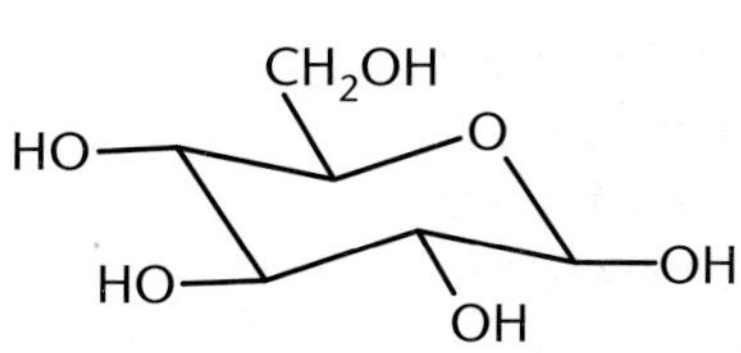

D.

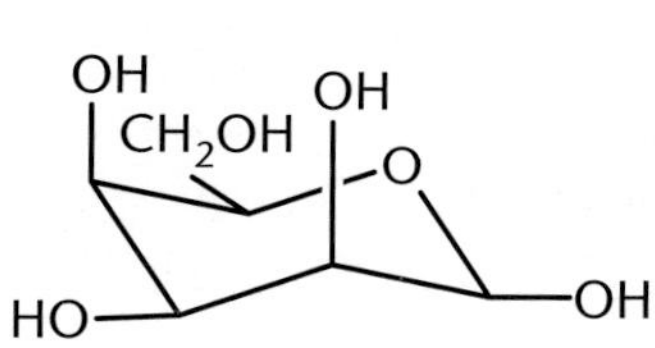

9. Why is the α-anomer of D-glucose less likely to form than the β-anomer?
   - **A.** The β-anomer is preferred for metabolism.
   - **B.** The β-anomer undergoes less electron repulsion.
   - **C.** The α-anomer is the more stable anomer.
   - **D.** The α-anomer forms more in L-glucose.

10. Which two polysaccharides share all of their glycosidic linkage types in common?
    - **A.** Cellulose and amylopectin
    - **B.** Amylose and glycogen
    - **C.** Amylose and cellulose
    - **D.** Glycogen and amylopectin

11. Which of the following is digestible by humans and is made up of only one type of monosaccharide?
    - **A.** Lactose
    - **B.** Sucrose
    - **C.** Maltose
    - **D.** Cellobiose

12. The reaction below is an example of one step in:

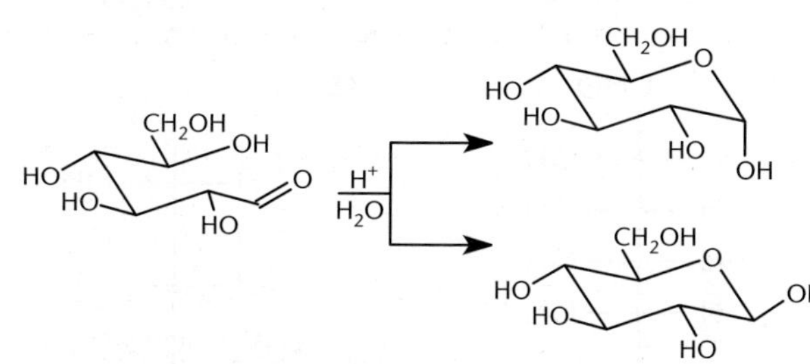

   - **A.** aldehyde formation.
   - **B.** hemiketal formation.
   - **C.** mutarotation.
   - **D.** glycosidic bond cleavage.

13. Galactose is the C-4 epimer of glucose, the structure of which is shown below. Which of the following structures is galactose?

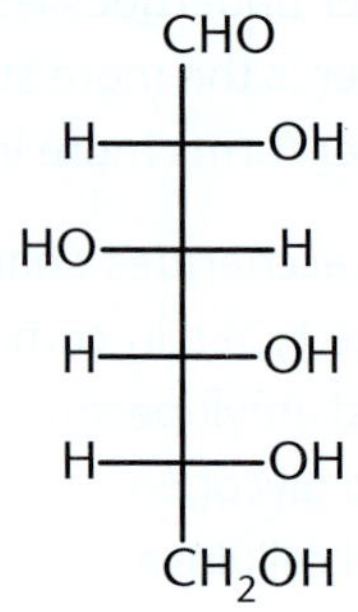

D-glucose

A.

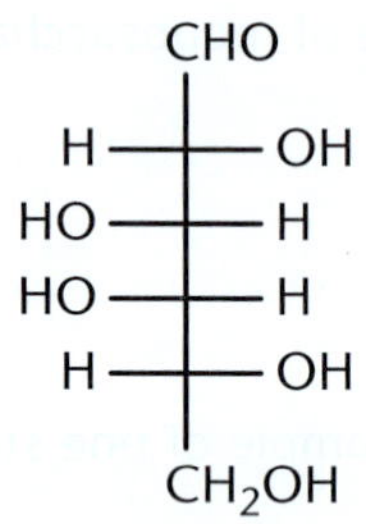

B.

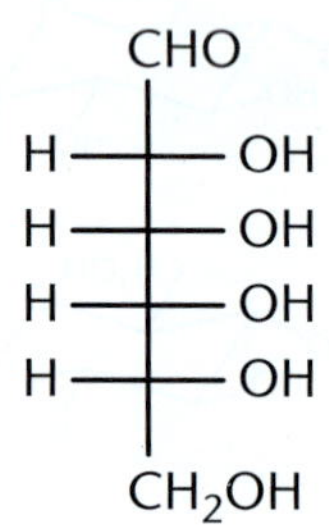

C.

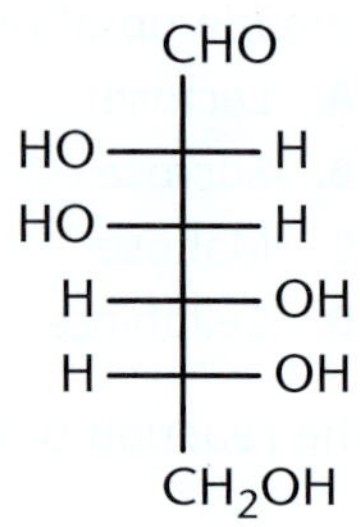

D.

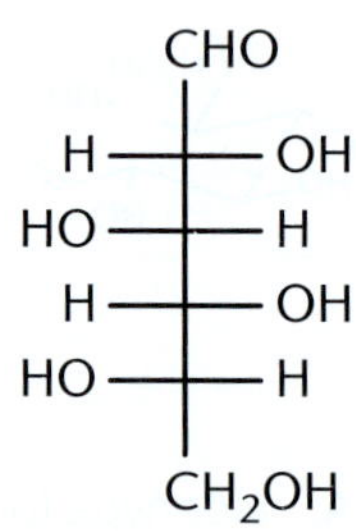

14. Andersen's disease (glycogen storage disease type IV) is a condition characterized by a deficiency in glycogen branching enzyme. Absence of this enzyme would be likely to cause all of the following effects EXCEPT:

A. decreased glycogen solubility in human cells.
B. slower action of glycogen phosphorylase.
C. less storage of glucose in the body.
D. glycogen devoid of α-1,4 linkages.

15. The cyclic forms of monosaccharides are:

I. hemiacetals.
II. hemiketals.
III. acetals.

A. I only
B. III only
C. I and II only
D. I, II, and III

Answer Key follows on next page.

Answer Key

1. **D** (See section 4.1)
2. **D** (See section 4.1)
3. **C** (See section 4.3)
4. **B** (See section 4.2)
5. **A** (See section 4.3)
6. **B** (See section 4.3)
7. **B** (See section 4.4)
8. **C** (See section 4.2)
9. **B** (See section 4.2)
10. **D** (See section 4.4)
11. **C** (See section 4.4)
12. **C** (See section 4.2)
13. **A** (See section 4.1)
14. **D** (See section 4.4)
15. **C** (See section 4.2)

The relevant section of the chapter to review for each question is given in parentheses after the correct answer. Detailed explanations can be found at the end of the chapter

CHAPTER 4

CARBOHYDRATE STRUCTURE AND FUNCTION

In This Chapter

CHAPTER PROFILE

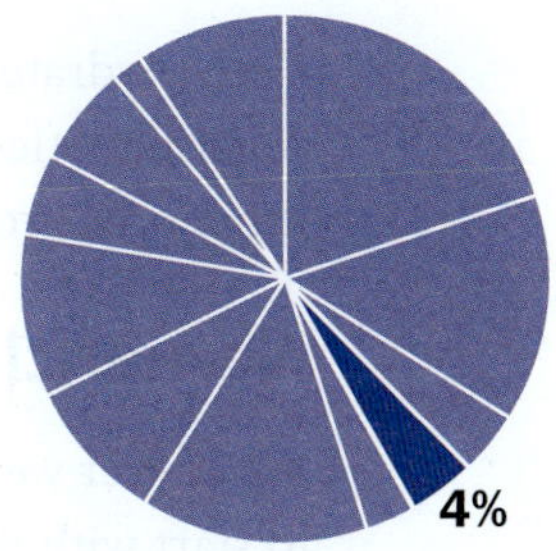

The content in this chapter should be relevant to about 4% of all questions about biochemistry on the MCAT.

This chapter covers material from the following AAMC content categories:

1D: Principles of bioenergetics and fuel molecule metabolism

5D: Structure, function, and reactivity of biologically-relevant molecules

Introduction

Carbohydrates (or, as they are known colloquially, *carbs*) have experienced a tumultuous few decades in American culinary culture. Remember the food pyramid, which advised that we consume 6 to 11 servings of carbohydrates—in the form of bread, cereal, rice, and pasta—per day? Nowadays, we're inundated with recommendations to cut down or even cut out carbs; still, carbohydrates make up most of the food and drink that continues to fill our refrigerators and cupboards. Whether or not this is healthy is debatable, as research on food choices continues. What is certain, however, is that carbohydrates are the most direct source of chemical energy for almost all organisms, ranging from single-celled protozoa to more complex organisms, such as plants and animals—including people.

From a molecular standpoint, carbohydrates used to be defined by the empirical formula $C_n(H_2O)_n$, but this definition is now considered antiquated. This formula only applies to simple monomeric sugars, which are also called monosaccharides. As simple sugars link to form complex sugars, water loss occurs, thus changing the empirical formula to $C_n(H_2O)_m$ for complex sugars.

In this chapter, we'll discuss how the various types of carbohydrates we utilize for metabolism are classified, the structures in which they exist, and the biochemical reactions they undergo.

4.1 Carbohydrate Classification

High Yield

LEARNING OBJECTIVES

After Chapter 4.1, you will be able to:

- Recognize common features of sugar nomenclature
- Apply principles of stereoisomerism to sugar nomenclature and structure
- Distinguish enantiomers from epimers
- Classify and name a simple sugar based on its structure

Carbohydrates come in many types. They can be classified by the number of sugar moieties that make them up, the number of carbons in each sugar, the functional groups present on the molecule, and the stereochemistry of the sugar.

MCAT EXPERTISE

The MCAT likes to present complex, novel molecules and then test you on the most basic information about them. Therefore, when dealing with carbohydrates on the exam, look for the functional groups we have seen before (aldehydes, ketones, and alcohols) and realize that they retain the same chemical properties that you already know.

Nomenclature

Whenever we discuss carbohydrates (or anything else in biology), it makes sense to start with the most basic structural units, which are **monosaccharides**. The simplest monosaccharides contain three carbon atoms and are called **trioses**. Carbohydrates with four, five, and six carbon atoms are called **tetroses**, **pentoses**, and **hexoses**, respectively. Carbohydrates that contain an aldehyde group as their most oxidized functional group are called **aldoses** and those with a ketone group as their most oxidized functional group are called **ketoses**. Taken together, a six-carbon sugar with an aldehyde group would be called an *aldohexose*, while a five-carbon sugar with a ketone group would be called a *ketopentose*. The basic structure of a monosaccharide is illustrated by the simple sugar ***glyceraldehyde***, which is an aldose as shown in Figure 4.1.

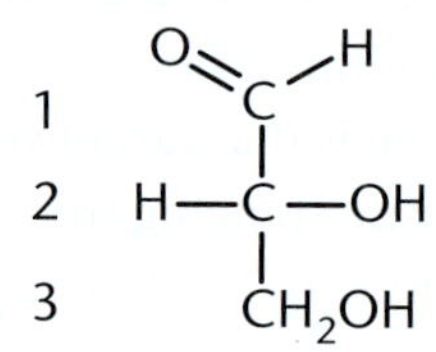

Figure 4.1 Glyceraldehyde
The simplest aldose (an aldotriose)

Glyceraldehyde is a polyhydroxylated aldehyde, or as described above, an aldose (aldehyde sugar). The numbering of carbon atoms in a monosaccharide follows the rules described in Chapter 1 of *MCAT Organic Chemistry Review*. The carbonyl carbon is the most oxidized, and therefore will always have the lowest possible number. In an aldose, the aldehyde carbon will always be carbon number one (C-1). The aldehyde carbon can participate in **glycosidic linkages**; sugars acting as substituents via this linkage are called *glycosyl* residues.

The simplest ketone sugar (ketose) is ***dihydroxyacetone***, shown in Figure 4.2. Again, the carbonyl carbon is the most oxidized; in this case, the lowest number it can be assigned is carbon number two (C-2). This is true, in fact, for most ketoses on the MCAT: the carbonyl carbon is C-2. Ketoses can also participate in glycosidic bonds at this carbon. Notice that on every monosaccharide, every carbon *other* than the carbonyl carbon will carry a hydroxyl group.

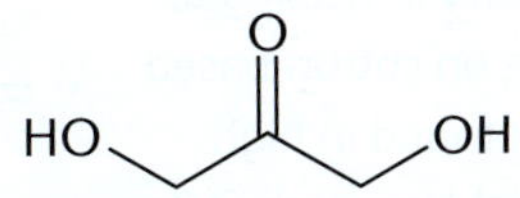

Figure 4.2 Dihydroxyacetone
The simplest ketose (a ketotriose)

Common Names

On the MCAT, a few sugars are tested by referencing their common names, or names that do not necessarily follow the nomenclature rules listed above. You should be familiar with the names of the important monosaccharides listed in Figure 4.3.

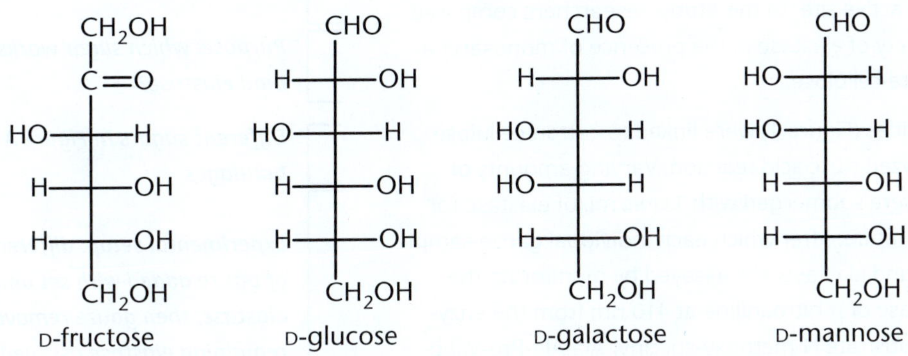

Figure 4.3 Common Names of Frequently Tested Sugars on the MCAT

BIOCHEMISTRY GUIDED EXAMPLE WITH EXPERT THINKING

Carbohydrate-based wound dressings have received increased attention in recent years for their occlusive and functionally interactive properties.

Topic: sugar-based bandages

They afford bacterial and odor protection, fluid balance, and elasticity. However, since all modern dressings had the same efficacy in healing as saline or paraffin gauze, there is opportunity to improve on cotton-based dressings.

Details about advantages, but want to make better

Proteases like human neutrophil elastase are found in high concentration in chronic wounds, which create considerable growth factor and extracellular matrix protein destruction, preventing the wound from healing.

Background about negative effects of elastase in wounds

Wound dressings that selectively sequester elastase from chronic wounds are built on the concept that the properties of the protease can be used to tailor the molecular design of the wound dressing.

We're interested in designing the sugar-based bandages to grab elastase

Elastase is a glycoprotein and contains a significant carbohydrate portion shown to be glycosamine-based. There is potential for carbohydrate–carbohydrate interactions between the protein and a monosaccharide conjugated to cellulose dressing. There may be additional carbohydrate–protein interactions through the active site.

Reasons why the researchers think that sugar-base bandages will work to bind elastase

In this study, researchers compared the preparation and activity of elastase in the presence of monosaccharides conjugated to citrate-cellulose.

Purpose: which sugar works best to bind elastase?

A series of monosaccharides (Figure 1) were linked to cotton-cellulose gauze with an acid-catalyzed citric acid reaction.

Different sugars in Figure A linked to bandages

Varying amounts of treated gauze samples were submerged with 1 unit/mL of elastase for one hour at room temperature, after which each individual gauze sample was removed. Any unbound elastase was assayed by monitoring the spectrophotometric release of p-nitroaniline at 410 nm from the enzymatic hydrolysis of the substrate N-methoxy-succinyl-Ala-Ala-Pro-Val-p-nitroanilide. The initial activity of remaining elastase for each monosaccharide at specific amounts of treated gauze was plotted below (Figure 2).

Experimental setup: different amounts of gauze added with set amount of elastase, then gauze removed; the remaining elastase assayed using spectrometry

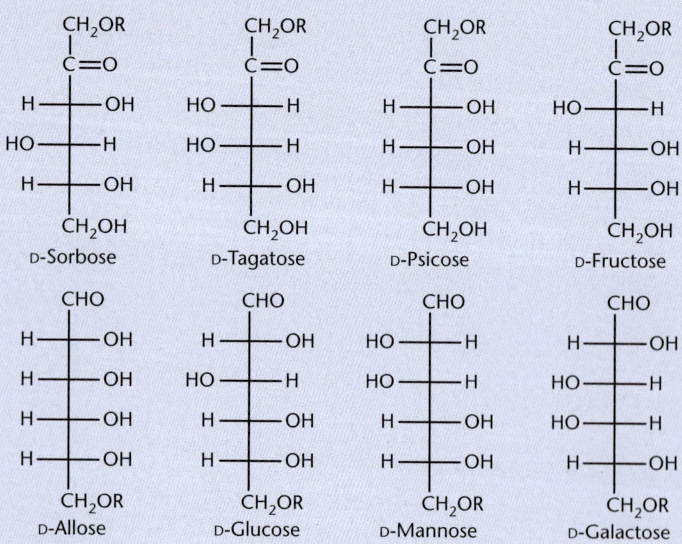

Figure 1

Sugar molecules—come back to this diagram if needed

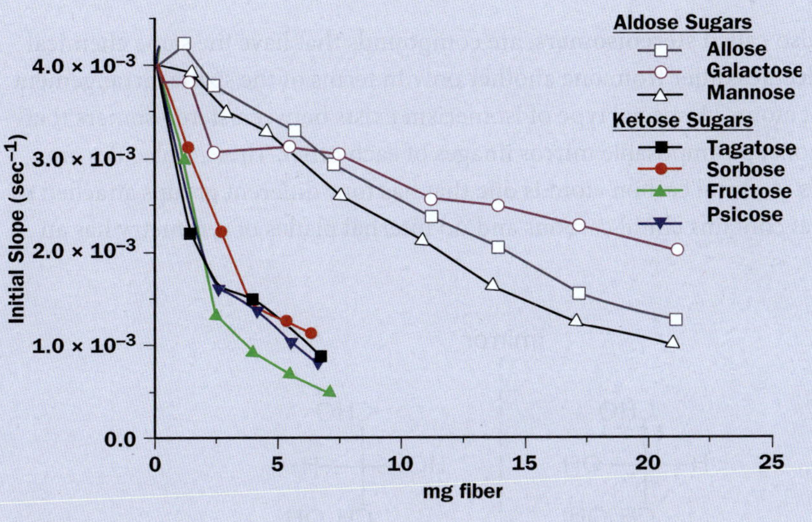

IVs: amount of gauze, type of sugar

DV: slope, which corresponds to initial elastase activity

Trend: galactose, allose, mannose have less steep lines compared to sorbose, tagalose, psicose, fructose

Figure 2

Adapted from Edwards, J. V., & Caston-Pierre, S. (2013). Citrate-linked keto- and aldo-hexose monosaccharide cellulose conjugates demonstrate selective human neutrophil elastase-lowering activity in cotton dressings. *Journal of Functional Biomaterials*, 4(2), 59-73. doi:10.3390/jfb4020059.

According to the data, which class of monosaccharide should be used in gauze to help prevent elastase-mediated wound damage?

The question asks us to select a type of monosaccharide to prevent elastase from doing damage, which means that it's important to understand the purpose of the passage and what the data tells us. The first paragraph describes how advantageous bandages currently are, but that researchers are interested in improving them by selectively binding proteases that prevent healing, like elastase.

Let's take a look at the experimental setup in paragraph 2. Since the sugar-linked bandages are soaked in a solution with elastase and then removed, the assumption is that the better the sugar binds elastase, the less elastase there is left over in the solution when the researchers assay it, after the bandage is removed. Therefore, the better the binding, the less activity there should be. The figure clearly has two sets of lines: galactose/allose/mannose have activity over a larger amount of fiber used, and, based on Figure 1, all three of these sugars are aldohexoses, which are sugars with an aldehyde at the C-1 position. Sorbose/tagatose/psicose/fructose, however, quickly drop in activity with increasing amounts of fiber, and, based on Figure 1, all four of these sugars are ketohexoses, which are sugars with a ketone at the C-2 position. To make the comparison a bit more clear, let's consider the activity for each set at 5 mg of fiber—ketohexoses have $\sim 1.5 \times 10^{-3}$ slope, and aldohexoses have $\sim 3.3 \times 10^{-3}$ slope. Since slope corresponds to activity, less activity is seen for ketohexoses with equivalent amounts of carbohydrate-bound bandage, therefore corresponding to more elastase binding.

Therefore, we can conclude that the researchers should investigate the usage of ketohexoses to help prevent elastase-mediated wound damage, since this class of sugar seems to bind elastase better than aldohexoses.

Stereochemistry

BRIDGE

Isomerism is discussed in detail in Chapter 2 of *MCAT Organic Chemistry Review.* The isomerism seen in carbohydrates is just an extension of that conversation; many sugars are related to each other as enantiomers or diastereomers.

Optical isomers, also called **stereoisomers**, are compounds that have the same chemical formula; these molecules differ from one another only in terms of the spatial arrangement of their component atoms. A special type of isomerism exists between stereoisomers that are nonidentical, nonsuperimposable mirror images of each other. These molecules are called **enantiomers**. A chiral carbon atom is one that has four different groups attached to it; any molecule that contains chiral carbons and no internal planes of symmetry has an enantiomer.

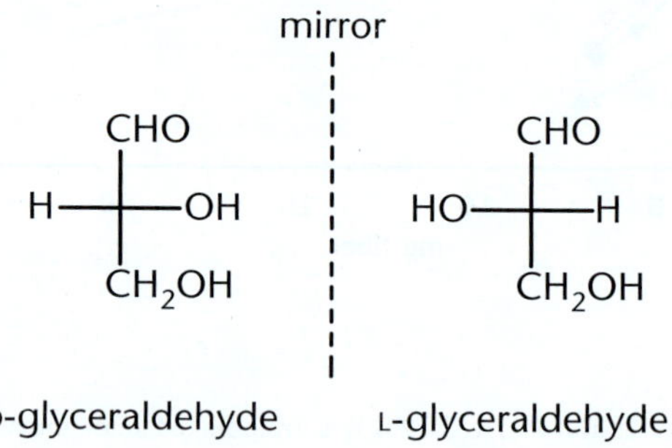

Figure 4.4 Enantiomers of Glyceraldehyde

KEY CONCEPT

The two systems for naming chiral carbons are not interchangeable! While some D-isomers are equivalent with (*R*), others are (*S*). When dealing with biomolecules like sugars, anticipate using the biochemists' method of nomenclature: D and L.

Figure 4.4 illustrates the two enantiomers of glyceraldehyde: D- and L-glyceraldehyde. The particular three-dimensional arrangement of the groups attached to the chiral carbon determines the compound's **absolute configuration**. While organic chemists use the newer (*R*) and (*S*) system when denoting absolute configuration, biochemists use the older D and L system. Notice in the figure above that D-glyceraldehyde and L-glyceraldehyde are mirror images of one another—this makes them enantiomers because they *must* have opposite absolute configurations. Because there is only one chiral carbon present, these are the only two stereoisomers that exist for glyceraldehyde. As the number of chiral carbons increases, so too does the number of possible stereoisomers because one compound may have many diastereomers. The number of possible stereoisomers of a compound can be calculated by:

KEY CONCEPT

When trying to figure out how many possible stereoisomers can exist for a multi-carbon compound, identify the number of chiral carbons (n) and plug into the formula 2^n. For example, $2^1 = 2$ stereoisomers and $2^2 = 4$ stereoisomers.

$$\text{Number of stereoisomers with common backbone} = 2^n$$

Equation 4.1

where n is the number of chiral carbons in the molecule.

Early in the twentieth century, scientists used glyceraldehyde to learn about the optical rotation of sugars. The results of this early study led to the **D** and **L** naming convention. D-Glyceraldehyde was later determined to exhibit a positive rotation (designated as D-(+)-glyceraldehyde), and L-glyceraldehyde a negative rotation (designated as L-(−)-glyceraldehyde). Note that the direction of rotation, (+) or (−), must be determined experimentally and cannot be determined from the D or L designation for the sugar.

KEY CONCEPT

D and L are based on the stereochemistry of glyceraldehyde. These are NOT directly related to the (+) and (−) designations denoting optical rotation.

On the MCAT, all monosaccharides are assigned the D or L configuration based on their relationship to glyceraldehyde. The **Fischer projection** is a simple two-dimensional drawing of stereoisomers. Recall that in a Fischer projection, the horizontal lines are wedges (out of the page), while vertical lines are dashes (into the page), as shown in Figure 4.5.

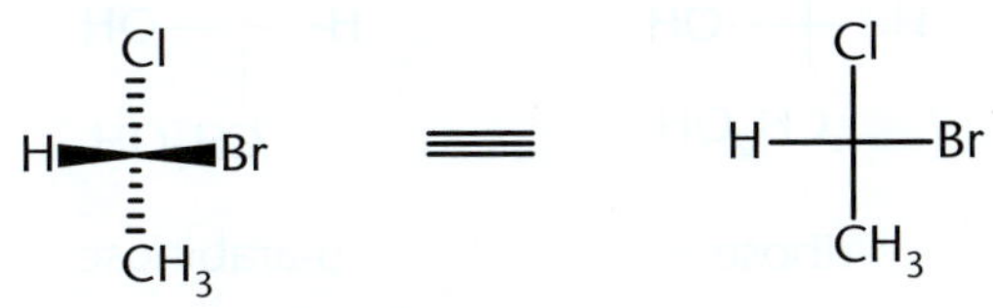

Figure 4.5 Fisher Projection
Horizontal lines are wedges (out of the page); vertical lines are dashes (into the page).

Fischer projections allow scientists to identify different enantiomers. Using this system of structural representation, all D-sugars have the hydroxide of their highest-numbered chiral center on the right, and all L-sugars have that hydroxide on the left. Because D-glucose and L-glucose are enantiomers, this means that *every* chiral center in D-glucose has the opposite configuration of L-glucose, as shown in Figure 4.6.

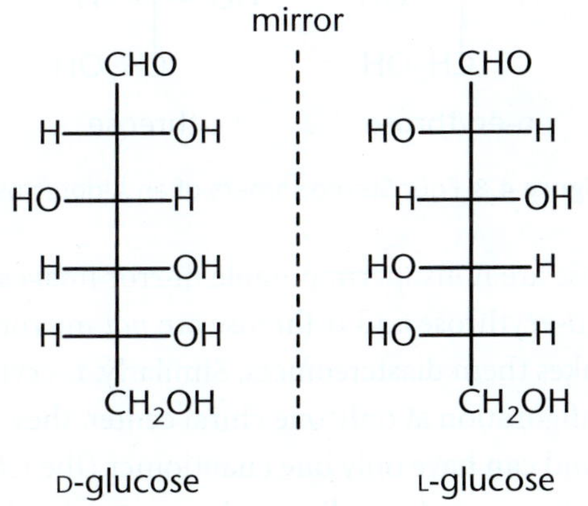

Figure 4.6 Enantiomers of Glucose

Make sure that you are familiar with these three types of stereoisomers:

1. The same sugars, in different optical families, are **enantiomers** (such as D-glucose and L-glucose).
2. Two sugars that are in the same family (both are either ketoses or aldoses, and have the same number of carbons) that are not identical and are not mirror images of each other are **diastereomers**.
3. A special subtype of diastereomers are those that differ in configuration at exactly one chiral center. These are defined as **epimers** (such as D-*ribose* and D-*arabinose*, which only differ at C-2, as shown in Figure 4.7).

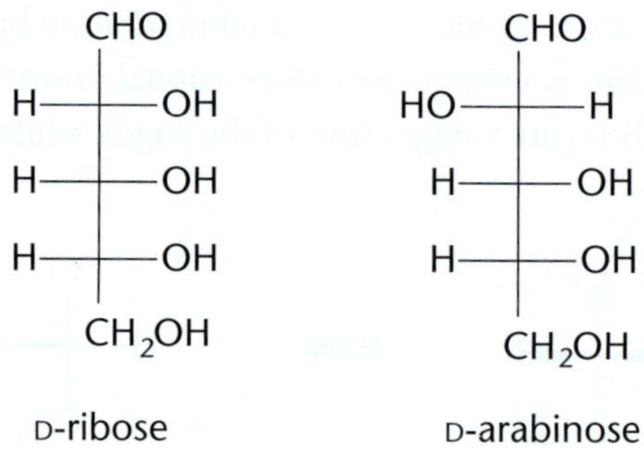

Figure 4.7 D-Ribose and D-Arabinose Are C-2 Epimers

A summary of these different types of isomers is provided in Figure 4.8, which shows four different stereoisomers of an aldotetrose, including two optical forms of *erythrose* and two optical forms of *threose*.

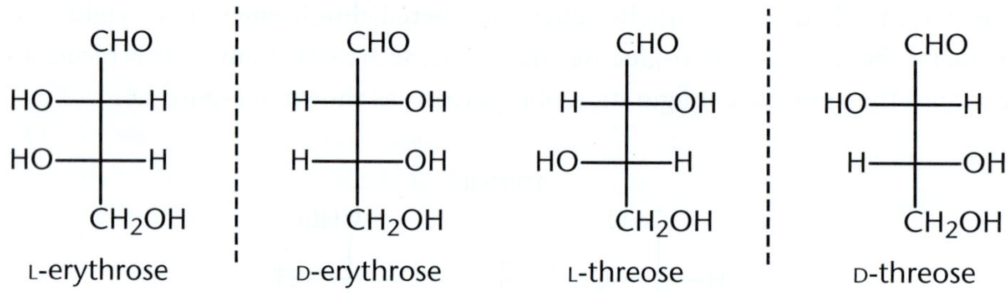

Figure 4.8 Four Stereoisomers of an Aldotetrose

Because D-erythrose and L-erythrose are nonsuperimposable mirror images of one another, they are enantiomers. On the other hand, while D-erythrose and D-threose are *not* mirror images of one another, they are still nonsuperimposable, which makes them diastereomers. Similarly, L-erythrose and D-threose are diastereomers. Because they differ in configuration at only one chiral center, they can also be defined as epimers of one another. Remember, a compound can have only one enantiomer (the left hand to its right hand, or vice versa), but may have multiple diastereomers, depending on how many (and which) chiral carbons are inverted between the two molecules.

MCAT CONCEPT CHECK 4.1

Before you move on, assess your understanding of the material with these questions.

1. What is the name for a five-carbon sugar with an aldehyde group? A six-carbon sugar with a ketone group?

____

2. Draw all of the possible D-stereoisomers of glucose in Fischer projection form.

3. Which of the diastereomers of glucose from the previous question are considered to be epimers of glucose? Enantiomers?

   - Epimers:

____

   - Enantiomers:

____

4.2 Cyclic Sugar Molecules

LEARNING OBJECTIVES

After Chapter 4.2, you will be able to:

- Convert between Haworth and Fischer projections
- Define and explain sugar-related concepts, including hemiacetal, hemiketal, pyranose, furanose, and anomeric carbon
- Predict the impact of mutarotation on conformation
- Identify the more stable anomer of a given sugar:

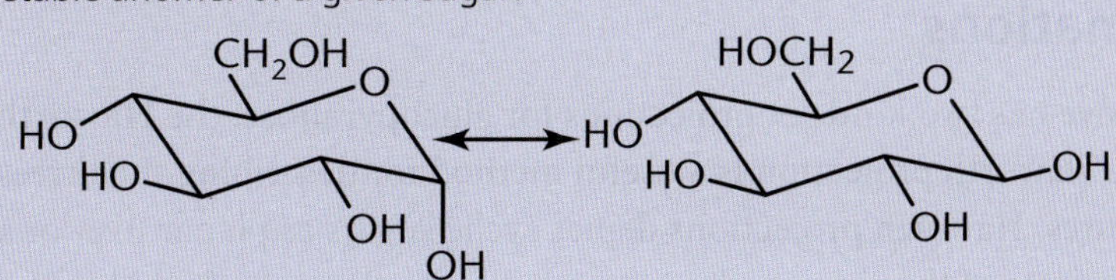

Monosaccharides contain both a hydroxyl group, which can serve as a nucleophile, and a carbonyl group, which is the most common electrophile on the MCAT. Therefore, they can undergo intramolecular reactions to form cyclic **hemiacetals** (from aldoses) and **hemiketals** (from ketoses). Due to ring strain, the only cyclic molecules that are stable in solution are six-membered **pyranose** rings or five-membered **furanose** rings. In fact, such sugars tend to exist predominantly in cyclic form. The hydroxyl group acts as the nucleophile during ring formation, so oxygen becomes a member of the ring structure. Regardless of whether hemiacetal or hemiketal is formed, the carbonyl carbon becomes chiral in this process, and is referred to as the **anomeric carbon**. Figure 4.9 demonstrates how the carbonyl containing C-1 and the hydroxyl group on C-5 of D-glucose undergo intramolecular hemiacetal formation. One of two ring forms can emerge during cyclization of a sugar molecule: α or β. Because these two molecules differ at the anomeric carbon, they are termed **anomers** of one another. In glucose, the **α-anomer** has the $-OH$ group of C-1 *trans* to the $-CH_2OH$ substituent (axial and down), whereas the **β-anomer** has the $-OH$ group of C-1 *cis* to the $-CH_2OH$ substituent (equatorial and up).

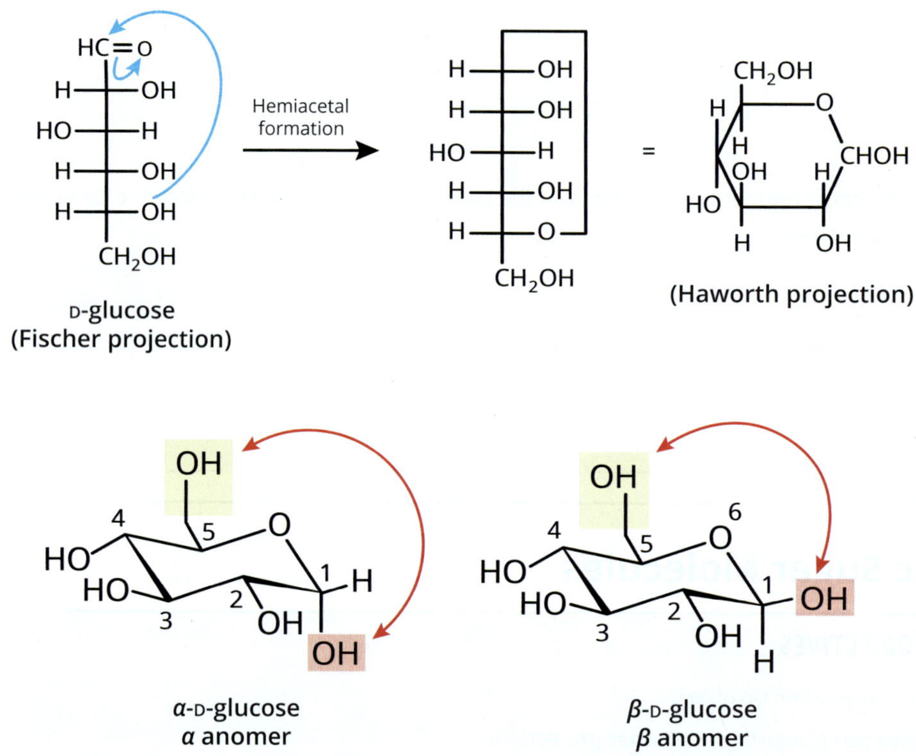

Figure 4.9 Cyclic Sugar Formation via Intramolecular Nucleophilic Addition
Glucose forms a six-membered ring with two anomeric forms: α (left) and β (right).

Hexose Conformations

Note how Figure 4.9 above has two kinds of projections for glucopyranose: the **Haworth projection** and the **Fischer projection**. The Haworth projection is a useful method for describing the three-dimensional conformations of cyclic structures. Haworth projections depict cyclic sugars as planar five- or six-membered rings with the top and bottom faces of the ring nearly perpendicular to the page. In reality the five-membered rings are very close to planar, but the pyranose rings adopt a chair-like configuration, and the substituents assume axial or equatorial positions to minimize steric hindrance. When we convert the monosaccharide from its straight-chain Fischer projection to the Haworth projection, any group on the right in the Fischer projection will point down.

Mutarotation

Exposing hemiacetal rings to water will cause them to spontaneously cycle between the open and closed form. Because the substituents on the single bond between C-1 and C-2 can rotate freely, either the α- or β-anomer can be formed, as demonstrated in Figure 4.10. This spontaneous change of configuration about C-1 is known as **mutarotation**, and occurs more rapidly when the reaction is catalyzed with an acid or base. Mutarotation results in a mixture that contains both α- and β-anomers at equilibrium concentrations (for glucose: 36% α, 64% β). In solution, the α-anomeric configuration is less favored because the hydroxyl group of the anomeric carbon is axial, adding to the steric strain of the molecule. In its solid state (not in solution), this preference can be mitigated by the anomeric effect, which helps stabilize the α-anomer, although this is outside the scope of the MCAT.

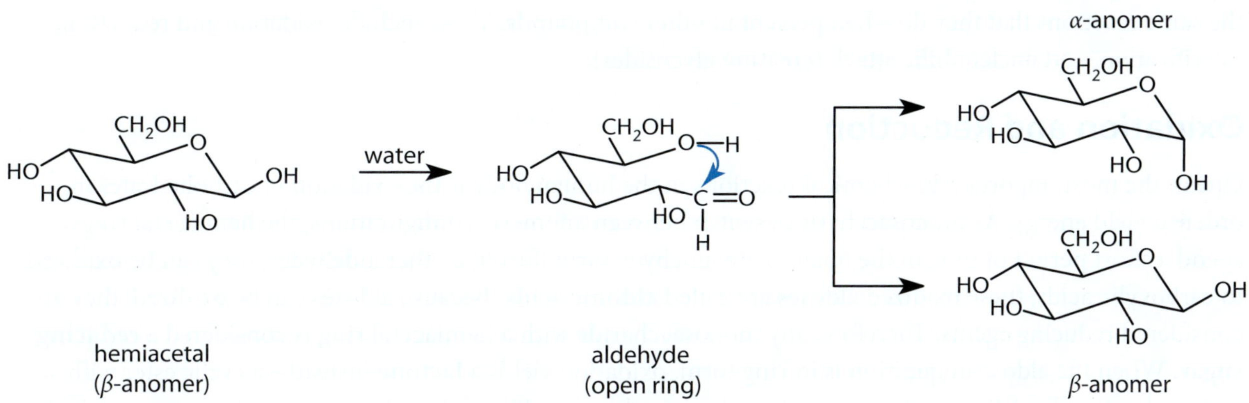

Figure 4.10 Mutarotation
Interconversion between the α- and β-anomers via ring opening and reclosing

MCAT CONCEPT CHECK 4.2

Before you move on, assess your understanding of the material with these questions.

1. Explain the relationship between the carbonyl carbon, anomeric carbon, and the alpha and beta forms of a sugar molecule.

2. Draw the less stable anomer of D-glucose in Haworth projection form.

3. Draw the less stable anomer of D-glucose in chair configuration.

4.3 Monosaccharides

LEARNING OBJECTIVES

After Chapter 4.3, you will be able to:

- Predict the products of sugar reactions, including oxidation, reduction, esterification, and glycosidic linkage formation
- Contrast Tollens' reagent and Benedict's reagent
- Apply reactions of sugars to biological contexts

Monosaccharides contain alcohols and either aldehydes or ketones. As such, these functional groups undergo the same reactions that they do when present in other compounds. These include oxidation and reduction, esterification, and nucleophilic attack (creating glycosides).

Oxidation and Reduction

One of the most important biochemical reactions in the human body is the oxidation of carbohydrates in order to yield energy. As monosaccharides switch between anomeric configurations, the hemiacetal rings spend a short period of time in the open-chain aldehyde form. Just like other aldehydes, they can be oxidized to carboxylic acids; these oxidized aldoses are called **aldonic acids**. Because aldoses can be oxidized, they are considered reducing agents. Therefore, any monosaccharide with a hemiacetal ring is considered a **reducing sugar**. When the aldose in question is in ring form, oxidation yields a **lactone** instead—a cyclic ester with a carbonyl group persisting on the anomeric carbon, as shown in Figure 4.11. Lactones, such as vitamin C, play an essential role in the human body.

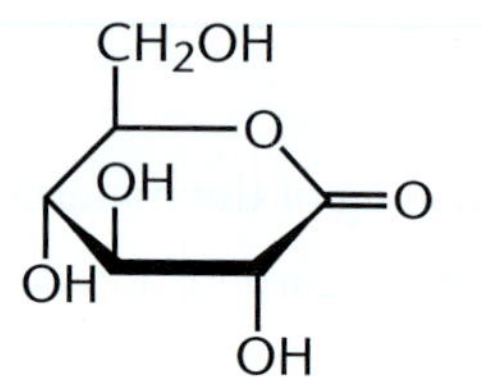

Figure 4.11 Lactone
Contains a cyclic ester

Two standard reagents are used to detect the presence of reducing sugars: Tollens' reagent and Benedict's reagent. **Tollens' reagent** must be freshly prepared, starting with silver nitrate ($AgNO_3$), which is mixed with NaOH to produce silver oxide (Ag_2O). Silver oxide is dissolved in ammonia to produce $[Ag(NH_3)_2]^+$, the actual Tollens' reagent. Tollens' reagent is reduced to produce a silvery mirror when aldehydes are present. When **Benedict's reagent** is used, the aldehyde group of an aldose is readily oxidized, indicated by a red precipitate of Cu_2O, as demonstrated in Figure 4.12. To test specifically for glucose, one may utilize the enzyme *glucose oxidase*, which does not react with other reducing sugars. A more powerful oxidizing agent, such as dilute nitric acid, will oxidize both the aldehyde and the primary alcohol (on C-6) to carboxylic acids.

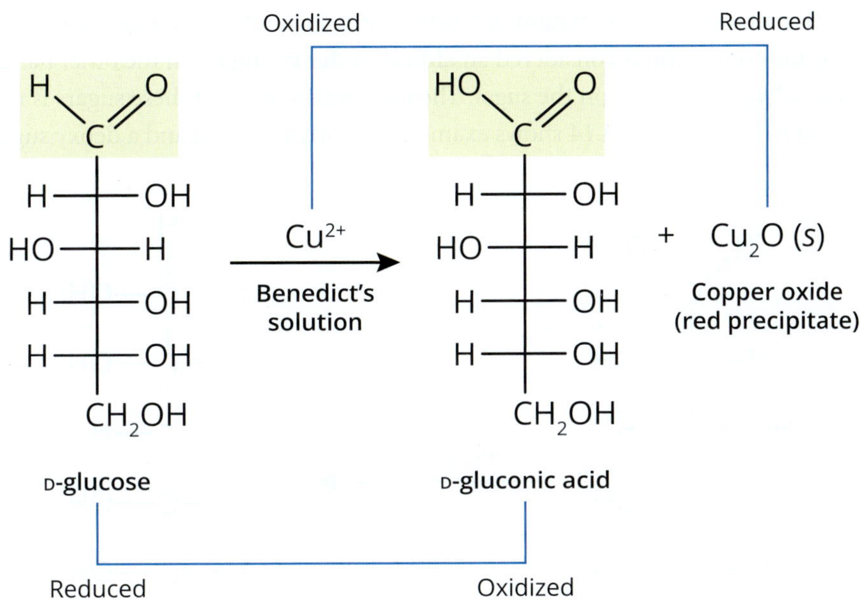

Figure 4.12 Positive Test for an Aldose Using Benedict's Reagent
Aldoses will react, forming copper(I) oxide; ketones may react more slowly.

An interesting phenomenon is that ketose sugars like fructose are also reducing sugars and give positive Tollens' and Benedict's tests. Although ketones cannot be oxidized directly to carboxylic acids, they can tautomerize to form aldoses under basic conditions, via *keto–enol* shifts. While in the aldose form, they can react with Tollens' or Benedict's reagents to form the carboxylic acid. **Tautomerization** refers to the rearrangement of bonds in a compound, usually by moving a hydrogen and forming a double bond. The tautomerization of fructose to glucose is shown in Figure 4.13. The ketone group picks up a hydrogen while the double bond is moved between two adjacent carbons, resulting in an **enol**: a compound with a double bond and an alcohol group. In this case, an enediol is the intermediate, which contains an alcohol on each of the two carbons. The enediol spontaneously rearranges to form glucose, an aldose.

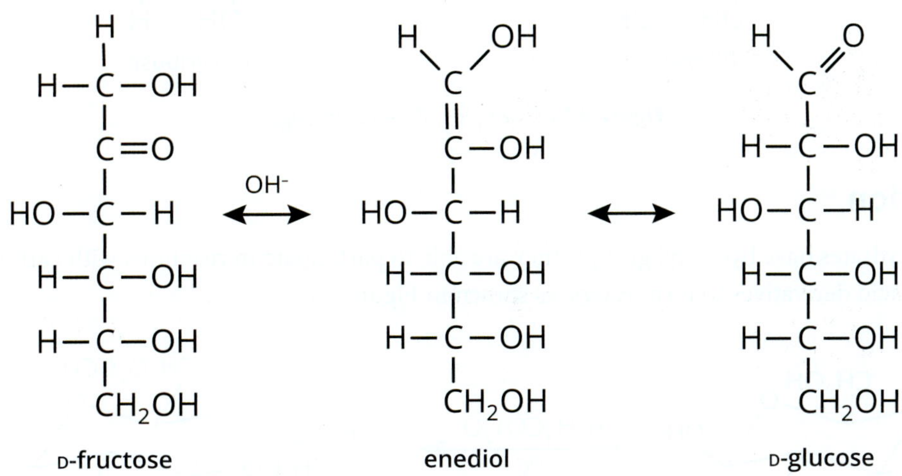

Figure 4.13 Tautomerization of Fructose to Glucose

Reduced sugars also play an essential role in human biochemistry. When the aldehyde group of an aldose is reduced to an alcohol, the compound is considered an **alditol**. A **deoxy sugar**, on the other hand, contains a hydrogen that replaces a hydroxyl group on the sugar. The most well-known of these sugars is D-2-deoxyribose, the carbohydrate found in DNA. Figure 4.14 shows examples of both an alditol and a deoxy sugar.

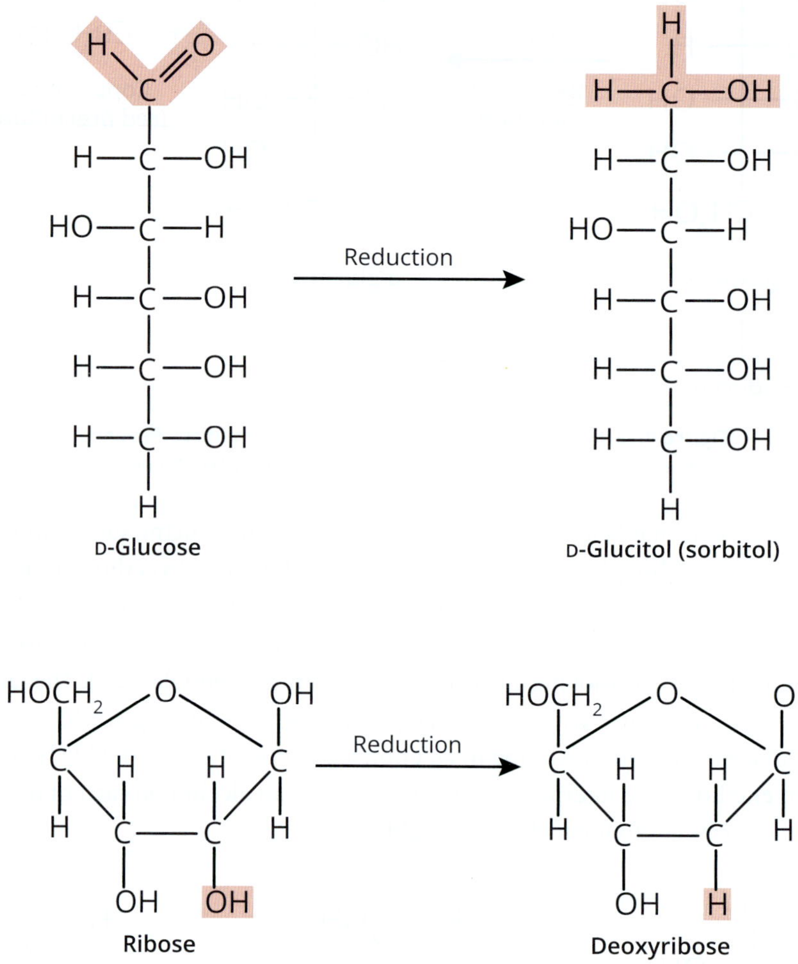

Figure 4.14 Examples of Reduced Sugars

Esterification

Because carbohydrates have hydroxyl groups, they are able to participate in reactions with carboxylic acids and carboxylic acid derivatives to form esters, as shown in Figure 4.15.

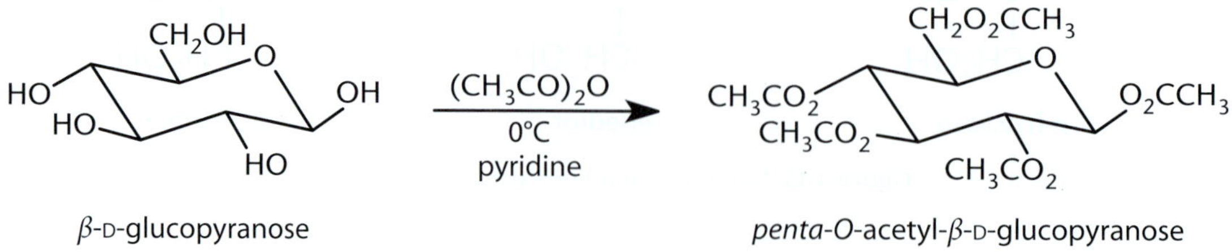

Figure 4.15 Esterification of Glucose
Acetic anhydride used as carboxylic acid derivative

In the body, esterification is very similar to the phosphorylation of glucose, in which a **phosphate ester** is formed. Phosphorylation of glucose is an extremely important metabolic reaction of glycolysis in which a phosphate group is transferred from ATP to glucose, thus phosphorylating glucose while forming ADP, as shown in Figure 4.16. *Hexokinase* (or *glucokinase*, in the liver and pancreatic β-islet cells) catalyzes this reaction.

BRIDGE

The action of hexokinase and glucokinase (as well as all the key glycolytic enzymes) is discussed in Chapter 9 of *MCAT Biochemistry Review*.

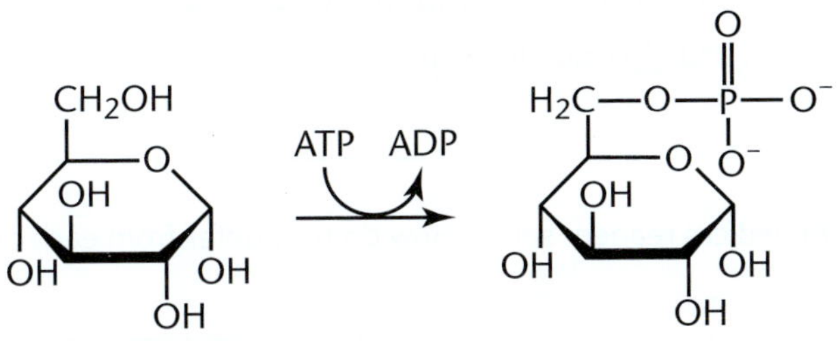

Figure 4.16 Phosphorylation of Glucose

Glycoside Formation

Hemiacetals are the anomeric carbons that result when sugars undergo intramolecular reactions. Hemiacetals can react with alcohols to form **acetals**. The anomeric hydroxyl group is transformed into an alkoxy group, yielding a mixture of α- and β-acetals (with water as a leaving group). The resulting carbon–oxygen (C—O) bonds are called **glycosidic bonds**, and the acetals formed are **glycosides**. An example is the reaction of glucose with ethanol shown in Figure 4.17. Equivalent reactions happen with hemiketals, forming ketals.

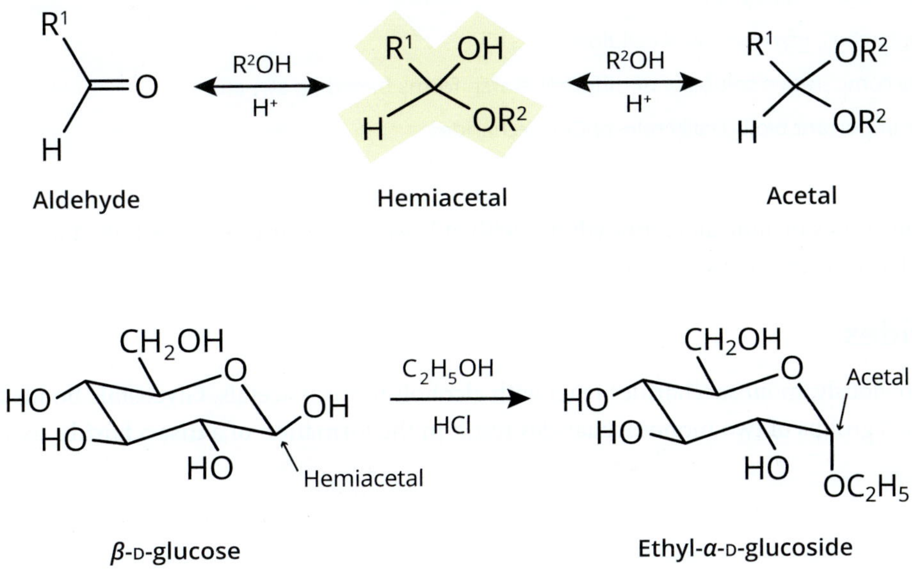

Figure 4.17 Glycosidic Linkage Formation
Hemiacetal (or hemiketal) sugars react with alcohols under acidic conditions to form acetals (or ketals).

Disaccharides and polysaccharides form as a result of glycosidic bonds between monosaccharides. Glycosides derived from furanose rings are referred to as **furanosides** and those derived from pyranose rings are called **pyranosides**. Note that glycoside formation is a dehydration reaction; thus, breaking a glycosidic bond requires hydrolysis.

MCAT CONCEPT CHECK 4.3

Before you move on, assess your understanding of the material with these questions.

1. Explain the difference between esterification and glycoside formation.

____

2. What purpose do Tollens' reagent and Benedict's reagent serve? How do they differ from each other?

____

3. From a metabolic standpoint, does it make sense for carbohydrates to get oxidized or reduced? What is the purpose of this process?

____

4.4 Complex Carbohydrates

LEARNING OBJECTIVES

After Chapter 4.4, you will be able to:

- Compare starches, glycogen, and cellulose
- Predict the comparative solubility of different starch forms based on structure
- Recognize important biologically relevant disaccharides

Complex carbohydrates include all carbohydrates with at least two sugar molecules linked together (disaccharides, oligosaccharides, and polysaccharides).

Disaccharides

As discussed previously, monosaccharides react with alcohols to form acetals. Glycosidic bonds formed between hydroxyl groups of two monosaccharides result in the formation of a **disaccharide**, as shown in Figure 4.18.

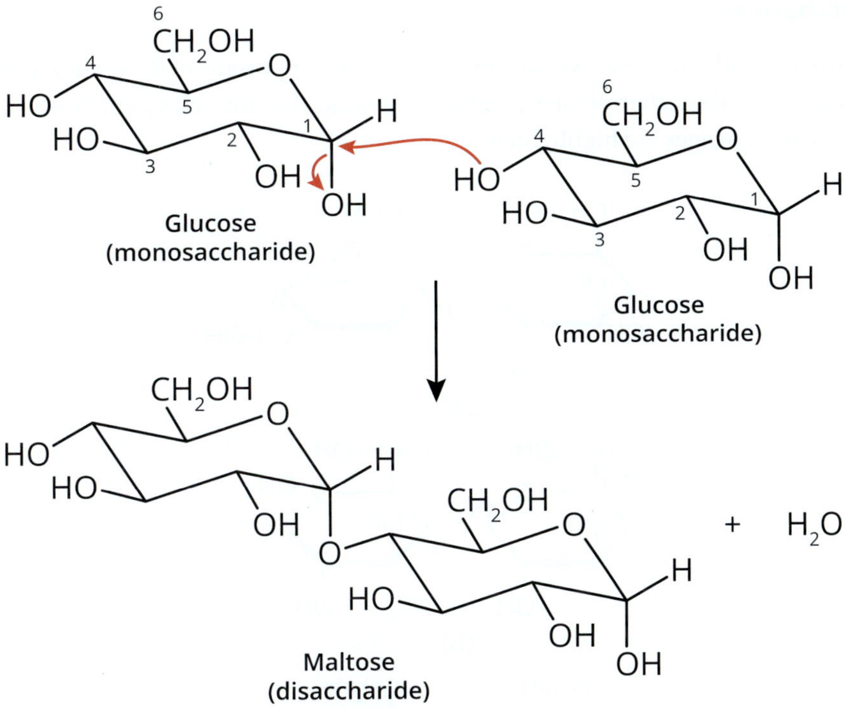

Figure 4.18 Disaccharide Formation
The hydroxyl group on the anomeric carbon reacts with the hydroxyl of another sugar to form an acetal (or ketal) with a 1,2; 1,4; or 1,6 glycosidic linkage.

Formation of an α- or β-glycosidic linkage is nonspecific in that the anomeric carbon of a cyclic sugar can react with any hydroxyl group on any other sugar molecule. The linkages are named for the configuration of the anomeric carbon and the numbers of the hydroxyl-containing carbons involved in the linkage. For example, in an α-1,6 glycosidic bond formation between two D-glucose molecules, the α-anomeric carbon of the first glucose (C-1) attaches to C-6 of the second glucose. Note that the second glucose could be either the α- or β-anomer. In the event that a glycosidic bond is formed between two anomeric carbons, this must be specified in the name. For example, a bond formed between the anomeric carbons of two α-D-glucose molecules would be termed an α,α-1,1 linkage, as demonstrated in Figure 4.19.

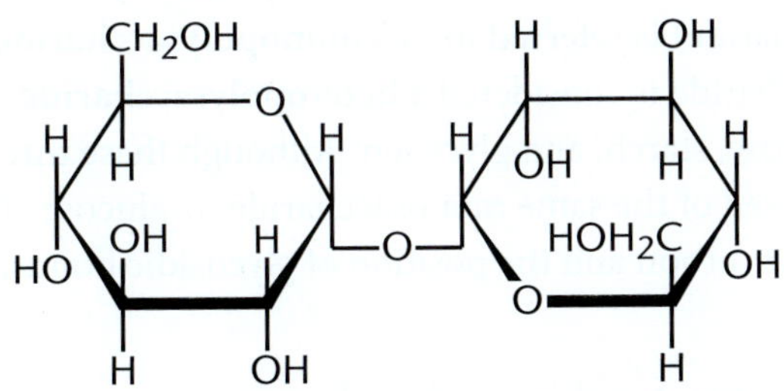

Figure 4.19 Trehalose
Example of a disaccharide with an α,α-1,1 linkage between the α-anomeric carbons of two glucose molecules

Various combinations of monosaccharides linked by glycosidic bonds result in the formation of different disaccharides. For instance, two glucose molecules linked by an α-1,4 glycosidic bond is called *maltose*, while two glucose molecules joined by a β-1,4 linkage is called *cellobiose*.

Important Disaccharides

When discussing disaccharides in a real-world context, the most important of these sugars are **sucrose**, **lactose**, and **maltose**. These disaccharides are commonly produced in the cell by enzymatic activity. Their molecular structures and linkages are highlighted in Figure 4.20.

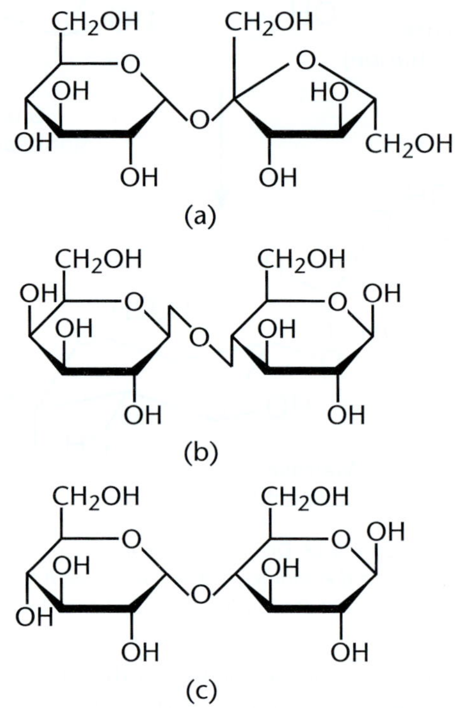

Figure 4.20 Important Disaccharides
(a) Sucrose (glucose-α-1,2-fructose), (b) Lactose (galactose-β-1,4-glucose), (c) Maltose (glucose-α-1,4-glucose)

Polysaccharides

Polysaccharides are long chains of monosaccharides linked together by glycosidic bonds. While glucose is the most frequently encountered monosaccharide, it is not the only one. A polysaccharide composed entirely of glucose (or any other monosaccharide) is referred to as a **homopolysaccharide**, while a polymer made up of more than one type of monosaccharide is considered a **heteropolysaccharide**. The three most important biological polysaccharides are cellulose, starch, and glycogen. Although these three polysaccharides have different functions, they are all composed of the same monosaccharide, D-glucose. These polysaccharides differ in configuration about the anomeric carbon and the position of glycosidic bonds, resulting in notable biological differences.

Because glycosidic bonding can occur at multiple hydroxyl groups in a monosaccharide, polymer formation can either be linear or branched. Branching happens when an internal monosaccharide in a polymer chain forms at least two glycosidic bonds, allowing branch formation. We'll take a closer look at how this is a key part of glycogen synthesis and glycogenolysis in Chapter 9 of *MCAT Biochemistry Review*.

Cellulose

Cellulose is the main structural component of plants. A homopolysaccharide, cellulose is a chain of β-D-glucose molecules linked by β-1,4 glycosidic bonds, with hydrogen bonds holding the actual polymer chains together for support. Humans are not able to digest cellulose because we lack the *cellulase* enzyme responsible for hydrolyzing cellulose to glucose monomers. Therefore, cellulose found in fruits and vegetables serves as a great source of fiber in our diet, drawing water into the gut. Cellulase is produced by some bacteria found in the digestive tract of certain animals, such as termites, cows, and goats, which enables them to digest cellulose. A portion of a cellulose chain can be seen in Figure 4.21 below.

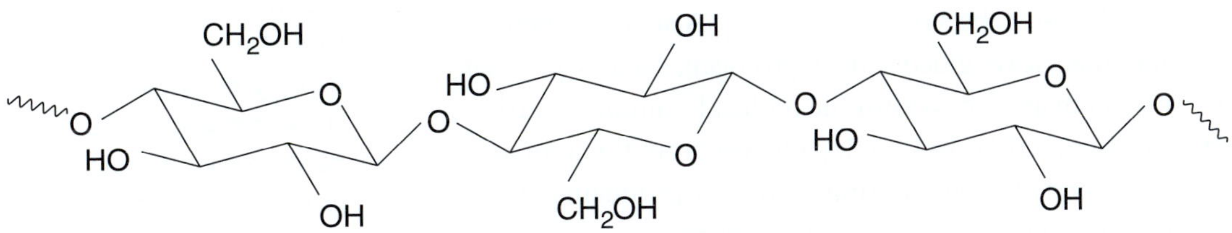

Figure 4.21 Cellulose Structure
Cellulose is a polymer of 1,4-linked β-D-glucose.

Starches

Starches are polysaccharides that are more digestible by humans because they are linked α-D-glucose monomers. Plants predominantly store starch as **amylose**, a linear glucose polymer linked via α-1,4 glycosidic bonds. Another type of starch is **amylopectin**, which starts off with the same type of linkage that amylose exhibits, but also contains branches via α-1,6 glycosidic bonds. Iodine is a well-known reagent that tests for the presence of starch and does so by fitting inside the helix conformation amylose typically makes, forming a starch–iodine complex. The structure of amylose is depicted in Figure 4.22.

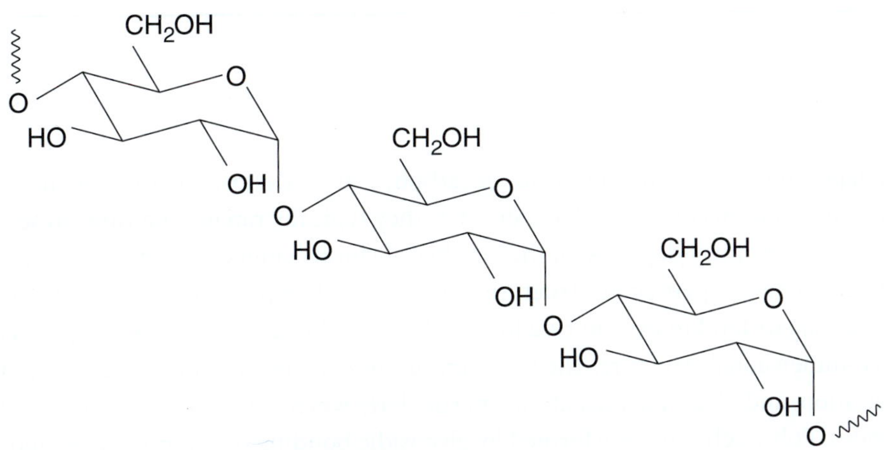

Figure 4.22 Starch Structure
Starches are polymers of 1,4-linked α-D-glucose.

BRIDGE

The contrast between cellulose and starch digestibility exemplifies the specificity of enzymes. A slight 109.5° rotation of the anomeric carbon to form β-linkages (instead of α-linkages) is enough to make the molecule indigestible by any enzymes in humans—even though they're both D-glucose polymers! Enzyme specificity is discussed in Chapter 2 of *MCAT Biochemistry Review.*

Starches like amylose and amylopectin are broken down by enzymes in the body and are used as a source of energy. Amylose is degraded by *α-amylase* and *β-amylase.* **β-Amylase** cleaves amylose at the nonreducing end of the polymer (the end with acetal) to yield maltose, while α-**amylase** cleaves randomly along the chain to yield shorter polysaccharide chains, maltose, and glucose. Because amylopectin is highly branched, debranching enzymes help degrade the polysaccharide chain.

Glycogen

Glycogen is a carbohydrate storage unit in animals. It is similar to starch, except that it has more α-1,6 glycosidic bonds (approximately one for every 10 glucose molecules, while amylopectin has approximately one for every 25), which makes it a highly branched compound. This branching optimizes the energy efficiency of glycogen and makes it more soluble in solution, thereby allowing more glucose to be stored in the body. Also, its branching pattern allows enzymes that cleave glucose from glycogen, such as *glycogen phosphorylase*, to work on many sites within the molecule simultaneously. **Glycogen phosphorylase** functions by cleaving glucose from the nonreducing end of a glycogen branch and phosphorylating it, thereby producing glucose 1-phosphate, which plays an important role in metabolism.

REAL WORLD

Hers disease, also known as glycogen storage disease (GSD) type VI, is a condition characterized by a deficiency in liver *glycogen phosphorylase*. Patients with this disease cannot break down glycogen in their livers and therefore have hepatomegaly (a swollen liver). They may also have hypoglycemia (low blood sugar) between meals because they cannot use glycogen to maintain blood glucose concentrations.

MCAT CONCEPT CHECK 4.4

Before you move on, assess your understanding of the material with these questions.

1. Which of the two forms of starch is more soluble in solution. Why?

____

2. Regarding glycogen and amylopectin, which of these two polymers should experience a higher rate of enzyme activity from enzymes that cleave side branches? Why?

____

Conclusion

This chapter examined, in depth, the unique characteristics of carbohydrates. Monosaccharides are the most basic form of carbohydrates, and in terms of human biochemistry, they typically range from three to seven carbon atoms. Classifying these monomers depends on the number of chiral centers present, which tells us the number of potential stereoisomers. Open-chain structures are most easily represented through Fischer projection diagrams; however, sugars tend to exist in ring form in biological systems, so Haworth projections are also used to depict three-dimensional structure. The most important reactions monosaccharides undergo are redox reactions, esterification, and glycoside formation—particularly when glycoside formation results in the formation of disaccharides. Polysaccharides are formed by glycosidic bonding of carbohydrates, and the polymers cellulose, starch, and glycogen are most commonly found in nature. Glycogen is the primary storage form of glucose in humans and other animals, and its unique branching structure allows for rapid access to these glucose stores.

The body has two primary energy-storage molecules: glycogen and triacylglycerols. Each has its own pros and cons—glycogen is more rapidly mobilized, but requires water of hydration, which increases its weight. Triacylglycerols serve as a long-term repository of energy, but take time to utilize. In the next chapter, we turn our attention to triacylglycerols, as well as the lipids used for structure and cell signaling.

GO ONLINE

You've reviewed the content, now test your knowledge and critical thinking skills by completing a test-like passage set in your online resources!

CONCEPT SUMMARY

Carbohydrate Classification

- Carbohydrates are organized by their number of carbon atoms and functional groups.
  - Common names are also frequently used when referring to sugars, such as glucose, fructose, and galactose.
  - Three-carbon sugars are trioses, four-carbon sugars are tetroses, and so on.
  - Sugars with aldehydes as their most oxidized group are **aldoses**; sugars with ketones as their most oxidized group are **ketoses**.
- The nomenclature of all sugars is based on the D- and L-forms of glyceraldehyde. Sugars with the highest-numbered chiral carbon with the –OH group on the right (in a Fischer projection) are D-sugars; those with the –OH on the left are L-sugars. D- and L-forms of the same sugar are **enantiomers**.
- **Diastereomers** are nonsuperimposable configurations of molecules with similar connectivity. They differ at at least one—but not all—chiral carbons. These also include epimers and anomers.
  - **Epimers** are a subtype of diastereomers that differ at exactly one chiral carbon.
  - **Anomers** are a subtype of epimers that differ at the anomeric carbon.

Cyclic Sugar Molecules

- Cyclization describes the ring formation of carbohydrates from their straight-chain forms.
- When rings form, the anomeric carbon can take on either an α- or β-conformation.
  - The **anomeric carbon** is the new chiral center formed in ring closure; it was the carbon containing the carbonyl in the straight-chain form.
  - **α-anomers** have the –OH on the anomeric carbon *trans* to the free $-CH_2OH$ group.
  - **β-anomers** have the –OH on the anomeric carbon *cis* to the free $-CH_2OH$ group.
- **Haworth projections** provide a good way to represent three-dimensional structure.
- Cyclic compounds can undergo **mutarotation**, in which they shift from one anomeric form to another with the straight-chain form as an intermediate.

Monosaccharides

- **Monosaccharides** are single carbohydrate units, with glucose as the most commonly observed monomer. They can undergo three main reactions: oxidation–reduction, esterification, and glycoside formation.
  - Aldoses can be oxidized to **aldonic acids** and reduced to **alditols**.
  - Sugars that can be oxidized are reducing agents (**reducing sugars**) themselves, and can be detected by reacting with **Tollens'** or **Benedict's reagents**.
  - Sugars with a –H replacing an –OH group are termed **deoxy sugars**.
  - Sugars can react with carboxylic acids and their derivatives, forming esters (**esterification**). **Phosphorylation** is a similar reaction in which a phosphate ester is formed by transferring a phosphate group from ATP onto a sugar.
  - **Glycoside formation** is the basis for building complex carbohydrates and requires the anomeric carbon to link to another sugar.

Complex Carbohydrates

- **Disaccharides** form as result of glycosidic bonding between two monosaccharide subunits; polysaccharides form by repeated monosaccharide or polysaccharide glycosidic bonding.
- Common disaccharides include **sucrose** (glucose-α-1,2-fructose), **lactose** (galactose-β-1,4-glucose), and **maltose** (glucose-α-1,4-glucose).
- Polysaccharides play various roles:
  - **Cellulose** is the main structural component for plant cell walls and is a main source of fiber in the human diet.
  - **Starches** (**amylose** and **amylopectin**) function as a main energy storage form for plants.
  - **Glycogen** functions as a main energy storage form for animals.

ANSWERS TO CONCEPT CHECKS

4.1

1. Aldopentose; ketohexose

2.

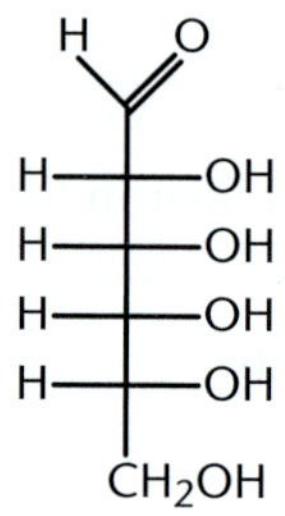

D-allose

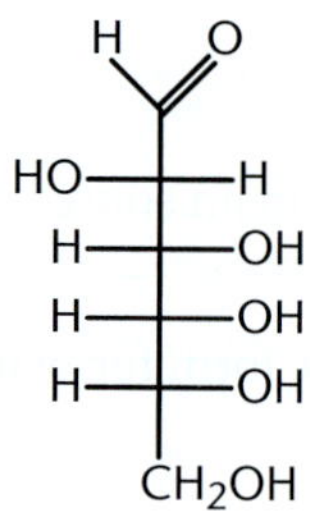

D-altrose

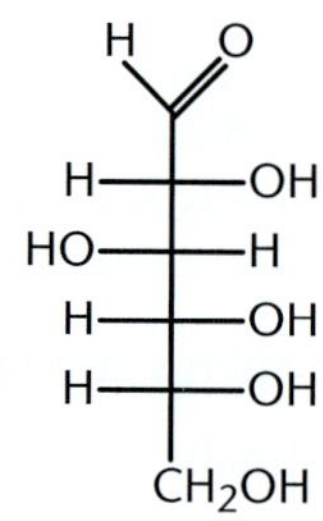

D-glucose

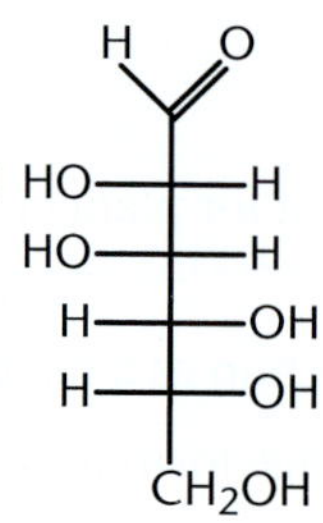

D-mannose

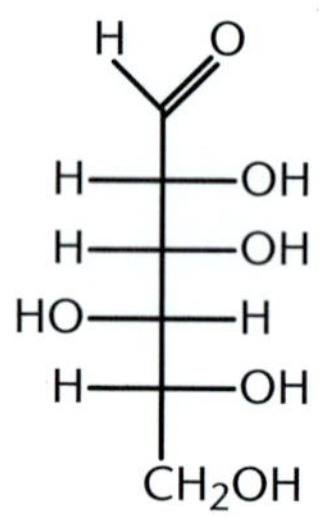

D-gulose

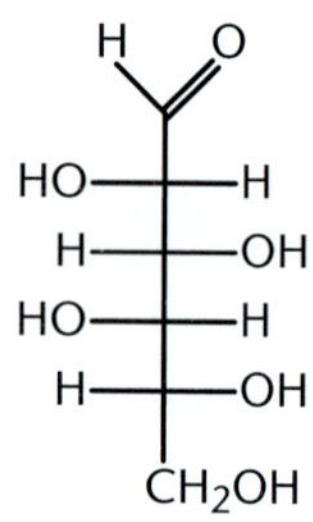

D-idose

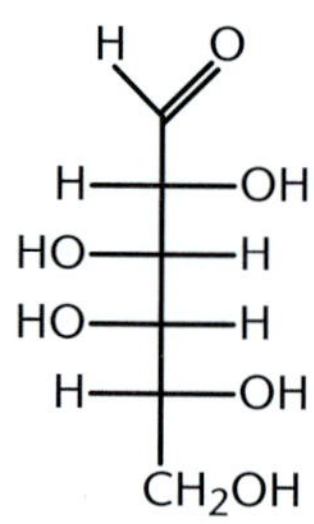

D-galactose

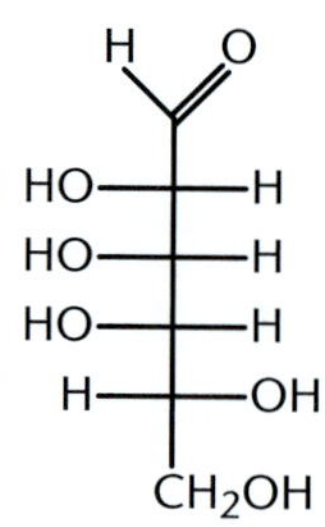

D-talose

3. D-Glucose's epimers are D-mannose (C-2), D-allose (C-3), and D-galactose (C-4). None of the D-stereoisomers is an enantiomer for glucose; L-glucose is the enantiomer of D-glucose.

4.2

1. During hemiacetal or hemiketal formation, the carbonyl carbon becomes chiral and is termed the anomeric carbon. The orientation of the –OH substituent on this carbon determines if the sugar molecule is the α- or β-anomer.

2.

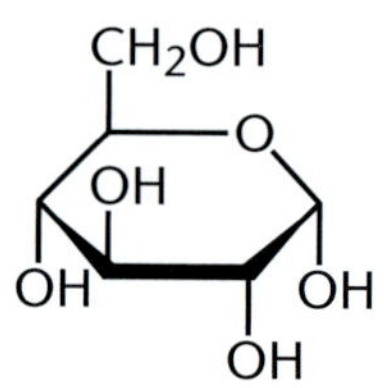

3.

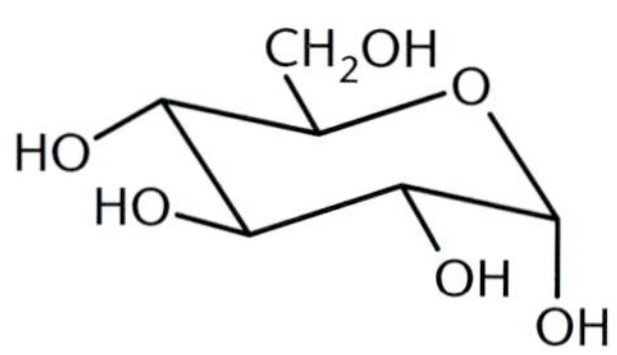

4.3

1. Esterification is the reaction by which a hydroxyl group reacts with either a carboxylic acid or a carboxylic acid derivative to form an ester. Glycoside formation refers to the reaction between an alcohol and a hemiacetal (or hemiketal) group on a sugar to yield an alkoxy group.
2. Tollens' reagent and Benedict's reagent are used to detect the presence of reducing sugars. Tollens' reagent is reduced to produce a silvery mirror when aldehydes are present whereas Benedict's reagent is indicated by a reddish precipitate of Cu_2O.
3. It makes sense for carbohydrates to become oxidized while reducing other groups. This is the case because aerobic metabolism requires reduced forms of electron carriers to facilitate processes such as oxidative phosphorylation. Because carbohydrates are a primary energy source, they are oxidized.

4.4

1. Amylopectin is more soluble in solution than amylose because of its branched structure. The highly branched structure of amylopectin decreases intermolecular bonding between polysaccharide polymers and increases interaction with the surrounding solution.
2. Glycogen has a higher rate of enzymatic branch cleavage because it contains significantly more branching than amylopectin.

SCIENCE MASTERY ASSESSMENT EXPLANATIONS

1. **D**

Glucose is an aldohexose, meaning that it has one aldehyde group and six carbons. Given this information, **(A)** and **(B)** can be eliminated. In aldose sugars, each nonterminal carbon is chiral. Therefore, glucose has four chiral centers, not five, as mentioned in **(C)**. The number of stereoisomers possible for a chiral molecule is 2^n, where n is the number of chiral carbons. Because glucose has four chiral centers, there are $2^4 = 16$ possible stereoisomers.

2. **D**

Epimers are monosaccharide diastereomers that differ in their configuration about only one carbon. As with all diastereomers, epimers have different chemical and physical properties, and their optical activities have no relation to each other. Enantiomers have equal but opposite optical activities. Therefore, **(D)** is the only statement that does not apply to epimers.

3. **C**

Aldonic acids form after the aldehyde group on a reducing sugar reduces another compound, becoming oxidized in the process.

4. **B**

Mutarotation is the interconversion between anomers of a compound. Enantiomerization and racemization, **(C)** and **(D)**, are related: enantiomerization is the formation of a mirror-image or optically inverted form of a compound, whereas racemization is moving a solution toward an equal concentration of both enantiomers. Glycosidation, **(A)**, is the addition of a sugar to another compound.

5. **A**

Ketose sugars undergo tautomerization, a rearrangement of bonds, to undergo *keto–enol* shifts. This forms an aldose, which then allows them to act as reducing sugars. A ketone group alone cannot be oxidized. Anomerization, mentioned in **(C)**, refers to ring closure of a monosaccharide, creating an anomeric carbon.

6. **B**

When glucose reacts with methanol under acid catalysis, the hemiacetal is converted to an acetal via replacement of the anomeric hydroxyl group with an alkoxy group. The result is a type of acetal known as a glycoside. This corresponds with **(B)**. The other choices all show alkoxy groups on the wrong carbon, or too many carbons.

7. **B**

β-Amylase cleaves amylose at the nonreducing end of the polymer to yield maltose exclusively, while α-amylase, **(A)**, cleaves amylose anywhere along the chain to yield short polysaccharides, maltose, and glucose. Debranching enzyme, **(C)**, removes oligosaccharides from a branch in glycogen or starches, while glycogen phosphorylase, **(D)**, yields glucose 1-phosphate.

8. **C**

Start by drawing out the Haworth projection. Recall that all the groups on the right in the Fischer projection will go on the bottom of the Haworth projection, and all the groups on the left will go on the top. Next, draw the chair structure, with the oxygen in the back right corner. Label the carbons in the ring 1 through 5, starting from the oxygen and moving clockwise around the ring. Now, draw in the lines for all the axial substituents, alternating above and below the ring. Remember to start on the anomeric C-1 carbon, where the axial substituent points down. Now start filling in the substituents. The substituent can be in either position on the anomeric carbon, so skip that one for now. The –OH groups on C-2 and C-4 should point downward while the –OH group on C-3 should point upward; **(C)**, the β-anomer of D-glucose, is the only one that matches.

9. **B**

The hydroxyl group on the anomeric carbon of the β-anomer is equatorial, thereby creating less nonbonded strain than the α-anomer, which has the hydroxyl group of the anomeric carbon in axial position.

10. **D**

Glycogen and amylopectin are the only polysaccharide forms that demonstrate branching structure, making them most similar in terms of linkage. Both glycogen and amylopectin use α-1,4 and α-1,6 linkages. Cellulose uses β-1,4 linkages and amylose does not contain α-1,6 linkages.

11. **C**

While maltose and cellobiose both have the same glucose subunits, only maltose is digestible by humans because the β-glycosidic linkages in cellobiose cannot be cleaved in the human body.

12. **C**

In solution, the hemiacetal ring of glucose will break open spontaneously and then re-form. When the ring is broken, bond rotation occurs between C-1 and C-2 to produce either the α- or the β-anomer. The reaction given in this question depicts the mutarotation of glucose. **(A)** is incorrect because the reactant is an aldehyde, not the product. **(B)** is incorrect because a hemiketal has an $-$OH group, an $-$OR group, and two $-$R groups. In addition, hemiketals are formed from ketones, and our starting reactant is an aldehyde. Finally, **(D)** is incorrect because there is no glycosidic bond in the starting reactant.

13. **A**

Galactose is a diastereomer of glucose, with the stereochemistry at C-4 (counting from the aldehyde) reversed. Being able to identify C-4 is enough to answer this question, even without looking at the glucose molecule. Because **(B)**, **(C)**, and **(D)** have identical stereochemistry at C-4, they are incorrect.

14. **D**

In Andersen's disease, glycogen is less branched than normal, thereby inducing lower solubility of glycogen. Branches reduce the interactions between adjacent chains of glycogen and encourage interactions with the aqueous environment. The smaller number of branches means that glycogen phosphorylase has fewer terminal glucose monomers on which to act, making enzyme activity slower than normal overall. Finally, without branches, the density of glucose monomers cannot be as high; therefore, the total glucose stored is lower than normal. Glycogen synthase is still functioning normally, so we would expect normal α-1,4 linkages in the glycogen of an individual with Andersen's disease but few (if any) α-1,6 linkages.

15. **C**

Monosaccharides can exist as hemiacetals or hemiketals, depending on whether they are aldoses or ketoses. When a monosaccharide is in its cyclic form, the anomeric carbon is attached to the oxygen in the ring and a hydroxyl group. Hence, it is only a hemiacetal or hemiketal because an acetal or ketal would require the $-$OH group to be converted to another $-$OR group.

GO ONLINE

Consult your online resources for additional practice.

EQUATIONS TO REMEMBER

(4.1) **Number of stereoisomers with common backbone** $= 2^n$

SHARED CONCEPTS

Biochemistry Chapter 9
Carbohydrate Metabolism I

Biochemistry Chapter 10
Carbohydrate Metabolism II

Organic Chemistry Chapter 1
Nomenclature

Organic Chemistry Chapter 2
Isomers

Organic Chemistry Chapter 5
Alcohols

Organic Chemistry Chapter 6
Aldehydes and Ketones I

CHAPTER 5

LIPID STRUCTURE AND FUNCTION

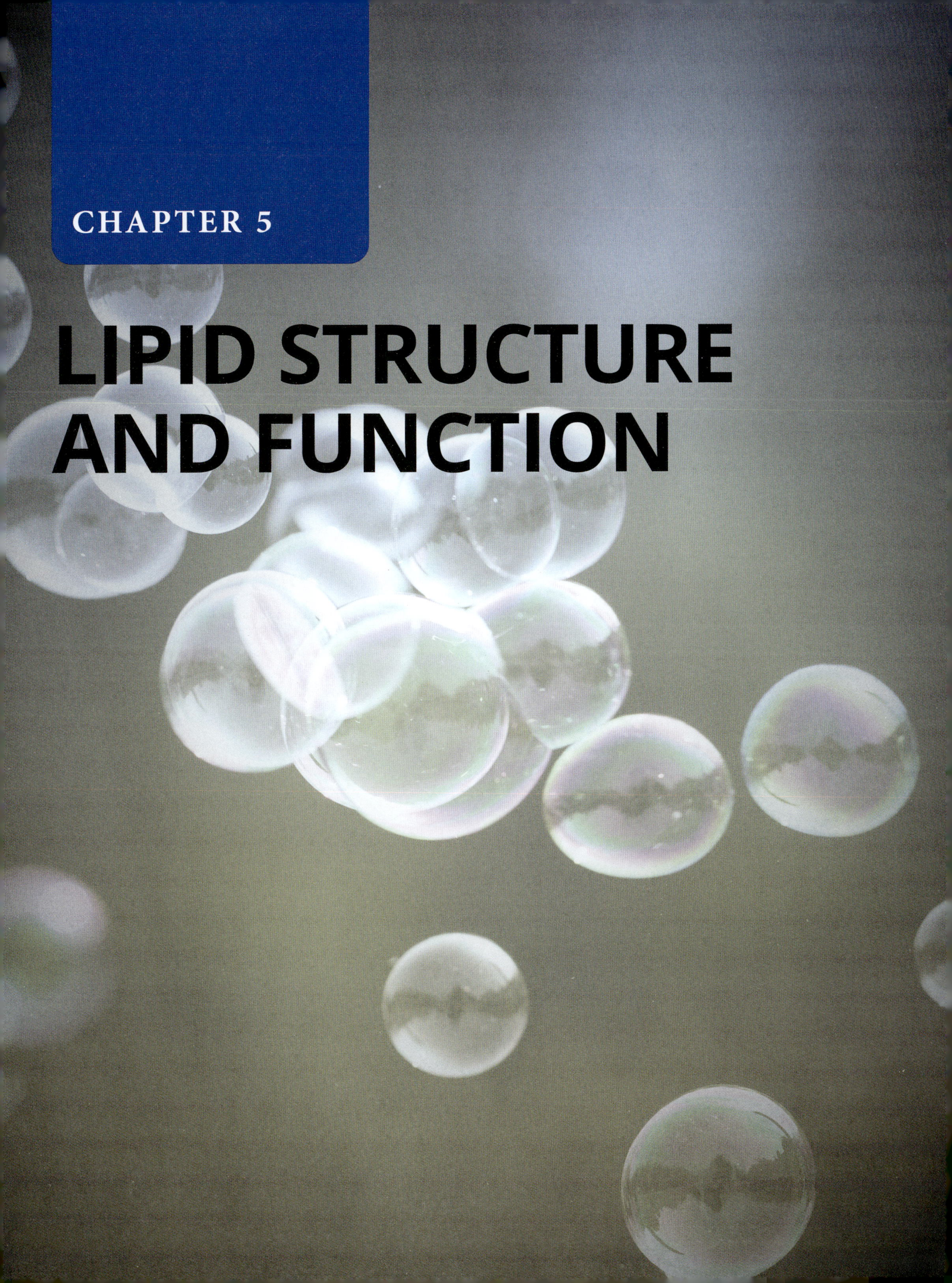

SCIENCE MASTERY ASSESSMENT

Every pre-med knows this feeling: there is so much content I have to know for the MCAT! How do I know what to do first or what's important?

While the high-yield badges throughout this book will help you identify the most important topics, this Science Mastery Assessment is another tool in your MCAT prep arsenal. This quiz (which can also be taken in your online resources) and the guidance below will help ensure that you are spending the appropriate amount of time on this chapter based on your personal strengths and weaknesses. Don't worry though—skipping something now does not mean you'll never study it. Later on in your prep, as you complete full-length tests, you'll uncover specific pieces of content that you need to review and can come back to these chapters as appropriate.

How to Use This Assessment

If you answer 0–7 questions correctly:

Spend about 1 hour to read this chapter in full and take limited notes throughout. Follow up by reviewing **all** quiz questions to ensure that you now understand how to solve each one.

If you answer 8–11 questions correctly:

Spend 20–40 minutes reviewing the quiz questions. Beginning with the questions you missed, read and take notes on the corresponding subchapters. For questions you answered correctly, ensure your thinking matches that of the explanation and you understand why each choice was correct or incorrect.

If you answer 12–15 questions correctly:

Spend less than 20 minutes reviewing all questions from the quiz. If you missed any, then include a quick read-through of the corresponding subchapters, or even just the relevant content within a subchapter, as part of your question review. For questions you got correct, ensure your thinking matches that of the explanation and review the Concept Summary at the end of the chapter.

1. Which of the following is NOT a type of glycolipid?
   - **A.** Cerebroside
   - **B.** Globoside
   - **C.** Ganglioside
   - **D.** Sphingomyelin

2. During saponification:
   - **A.** triacylglycerols undergo a condensation reaction.
   - **B.** triacylglycerols undergo ester hydrolysis.
   - **C.** fatty acid salts are produced using a strong acid.
   - **D.** fatty acid salts are bound to albumin.

3. Which of the following best describes the structure of steroids?
   - **A.** Three cyclopentane rings, one cyclohexane ring
   - **B.** Three cyclohexane rings, one cyclopentane ring
   - **C.** Four carbon rings, differing in structure for each steroid
   - **D.** Three cyclic carbon rings and a functional group

4. Soap bubbles form because fatty acid salts organize into:
   - **A.** lysosomes.
   - **B.** micelles.
   - **C.** phospholipid bilayers.
   - **D.** hydrogen bonds.

5. Steroid hormones are steroids that:
   - **I.** have specific high-affinity receptors.
   - **II.** travel in the bloodstream from endocrine glands to distant sites.
   - **III.** affect gene transcription by binding directly to DNA.
   - **A.** I only
   - **B.** III only
   - **C.** I and II only
   - **D.** I and III only

6. Why are triacylglycerols used in the human body for energy storage?
   - **A.** They are highly hydrated and therefore can store lots of energy.
   - **B.** They always have short fatty acid chains for easy access by metabolic enzymes.
   - **C.** The carbon atoms of the fatty acid chains are highly reduced and therefore yield more energy upon oxidation.
   - **D.** Polysaccharides, which would actually be a better energy storage form, would dissolve in the body.

7. Which of the following is correct about fat-soluble vitamins?
   - **I.** Vitamin E is important for calcium regulation.
   - **II.** Vitamin D protects against cancer because it is a biological antioxidant.
   - **III.** Vitamin K is necessary for the posttranslational introduction of calcium-binding sites.
   - **IV.** Vitamin A is metabolized to retinal, which is important for sight.
   - **A.** III only
   - **B.** I and II only
   - **C.** III and IV only
   - **D.** II, III, and IV only

8. Which of the following is true of amphipathic molecules?
   - **A.** They form protective spheres in any solvent, with hydrophobic molecules interior and hydrophilic molecules exterior.
   - **B.** They have two fatty acid chains and a polar head group.
   - **C.** They are important to the formation of the phospholipid bilayer and soap bubbles.
   - **D.** They have a glycerol base.

9. Which of the following is/are true about sphingolipids?
   I. They are all phospholipids.
   II. They all contain a sphingosine backbone.
   III. They can have either phosphodiester or glycosidic linkages to their polar head groups.
   A. I only
   B. III only
   C. II and III only
   D. I, II, and III

10. Which of the following statements about saturation is FALSE?
    A. It can describe the number of double or triple bonds in a fatty acid tail.
    B. It determines at least one of the properties of membranes.
    C. More saturated fatty acids make for a more fluid solution.
    D. Fully saturated fatty acids have only single bonds.

11. Which of the following is true about glycerophospholipids?
    A. Glycerophospholipids can sometimes be sphingolipids, depending on the bonds in their head groups.
    B. Glycerophospholipids are merely a subset of phospholipids.
    C. Glycerophospholipids are used in the ABO blood typing system.
    D. Glycerophospholipids have one glycerol, one polar head group, and one fatty acid tail.

12. Which of the following statements about terpenes is FALSE?
    A. Terpenes are strongly scented molecules that sometimes serve protective functions.
    B. Terpenes are steroid precursors.
    C. A triterpene is made of three isoprene moieties, and therefore has 15 carbons.
    D. Terpenes are made by plants and insects.

13. Which of the following is true about cholesterol?
    A. Cholesterol always increases membrane fluidity in cells.
    B. Cholesterol is a steroid hormone precursor.
    C. Cholesterol is a precursor for vitamin A, which is produced in the skin.
    D. Cholesterol interacts only with the hydrophobic tails of phospholipids.

14. Which of the following statements regarding prostaglandins is FALSE?
    A. Prostaglandins regulate the synthesis of cAMP.
    B. Prostaglandin synthesis is inhibited by NSAIDs.
    C. Prostaglandins affect pain, inflammation, and smooth muscle function.
    D. Prostaglandins are endocrine hormones, like steroid hormones.

15. Which of the statements regarding waxes is FALSE?
    A. Waxes generally have melting points above room temperature.
    B. Waxes are produced only in plants and insects and therefore must be consumed by humans.
    C. Waxes protect against dehydration and parasites.
    D. Waxes are esters of long-chain fatty acids and long-chain alcohols.

Answer Key

1. **D** (See section 5.1)
2. **B** (See section 5.3)
3. **B** (See section 5.2)
4. **B** (See section 5.3)
5. **C** (See section 5.2)
6. **C** (See section 5.3)
7. **C** (See section 5.2)
8. **C** (See section 5.1)
9. **B** (See section 5.1)
10. **C** (See section 5.1)
11. **B** (See section 5.1)
12. **C** (See section 5.2)
13. **B** (See section 5.2)
14. **D** (See section 5.2)
15. **B** (See section 5.1)

The relevant section of the chapter to review for each question is given in parentheses after the correct answer. Detailed explanations can be found at the end of the chapter.

CHAPTER 5

LIPID STRUCTURE AND FUNCTION

In This Chapter

CHAPTER PROFILE

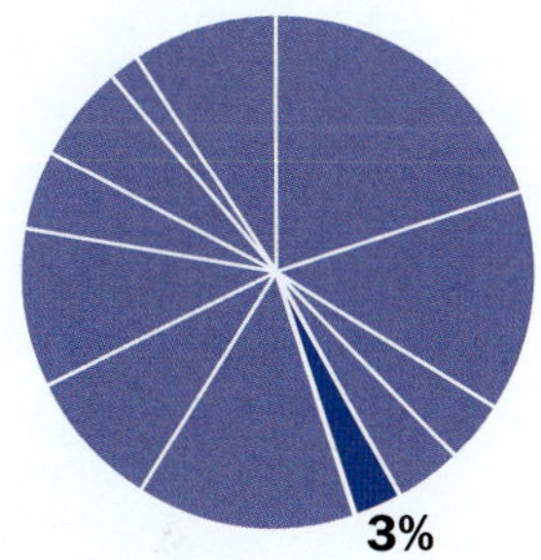

The content in this chapter should be relevant to about 3% of all questions about biochemistry on the MCAT.

This chapter covers material from the following AAMC content categories:

1D: Principles of bioenergetics and fuel molecule metabolism

3A: Structure and functions of the nervous and endocrine systems, and ways in which these systems coordinate the organ systems

5D: Structure, function, and reactivity of biologically-relevant molecules

Introduction

What do beer, human eyes, and sperm whales have in common? For all of these, lipids play a key role in some of their most interesting characteristics. The taste and smell of hops comes from lipids called *terpenes*. The ability of the human eye to respond to light (and therefore see) relies heavily on *retinal*, a lipid derived from vitamin A. Sperm whales use an enormous reservoir of *spermaceti* to dive to a depth of up to three kilometers to hunt giant squid. Spermaceti is a lipid with a density that changes dramatically with temperature—effectively allowing sperm whales to adjust their density with depth so that they can stay submerged without having to constantly fight buoyancy.

Lipids, as a class, are characterized by insolubility in water and solubility in nonpolar organic solvents. Aside from this shared feature, lipids diverge dramatically in their structural organization and biological functions, serving vital structural, signaling, and energy storage roles. In this chapter, we will explore the structural and functional characteristics of each of the major categories of lipids tested on the MCAT.

As structural building blocks, we will investigate *phospholipids* and *sterols*, which make up vesicles, liposomes, and membranes. When it comes to signaling, we will note that lipids serve multiple roles, from enzyme cofactors to light-absorbing pigments, and from intracellular messengers to hormones. Finally, we will see that lipids are the workhorse of energy storage, giving the most "bang" for the metabolic "buck" by weight.

5.1 Structural Lipids

LEARNING OBJECTIVES

After Chapter 5.1, you will be able to:

- Recall the major structural traits of phospholipids, glycerophospholipids, and sphingolipids
- Recognize how membrane lipid structure contributes to overall membrane structure and function
- Distinguish between the three types of sphingolipids
- Identify the polar and nonpolar regions of lipids:

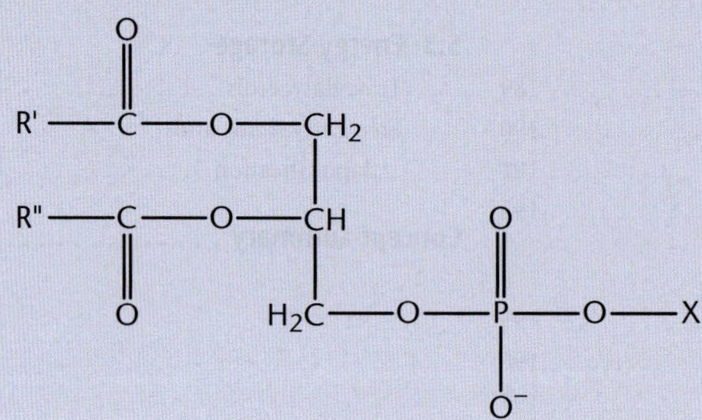

Lipids are the major component of the phospholipid bilayer, one of the most important structural parts of the cell. The unique ability of phospholipids to form a bilayer allows our cells to function as they do, separating the cell interior from the surrounding environment. We will first take a close look at the structure and role of phospholipids, glycerophospholipids, and sphingolipids. Finally, we will review the gross structural characteristics of the unique class called waxes.

Each of the membrane components is an **amphipathic** molecule, meaning that it has both hydrophilic and hydrophobic regions. For these membrane lipids, the polar head is the hydrophilic region, whereas the fatty acid tails are the hydrophobic region. When placed in aqueous solution, these molecules spontaneously form structures that allow the hydrophobic regions to group internally while the hydrophilic regions interact with water. This leads to the formation of various structures, including liposomes, micelles, and the phospholipid bilayer, shown in Figure 5.1.

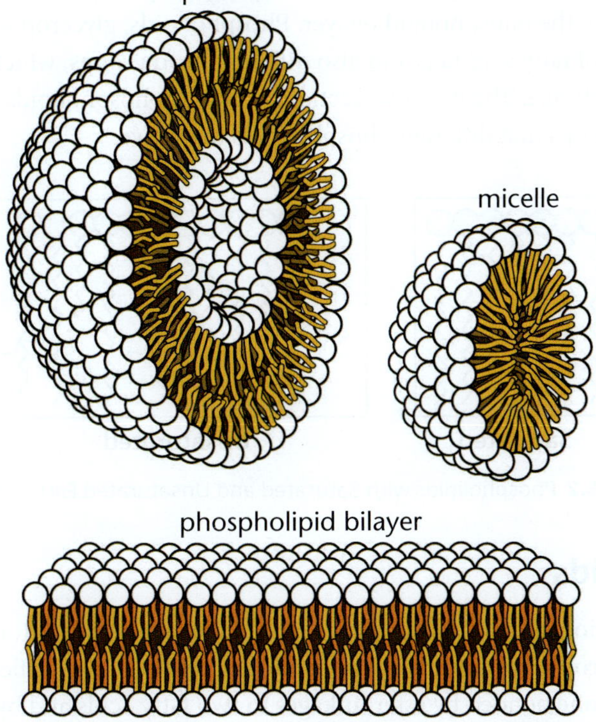

Figure 5.1 Membrane Lipids Form Various Structures in Aqueous Solutions

Phospholipids

Phospholipids contain the following elements: a phosphate and alcohol that comprise the polar head group, joined to a hydrophobic fatty acid tail by phosphodiester linkages. One or more fatty acids are attached to a backbone to form the hydrophobic tail region. Phospholipids can be further classified according to the backbone on which the molecule is built. For example, ***glycerol***, a three-carbon alcohol, forms *phosphoglycerides* or *glycerophospholipids*, and *sphingolipids* have a *sphingosine* backbone. One important thing to note, however, is that not all sphingolipids are phospholipids, as described later in this chapter.

One thing that these lipids do all share in common is a tail composed of long-chain fatty acids. These hydrocarbon chains vary by their degree of **saturation** and length. These two properties determine how the overall molecule will behave. Fully **saturated fatty acid** tails will have only single bonds; the carbon atom is considered saturated when it is bonded to four other atoms, with no π bonds. Saturated fatty acids, such as those in butter, have greater van der Waals forces and a more stable overall structure. Therefore, they form solids at room temperature. An **unsaturated fatty acid** includes one or more double bonds. Double bonds introduce kinks into the fatty acid chain, which makes it difficult for them to stack and solidify. This contrast with phospholipids that have saturated fatty acid tails is depicted in Figure 5.2. As a consequence of this difficulty stacking, unsaturated fats—like olive oil—tend to be liquids at room

BRIDGE

Although phospholipids are indeed the largest component of the phospholipid bilayer, nonphospholipids like glycolipids also play a role—and can be an important part of processes like cell recognition and signaling, discussed in Chapter 3 of *MCAT Biochemistry Review.*

KEY CONCEPT

Lipid properties—for all categories of lipids—are determined by the degree of saturation in fatty acid chains and the functional groups to which the fatty acid chains are bonded.

temperature. The same rules apply in the phospholipid bilayer: phospholipids with unsaturated fatty acid tails make up more fluid regions of the phospholipid bilayer. Phospholipids, glycerophospholipids, and sphingolipids can have any of a variety of fatty acid tails and also different head groups, which determine their properties at the surface of the cell membrane. The next two sections—glycerophospholipids and sphingolipids—focus on the various polar head groups that different phospholipids may have.

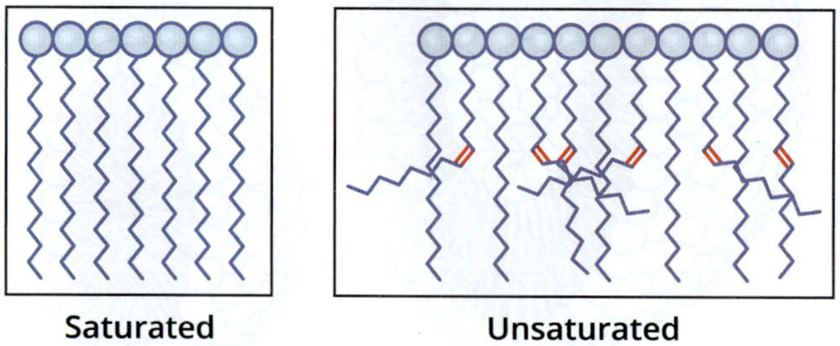

Figure 5.2 Phospholipids with Saturated and Unsaturated Fatty Acid Tails

Glycerophospholipids

As mentioned in the last section, glycerophospholipids are all phospholipids; yet, not all phospholipids are glycerophospholipids! **Glycerophospholipids** (or **phosphoglycerides**) are specifically those phospholipids that contain a glycerol backbone bonded by ester linkages to two fatty acids and by a phosphodiester linkage to a highly polar head group, as shown in Figure 5.3. Because the head group determines the membrane surface properties, glycerophospholipids are named according to their head group. For example, ***phosphatidylcholine*** is the name of a glycerophospholipid with a *choline* head group, and ***phosphatidylethanolamine*** is one with an *ethanolamine* head group. The head group can be positively charged, negatively charged, or neutral. The membrane surface properties of these molecules make them very important to cell recognition, signaling, and binding. Within each subtype, the fatty acid chains can vary in length and saturation, resulting in an astounding variety of functions that are the focus of active scientific research.

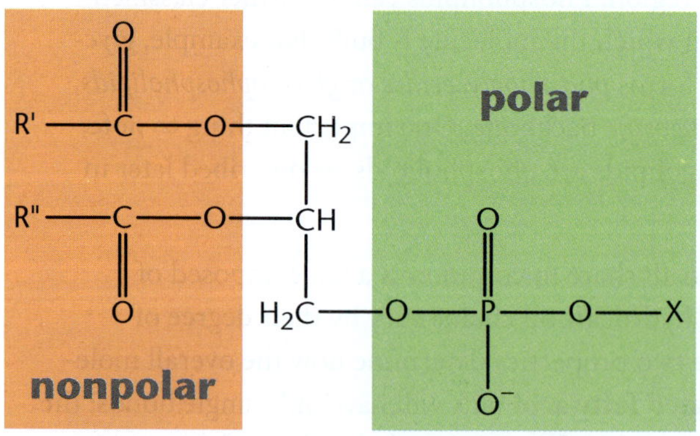

Figure 5.3 Structure of a Glycerophospholipid
X denotes the head group connected to the glycerol backbone by a phosphodiester linkage.

Sphingolipids

Blood typing makes it possible to give life-saving blood transfusions without risking potentially fatal acute hemolytic reactions. The ABO blood typing system is based on cell-surface antigens on red blood cells. These cell-surface antigens are some of the most well-known sphingolipids. Like glycerophospholipids, sphingolipids are also sites of biological recognition at the cell surface and can be bonded to various head groups and fatty acids.

Sphingolipids have a **sphingosine** or **sphingoid** (sphingosine-like) backbone, as opposed to the glycerol backbone of glycerophospholipids. These molecules also have long-chain, nonpolar fatty acid tails and polar head groups. Many sphingolipids are also phospholipids because they contain a phosphodiester linkage. However, other sphingolipids contain glycosidic linkages to sugars; any lipid linked to a sugar can be termed a ***glycolipid***. Sphingolipids are divided into four major subclasses, differing by their head group.

The simplest sphingolipid is ***ceramide***, which has a single hydrogen atom as its head group.

Sphingomyelins are the major class of sphingolipids that are also phospholipids (**sphingophospholipids**). These molecules have either phosphocholine or phosphoethanolamine as a head group, and thus contain a phosphodiester bond. Sphingomyelin head groups have no net charge. As the name implies, sphingomyelins are major components in the plasma membranes of cells producing myelin (oligodendrocytes and Schwann cells), the insulating sheath for axons.

Sphingolipids with head groups composed of sugars bonded by glycosidic linkages are considered glycolipids, as mentioned above, or, more specifically, ***glycosphingolipids***. These molecules are not phospholipids because they contain no phosphodiester linkage. Glycosphingolipids are found mainly on the outer surface of the plasma membrane and can be further classified as *cerebrosides* or *globosides*. **Cerebrosides** have a single sugar, whereas **globosides** have two or more. These molecules are also referred to as neutral glycolipids because they have no net charge at physiological pH.

The final group is composed of the most complex sphingolipids. ***Gangliosides*** are glycolipids that have polar head groups composed of oligosaccharides with one or more ***N-acetylneuraminic acid*** (**NANA**; also called **sialic acid**) molecules at the terminus and a negative charge. These molecules are also considered glycolipids because they have a glycosidic linkage and no phosphate group. Gangliosides play a major role in cell interaction, recognition, and signal transduction.

A summary of the different types of sphingolipids is provided in Figure 5.4.

REAL WORLD

Although experiments in blood transfusion are recorded as early as the 17th century, blood typing wasn't developed until the 20th century. With the advent of the ABO and Rh factor blood typing systems, blood transfusions could now be successfully administered to patients with hemophilia (a clotting disorder that causes significant bleeding), during surgery, and in a number of other applications.

REAL WORLD

Sphingolipid accumulation is associated with numerous pathological conditions. Sphingomyelins found in the myelin sheath help in signal transduction. Accumulation of sphingomyelin, resulting from lack of the enzyme *sphingomyelinase*, can result in *Niemann–Pick disease*. Symptoms can include intellectual disability and seizures. *Sulfatides* are sulfated cerebrosides associated with Alzheimer's disease.

MNEMONIC

Gangliosides are the "**gangly**" sphingolipids, with the most complex structure and functional groups (oligosaccharides and NANA) in all directions.

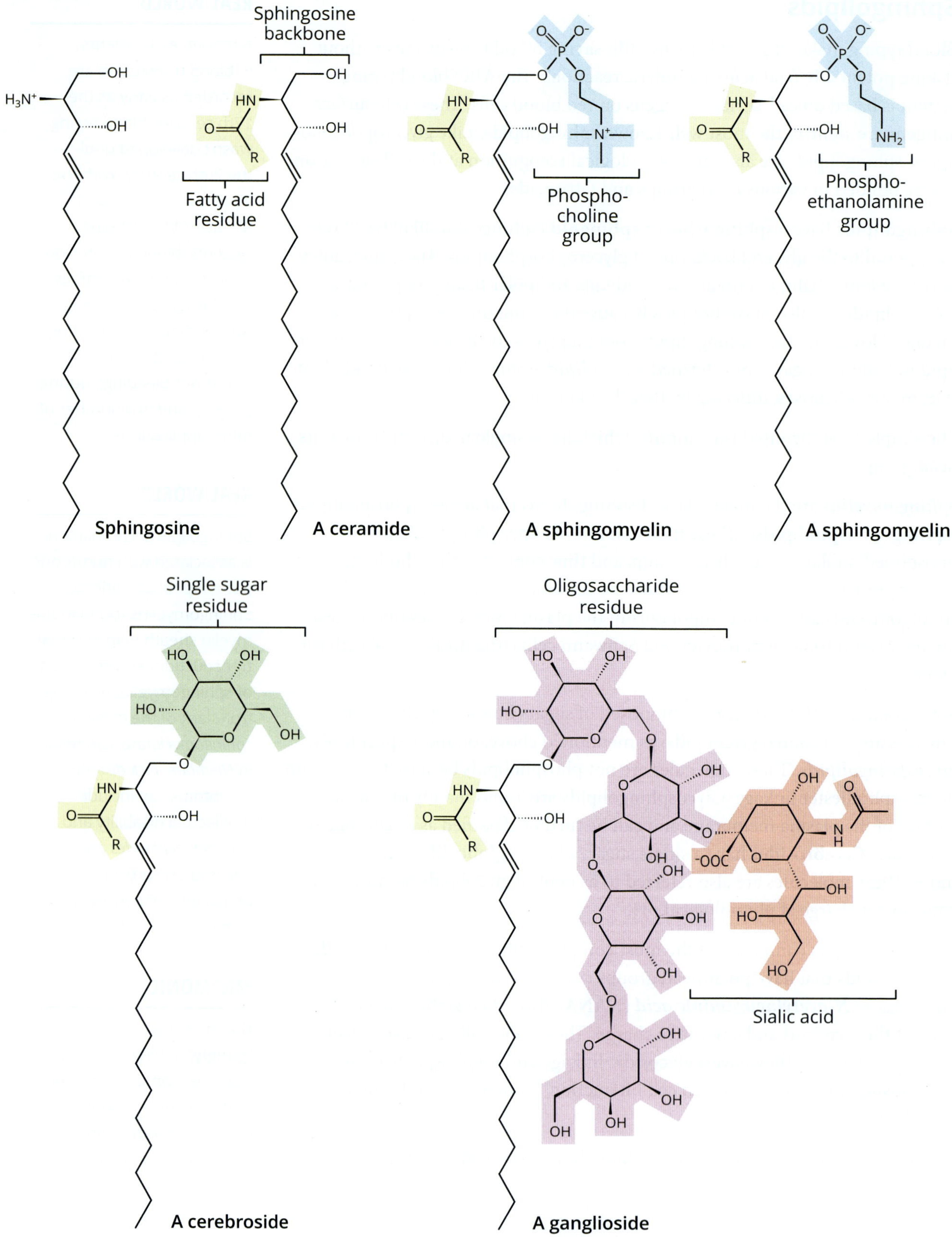

Figure 5.4 Types of Sphingolipids

Waxes

Waxes are esters created from long-chain fatty acids and long-chain alcohols. As one might expect, they form pliable solids at room temperature (what we generally think of as *wax*). Biologically, they function as protection for both plants and animals. In plants, waxes are secreted as a surface coating to prevent excessive evaporation and to protect against parasites. In animals, waxes are secreted to prevent dehydration, as a water-repellant to keep skin and feathers dry, and as lubricant. For example, *carnauba wax* is made from the leaves of the *Copernicia prunifera* palm and is used to coat candies and wax cars. Bees secrete waxes to construct shelter, as shown in Figure 5.5.

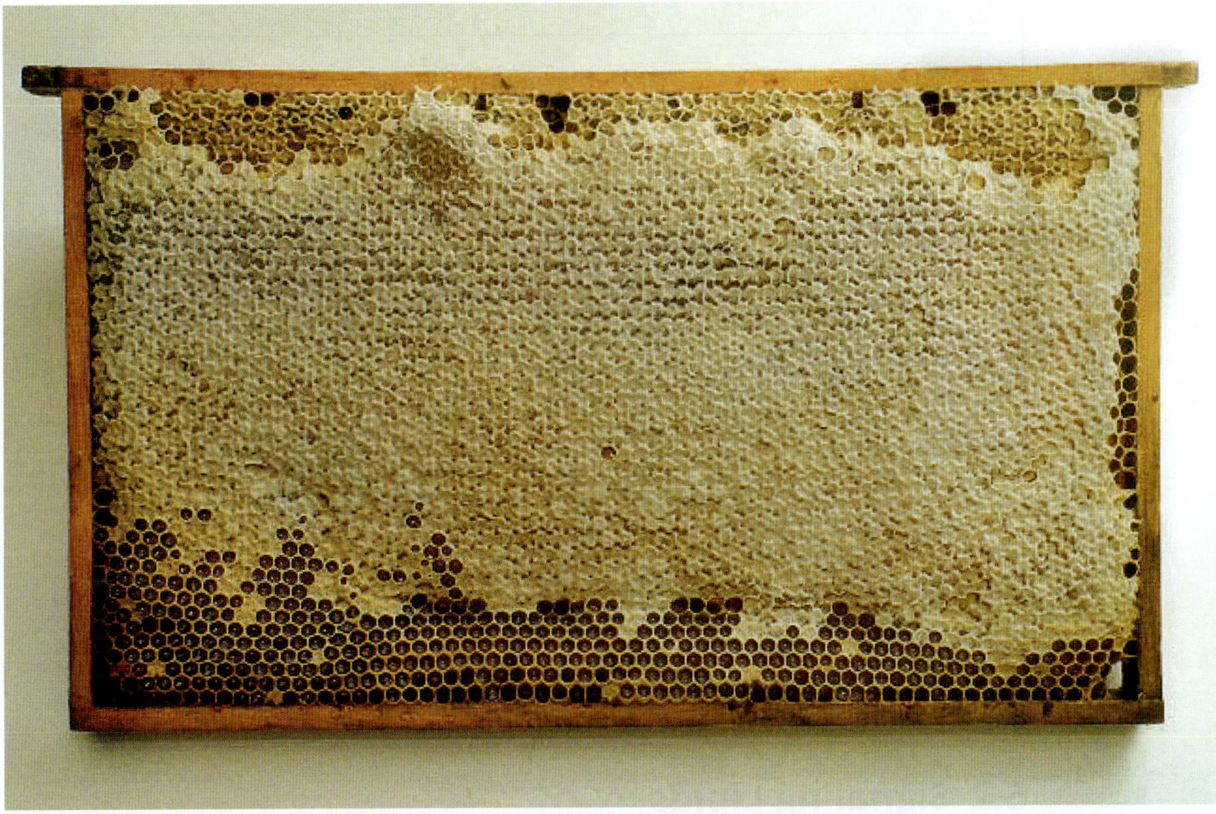

Figure 5.5 Honeycomb Structure Made from Beeswax
The solid and plastic nature of waxes, which contain esters with long alkyl chains, permits their use for structure building.

MCAT CONCEPT CHECK 5.1

Before you move on, assess your understanding of the material with these questions.

1. Which components of membrane lipids contribute to their structural role in membranes? Which components contribute to function?
   - Structure:

   ____

   - Function:

   ____

2. What is the difference between a sphingolipid that is also a phospholipid and one that is NOT?

   ____

3. Name the three main types of sphingolipids and their characteristics.

Type	Phospholipid or Glycolipid?	Functional Group(s)

4. What would happen if an amphipathic molecule were placed in a nonpolar solvent rather than an aqueous solution?

   ____

5.2 Signaling Lipids

LEARNING OBJECTIVES

After Chapter 5.2, you will be able to:

- Recall the structural features of terpenes, steroids, and prostaglandins
- Differentiate steroids from steroid hormones
- Connect prostaglandins to the symptoms associated with their presence, such as pain and inflammation
- Explain the importance of fat-soluble vitamins: A, D, E, and K

BRIDGE

Remember from Chapter 2 of *MCAT Biochemistry Review* that a coenzyme is an organic, nonprotein factor bound to an enzyme and required for its normal activity.

In addition to passive roles in structure, lipids also perform active roles in cellular signaling and as coenzymes. Lipids serve as coenzymes in the electron transport chain and in glycosylation reactions. Lipids also function as hormones that transmit signals over long distances and as intracellular messengers responding to extracellular signals. Certain special lipids with conjugated double bonds absorb light, which is extremely important for vision; others act as pigments in plants and animals. Here, we will focus on three important categories of signaling lipids: steroids, prostaglandins, and fat-soluble vitamins, as well as important precursors like terpenes.

Terpenes and Terpenoids

Before we delve into the details of downstream lipid signaling molecules, we must first turn our attention to *terpenes*. These odiferous chemicals are the metabolic precursors to steroids and other lipid signaling molecules, and have varied independent functions. **Terpenes** are a class of lipids built from ***isoprene*** (C_5H_8) moieties and share a common structural pattern with carbons grouped in multiples of five, as shown in Figure 5.6.

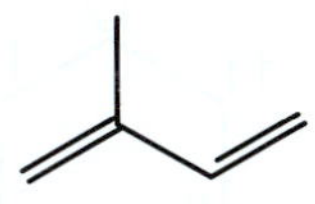

Figure 5.6 Isoprene

Terpenes are produced mainly by plants and also by some insects. They are generally strongly scented. In some cases, these pungent chemicals are part of the plant or insect's protective mechanism. The strong smell of turpentine, a derivative of resin, comes from the monoterpenes that are resin's major components; terpenes actually get their name from their original discovery in turpentine. Terpenes are also the primary components of much more pleasant-smelling essential oils extracted from plants.

Terpenes are grouped according to the number of isoprene units present; a single terpene unit contains two isoprene units. ***Monoterpenes*** ($C_{10}H_{16}$), which are abundant in both essential oils and turpentine as described above, contain two isoprene units. ***Sesquiterpenes*** (*sesqui–* meaning one-and-a-half) contain three isoprene units, and ***diterpenes*** contain four. Vitamin A, which will be discussed later in this chapter, is a diterpene from which *retinal*, a visual pigment vital for sight, is derived. ***Triterpenes***, with six isoprene units, can be converted to cholesterol and various steroids, also discussed later in this chapter. ***Carotenoids***, like *β-carotene* and *lutein*, are ***tetraterpenes*** and have eight isoprene units. Natural rubber has isoprene chains between 1000 and 5000 units long and is therefore considered a polyterpene.

Terpenoids, also sometimes referred to as isoprenoids, are derivatives of terpenes that have undergone oxygenation or rearrangement of the carbon skeleton. These compounds are further modified, as are terpenes, by the addition of an extensive variety of functional groups. Terpenoids share similar characteristics with terpenes in terms of both biological precursor function and aromatic properties, contributing to steroid biosynthesis, as well as the scents of cinnamon, eucalyptus, camphor, turmeric, and numerous other compounds. Terpenoids are named in an analogous fashion, with diterpenoids deriving from four isoprene units and so on. Terpenes and terpenoids are precursor molecules that feed into various biosynthesis pathways that produce important products, including steroids, which have widespread effects on biological function, and vitamin A, which is vital to sight.

Steroids

The term steroid probably brings to mind muscle–bound body builders or home run–hitting professional athletes. In science, and on the MCAT, steroid refers not just to the infamously abused anabolic steroids, but also to a broader class of molecules defined by their structure.

Structurally, **steroids**, shown in Figure 5.7, are metabolic derivatives of terpenes and are very different from the lipids mentioned earlier in this chapter in both structure and function. Steroids are characterized by having four cycloalkane rings fused together: three cyclohexane and one cyclopentane. Steroid functionality is determined by the oxidation status of these rings, as well as the functional groups they carry. It is important to note that the large number of carbons and hydrogens make steroids nonpolar, like the other lipids mentioned.

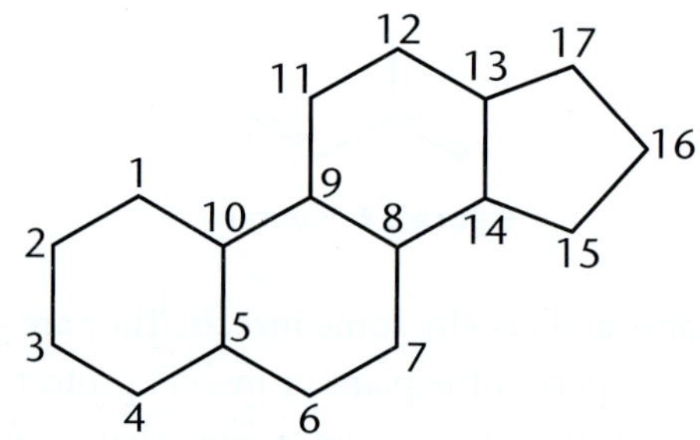

Figure 5.7 Common Steroid Structure

Keep in mind the terminology difference between steroids and steroid hormones. Steroid refers to a group defined by a particular chemical structure, demonstrated above. **Steroid hormones** are steroids that act as hormones, meaning that they are secreted by endocrine glands into the bloodstream and then travel on protein carriers to distant sites, where they can bind to specific high-affinity receptors and alter gene expression levels. Steroid hormones are potent biological signals that regulate gene expression and metabolism, affecting a wide variety of biological systems even at low concentrations. Some important steroid hormones include testosterone, various estrogens, cortisol, and aldosterone, which are discussed in Chapter 5 of *MCAT Biology Review*. Plants, like animals, also use steroids as signaling molecules.

Cholesterol, shown in Figure 5.8, is a steroid of primary importance. Cholesterol is a major component of the phospholipid bilayer and is responsible for mediating membrane fluidity. Cholesterol, like a phospholipid, is an amphipathic molecule containing both hydrophilic and hydrophobic components. Interactions with both the hydrophobic tails and hydrophilic heads of phospholipids allows cholesterol to maintain relatively constant fluidity in cell membranes. At low temperatures, it keeps the cell membrane from solidifying; at high temperatures, it holds the membrane intact and prevents it from becoming too permeable. Cholesterol also serves as a precursor to many important molecules, including steroid hormones, bile acids, and vitamin D.

BRIDGE

Hormone types, including steroid hormones, are the focus of Chapter 5 of *Kaplan MCAT Biology Review*.

REAL WORLD

Cholesterol can be produced *de novo* or absorbed from dietary sources. *Hypercholesterolemia*, or high cholesterol, is a condition that is strongly correlated with heart disease, in which the combination of these two cholesterol sources is excessive. Accumulation of cholesterol in arterial walls results in atherosclerosis, a hardening of the wall.

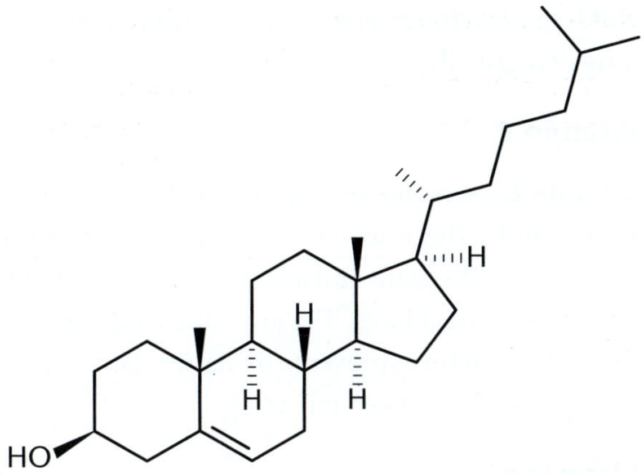

Figure 5.8 Cholesterol

Prostaglandins

Prostaglandins acquired their name because they were first thought to be produced by the prostate gland, but have since been determined to be produced by almost all cells in the body. These 20-carbon molecules are unsaturated carboxylic acids derived from ***arachidonic acid*** and contain one five-carbon ring. They act as paracrine or autocrine signaling molecules. In many tissues, the biological function of prostaglandins is to regulate the synthesis of cyclic adenosine monophosphate (cAMP), which is a ubiquitous intracellular messenger. In turn, cAMP mediates the actions of many other hormones. Downstream effects of prostaglandins include powerful effects on smooth muscle function, influence over the sleep–wake cycle, and the elevation of body temperature associated with fever and pain. Nonsteroidal anti-inflammatory drugs (NSAIDs) like aspirin inhibit the enzyme *cyclooxygenase* (COX), which aids in the production of prostaglandins.

Fat-Soluble Vitamins

A **vitamin** is an essential nutrient that cannot be adequately synthesized by the body and therefore must be consumed in the diet. Vitamins are commonly divided into water-soluble and lipid-soluble categories. Lipid-soluble vitamins can accumulate in stored fat, whereas excess water-soluble vitamins are excreted through the urine. The fat-soluble vitamins include A, D, E, and K. Each of these has important and varied functions.

Vitamin A

Vitamin A, or ***carotene***, is an unsaturated hydrocarbon that is important in vision, growth and development, and immune function. The most significant metabolite of vitamin A is the aldehyde form, ***retinal***, which is a component of the light-sensing molecular system in the human eye. ***Retinol***, the storage form of vitamin A, is also oxidized to ***retinoic acid***, a hormone that regulates gene expression during epithelial development.

MNEMONIC

One way to remember **carotene** is to remember that **carrots** are high in **vitamin A**, which is why eating carrots is colloquially suggested to improve **vision**. To remember that **vitamin D** regulates calcium, remember that it is frequently added to **milk** in order to aid in the absorption of **calcium**.

Vitamin D

Vitamin D, or ***cholecalciferol***, can be consumed or formed in a UV light–driven reaction in the skin. In the liver and kidneys, vitamin D is converted to ***calcitriol*** (1,25-$(OH)_2D_3$), the biologically active form of vitamin D. Calcitriol increases calcium and phosphate uptake in the intestines, which promotes bone production. A lack of vitamin D can result in **rickets**, a condition seen in children and characterized by underdeveloped, curved long bones as well as impeded growth.

MNEMONIC

Vitamin **K** is for **K**oagulation.

REAL WORLD

The anticoagulant *warfarin* works by blocking the recycling of vitamin K, causing a deficiency or lowering of the active amount of vitamin K. Therefore, patients taking warfarin are recommended to stay away from food containing high amounts of vitamin K, such as green leafy vegetables.

Vitamin E

Vitamin E characterizes a group of closely related lipids called ***tocopherols*** and ***tocotrienols***. These are characterized by a substituted aromatic ring with a long isoprenoid side chain and are characteristically hydrophobic. Tocopherols are biological antioxidants. The aromatic ring reacts with free radicals, destroying them. This, in turn, prevents oxidative damage, an important contributor to the development of cancer and aging.

Vitamin K

Vitamin K is actually a group of compounds, including ***phylloquinone*** (K_1) and the ***menaquinones*** (K_2). Vitamin K is vital to the posttranslational modifications required to form *prothrombin*, an important clotting factor in the blood. The aromatic ring of vitamin K undergoes a cycle of oxidation and reduction during the formation of prothrombin. Vitamin K is also required to introduce calcium-binding sites on several calcium-dependent proteins.

MCAT CONCEPT CHECK 5.2

Before you move on, assess your understanding of the material with these questions.

1. How many carbons are in a diterpene?

___

2. What is the difference between a steroid and a steroid hormone?

___

3. NSAIDs block prostaglandin production in order to reduce pain and inflammation. What do prostaglandins do to bring about these symptoms?

___

4. What are the names and functions of the four fat-soluble vitamins?

Name	Function

5.3 Energy Storage

LEARNING OBJECTIVES

After Chapter 5.3, you will be able to:

- Explain why energy is more optimally stored as fat than as sugar
- Recall the structure and function of triacylglycerols
- Predict the products of saponification reactions:

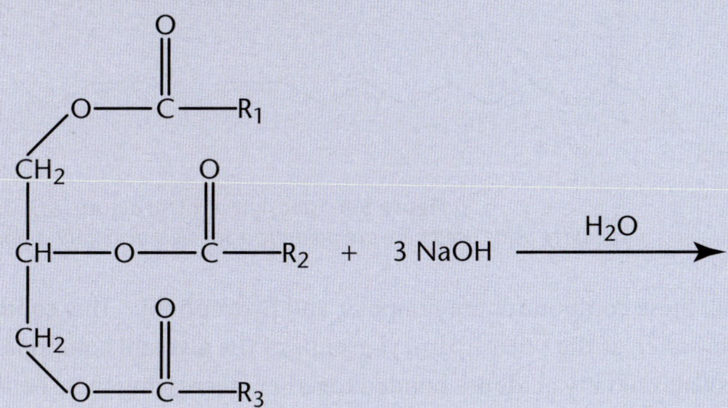

Triacylglycerols are a class of lipids specifically used for energy storage. From the body's point of view, lipids in general are a fantastic way to store energy. This is true for two major reasons. First, the carbon atoms of fatty acids are more reduced than those of sugars, which contain numerous alcohol groups. The result of this is that the oxidation of triacylglycerols yields twice the amount of energy per gram as carbohydrates, making this a far more energy-dense storage mechanism compared to polysaccharides like glycogen. Second, triacylglycerols are hydrophobic. They do not draw in water and do not require hydration for stability. This helps decrease their weight, especially in comparison to hydrophilic polysaccharides. One final perk for vertebrates surviving in colder temperatures (like penguins, polar bears, and arctic explorers) is that the layer of lipids serves a dual purpose of energy storage and insulation—it helps to retain body heat so that less energy is required to maintain a constant internal temperature.

Triacylglycerols

Triacylglycerols, also called **triglycerides**, are composed of three fatty acids bonded by ester linkages to glycerol, as shown in Figure 5.9. For most naturally occurring triacylglycerols, it is rare for all three fatty acids to be the same.

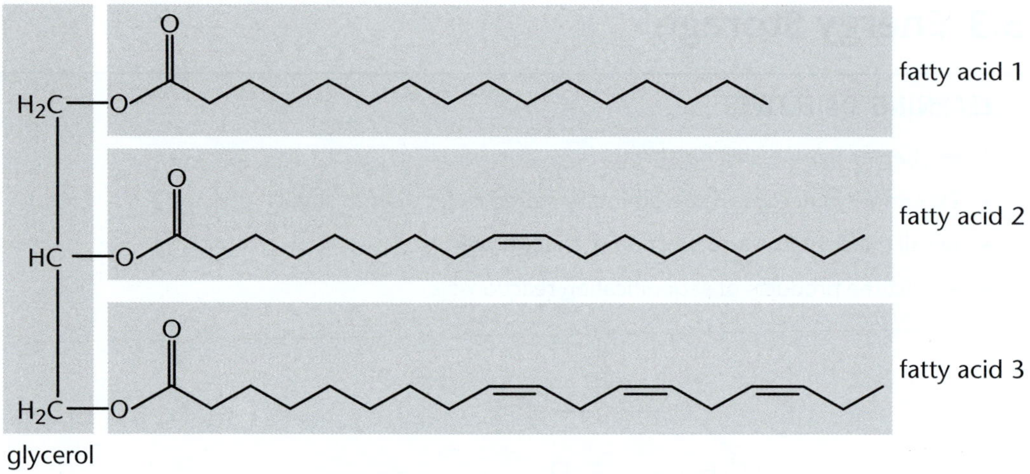

Figure 5.9 Triacylglycerol Structure
The fatty acids used here are palmitic acid, oleic acid, and α-linolenic acid.

Overall, these compounds are nonpolar and hydrophobic. This contributes to their insolubility in water, as the polar hydroxyl groups of the glycerol component and the polar carboxylates of fatty acids are bonded together, decreasing their polarity.

Triacylglycerol deposits can be observed in cells as oily droplets in the cytosol. These serve as depots of metabolic fuel that can be recruited when the cell needs additional energy to divide or survive when other fuel supplies are low. Special cells in animals, known as **adipocytes**, store large amounts of fat and are found primarily under the skin, around mammary glands, and in the abdominal cavity. In plants, triacylglycerol deposits are also found in seeds as oils. Triacylglycerols travel bidirectionally in the bloodstream between the liver and adipose tissue. The physical characteristics of triacylglycerols are primarily determined by the saturation (or unsaturation) of the fatty acid chains that make them up, much like phospholipids.

Free Fatty Acids and Saponification

Free fatty acids are unesterified fatty acids with a free carboxylate group. In the body, these circulate in the blood bonded noncovalently to serum albumin. Fatty acids also make up what we know as soap, which can be produced through a process called saponification.

Saponification is the ester hydrolysis of triacylglycerols using a strong base. Traditionally, the base that is used is **lye**, the common name for sodium or potassium hydroxide. The result is the basic cleavage of the fatty acid, leaving the sodium salt of the fatty acid and glycerol, as shown in Figure 5.10. The fatty acid salt is what we know as soap.

REAL WORLD

The two main methods of energy storage in the body are as triacylglycerols in adipose tissue or as carbohydrates in glycogen. Each method has its advantages and disadvantages. For example, glycogen offers access to metabolic energy in a faster water-soluble form; however, because of its low energy density, glycogen can only provide energy for a bit less than one day. In contrast, an individual who is moderately obese with 15 to 20 kg of stored triacylglycerols in adipocytes could draw upon fat stores for months, but it takes more time to mobilize this energy.

REAL WORLD

Saponification also occurs naturally, although more slowly, in corpses and oil paintings, as the triacylglycerols are hydrolyzed by naturally occurring bases. In corpses, the result of this process is known as *adipocere*, or grave wax.

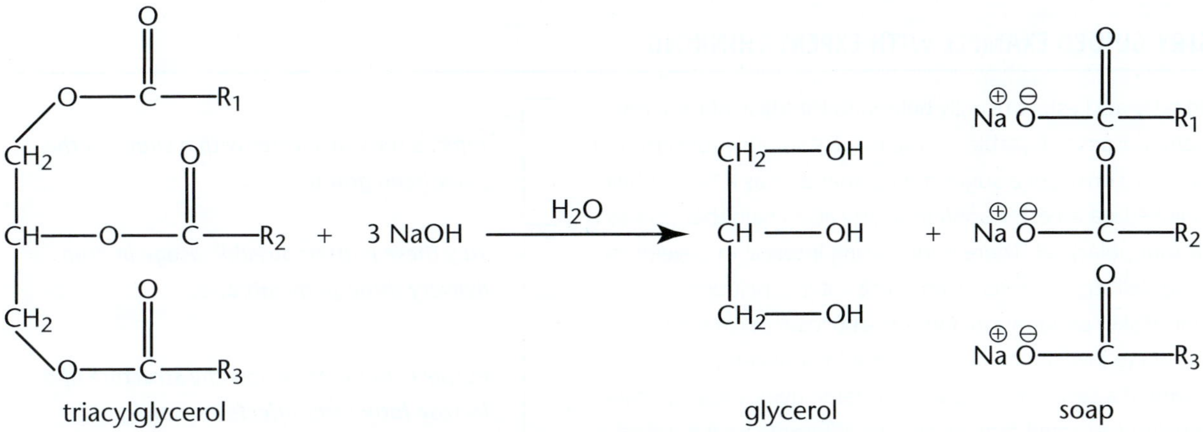

Figure 5.10 Saponification
Ester hydrolysis of a triacylglycerol using lye (NaOH)

Soaps can act as surfactants. A **surfactant** lowers the surface tension at the surface of a liquid, serving as a detergent or emulsifier. This is important to how soap works. If we try to combine an aqueous solution and oil, as with vinegar and olive oil in salad dressing, these solutions will remain in separate phases. If we were to add a soap, however, the two phases would appear to combine into a single phase, forming a **colloid**. This occurs because of the formation of **micelles**: tiny aggregates of soap with the hydrophobic tails turned inward and the hydrophilic heads turned outward, thereby shielding the hydrophobic lipid tails and allowing for overall solvation, as shown in Figure 5.11. We saw these earlier when we discussed membrane lipids.

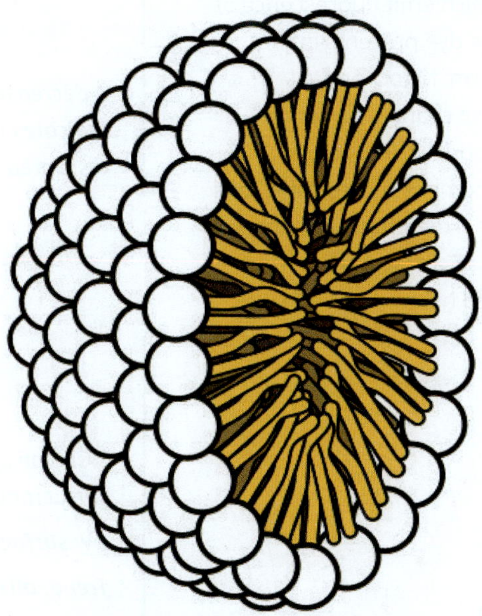

Figure 5.11 Cross-Section of a Micelle
Micelles organize in aqueous solution by forcing hydrophobic tails to the interior, allowing the hydrophilic heads to interact with water in the environment.

BIOCHEMISTRY GUIDED EXAMPLE WITH EXPERT THINKING

Sugar-based fatty acid esters usually belong to the class of non-ionic surfactants and possess desirable characteristics suitable for different applications. They consist of a sugar moiety that acts as a hydrophilic (polar) head linked via an ester bond to a fatty acid chain that acts as a hydrophobic (nonpolar) tail. There is increasing interest in developing advanced drug delivery systems using these esters, including enhancement of skin penetration and transmucosal permeability. This study aimed to investigate the relationship between the structure and activity of a series of lactose ester derivatives, enzymatically synthesized using saturated fatty acids with different chain lengths (C10–caprate; C12–laurate; C14–myristate; C16–palmitate).

Topic: a fatty acid ester with a sugar as the polar head group

Why these matter: possible usage in drug delivery through membranes

Purpose: to examine how the structure of a lactose fatty ester affects its activity

Solutions of each surfactant in water were prepared at varying concentrations and the surface tension was measured using a K100-Krüss force tensiometer with a platinum cylindrical rod probe of wetted length 1.6 mm at room temperature. The results are plotted in Figure 1 below. To examine the effect of lactose surfactants on the variation of mitochondrial membrane potential, the ratiometric dye JC-1 assay was employed. The JC-1 dye readily permeates across the cell plasma membrane where it specifically accumulates in active mitochondria, in a potential-dependent way. When present in the mitochondria, the dye forms J-aggregates, which emit fluorescence at a wavelength distinct from the wavelength the dye presents in the cytoplasm, where it remains in monomeric form. Mitochondrial depolarization, due to the dissipation of negative charges across the mitochondrial membrane because of mitochondrial disruption, is indicated by a decrease in the J-aggregate/monomer intensity ratio, thus representing an arbitrary value for mitochondrial membrane potential. The effect of different concentrations of lactose surfactants on the mitochondrial membrane potential is reported below (Figure 2).

They measured the surface tension of the different surfactants and plotted it in Fig 1

Mitochondrial membrane potential was measured in the presence of the different surfactants

A decrease in aggregate/monomer ratio indicates that the mitochondria has been disrupted

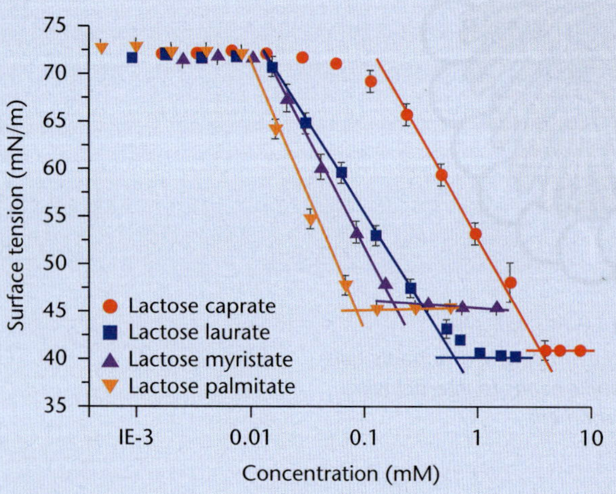

Figure 1

IVs: type of surfactant, concentration of surfactant; x-axis is a log-scale

DV: surface tension

Trend: all lines are a negative S-shaped curve; the greater the number of carbons, the lower the concentration required to decrease surface tension

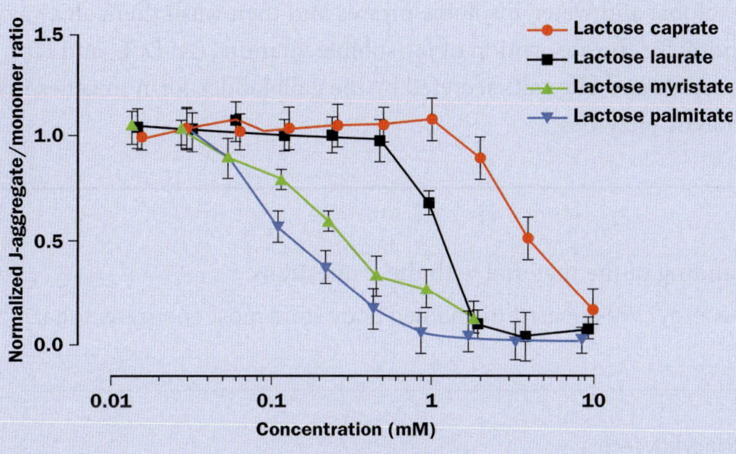

IVs: type of surfactant, concentration of surfactant; x-axis is again log-scale

DV: aggregate/monomer ratio

Trend: lines seem roughly negative S-shaped; the greater the number of carbons, the lower the concentration required to decrease the aggregate/monomer ratio

Figure 2

Adapted from Lucarini, S., Fagioli, L., Cavanagh, R., Liang, W., Perinelli, D. R., Campana, M., Stolnik, S., … Duranti, A. (2018). Synthesis, structure-activity relationships and in vitro toxicity profile of lactose-based fatty acid monoesters as possible drug permeability enhancers. *Pharmaceutics*, 10(3), 81. doi:10.3390/pharmaceutics10030081.

If the researchers were to examine cell viability in future experiments, which of the four surfactants would be expected to be the most cytotoxic?

The question asks us to predict the outcome of a future experiment, which indicates that we need to understand the results of the current experiment in order to predict future events. In the first paragraph, we see that the purpose of the passage is to discuss how these surfactants work as a function of the number of carbons attached to the sugar head group. From our outside knowledge we want to recall that surfactants have polar head groups, fatty acid tails, and often form micelles, allowing for nonpolar compounds (like many drugs!) to dissolve in the hydrophobic interior, while the surface-exposed portion of the micelle is water-soluble. Since the question specifically asks about the cytotoxic effects of the surfactants, we can mostly ignore Figure 1, as information about surface tension would not tell us if the surfactant was cytotoxic. Quickly assessing whether or not a figure is useful is an important skill for Test Day: not all of the figures will be valuable in answering every question. The measured variable in Figure 2 is the J-aggregate/monomer ratio, and the passage tells us that a drop in this ratio indicates that the potential across the mitochondrial membrane has been disrupted. We know from our content background that a proton gradient must be built across the inner mitochondrial membrane in order for ATP to be synthesized, and without that proton gradient the cell will quickly die due to a lack of energy. It's possible that the amphiphilic nature of the surfactant is "poking" holes into the inner mitochondrial membrane, allowing for the proton gradient to dissipate without moving through ATP synthase.

Figure 2 shows that increasing carbon number in the fatty acid tail corresponds with decreasing concentration required to dissipate the mitochondrial potential. Thus, we can predict that a longer fatty acid tail will be linked with greater cytotoxic activity. Specifically, we would expect lactose palmitate to be the most cytotoxic of the four surfactants studied in the current experiment.

Nonpolar compounds can dissolve in the hydrophobic interior of the water-soluble micelle, meaning that our cleaning agents can dissolve both water-soluble and water-insoluble messes and then wash them all away together. Micelles are also important in the body for the absorption of fat-soluble vitamins (A, D, E, and K) and complicated lipids such as *lecithins*. Fatty acids and bile salts secreted by the gallbladder form micelles that can increase the surface area available for lipolytic enzymes.

MCAT CONCEPT CHECK 5.3

Before you move on, assess your understanding of the material with these questions.

1. How does the human body store spare energy? Why doesn't the human body store most energy as sugar?

 ____

2. Describe the structure and function of triacylglycerols.

 ____

3. What bonds are broken during saponification?

 ____

4. Why does soap appear to dissolve in water, and how is this fact important to cleaning?

 ____

Conclusion

In this chapter, we examined the myriad biological functions performed by lipids. We first learned the structural functions of lipids, looking at the phospholipids that are the primary component of the phospholipid bilayer and other membrane lipids. Making our way through terpenes, we looked at the structure and function of signaling lipids, examining steroid hormones in particular. We looked into the fat-soluble vitamins and their downstream functions in the body. Finally, we summarized energy storage in the form of triacylglycerols and applied our acid–base chemistry knowledge to the formation of soap. In the next chapter, we turn our attention to the final class of biomolecules: nucleic acids.

GO ONLINE

You've reviewed the content, now test your knowledge and critical thinking skills by completing a test-like passage set in your online resources!

CONCEPT SUMMARY

Structural Lipids

- Lipids are insoluble in water and soluble in nonpolar organic solvents.
- **Phospholipids** are amphipathic and form the bilayer of biological membranes.
  - They contain a hydrophilic (polar) head group and hydrophobic (nonpolar) tails.
  - The head group is attached by a **phosphodiester linkage** and, because it interacts with the environment, determines the function of the phospholipid.
  - The **saturation** of the fatty acid tails determines the fluidity of the membrane; saturated fatty acids are less fluid than unsaturated ones. Fatty acids form most of the structural thickness of the phospholipid bilayer.
  - **Glycerophospholipids** are phospholipids that contain a glycerol backbone.
- **Sphingolipids** contain a sphingosine or sphingoid backbone.
  - Many (but not all) sphingolipids are also phospholipids, containing a phosphodiester bond; these are termed **sphingophospholipids**.
  - **Sphingomyelins** are the major class of sphingophospholipids and contain a phosphatidylcholine or phosphatidylethanolamine head group. They are a major component of the myelin sheath.
  - **Glycosphingolipids** are attached to sugar moieties instead of a phosphate group. **Cerebrosides** have one sugar connected to sphingosine; **globosides** have two or more.
  - **Gangliosides** contain oligosaccharides with at least one terminal ***N*-acetylneuraminic acid** (**NANA**; also called **sialic acid**).
- **Waxes** contain long-chain fatty acids esterified to long-chain alcohols. They are used as protection against evaporation and parasites in plants and animals.

Signaling Lipids

- **Terpenes** are odiferous steroid precursors made from **isoprene**, a five-carbon molecule.
  - One terpene unit (a **monoterpene**) contains two isoprene units.
  - **Terpenoids** are derived from terpenes via oxygenation or backbone rearrangement. They have similar odorous characteristics.
- **Steroids** contain three cyclohexane rings and one cyclopentane ring. Their oxidation state and functional groups may vary.
  - **Steroid hormones** have high-affinity receptors, work at low concentrations, and affect gene expression and metabolism.
  - **Cholesterol** is a steroid important to membrane fluidity and stability; it serves as a precursor to a host of other molecules.
- **Prostaglandins** are autocrine and paracrine signaling molecules that regulate cAMP levels. They have powerful effects on smooth muscle contraction, body temperature, the sleep–wake cycle, fever, and pain.
- The fat-soluble vitamins include vitamins A, D, E, and K.
  - **Vitamin A** (**carotene**) is metabolized to **retinal** for vision and **retinoic acid** for gene expression in epithelial development.

- **Vitamin D** (**cholecalciferol**) is metabolized to **calcitriol** in the kidneys and regulates calcium and phosphorus homeostasis in the intestines (increasing calcium and phosphate absorption), promoting bone formation. A deficiency of vitamin D causes **rickets**.
- **Vitamin E** (**tocopherols**) act as biological antioxidants. Their aromatic rings destroy free radicals, preventing oxidative damage.
- **Vitamin K** (**phylloquinone** and **menaquinones**) is important for formation of prothrombin, a clotting factor. It performs posttranslational modifications on a number of proteins, creating calcium-binding sites.

Energy Storage

- **Triacylglycerols** (**triglycerides**) are the preferred method of storing energy for long-term use.
  - They contain one glycerol attached to three fatty acids by ester bonds. The fatty acids usually vary within the same triacylglycerol.
  - The carbon atoms in lipids are more reduced than carbohydrates, giving twice as much energy per gram during oxidation.
  - Triacylglycerols are very hydrophobic, so they are not hydrated by body water and do not carry additional water weight.
- Animal cells specifically used for storage of large triacylglycerol deposits are called **adipocytes**.
- Free fatty acids are unesterified fatty acids that travel in the bloodstream. Salts of free fatty acids are **soaps** and can be synthesized in saponification.
  - **Saponification** is the ester hydrolysis of triacylglycerols using a strong base, like sodium or potassium hydroxide.
  - Soaps act as surfactants, forming micelles. A **micelle** can dissolve a lipid-soluble molecule in its fatty acid core, and washes away with water because of its shell of carboxylate head groups.

ANSWERS TO CONCEPT CHECKS

5.1

1. Membrane lipids are amphipathic: they have hydrophilic heads and hydrophobic tails, allowing for the formation of bilayers in aqueous solution. The fatty acid tails form the bulk of the phospholipid bilayer, and play a predominantly structural role. On the other hand, the functional differences between membrane lipids are determined by the polar head group, due to its constant exposure to the exterior environment of the phospholipid bilayer (remember, this can be either the inside or outside of the cell). The degree of unsaturation of fatty acid tails can also play a small role in function.
2. The difference is the bond between the sphingosine backbone and the head group. When this is a phosphodiester bond, it's a phospholipid (note the *phospho–* prefixes). Nonphospholipid sphingolipids include glycolipids, which contain a glycosidic linkage to a sugar.
3.

Type	Phospholipid or Glycolipid?	Functional Group(s)
Sphingomyelin	Phospholipid	Phosphatidylethanolamine/ phosphatidylcholine
Glycosphingolipid	Glycolipid	Sugars (mono- or polysaccharide)
Ganglioside	Glycolipid	Oligosaccharides and *N*-acetylneuraminic acid (NANA)

4. In a nonpolar solvent, we would see the opposite of what happens in a polar solvent like water: the hydrophilic, polar part of the molecules would be sequestered inside, while the nonpolar, hydrophobic part of the molecules would be found on the exterior and exposed to the solvent.

5.2

1. A diterpene has 20 carbon molecules in its backbone. One terpene unit is made from two isoprene units, each of which has five carbons.
2. A steroid is defined by its structure: it includes three cyclohexane rings and a cyclopentane ring. A steroid hormone is a molecule within this class that also functions as a hormone, meaning that it travels in the bloodstream, is active at low concentrations, has high-affinity receptors, and affects gene expression and metabolism.
3. Prostaglandins regulate the synthesis of cAMP, which is involved in many pathways, including those that drive pain and inflammation.

4.

Name	Function
A (carotene)	As retinal: vision; as retinoic acid: epithelial development
D (cholecalciferol)	As calcitriol: calcium and phosphate regulation
E (tocopherols)	Antioxidants, using aromatic ring
K (phylloquinone and menaquinones)	Posttranslational modification of prothrombin, addition of calcium-binding sites on many proteins

5.3

1. The human body stores energy as glycogen and triacylglycerols. Triacylglycerols are preferred because their carbons are more reduced, resulting in a larger amount of energy yield per unit weight. In addition, due to their hydrophobic nature, triacylglycerols do not need to carry extra weight from hydration.
2. Triacylglycerols, also called triglycerides, are composed of a glycerol backbone esterified to three fatty acids. They are used for energy storage.
3. The ester bonds of triacylglycerols are broken to form a glycerol molecule and the salts of fatty acids (soap).
4. Soap appears to dissolve in water because amphipathic free fatty acid salts form micelles, with hydrophobic fatty acid tails toward the center and carboxylate groups facing outward toward the water. Fat-soluble particles can then dissolve inside micelles in the soap–water solution and wash away. Water-soluble compounds can freely dissolve in the water.

SCIENCE MASTERY ASSESSMENT EXPLANATIONS

1. **D**

Glycolipids contain sugar moieties connected to their backbone. Sphingomyelin is not a glycolipid, but rather a phospholipid. This class can either have phosphatidylcholine or phosphatidylethanolamine as a head group and therefore contains a phosphodiester, not glycosidic, bond.

2. **B**

Saponification is the ester hydrolysis of triacylglycerol using a strong base like sodium or potassium hydroxide to form glycerol and fatty acid salts. This is not a condensation reaction, as in **(A)**, but a cleavage reaction. Fatty acids do travel in the body bonded to serum albumin, as in **(D)**, but that is unrelated to the process of saponification.

3. **B**

The basic backbone of steroid structure contains three cyclohexane rings and one cyclopentane ring. Although the oxidation status of these rings varies for different steroids, the overall structure does not, as in **(C)**.

4. **B**

Fatty acid salt micelles are responsible for the formation of soap bubbles. While phospholipids can form bilayers, as in **(C)**, the fatty acids in soap are free fatty acids, not phospholipids.

5. **C**

Steroid hormones are produced in endocrine glands and travel in the bloodstream to bind high-affinity receptors in the nucleus. The hormone's receptor binds to DNA as part of the hormone–receptor complex, but the hormone itself does not.

6. **C**

Triacylglycerols are highly hydrophobic and therefore not highly hydrated (which would add extra weight from the water of hydration, taking away from the energy density of these molecules), eliminating **(A)**. The fatty acid chains produce twice as much energy as polysaccharides during oxidation because they are highly reduced. The fatty acid chains vary in length and saturation.

7. **C**

Vitamin A is metabolized to retinal, which is important for sight. Vitamin D is metabolized to calcitriol, which is important for calcium regulation. Vitamin E is made up of tocopherols, which are biological antioxidants. Vitamin K is necessary for the introduction of calcium binding sites, such as during the posttranslational modification of prothrombin.

8. **C**

Phospholipids are amphipathic, as are fatty acid salts. Although amphipathic molecules take spherical forms with hydrophobic molecules interior in aqueous solution, as in **(A)**, the opposite would be true in a nonpolar solvent. **(B)** describes phospholipids and sphingolipids, and **(D)** describes triacylglycerols and phospholipids; both groups do not include fatty acid salts.

9. **B**

Sphingolipids can either have a phosphodiester bond, and therefore be phospholipids, or have a glycosidic linkage and therefore be glycolipids. Not all sphingolipids have a sphingosine backbone, as in statement II; some have related (sphingoid) compounds as backbones instead.

10. **C**

More saturated fatty acids make for a less fluid solution. This is because they can pack more tightly and form more noncovalent bonds, resulting in more energy being needed to disrupt the overall structure.

11. **B**

Glycerophospholipids are a subset of phospholipids, as are sphingomyelins. Glycerophospholipids are never sphingolipids because they contain a glycerol backbone (rather than sphingosine or a sphingoid backbone), eliminating **(A)**. Sphingolipids are used in the ABO blood typing system, eliminating **(C)**. Glycerophospholipids have a polar head group, glycerol, and two fatty acid tails, not one, as in **(D)**.

12. **C**

A triterpene is made of six isoprene moieties (remember, one terpene unit contains two isoprene units), and therefore has a 30-carbon backbone.

13. **B**

Cholesterol is a steroid hormone precursor that has variable effects on membrane fluidity depending on temperature, eliminating **(A)**. It interacts with both the hydrophobic tails and the hydrophilic heads of membrane lipids, nullifying **(D)**. It is also a precursor for vitamin D (not vitamin A), which can be produced in the skin in a UV-driven reaction, eliminating **(C)**.

14. **D**

Prostaglandins are paracrine or autocrine signaling molecules, not endocrine—they affect regions close to where they are produced, rather than affecting the entire body. Think of the swelling that happens when you bash your knee into your desk: your knee will swell, become discolored, and possibly bruise. Luckily, however, your entire body won't swell as well.

15. **B**

Waxes are also produced in animals for similar protective functions. Cerumen, or earwax, is a prime example in humans.

GO ONLINE

Consult your online resources for additional practice.

SHARED CONCEPTS

Biochemistry Chapter 2
Enzymes

Biochemistry Chapter 8
Biological Membranes

Biochemistry Chapter 11
Lipid and Amino Acid Metabolism

Biology Chapter 5
The Endocrine System

Biology Chapter 9
The Digestive System

Organic Chemistry Chapter 8
Carboxylic Acids

CHAPTER 6

DNA AND BIOTECHNOLOGY

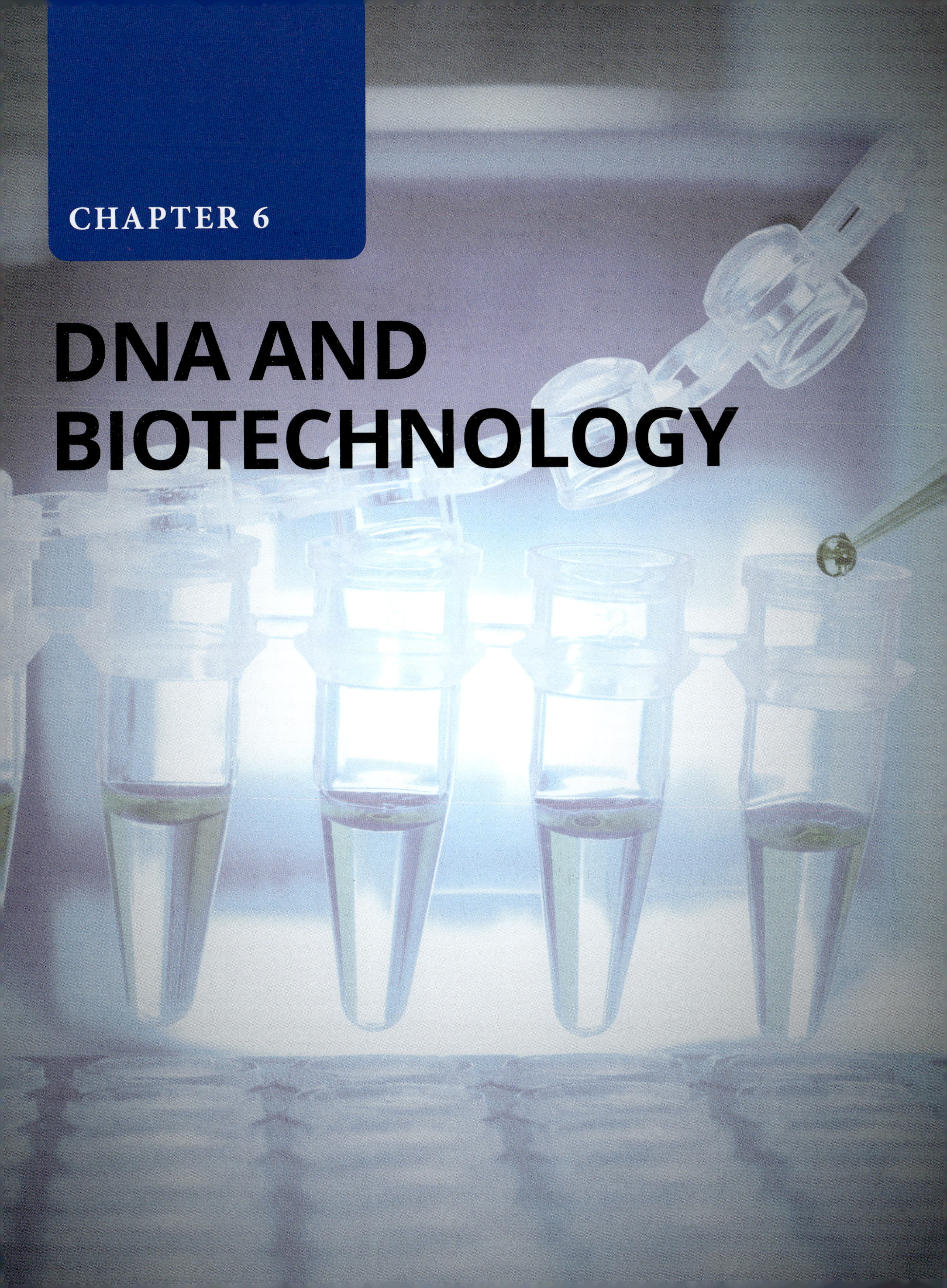

SCIENCE MASTERY ASSESSMENT

Every pre-med knows this feeling: there is so much content I have to know for the MCAT! How do I know what to do first or what's important?

While the high-yield badges throughout this book will help you identify the most important topics, this Science Mastery Assessment is another tool in your MCAT prep arsenal. This quiz (which can also be taken in your online resources) and the guidance below will help ensure that you are spending the appropriate amount of time on this chapter based on your personal strengths and weaknesses. Don't worry though—skipping something now does not mean you'll never study it. Later on in your prep, as you complete full-length tests, you'll uncover specific pieces of content that you need to review and can come back to these chapters as appropriate.

How to Use This Assessment

If you answer 0–7 questions correctly:

Spend about 1 hour to read this chapter in full and take limited notes throughout. Follow up by reviewing **all** quiz questions to ensure that you now understand how to solve each one.

If you answer 8–11 questions correctly:

Spend 20–40 minutes reviewing the quiz questions. Beginning with the questions you missed, read and take notes on the corresponding subchapters. For questions you answered correctly, ensure your thinking matches that of the explanation and you understand why each choice was correct or incorrect.

If you answer 12–15 questions correctly:

Spend less than 20 minutes reviewing all questions from the quiz. If you missed any, then include a quick read-through of the corresponding subchapters, or even just the relevant content within a subchapter, as part of your question review. For questions you got correct, ensure your thinking matches that of the explanation and review the Concept Summary at the end of the chapter.

1. In a single strand of a nucleic acid, nucleotides are linked by:
   - **A.** hydrogen bonds.
   - **B.** phosphodiester bonds.
   - **C.** ionic bonds.
   - **D.** van der Waals forces.

2. Which of the following statements regarding differences between DNA and RNA is FALSE?
   - **A.** In cells, DNA is double-stranded, whereas RNA is single-stranded.
   - **B.** DNA uses the nitrogenous base thymine; RNA uses uracil.
   - **C.** The sugar in DNA is deoxyribose; the sugar in RNA is ribose.
   - **D.** DNA strands replicate in a 5′ to 3′ direction, whereas RNA is synthesized in a 3′ to 5′ direction.

3. Which of the following DNA sequences would have the highest melting temperature?
   - **A.** CGCAACCATCCG
   - **B.** CGCAATAATACA
   - **C.** CGTAATAATACA
   - **D.** CATAACAAATCA

4. Which of the following biomolecules is LEAST likely to contain an aromatic ring?
   - **A.** Proteins
   - **B.** Purines
   - **C.** Carbohydrates
   - **D.** Pyrimidines

5. For a compound to be aromatic, all of the following must be true EXCEPT:
   - **A.** the molecule is cyclic.
   - **B.** the molecule contains $4n + 2$ π electrons.
   - **C.** the molecule contains alternating single and double bonds.
   - **D.** the molecule is planar.

6. Which of the following enzymes is NOT involved in DNA replication?
   - **A.** Primase
   - **B.** DNA ligase
   - **C.** RNA polymerase I
   - **D.** Telomerase

7. How is cDNA best characterized?
   - **A.** cDNA results from a DNA transcript with noncoding regions removed.
   - **B.** cDNA results from the reverse transcription of processed mRNA.
   - **C.** cDNA is the abbreviation for deoxycytosine.
   - **D.** cDNA is the circular DNA molecule that forms the bacterial genome.

8. Which of the following statements regarding polymerase chain reaction is FALSE?
   - **A.** Human DNA polymerase is used because it is the most accurate.
   - **B.** A primer must be prepared with a complementary sequence to part of the DNA of interest.
   - **C.** Repeated heating and cooling cycles allow the enzymes to act specifically and replaces helicase.
   - **D.** Each cycle of the polymerase chain reaction doubles the amount of DNA of interest.

9. Endonucleases are used for which of the following?
   - **I.** Gene therapy
   - **II.** Southern blotting
   - **III.** DNA repair
   - **A.** I only
   - **B.** II only
   - **C.** II and III only
   - **D.** I, II, and III

10. How does prokaryotic DNA differ from eukaryotic DNA?

I. Prokaryotic DNA lacks nucleosomes.

II. Eukaryotic DNA has telomeres.

III. Prokaryotic DNA is replicated by a different DNA polymerase.

IV. Eukaryotic DNA is circular when not restricted by centromeres.

A. I only
B. IV only
C. II and III only
D. I, II, and III only

11. Why might uracil be excluded from DNA but NOT RNA?

A. Uracil is much more difficult to synthesize than thymine.
B. Uracil binds adenine too strongly for replication.
C. Cytosine degradation results in uracil.
D. Uracil is used as a DNA synthesis activator.

12. Tumor suppressor genes are most likely to result in cancer through:

A. loss of function mutations.
B. gain of function mutations.
C. overexpression.
D. proto-oncogene formation.

13. Which of the following is an ethical concern of gene sequencing?

A. Gene sequencing is invasive, thus the potential health risks must be thoroughly explained.
B. Gene sequencing impacts relatives, thus privacy concerns may be raised.
C. Gene sequencing is very inaccurate, which increases anxiety related to findings.
D. Gene sequencing can provide false-negative results, giving a false sense of security.

14. Which of the following is NOT a difference between heterochromatin and euchromatin?

A. Euchromatin has areas that can be transcribed, whereas heterochromatin is silent.
B. Heterochromatin is tightly packed, whereas euchromatin is less dense.
C. Heterochromatin stains darkly, whereas euchromatin stains lightly.
D. Heterochromatin is found in the nucleus, whereas euchromatin is in the cytoplasm.

15. During which phase of the cell cycle are DNA repair mechanisms least active?

A. G_1
B. S
C. G_2
D. M

Answer Key

1. **B** (See section 6.1)
2. **D** (See section 6.1)
3. **A** (See section 6.1)
4. **C** (See section 6.1)
5. **C** (See section 6.1)
6. **C** (See section 6.3)
7. **B** (See section 6.5)
8. **A** (See section 6.5)
9. **D** (See section 6.5)
10. **D** (See section 6.2)
11. **C** (See section 6.4)
12. **A** (See section 6.4)
13. **B** (See section 6.5)
14. **D** (See section 6.2)
15. **D** (See section 6.3)

The relevant section of the chapter to review for each question is given in parentheses after the correct answer. Detailed explanations can be found at the end of the chapter.

CHAPTER 6

DNA AND BIOTECHNOLOGY

In This Chapter

CHAPTER PROFILE

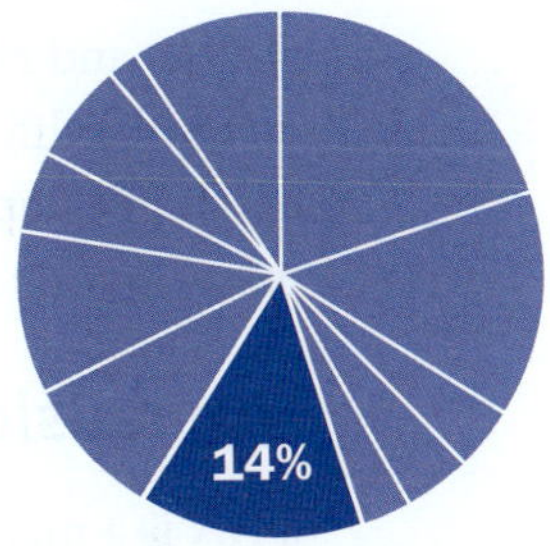

The content in this chapter should be relevant to about 14% of all questions about biochemistry on the MCAT.

This chapter covers material from the following AAMC content categories:

1B: Transmission of genetic information from the gene to the protein

5D: Structure, function, and reactivity of biologically-relevant molecules

Introduction

How do all of the cells of our body know what job to do? The cells that make up the human body have nucleic acids that instruct the cell on how to function. The nucleic acid *deoxyribonucleic acid* (DNA) stores the information in our cells and selectively shares that information when appropriate. DNA is a molecule that can be passed from generation to generation. DNA can be replicated in a carefully regulated process designed to keep the genome safe from degradation and free from errors. Seemingly small changes in the genetic code can result in life-threatening and even life-incompatible alterations to protein structure and function. In this chapter, the unique structure of DNA will be discussed, along with replication and repair processes. The primary focus will be on eukaryotic processes, but there will be some review of prokaryotic genetics to help us better understand the molecular basis of life.

Much of the advancement of medicine in the past two decades has been due to our increased understanding of molecular genetics, which has led to the creation of an entire biotechnology industry centered around genomics and the utilization of nucleic acids for various diagnostic tests and therapeutic interventions. We will also take a look at some of these important principles in this chapter.

6.1 DNA Structure High Yield

LEARNING OBJECTIVES

After Chapter 6.1, you will be able to:

- Identify the structures of, and distinguish the differences between, nucleotides and nucleosides
- Recognize the key features and rules of purine and pyrimidine structure and pairing
- Recall the structural differences between DNA and RNA molecules

There are two chemically distinct forms of nucleic acids within eukaryotic cells. **Deoxyribonucleic acid (DNA)** and **ribonucleic acid (RNA)** are polymers, each with distinct roles, that together create the molecules integral to life in all living organisms. DNA is the focus of this chapter and RNA will be discussed in more detail in Chapter 7 of *MCAT Biochemistry Review*. The bulk of DNA is found in chromosomes in the nucleus of eukaryotic cells, although some is also present in mitochondria and chloroplasts.

Nucleosides and Nucleotides

DNA is a macromolecule and it is essential to understand how this molecule is constructed. DNA is a *polydeoxyribonucleotide* that is composed of many *monodeoxyribonucleotides* linked together. The nomenclature of nucleic acids can be complicated, so the terms have been defined here:

- **Nucleosides** are composed of a five-carbon sugar (*pentose*) bonded to a nitrogenous base and are formed by covalently linking the base to C-1′ of the sugar, as shown in Figure 6.1. Note that the carbon atoms in the sugar are labeled with a prime symbol to distinguish them from the carbon atoms in the nitrogenous base.
- **Nucleotides** are formed when one or more phosphate groups are attached to C-5′ of a nucleoside. Often these molecules are named according to the number of phosphates present. Adenosine di- and triphosphate (ADP and ATP), for example, gain their names from the number of phosphate groups attached to the nucleoside adenosine. These are high-energy compounds because of the energy associated with the repulsion between closely associated negative charges on the phosphate groups, as shown in Figure 6.2. Nucleotides are the building blocks of DNA.

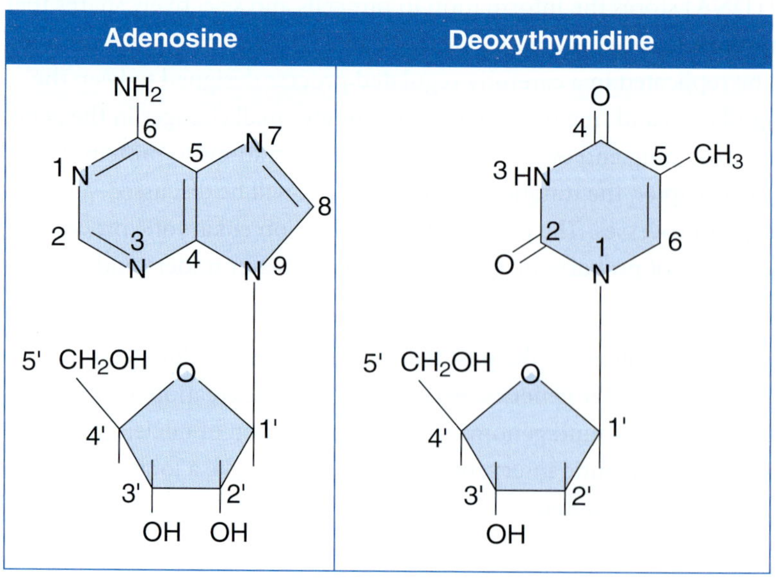

Figure 6.1 Examples of Nucleosides

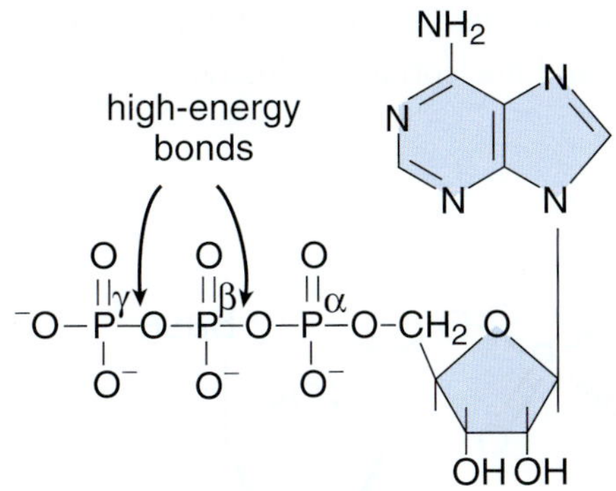

Figure 6.2 High-Energy Bonds in Adenosine Triphosphate, a Nucleotide

Nucleic acids are classified according to the pentose they contain, as shown in Figure 6.3. If the pentose is **ribose**, the nucleic acid is RNA; if the pentose is **deoxyribose** (ribose with the 2′ –OH group replaced by –H), then it is DNA.

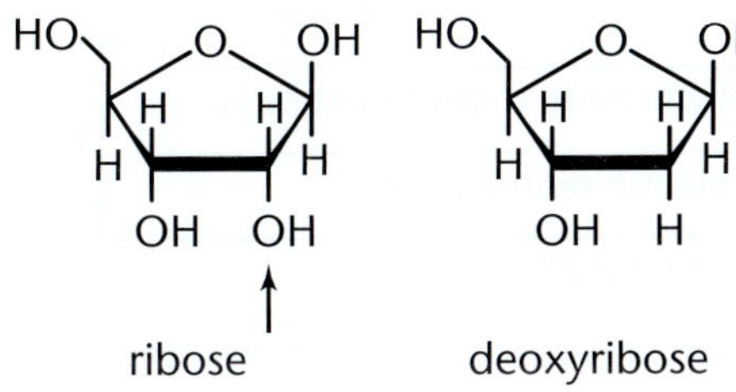

Figure 6.3 Ribose and Deoxyribose
Ribose has an –OH group at C-2; deoxyribose has an –H.

BRIDGE

In Chapter 3 of *MCAT General Chemistry Review*, we learned that bond breaking is usually endothermic and bond making is usually exothermic. ATP offers a biologically relevant—and MCAT tested—exception to this rule. Due to all the negative charges in close proximity, removing the terminal phosphate from ATP actually releases energy, which powers our cells.

The nomenclature for the common bases, nucleosides, and nucleotides is shown in Table 6.1.

Base	RNA Names (Nucleoside/ Nucleotide)	RNA Acronyms	DNA Names (Nucleoside/ Nucleotide)	DNA Acronyms
Adenine	Adenosine/ Adenylate	AMP, ADP, ATP	Deoxyadenosine/ Deoxyadenylate	dAMP, dADP, dATP
Guanine	Guanosine/ Guanylate	GMP, GDP, GTP	Deoxyguanosine/ Deoxyguanylate	dGMP, dGDP, dGTP
Cytosine	Cytidine/Cytidylate	CMP, CDP, CTP	Deoxycytidine/ Deoxycytidylate	dCMP, dCDP, dCTP
Uracil	Uridine/Uridylate	UMP, UDP, UTP	N/A	N/A
Thymine	N/A	N/A	Deoxythymidine/ Deoxythymidylate	dTMP, dTDP, dTTP

Table 6.1 Nomenclature of Important Bases, Nucleosides, and Nucleotides

Note that there is no *thymidine* listed (only *deoxythymidine*) because thymine appears almost exclusively in DNA. A structural comparison of nucleosides and nucleotides is illustrated in Figure 6.4.

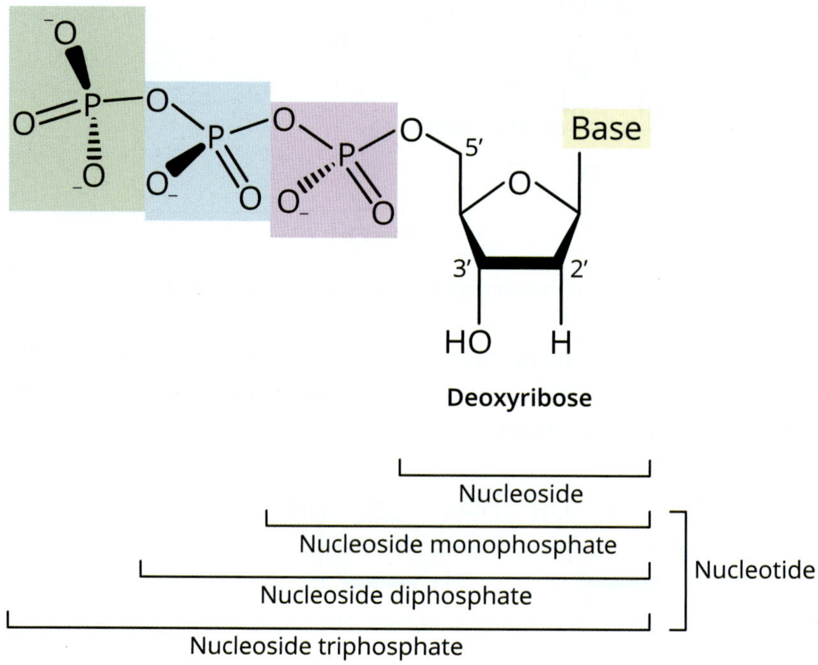

Figure 6.4 Structure of Nucleosides and Nucleotides

Sugar–Phosphate Backbone

The backbone of DNA is composed of alternating sugar and phosphate groups; it determines the directionality of the DNA and is always read from 5′ to 3′. It is formed as nucleotides are joined by 3′–5′ phosphodiester bonds. That is, a phosphate group links the 3′ carbon of one sugar to the 5′ phosphate group of the next incoming sugar in the chain. Phosphates carry a negative charge; thus, DNA and RNA strands have an overall negative charge.

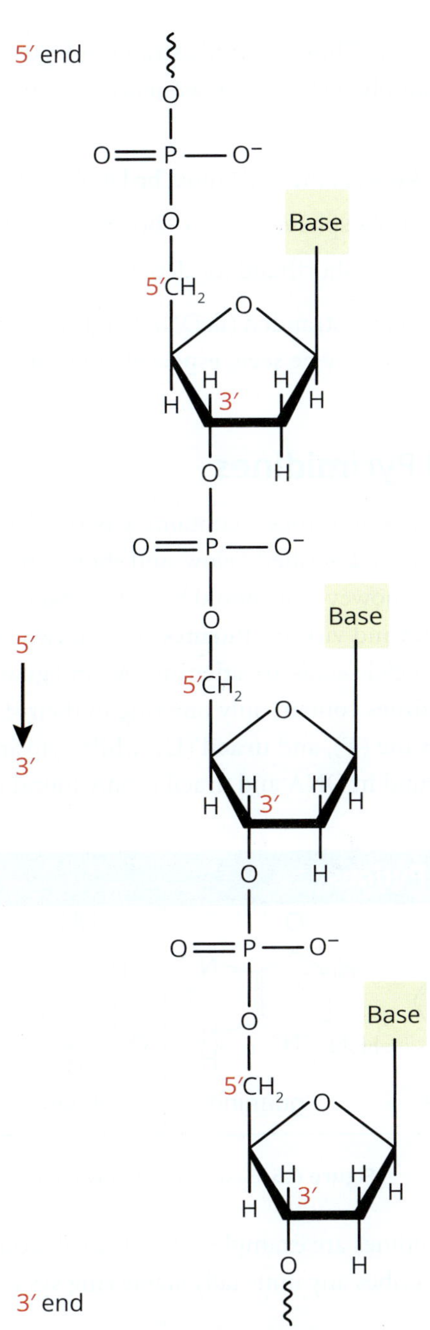

Figure 6.5 DNA Strand Polarity
DNA strands run antiparallel to one another; enzymes that replicate and transcribe DNA only work in the 5' to 3' direction.

Each strand of DNA has distinct 5′ and 3′ ends, creating polarity within the backbone, as shown in Figure 6.5. The 5′ end of DNA, for instance, will have an –OH or phosphate group bonded to C-5′ of the sugar, while the 3′ end has a free –OH on C-3′ of the sugar. The base sequence of a nucleic acid strand is both written and read in the 5′ to 3′ direction. Thus, the DNA strand in Figure 6.5 must be written: 5′—ATG—3′ (or simply ATG). DNA sequences can also be written in slightly different ways:

- If written backwards, the ends must be labeled: 3′—GTA—5′
- The position of phosphates may be shown: pApTpG
- "d" may be used as shorthand for deoxyribose: dAdTdG

DNA is generally double-stranded (dsDNA) and RNA is generally single-stranded (ssRNA). Exceptions to this rule may be seen, especially in viruses, as described in Chapter 1 of *MCAT Biology Review*.

MCAT EXPERTISE

On the MCAT, always check nucleic acids for polarity. One of the easiest ways to generate incorrect answers is to simply reverse the reading frame: 3′—GATTACA—5′ is not the same as 3′—ACATTAG—5′.

Purines and Pyrimidines

There are two families of nitrogen-containing bases found in nucleotides: purines and pyrimidines. The bases described below, and shown in Figure 6.6, represent the common bases in eukaryotes; however, it should be noted that exceptions may be seen in tRNA and in some prokaryotes and viruses. **Purines** contain two rings in their structure. The two purines found in nucleic acids are **adenine** (**A**) and **guanine** (**G**); both are found in DNA and RNA. **Pyrimidines** contain only one ring in their structure. The three pyrimidines are **cytosine** (**C**), **thymine** (**T**), and **uracil** (**U**); while cytosine is found in both DNA and RNA, thymine is only found in DNA and uracil is only found in RNA.

MNEMONIC

To remember the types and structures of these two classes of nitrogenous bases, remember to **CUT** the **PY**e (as **C, U,** and **T** are **py**rimidines). You can also note that pie has one ring of crust, and pyrimidines have only one ring in their structure. You can also remember **PUR**e **A**s **G**old (as **A** and **G** are **pur**ines); think of gold wedding rings. It takes two gold rings at a wedding, just like purines have two rings in their structure.

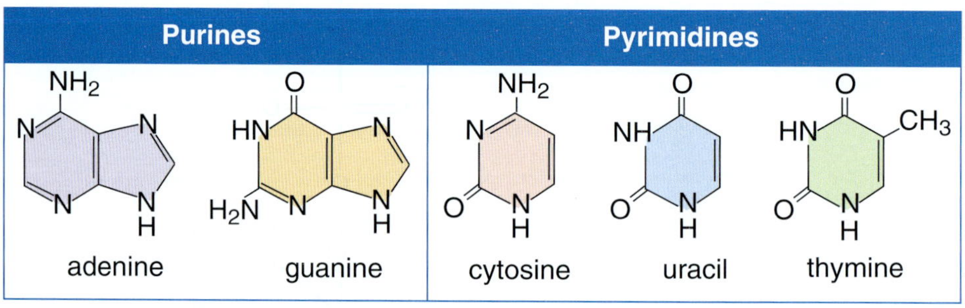

Figure 6.6 Bases Commonly Found in Nucleic Acids

Purines and pyrimidines are examples of biological aromatic heterocycles. In chemistry, the term **aromatic** describes any unusually stable ring system that adheres to the following four specific rules:

1. The compound is cyclic.
2. The compound is planar.
3. The compound is conjugated (has alternating single and multiple bonds, or lone pairs, creating at least one unhybridized *p*-orbital for each atom in the ring).
4. The compound has $4n + 2$ (where n is any integer) π electrons. This is called **Hückel's rule**.

The most common example of an aromatic compound is benzene, but many different structures obey these rules. In an aromatic compound, the extra stability is due to the delocalized π electrons, which can travel throughout the entire compound using available molecular orbitals. All six of the carbon atoms in benzene are sp^2-hybridized, and each of the six orbitals overlaps equally with its two neighbors. As a result, the delocalized electrons form two π electron clouds (one above and one below the plane of the ring), as shown in Figure 6.7. This delocalization is characteristic of all aromatic molecules, and because of this, aromatic molecules are fairly unreactive.

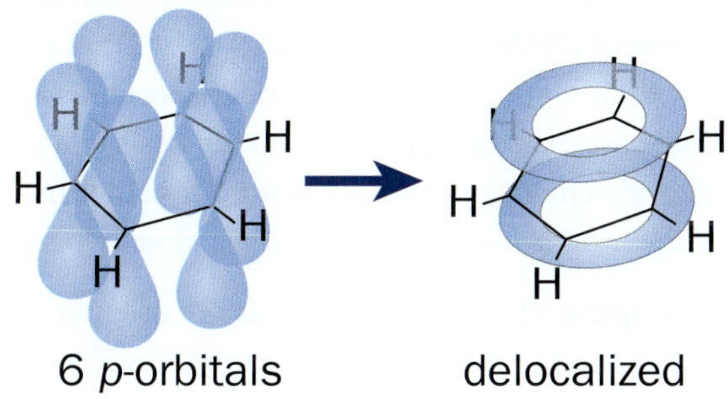

Figure 6.7 Delocalization of π Electrons in Benzene

Heterocycles are ring structures that contain at least two different elements in the ring. As shown in Figure 6.6 earlier, both purines and pyrimidines contain nitrogen in their aromatic rings. Nucleic acids are thus imbued with exceptional stability. This helps to explain the utility of nucleotides as the molecule for storing genetic information. A **furan** is a heterocyclic compound that is a five-membered aromatic ring containing one oxygen atom and four carbon atoms. Compounds that contain these rings are referred to as furans. **Pyridine** is another type of heterocyclic compound, but has the chemical formula C_5H_5N. The molecule is similar in structure to benzene, with one of the carbons in the ring substituted with a nitrogen atom instead.

Nucleotides can also undergo **pi stacking**, which is a type of non-covalent attractive interaction between two aromatic rings. The most commonly observed types of pi stacking, which are shown in Figure 6.8, are **staggered stacking** (also called **parallel displaced**) and **pi-teeing** (also called **T-shaped**). In staggered stacking, the aromatic rings are parallel to one another but are not directly overlapping, with one aromatic ring slightly offset from the other. In this formation, carbon atoms that have a partial negative charge are placed above hydrogen atoms with a partial positive charge, leading to an attractive electrostatic interaction. In pi-teeing, one aromatic ring is perpendicular to the other aromatic ring to form a T shape, which similarly aligns partially-negative carbon atoms with partially-positive hydrogen atoms.

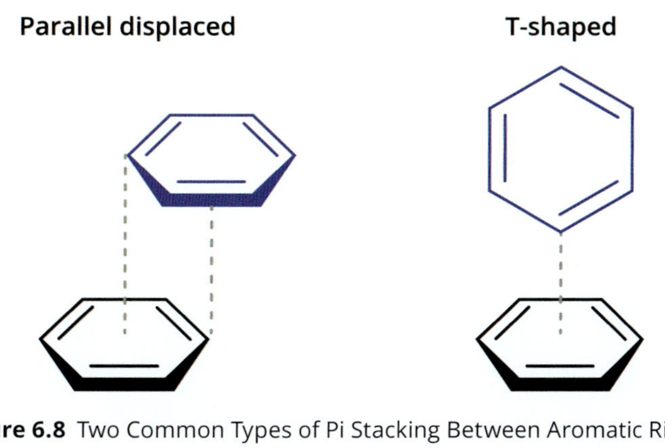

Figure 6.8 Two Common Types of Pi Stacking Between Aromatic Rings

The staggered formation is an important contributor of nucleobase stacking within DNA and RNA polynucleotide strands, which increases structural stability. Staggered stacking and pi-teeing formations are also commonly found between amino acids with aromatic side chains, which, along with other types of molecular interactions, can help drive protein folding.

Watson–Crick Model

Putting this information together, we can start looking at the **Watson–Crick model** of DNA structure. In 1953, James Watson and Francis Crick presented one of the landmark findings of modern biology and medicine: the three-dimensional structure of DNA. With X-ray patterns of DNA produced by Rosalind Franklin laying the necessary foundation for their work, Watson and Crick were able to deduce the double-helical nature of DNA and propose specific base-pairing that would be the basis of a copying mechanism. In the **double helix**, two linear polynucleotide chains of DNA are wound together in a spiral orientation along a common axis. The key features of the model—some of which have already been mentioned—are:

- The two strands of DNA are antiparallel; that is, the strands are oriented in opposite directions. When one strand has polarity 5′ to 3′ *down* the page, the other strand has 5′ to 3′ polarity *up* the page.
- The sugar–phosphate backbone is on the outside of the helix with the nitrogenous bases on the inside.
- There are specific base-pairing rules, often referred to as **complementary base-pairing**, as shown in Figure 6.9. An adenine (A) is always base-paired with a thymine (T) via two hydrogen bonds. A guanine (G) always pairs with cytosine (C) via three hydrogen bonds. The three hydrogen bonds make the G–C base pair interaction stronger. These hydrogen bonds, and the hydrophobic interactions between bases, provide stability to the double helix structure. Thus, the base sequence on one strand defines the base sequence on the other strand.
- Because of the specific base-pairing, the amount of A equals the amount of T, and the amount of G equals the amount of C. Thus, total purines will be equal to total pyrimidines overall. These properties are known as **Chargaff's rules**.

KEY CONCEPT

When writing a complementary strand of DNA, it is important to not only remember the base-pairing rules but to also keep track of the 5′ and 3′ ends. Remember that the sequences need to be both complementary and antiparallel. For example, 5′—ATCG—3′ will be complementary to 5′—CGAT—3′.

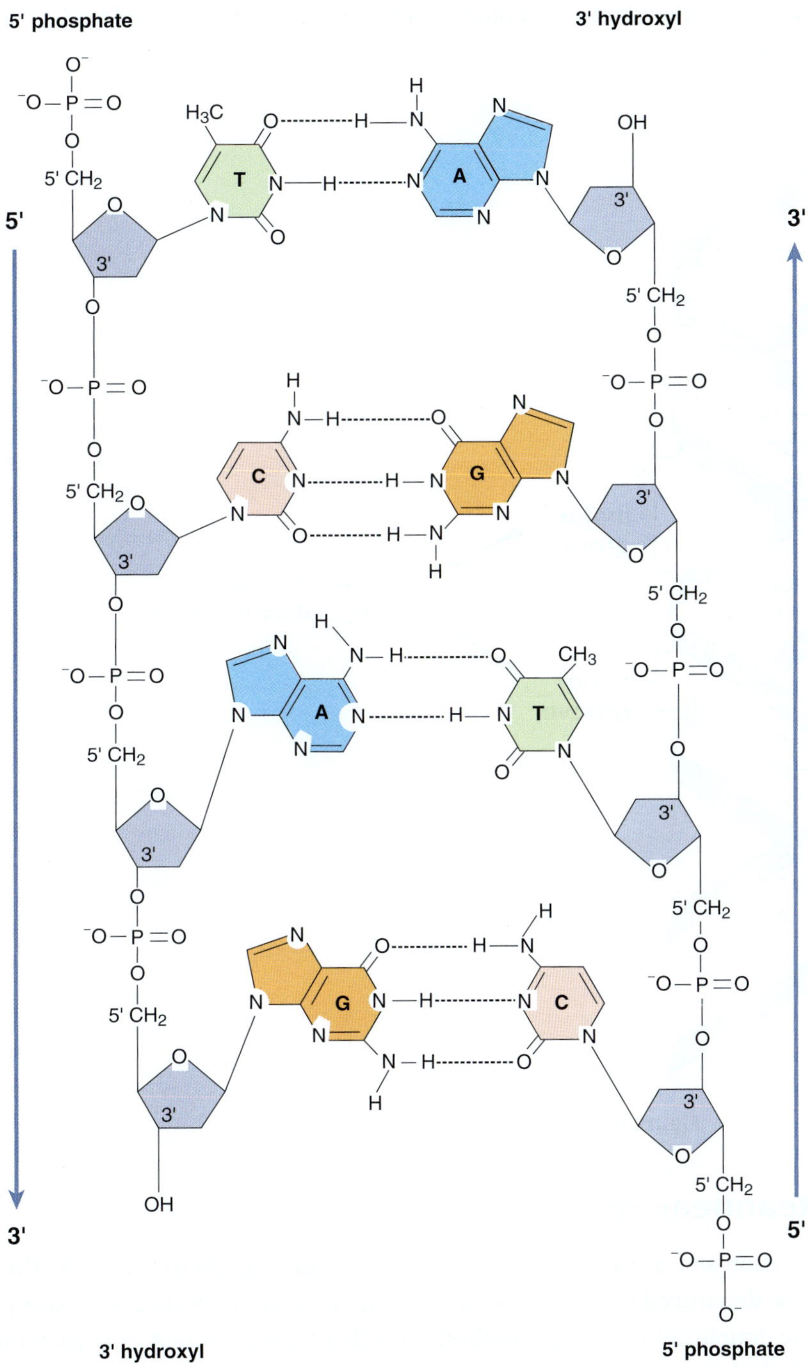

Figure 6.9 Base-Pairing in DNA

MCAT EXPERTISE

Using Chargaff's rules:

In double-stranded DNA, purines = pyrimidines:

- %A = %T
- %G = %C

If a sample of DNA has 10% G, what is the % of T?

10% G = 10% C, thus

%G + %C = 20%

%A + %T = 80%, thus

%T = 40%.

The double helix of most DNA is a right-handed helix, forming what is called **B-DNA**, as shown in Figure 6.10. The helix in B-DNA makes a turn every 3.4 nm and contains about 10 bases within that span. Major and minor grooves can be identified between the interlocking strands and are often the site of protein binding. Another form of DNA is called **Z-DNA** for its zigzag appearance; it is a left-handed helix that has a turn every 4.6 nm and contains 12 bases within each turn. A high GC-content or a high salt concentration may contribute to the formation of this form of DNA. No biological activity has been attributed to Z-DNA partly because it is unstable and difficult to research.

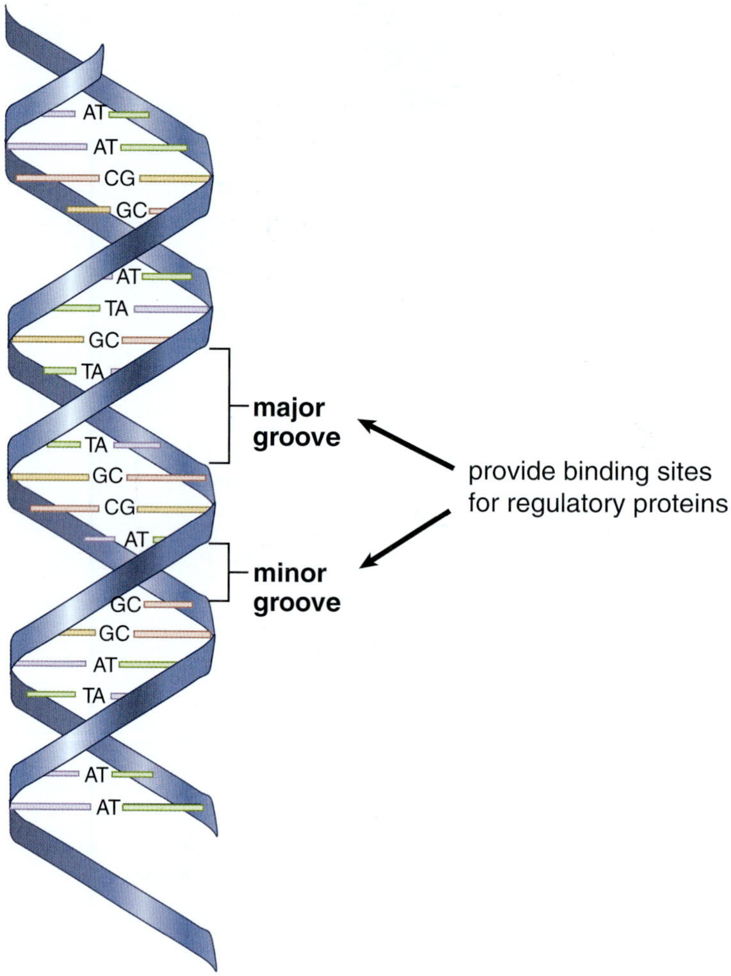

Figure 6.10 The B-DNA Double Helix

Denaturation and Reannealing

During processes such as replication and transcription, it is necessary to gain access to the DNA. The double helical nature of DNA can be **denatured** by conditions that disrupt hydrogen bonding and base-pairing, resulting in the "melting" of the double helix into two single strands that have separated from each other. Notably, none of the covalent links between the nucleotides in the backbone of the DNA break during this process. Heat, alkaline pH, and chemicals like formaldehyde and urea are commonly used to denature DNA.

Denatured, single-stranded DNA can be **reannealed** (brought back together) if the denaturing condition is slowly removed. If a solution of heat-denatured DNA is slowly cooled, for example, then the two complementary strands can become paired again, as shown in Figure 6.11.

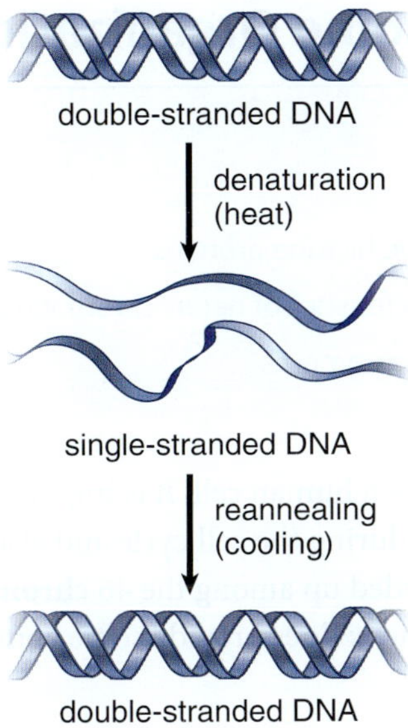

Figure 6.11 Denaturation and Reannealing of DNA

Such annealing of complementary DNA strands is also an important step in many laboratory processes, such as polymerase chain reactions (PCR) and in the detection of specific DNA sequences. In these techniques, a well-characterized **probe DNA** (DNA with known sequence) is added to a mixture of target DNA sequences. When probe DNA binds to target DNA sequences, this may provide evidence of the presence of a gene of interest. This binding process is called hybridization and is described in further detail later in this chapter.

MCAT CONCEPT CHECK 6.1

Before you move on, assess your understanding of the material with these questions.

1. What is the difference between a nucleoside and a nucleotide?

____

2. What are the base-pairing rules according to the Watson–Crick model?

____

3. What are the three major structural differences between DNA and RNA?

    1. ______________________________
    2. ______________________________
    3. ______________________________

4. How does the aromaticity of purines and pyrimidines underscore their genetic function?

____

5. If a strand of RNA contained 15% cytosine, 15% adenine, 35% guanine, and 35% uracil, would this violate Chargaff's rules? Why or why not?

____

6.2 Eukaryotic Chromosome Organization

LEARNING OBJECTIVES

After Chapter 6.2, you will be able to:

- Recall the names and the role of the five histone proteins
- Differentiate between the major characteristics of heterochromatin and euchromatin
- Describe the traits of telomeres and centromeres

There are over 6 billion bases of DNA in each human cell. It is important for the cell to organize these bases effectively. These bases must be replicated during the cell cycle and also utilized in gene expression for normal cellular functions. In humans, DNA is divided up among the 46 **chromosomes** found in the nucleus of the cell. The supercoiling of the DNA double helix does provide some compaction, but much more is necessary.

Histones

The DNA that makes up a chromosome is wound around a group of small lysine- and arginine-rich proteins called **histones**, forming **chromatin**. The positive charge on the sidechain of lysine and arginine residues interact favorably with the negatively charged phosphate backbone of DNA. There are five histone proteins found in eukaryotic cells. Two copies each of the histone proteins H2A, H2B, H3, and H4 form a histone core and about 200 base pairs of DNA are wrapped around this protein complex, forming a **nucleosome**, as shown in Figure 6.12. Under an electron microscope, the nucleosomes look like beads on a string. The last histone, H1, seals off the DNA as it enters and leaves the nucleosome, adding stability to the structure. Together, the nucleosomes create a much more organized and compacted DNA.

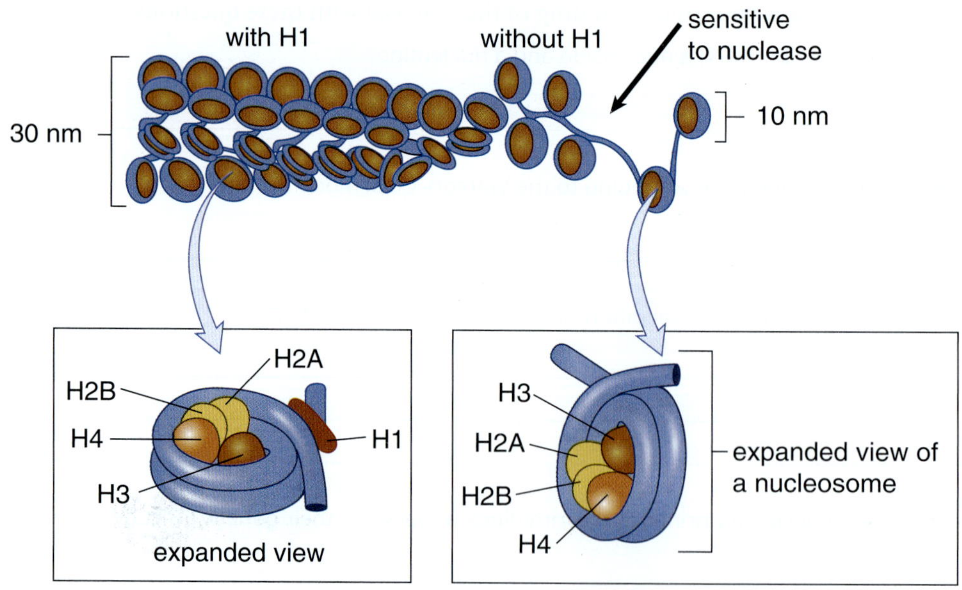

Figure 6.12 Nucleosome Structure
Nucleosomes are composed of DNA wrapped around histone proteins.

Histones are one example of **nucleoproteins** (proteins that associate with DNA). Most other nucleoproteins are acid-soluble and tend to stimulate processes such as transcription. **Histone acetyltransferases** are enzymes that can modify lysine residues on histones by masking the positive charge on the sidechain of lysine residues through the addition of an acetyl group. As illustrated in Figure 6.13, this loss of the positive charge on the lysine side chain, which typically interacts with the negatively-charged DNA wound around the histones, leads to the release of the DNA due to the weakened interaction. Post-translational modifications by histone acetyltransferases are often associated with transcriptional activation, whereas **histone deacetylases (HDACs)** usually repress the transcription of specific genes. Similarly, **histone methyltransferases** are enzymes that add methyl groups to lysine and arginine residues. Because methylation preserves the positive charges on lysine and arginine, histone methylation tends to be associated with decreased transcription.

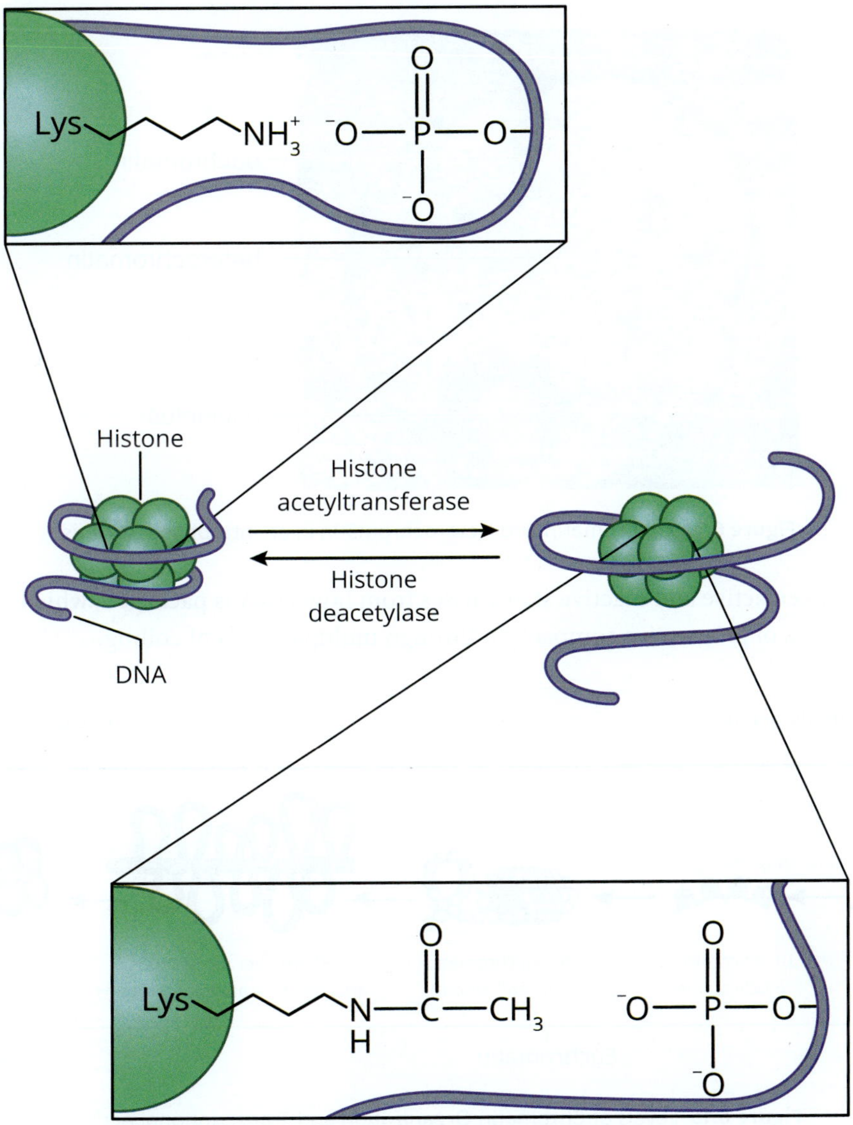

Figure 6.13 Histone Acetylation and Deacetylation
Acetylation removes the positive charge on the lysine side chain, loosening the interaction between histones and DNA.

Heterochromatin and Euchromatin

The chromosomes have a diffuse configuration during interphase of the cell cycle. The cell will undergo DNA replication during the S phase of interphase and having the DNA uncondensed and accessible makes the process more efficient. A small percentage of the chromatin remains compacted during interphase and is referred to as **heterochromatin**. Heterochromatin appears dark under light microscopy and is transcriptionally silent. Heterochromatin often consists of DNA with highly repetitive sequences. In contrast, the dispersed chromatin is called **euchromatin**, which appears light under light microscopy. Euchromatin contains genetically active DNA. Both heterochromatin and euchromatin can be seen in the nucleus in Figure 6.14.

KEY CONCEPT

Heterochromatin is dark, dense, and silent. Euchromatin is light, uncondensed, and expressed.

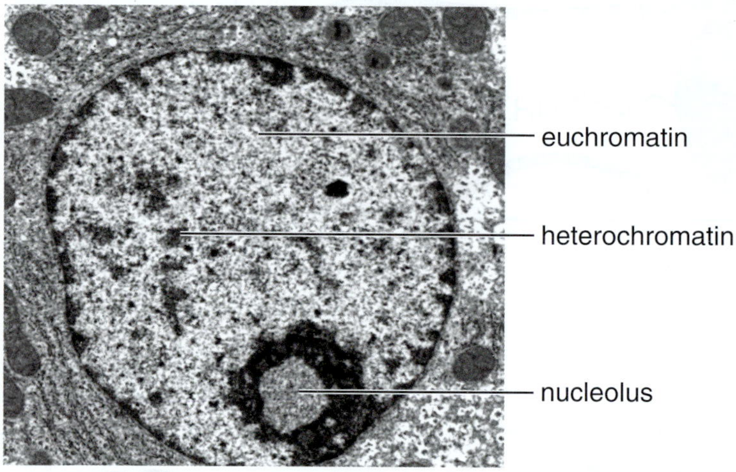

Figure 6.14 Euchromatin and Heterochromatin in an Interphase Nucleus

This distinction between active and inactive states arises from how DNA is packaged, which, as shown in Figure 6.15, is a process of progressive compaction through multiple levels of coiling.

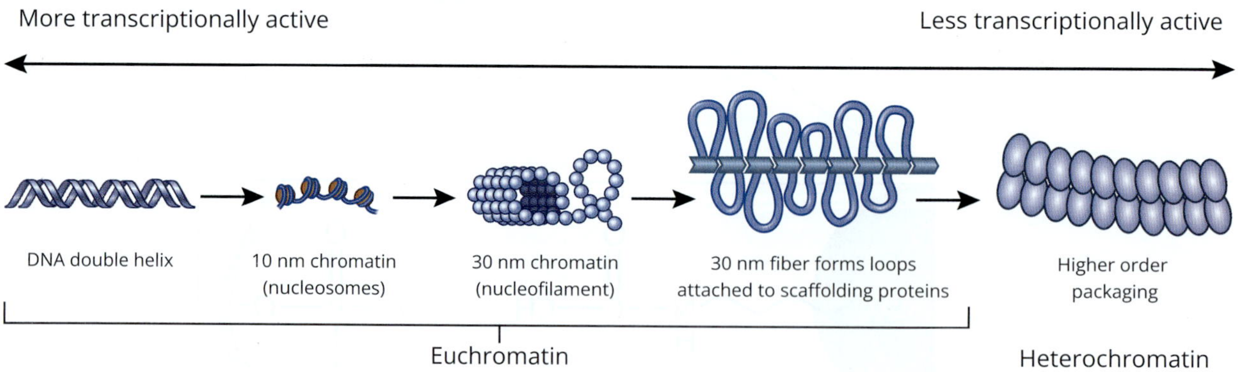

Figure 6.15 Levels of Chromatin Organization and Transcriptional Activity

Telomeres and Centromeres

As described later in this chapter, DNA replication cannot extend all the way to the end of a chromosome. This will result in losing sequences and information with each round of replication. The solution for our cells is a simple repeating unit (TTAGGG) at the end of the DNA, forming a **telomere**, as shown in Figure 6.16. Some of the sequence is lost in each round of replication and can be replaced by the enzyme ***telomerase***. Telomerase is more highly expressed in rapidly dividing cells. Animal studies indicate that there are a set number of replications possible, and that the progressive shortening of telomeres contributes to aging. Telomeres also serve a second function: their high GC-content creates exceptionally strong strand attractions at the end of chromosomes to prevent unraveling; think of telomeres as "knotting off" the end of the chromosome.

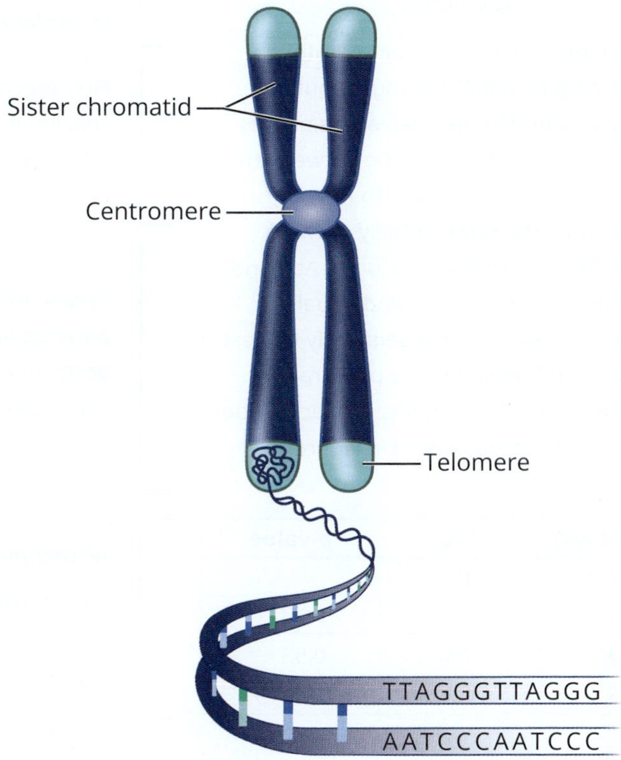

Figure 6.16 Telomere

Centromeres, as their name suggests, are a region of DNA found in the center of chromosomes. They are often referred to as sites of constriction because they form noticeable indentations. This part of the chromosome is composed of heterochromatin, which is in turn composed of tandem repeat sequences that also contain high GC-content. During cell division, the two sister chromatids can therefore remain connected at the centromere until microtubules separate the chromatids during anaphase.

BIOCHEMISTRY GUIDED EXAMPLE WITH EXPERT THINKING

Cisplatin is an effective chemotherapeutic agent against a number of cancers, including notoriously difficult to treat head and neck cancers. Cisplatin acts by binding DNA, which then irreversibly binds repair complexes, preventing effective repair. Cisplatin exhibits two major drawbacks that limit its application in cancer therapy—severe side effects and the rapid development of drug resistance. They are mutually connected, as adverse side effects restrict the administration of high doses, while underdosing leads to development of resistance in the cancerous cells. For this reason, drugs that sensitize cancer cells towards cisplatin could increase its therapeutic efficacy.

Topic: cisplatin is a drug used in chemotherapy; it inhibits DNA repair

Problem: cisplatin has bad side effects and cancer cells can develop resistance

Purpose: looking for a drug that makes cancer cells more susceptible to cisplatin

Four groups of mice were transfected with tumor cells by an intraperitoneal injection; 24 hours later they received 5 mg/kg cisplatin, 166 mg/kg butyrate, both cisplatin and butyrate, or a sham treatment. The life span of the mice is noted below in Table 1 along with the T/C ratio, which is the ratio between the mean life spans of the treated animals (T) and the controls (C). To further investigate the mechanism by which butyrate acts, exponentially growing HeLa cells were treated with 5 mM butyrate, 8 μM cisplatin, or both. At 4 and 24 hours after treatment, total histone fraction was isolated and equal quantities of histones were subjected to SDS-PAGE, and subsequently to western blot with anti-acetylated histone antibody. Acetylation is a post-translational modification added to lysine groups on histone proteins. The acetylation levels are expressed as a percentage of the untreated control in Figure 1 below.

First experiment: the life span of cancerous mice were measured with different treatments

Second experiment: how does butyrate act? The histone acetylation levels were measured with different treatments

Treatment	Life span (days)	T/C	*p*-value
Control	10.8 ± 2.0	1	
Butyrate	14.0 ± 4.5	1.3	0.19
Cisplatin	12.0 ± 3.5	1.1	0.53
Cisplatin + Butyrate	19.0 ± 3.4	1.8	0.0019

Table 1

IV: treatment

DV: life span

Trend: cisplatin + butyrate-treated mice had significantly longer life span

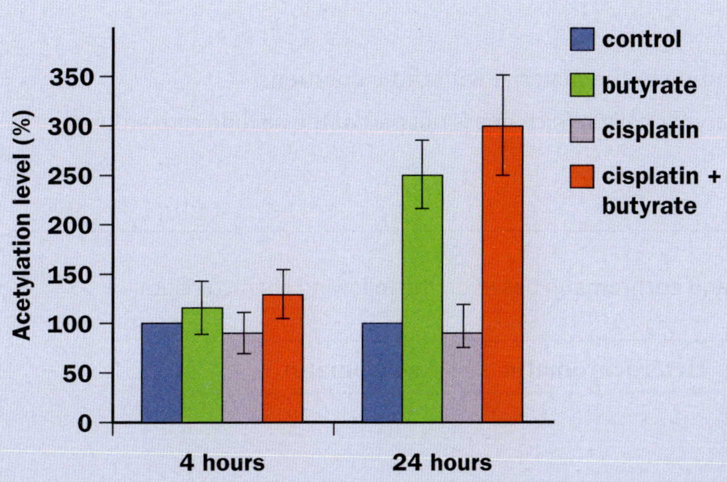

IVs: treatment, time of treatment

DV: histone acetylation

Trend: butyrate and cisplatin + butyrate had significantly higher levels of acetylation after 24 hours

Figure 1

Adapted from Koprinarova, M., Markovska, P., Iliev, I., Anachkova, B., & Russev, G. (2010). Sodium butyrate enhances the cytotoxic effect of cisplatin by abrogating the cisplatin imposed cell cycle arrest. *BMC Molecular Biology*, 11, 49. doi:10.1186/1471-2199-11-49.

Given the fact that histones are enriched with surface-exposed basic amino acids, how does butyrate enhance the cytotoxic effect of cisplatin on tumor cells?

The question stem asks us to explain the action of butyrate in conjunction with cisplatin, which means we need to dig into the experiment and results of the passage. The first paragraph tells us that cisplatin blocks DNA repair, and when targeting cancerous cells, cisplatin would likely cause cell death. Table 1 clearly shows that cisplatin alone doesn't increase the life span of mice with cancer, but coupling cisplatin with butyrate does. However, this result doesn't tell us how this paired treatment works (just that it does work), which means that we need to find this information in Figure 1. The treatments do not differ from the control after 4 hours, but butyrate and cisplatin + butyrate do increase the levels of histone acetylation. The passage tells us that histone acetylation is a post-translational addition of an acetyl group on to lysines. We know from the structure of amino acids that lysines are positively charged, so adding an acetyl group would mask the positive charge. We're also told that histones have many surface-exposed basic amino acids, and basic amino acids (like lysine and arginine) are positively charged at physiological pH. Let's also recall that when DNA is wrapped tightly around histone proteins, it is referred to as heterochromatin, which means the DNA is transcriptionally silent. Since DNA has a negative charge due to the phosphodiester backbone, acetylating the lysines on histones will remove some of the positive charge. Without that positive charge binding the negatively charged DNA, the histones will no longer be held tightly to the DNA, meaning they will dissociate from the DNA. DNA that is not tightly bound to histones forms euchromatin, which is genetically active: those genes can now be transcribed and translated. The DNA will then also be accessible to cisplatin, which will bind and stop DNA repair complexes. A build up of unrepaired DNA often causes cells to die, usually through apoptotic mechanisms.

In summary, butyrate causes DNA to separate from histones, allowing for cisplatin to bind and stop DNA repair complexes from fixing errors in the DNA, leading to eventual cell death.

MCAT CONCEPT CHECK 6.2

Before you move on, assess your understanding of the material with these questions.

1. What are the five histone proteins in eukaryotic cells? Which one is not part of the histone core around which DNA wraps to form chromatin?

____

2. Compare and contrast heterochromatin and euchromatin based on the following characteristics:

Characteristic	Heterochromatin	Euchromatin
Density of chromatin packing		
Appearance under light microscopy		
Transcriptional activity		

3. What property of telomeres and centromeres allows them to stay tightly raveled, even when the rest of DNA is uncondensed?

____

6.3 DNA Replication

LEARNING OBJECTIVES

After Chapter 6.3, you will be able to:

- List the names and functions of the major enzymes of DNA synthesis in prokaryotes and eukaryotes
- Differentiate between synthesis of the leading and lagging strands
- Explain the role of telomerase and the function of the telomere

The DNA is an organism's "blueprint" that provides not only the ability to sustain activities of life but also insight into our evolutionary past. The process of DNA replication is highly regulated to ensure as close to 100 percent perfection when making a copy of our genome as possible. DNA replication is necessary for the reproduction of a species and for any dividing cell.

Strand Separation and Origins of Replication

The human genome has about 3 billion base pairs packed into multiple chromosomes. The **replisome** or **replication complex** is a set of specialized proteins that assist the DNA polymerases. To begin the process of replication, DNA unwinds at points called **origins of replication**. The generation of new DNA proceeds in both directions, creating **replication forks** on both sides of the origin, as shown in Figure 6.17.

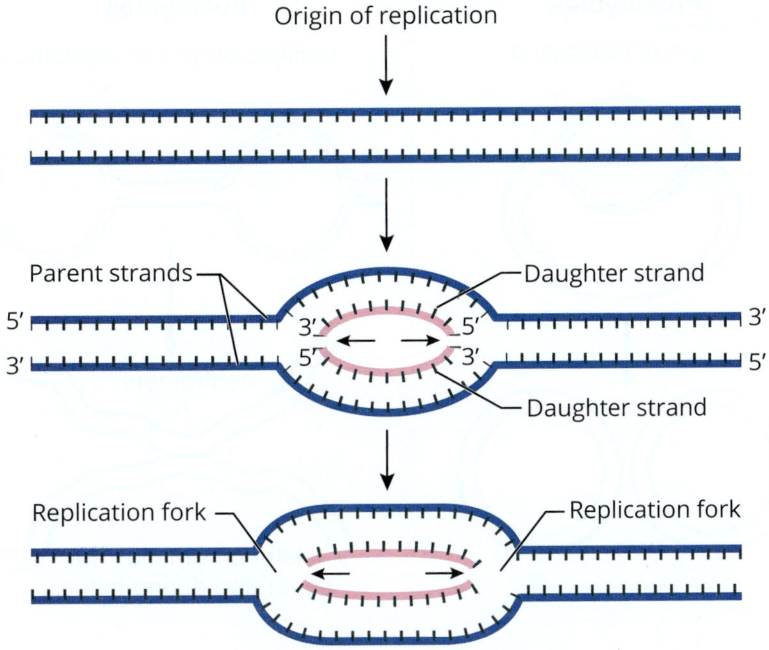

Figure 6.17 Origins of Replication
Replication forks form on both sides of the origin, increasing the efficiency of replication.

The bacterial chromosome is a closed, double-stranded circular DNA molecule with a single origin of replication. Thus, there are two replication forks that move away from each other in opposite directions around the circle. The two replication forks eventually meet, resulting in the production of two identical circular molecules of DNA.

Eukaryotic replication must copy many more bases compared to prokaryotic and is a slower process. In order to duplicate all of the chromosomes efficiently, each eukaryotic chromosome contains one linear molecule of double-stranded DNA having multiple origins of replication. As the replication forks move toward each other and **sister chromatids** are created, the chromatids will remain connected at the **centromere**. The differences between prokaryotic and eukaryotic replication patterns are shown in Figure 6.18.

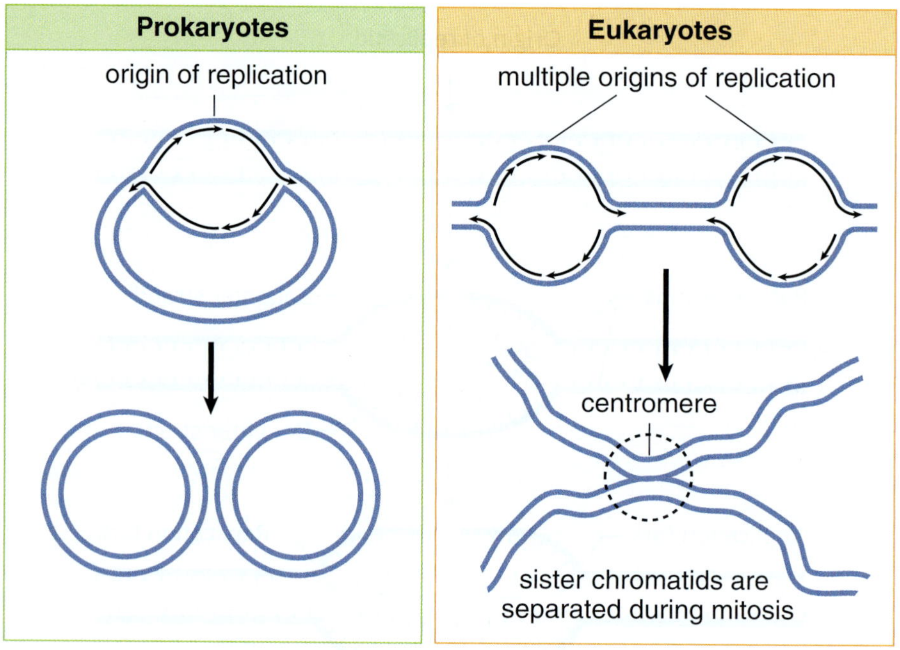

Figure 6.18 DNA Replication in Prokaryotes and Eukaryotes

Helicase is the enzyme responsible for unwinding the DNA, generating two single-stranded template strands ahead of the polymerase. Once opened, the unpaired strands of DNA are very sticky, in a molecular sense. The free purines and pyrimidines seek out other molecules with which to hydrogen bond. Proteins are therefore required to hold the strands apart: **single-stranded DNA-binding proteins** will bind to the unraveled strand, preventing both the reassociation of the DNA strands and the degradation of DNA by ***nucleases***. As the helicase unwinds the DNA, it will cause positive supercoiling that strains the DNA helix. **Supercoiling** is a wrapping of DNA on itself as its helical structure is pushed ever further toward the telomeres during replication; picture an old-fashioned telephone cord that's become tangled on itself. To alleviate this torsional stress and reduce the risk of strand breakage, ***DNA topoisomerases*** introduce negative supercoils. They do so by working ahead of helicase, nicking one or both strands, allowing relaxation of the torsional pressure, and then resealing the cut strands.

REAL WORLD

Any antibiotic ending with *–floxacin* (ciprofloxacin, moxifloxacin, and so on) is called a *fluoroquinolone* and targets the prokaryotic topoisomerase *DNA gyrase*. This stops bacterial replication and slows the infection. Fluoroquinolones are routinely used for pneumonia and certain infections of the genitourinary system.

During replication, these **parental strands** will serve as templates for the generation of new **daughter strands**. The replication process is termed **semiconservative** because one parental strand is retained in each of the two resulting identical double-stranded DNA molecules, as shown in Figure 6.19.

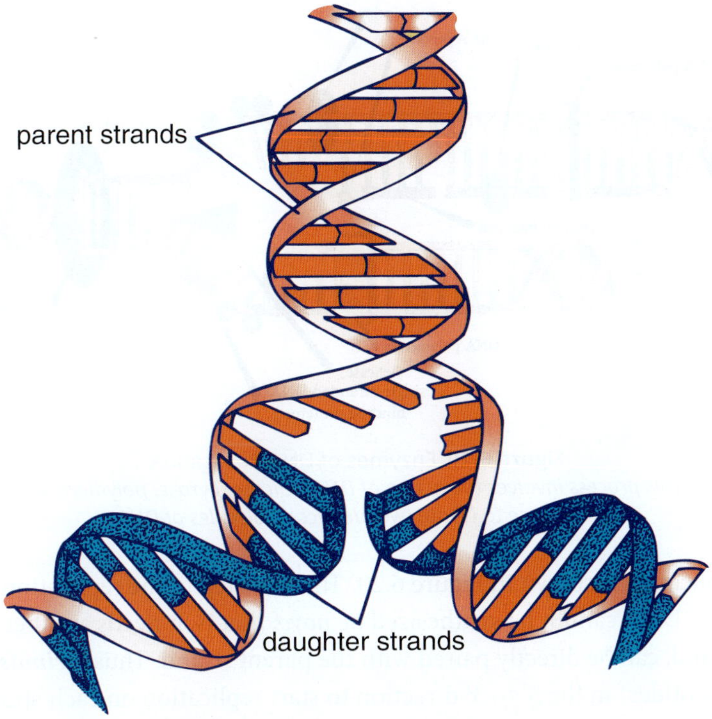

Figure 6.19 Semiconservative Replication
A new double helix is made of one old parent strand and one new daughter strand.

Synthesis of Daughter Strands

DNA polymerases are responsible for reading the DNA template, or parental strand, and synthesizing the new daughter strand. The DNA polymerase can read the template strand in a 3′ to 5′ direction while synthesizing the complementary strand in the 5′ to 3′ direction. This will result in a new double helix of DNA that has the required antiparallel orientation. Due to this directionality of the DNA polymerase, certain constraints arise. Remember that the two separated parental strands of the helix are also antiparallel to each other. Thus, at each replication fork, one strand is oriented in the correct direction for DNA polymerase; the other strand is antiparallel.

KEY CONCEPT

With the exception of DNA polymerase's *reading* direction (and a few untested endonucleases), everything in molecular biology is 5′ to 3′. DNA polymerase reads 3′ to 5′, but the following processes occur 5′ to 3′:

- DNA synthesis
- DNA repair
- RNA transcription
- RNA translation (reading of codons)

The **leading strand** in each replication fork is the strand that is copied in a continuous fashion, in the same direction as the advancing replication fork. This parental strand will be read 3′ to 5′ and its complement will be synthesized in a 5′ to 3′ manner, as discussed above.

The **lagging strand** is the strand that is copied in a direction opposite the direction of the replication fork. On this side of the replication fork, the parental strand has 5′ to 3′ polarity. DNA polymerase cannot simply read and synthesize on this strand. How does it solve this problem? Because DNA polymerase can only synthesize in the 5′ to 3′ direction from a 3′ to 5′ template, small strands called **Okazaki fragments** are produced. As the replication fork continues to move forward, it clears additional space that DNA polymerase must fill in. Each time DNA polymerase completes an Okazaki fragment, it turns around to find another gap that needs to be filled in.

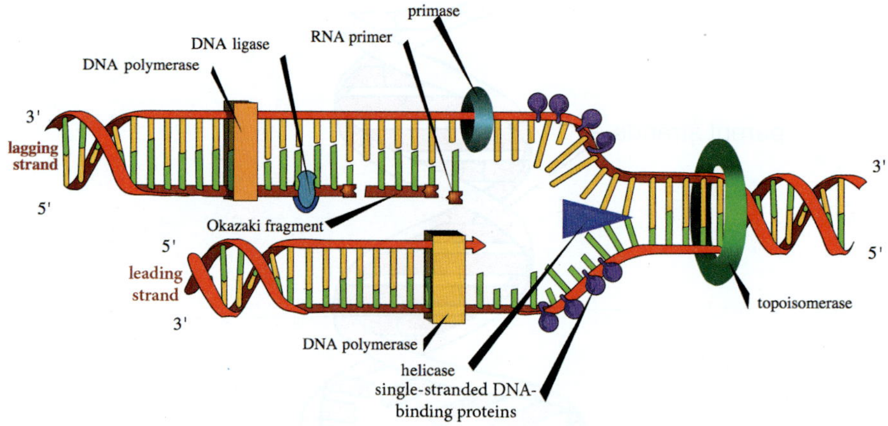

Figure 6.20 Enzymes of DNA Replication
This process involves the action of DNA helicase, gyrase, polymerase, and ligase to create two identical molecules of DNA.

The process of DNA replication is shown in Figure 6.20. The first step in the replication of DNA is actually to lay down an RNA primer. DNA cannot be synthesized *de novo*; that is, it needs another molecule to "hook on" to. RNA, on the other hand, can be directly paired with the parent strand. Thus, ***primase*** synthesizes a short primer (roughly 10 nucleotides) in the 5′ to 3′ direction to start replication on each strand. These short RNA sequences are constantly being added to the lagging strand because each Okazaki fragment must start with a new primer. In contrast, the leading strand requires only one, in theory (in reality, there are usually a few primers on the leading strand). ***DNA polymerase III*** (prokaryotes) or ***DNA polymerases*** α, δ, and ε (eukaryotes) will then begin synthesizing the daughter strands of DNA in the 5′ to 3′ manner. The incoming nucleotides are 5′ deoxyribonucleotide triphosphates: dATP, dCTP, dGTP, and dTTP. As the new phosphodiester bond is made, a free *pyrophosphate* (PP_i) is released.

The RNA must eventually be removed to maintain integrity of the genome. This is accomplished by the enzyme ***DNA polymerase I*** (prokaryotes) or ***RNase H*** (eukaryotes). Then, ***DNA polymerase I*** (prokaryotes) or ***DNA polymerase*** δ (eukaryotes) adds DNA nucleotides where the RNA primer had been. ***DNA ligase*** seals the ends of the DNA molecules together, creating one continuous strand of DNA.

While prokaryotic DNA synthesis has been worked out in great detail, and eukaryotic synthesis is considered to be very similar, there are a few differences in the enzymes involved. There are five "classic" DNA polymerases in eukaryotic cells, which are designated with the Greek letters α, β, γ, δ, and ε. Further research has revealed more polymerases named ζ through μ, but these are outside the scope of the MCAT. Table 6.2 highlights differences in the names of the enzymes associated with DNA replication in prokaryotic vs. eukaryotic cells; special attention should be paid to the eukaryotic DNA polymerases:

- DNA polymerases α, δ, and ε work together to synthesize both the leading and lagging strands; DNA polymerase δ also fills in the gaps left behind when RNA primers are removed
- DNA polymerase γ replicates mitochondrial DNA

- DNA polymerases β and ε are important to the process of DNA repair
- DNA polymerases δ and ε are assisted by the *PCNA* protein, which assembles into a trimer to form the **sliding clamp**. The clamp helps to strengthen the interaction between these DNA polymerases and the template strand

Step in Replication	Prokaryotic Cells	Eukaryotic Cells (Nuclei)
Origin of replication	One per chromosome	Multiple per chromosome
Unwinding of DNA double helix	Helicase	Helicase
Stabilization of unwound template strands	Single-stranded DNA-binding protein	Single-stranded DNA-binding protein
Synthesis of RNA primers	Primase	Primase
Synthesis of DNA	DNA polymerase III	DNA polymerases α, δ, *and* ε
Removal of RNA primers	DNA polymerase I ($5' \rightarrow 3'$ exonuclease)	RNase H ($5' \rightarrow 3'$ exonuclease)
Replacement of RNA with DNA	DNA polymerase I	DNA polymerase δ
Joining of Okazaki fragments	DNA ligase	DNA ligase
Removal of positive supercoils ahead of advancing replication forks	DNA topoisomerases (DNA gyrase)	DNA topoisomerases
Synthesis of telomeres	Not applicable	Telomerase

Table 6.2 Steps and Proteins Involved in DNA Replication

Replicating the Ends of Chromosomes

While DNA polymerase does an excellent job of synthesizing DNA, it unfortunately cannot complete synthesis of the $5'$ end of the strand. Thus, each time DNA synthesis is carried out, the chromosome becomes a little shorter. To lengthen the time that cells can replicate and synthesize DNA before necessary genes are damaged, chromosomes contain **telomeres**. As described earlier, telomeres are located at the very tips of the chromosome and consist of repetitive sequences with a high GC-content. This repetition means that telomeres can be slightly degraded between replication cycles without loss of function.

MCAT CONCEPT CHECK 6.3

Before you move on, assess your understanding of the material with these questions.

1. For each of the enzymes listed below, list the function of the enzyme and if it is found in prokaryotes, eukaryotes, or both.

Enzyme	Prokaryotes/ Eukaryotes/Both	Function
Helicase		
Single-stranded DNA-binding protein		
Primase		
DNA polymerase III		
DNA polymerase α		
DNA polymerase I		
RNase H		
DNA ligase		
DNA topoisomerases		

2. Between the leading strand and lagging strand, which is more prone to mutations? Why?

____

3. What is the function of a telomere?

____

6.4 DNA Repair

LEARNING OBJECTIVES

After Chapter 6.4, you will be able to:

- Describe the major DNA repair processes, including proofreading, mismatch repair, and excision repair
- Recognize the key components and locations of each DNA repair process, including both mismatch and excision processes
- Identify major traits of oncogenes and tumor suppressor genes

The structure of DNA can be damaged in a number of ways such as exposure to chemicals or radiation. DNA is very susceptible to damage and if the damage is not corrected, it will subsequently be copied and passed on to daughter cells. Damage can include breaking of the DNA backbone, structural or spontaneous alterations of bases, or incorporation of the incorrect base during replication. Any defect in the genetic code can cause an increased risk of cancer, so the cell has multiple processes in place to catch and correct genetic errors. This helps maintain the integrity and stability of the genome from cell to cell, and from generation to generation.

Oncogenes and Tumor Suppressor Genes

Certain genes, when mutated, can lead to cancer. **Cancer** cells proliferate excessively because they are able to divide without stimulation from other cells and are no longer subject to the normal controls on cell proliferation. By definition, cancer cells are able to migrate by local invasion or **metastasis**, a migration to distant tissues by the bloodstream or lymphatic system. Over time, cancer cells tend to accumulate mutations.

Mutated genes that cause cancer are termed **oncogenes**. Oncogenes primarily encode cell cycle–related proteins. Before these genes are mutated, they are often referred to as **proto-oncogenes**. The first gene in this category to be discovered was *src* (named after *sarcoma*, a category of connective tissue cancers). The abnormal alleles encode proteins that are more active than normal proteins, promoting rapid cell cycle advancement. Typically, a mutation in only one copy is sufficient to promote tumor growth and is therefore considered dominant.

Tumor suppressor genes, like *p53* or *Rb* (*retinoblastoma*), encode proteins that inhibit the cell cycle or participate in DNA repair processes. They normally function to stop tumor progression, and are sometimes called **antioncogenes**. Mutations of these genes result in the loss of tumor suppression activity, and therefore promote cancer. Inactivation of both alleles is necessary for the loss of function because, in most cases, even one copy of the normal protein can function to inhibit tumor formation. In this example, multiple mutations or "hits" are required.

KEY CONCEPT

While the outcome of oncogenes and mutated tumor suppressor genes is the same (cancer), the actual cause is different. Oncogenes promote the cell cycle while mutated tumor suppressors can no longer slow the cell cycle. Oncogenes are like stepping on the gas pedal; mutated tumor suppressors are like cutting the brakes.

Proofreading and Mismatch Repair

DNA polymerase moves along a single strand of DNA, building the complementary strand as it goes. While DNA polymerase is almost 100 percent accurate, it does occasionally make errors.

Proofreading

During synthesis, the two double-stranded DNA molecules will pass through a part of the DNA polymerase enzyme for **proofreading**. When the complementary strands have incorrectly paired bases, the hydrogen bonds between the strands can be unstable, and this lack of stability is detected as the DNA passes through this part of the polymerase. The incorrect base is excised and can be replaced with the correct one, as shown in Figure 6.21. If both the parent and daughter strands are simply DNA, how does the enzyme discriminate which is the template strand, and which is the incorrectly paired daughter strand? It looks at the level of methylation: the template strand has existed in the cell for a longer period of time, and therefore is more heavily methylated. Methylation also plays a role in the transcriptional activity of DNA, as described in Chapter 7 of *MCAT Biochemistry Review*. This system is very efficient, correcting most of the errors put into the sequence during replication. DNA ligase, which closes the gaps between Okazaki fragments, lacks proofreading ability. Thus, the likelihood of mutations in the lagging strand is considerably higher than the leading strand.

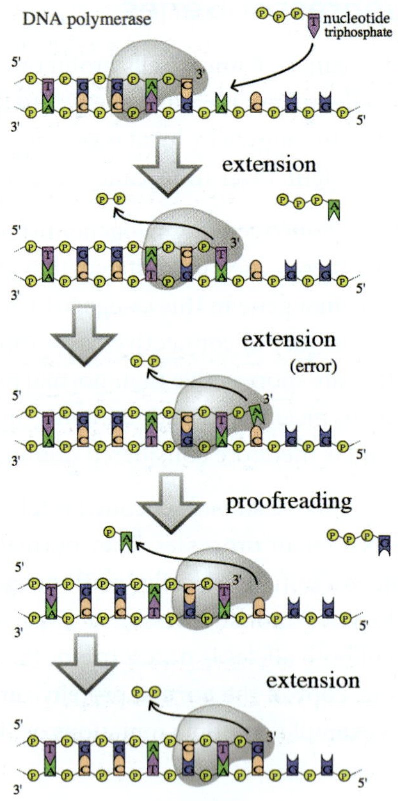

Figure 6.21 Proofreading by DNA Polymerase

Mismatch Repair

Cells also have machinery in the G_2 phase of the cell cycle for **mismatch repair**; these enzymes are encoded by genes *MSH2* and *MLH1*, which detect and remove errors introduced in replication that were missed during the S phase of the cell cycle. These enzymes are homologues of *MutS* and *MutL* in prokaryotes, which serve a similar function.

Nucleotide and Base Excision Repair

Most of the repair mechanisms involve proteins that recognize damage or a lesion, remove the damage, and then use the complementary strand as a template to fill in the gap. Our cell machinery recognizes two specific types of DNA damage in the G_1 and G_2 cell cycle phases and fixes them through nucleotide excision repair or base excision repair.

Nucleotide Excision Repair

Ultraviolet light induces the formation of dimers between adjacent thymine residues in DNA. The formation of thymine dimers interferes with DNA replication and normal gene expression, and distorts the shape of the double helix. Thymine dimers are eliminated from DNA by a **nucleotide excision repair** (**NER**) mechanism, which is a cut-and-patch process, as shown in Figure 6.22. First, specific proteins scan the DNA molecule and recognize the lesion because of a bulge in the strand. An ***excision endonuclease*** then makes nicks in the phosphodiester backbone of the damaged strand on both sides of the thymine dimer and removes the defective oligonucleotide. DNA polymerase can then fill in the gap by synthesizing DNA in the 5′ to 3′ direction, using the undamaged strand as a template. Finally, the nick in the strand is sealed by DNA ligase.

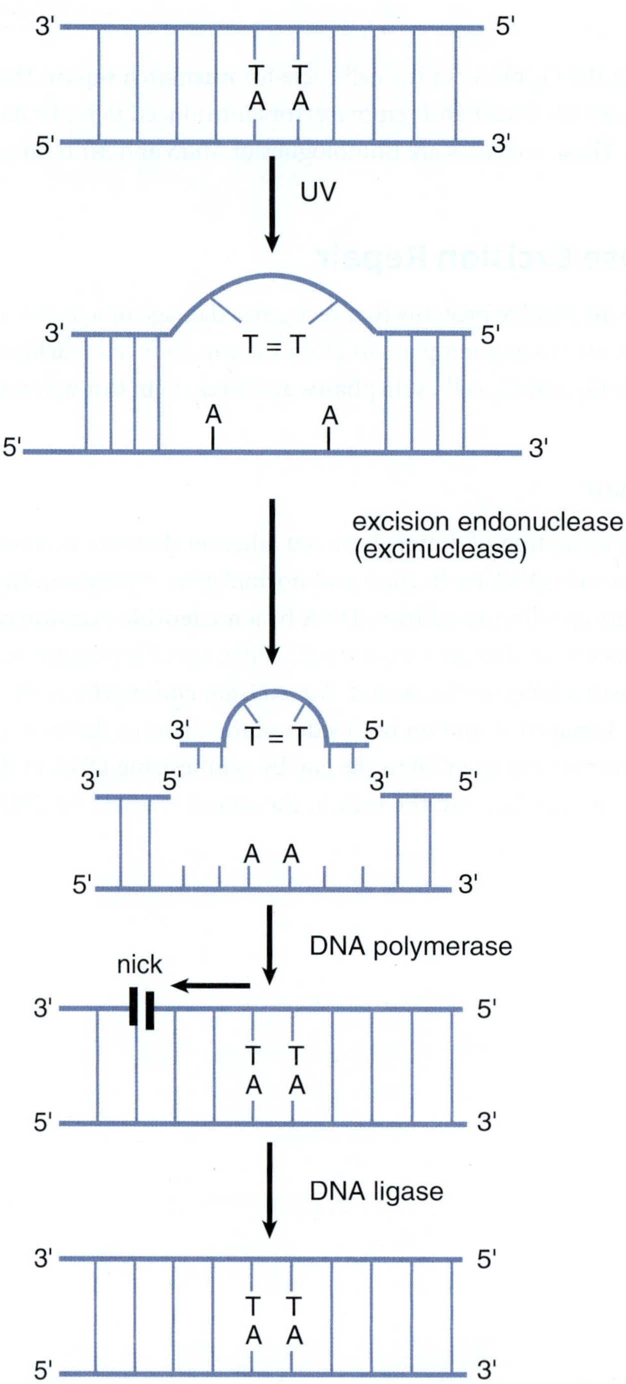

Figure 6.22 Thymine Dimer Formation and Nucleotide Excision Repair

Base Excision Repair

Alterations to bases can occur with other cellular insults. For example, thermal energy can be absorbed by DNA and may lead to cytosine deamination. This is the loss of an amino group from cytosine and results in the conversion of cytosine to uracil. Uracil should not be found in a DNA molecule and is thus easily detected as an error; however, detection systems exist for small, non-helix-distorting mutations in other bases as well. These are repaired by **base excision repair**, the steps of which are depicted in Figure 6.23. First, the affected base is recognized and removed by a glycosylase enzyme, leaving behind an **apurinic/apyrimidinic (AP) site**, also called an **abasic site**. The AP site is recognized by an ***AP endonuclease*** that removes the damaged sequence from the DNA. DNA polymerase and DNA ligase can then fill in the gap and seal the strand, as described above.

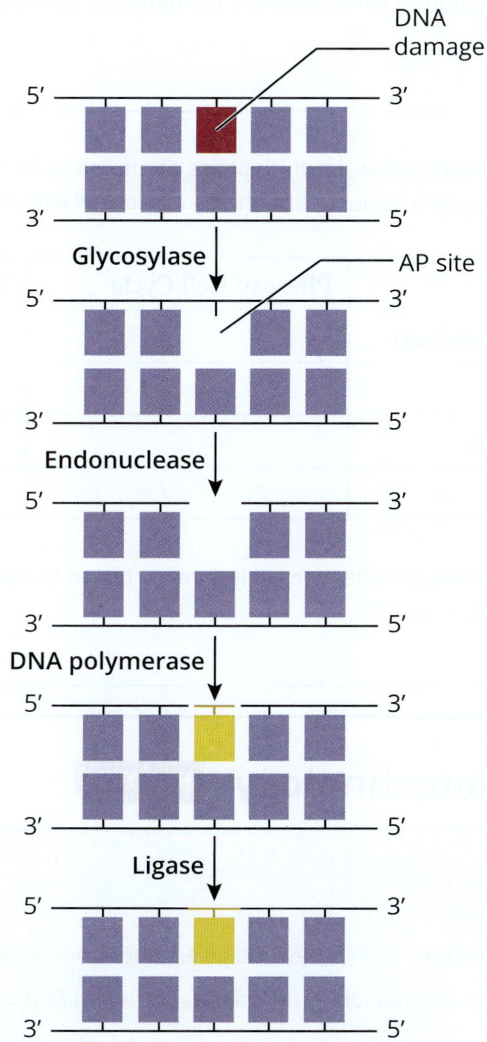

Figure 6.23 Steps of Base Excision Repair

MCAT CONCEPT CHECK 6.4

Before you move on, assess your understanding of the material with these questions.

1. What is the difference between an oncogene and a tumor suppressor gene?

2. How does DNA polymerase recognize which strand is the template strand once the daughter strand is synthesized?

3. For each of the repair mechanisms below, in which phase of the cell cycle does the repair mechanism function? What are the key enzymes or genes specifically associated with each mechanism?

Repair Mechanism	Phase of Cell Cycle	Key Enzymes/Genes
DNA polymerase (proofreading)		
Mismatch repair		
Nucleotide excision repair		
Base excision repair		

4. What is the key structural difference in the types of lesions corrected by nucleotide excision repair vs. those corrected by base excision repair?

6.5 Recombinant Biotechnology High Yield

LEARNING OBJECTIVES

After Chapter 6.5, you will be able to:

- Predict the most effective DNA library technique for a given laboratory application
- Recall the inputs and outputs of biotechnology techniques, including PCR, Southern blotting, and sequencing
- Describe the differences between transgenic mice and knockout mice

Now that we have reviewed the basics of DNA structure and function, we can discuss how this knowledge has been harnessed for a variety of research and treatment innovations. Recombinant DNA technology allows for the creation of **recombinant DNA**, which is DNA that is created from combining pieces of DNA from different sources together to make one new molecule, and then multiplication of the recombinant sequence through either gene cloning or polymerase chain reaction (PCR). This provides a means of analyzing and altering genes and proteins. It also provides the reagents necessary for genetic testing, such as carrier detection (detecting heterozygote status for a particular disease) and prenatal diagnosis of genetic diseases; it is also useful for gene therapy. Additionally, this technology can provide a source of a specific protein, such as recombinant human insulin, in almost unlimited quantities.

Molecular Cloning and Restriction Enzymes

Molecular cloning is a technique that is used to create recombinant DNA and produce large amounts of it using host organisms. Cloning conventionally starts with the desired sequence of DNA being inserted into a **vector backbone** to create a **recombinant vector**. The recombinant vector is then transferred to a host bacterium that is then allowed to grow into colonies. Colonies that contain the recombinant vector are isolated and grown in large quantities. Depending on the investigator's goal and experimental setup, the bacteria can then be lysed to purify the recombinant vectors or any proteins expressed from the recombinant sequence.

DNA vector backbones, often referred to as simply vectors, are particles used to carry foreign DNA sequences. The most commonly used (and most likely to be tested) type of vector on the MCAT are **plasmids**, which are small circular DNA molecules. Plasmids that are used as vectors tend to have specific sequences that make them ideal for molecular cloning, including a promoter, origin of replication, **multiple cloning site (MCS)** (also known as a **polylinker**), and selectable marker, as shown in the plasmid map in Figure 6.24. These components are described in further detail below.

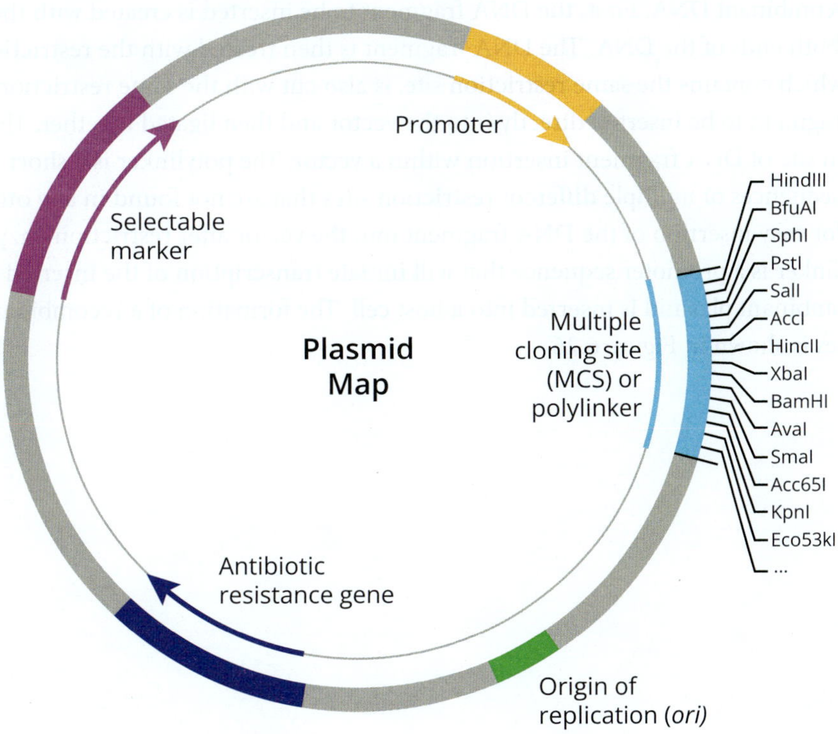

Figure 6.24 Plasmid Map for Molecular Cloning

Restriction enzymes (**restriction endonucleases**) are used in molecular cloning that recognize specific double-stranded DNA sequences called **restriction sites**. These sequences are palindromic, meaning that the 5′ to 3′ sequence of one strand is identical to the 5′ to 3′ sequence of the other strand (in antiparallel orientation). Restriction enzymes are isolated from bacteria, which are their natural source. In bacteria, they act as part of the *restriction modification system* that protects the bacteria from infection by DNA viruses. Once the specific restriction site has been identified, the restriction enzyme can cut through the backbones of the double helix. Thousands of restriction enzymes have been studied and many are commercially available to laboratories, allowing scientists to process DNA in very specific ways. Some restriction enzymes produce offset cuts, yielding single-stranded "sticky ends" on the DNA fragments, as shown in Figure 6.25.

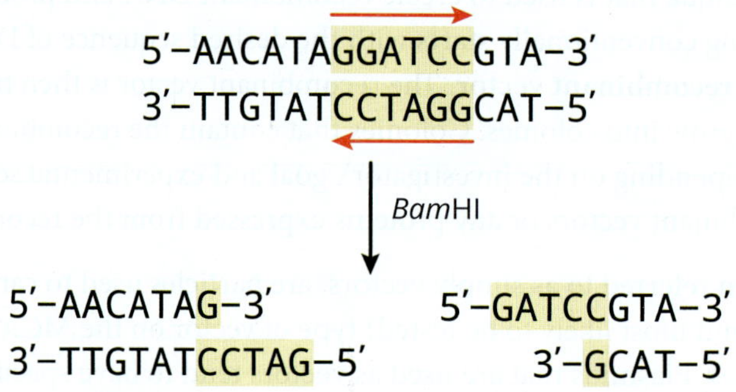

Figure 6.25 A Restriction Enzyme (*Bam*HI) Creating Sticky Ends
Restriction enzymes cut at palindromic sequences, such as BamHI, which cuts the sequence GGATCC.

Sticky ends generated from restriction enzymes are advantageous in facilitating the insertion of DNA into a vector to create recombinant DNA. First, the DNA fragment to be inserted is created with the chosen restriction site flanking both ends of the DNA. The DNA fragment is then treated with the restriction enzyme. The vector of choice, which contains the same restriction site, is also cut with the same restriction enzyme, which allows the DNA fragment to be inserted directly into the vector and then ligated together. The polylinker, or MCS, is a common site of DNA fragment insertion within a vector. The polylinker is a short segment of DNA that contains the sequences of multiple different restriction sites that are not found in any other parts of the plasmid to allow for easy insertion of the DNA fragment into the vector after restriction enzyme digestion. Just 5′ of the polylinker is a promoter sequence that will initiate transcription of the inserted DNA fragment after the final recombinant plasmid is inserted into a host cell. The formation of a recombinant plasmid using restriction enzymes is shown in Figure 6.26.

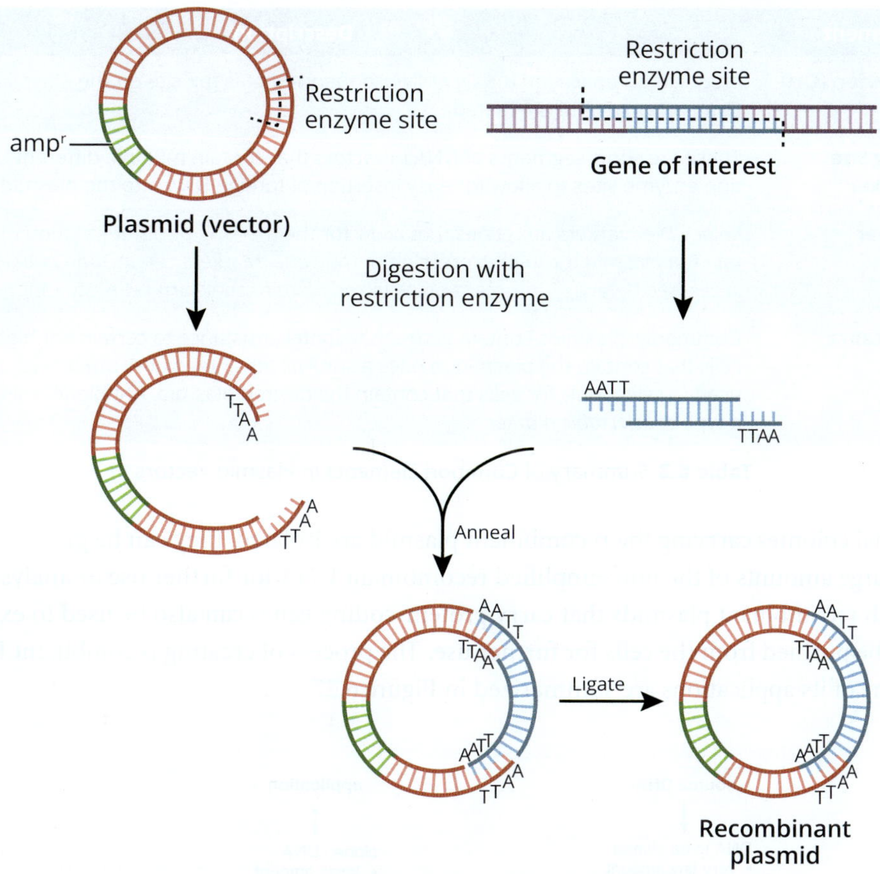

Figure 6.26 Formation of a Recombinant Plasmid Vector
amp^r: gene for resistance to ampicillin (an antibiotic)

Once the DNA sequence of interest is inserted into the vector backbone, the recombinant plasmid can be inserted into a host, such as certain strains of the bacterium *E. coli*. The recombinant plasmid is inserted into the bacteria through transformation (a process described in further detail in Chapter 1 of *MCAT Biology Review*). Once inside the host bacteria, the origin of replication (ori) within the recombinant plasmid allows for its duplication. The bacteria are then spread onto plates containing a solid growth medium and allowed to form colonies. The selection marker of the plasmid aids in allowing for the isolation of bacteria that contain the recombinant plasmid. For example, plasmids that contain antibiotic resistance genes confer antibiotic resistance to the host bacteria, so when the transformed bacteria are spread onto plates whose growth media contain that antibiotic, only the bacteria that carry the plasmid with the resistance gene can grow. A summary of common key sequences found in vectors used in molecular cloning are summarized below in Table 6.3.

Plasmid Element	Description
Origin of Replication (Ori)	An origin of replication (ori) is a DNA sequence that is the site on the plasmid where replication of the plasmid is initiated.
Multiple Cloning Site (MCS) or Polylinker	These are short segments of DNA in vectors that contain multiple different unique restriction enzyme sites to allow for easy insertion of foreign DNA into the plasmid.
Selectable Marker	Selectable markers are genes that allow for the marking or differentiation of cells that contain the plasmid through expression of the gene. Markers can include *antibiotic resistance genes* (see below), fluorescent proteins, or proteins that turn cells into different colors.
Antibiotic Resistance Gene	Commonly, plasmids contain genes that confer resistance to certain antibiotics. This allows cells that contain the plasmid to have a survival advantage over other cells, and can thus be used to select only for cells that contain the desired plasmid. Antibiotic resistance genes are a type of *selectable marker.*

Table 6.3 Summary of Common Elements in Plasmid Vectors

Once the bacterial colonies carrying the recombinant plasmid are isolated, they can be grown in large quantities to isolate large amounts of the now-amplified recombinant DNA for further use or analysis. Bacteria transformed with recombinant plasmids that carry protein-coding genes can also be used to express the protein, which can be purified from the cells for further use. The process of creating recombinant DNA by gene cloning and some of its applications are summarized in Figure 6.27.

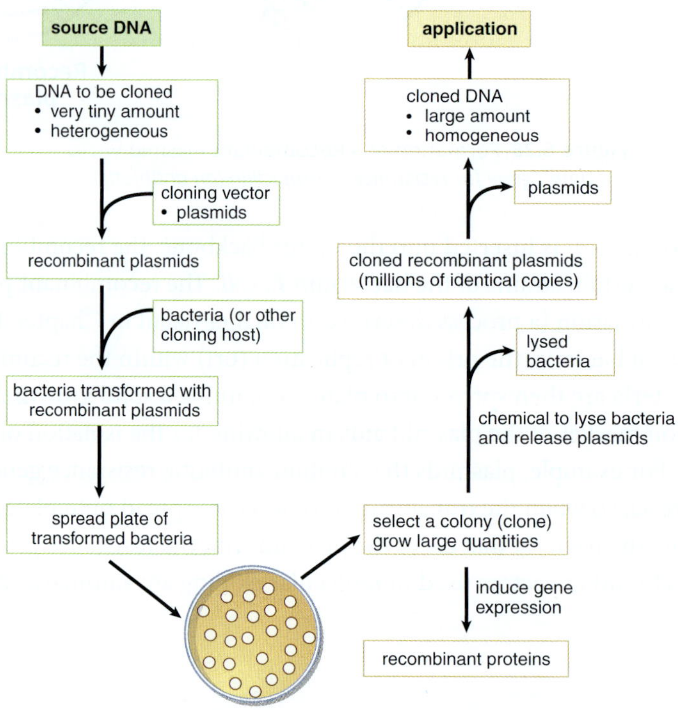

Figure 6.27 Cloning Recombinant DNA
Cloning allows production of recombinant proteins, or identification and characterization of DNA by increasing its volume and purity.

DNA Libraries and cDNA

DNA cloning can be used to produce DNA libraries. **DNA libraries** are large collections of known DNA sequences; in sum, these sequences could equate to the genome of an organism. To make a DNA library, DNA fragments, often digested randomly, are cloned into vectors and can be utilized for further study. Libraries can consist of either genomic DNA or cDNA. **Genomic libraries** contain large fragments of DNA, and include both coding (exon) and noncoding (intron) regions of the genome. **cDNA** (**complementary DNA**) libraries are constructed by reverse-transcribing processed mRNA, as shown in Figure 6.28. As such, cDNA lacks non-coding regions, such as introns, and only includes the genes that are expressed in the tissue from which the mRNA was isolated. For that reason, these libraries are sometimes called **expression libraries**. While genomic libraries contain the entire genome of an organism, genes may by chance be split into multiple vectors. Therefore, only cDNA libraries can be used to reliably sequence specific genes and identify disease-causing mutations, produce recombinant proteins (such as insulin, clotting factors, or vaccines), or produce transgenic animals. Several of these applications are discussed in more detail in subsequent sections of this chapter. Table 6.4 contrasts some of the characteristics of genomic and cDNA libraries.

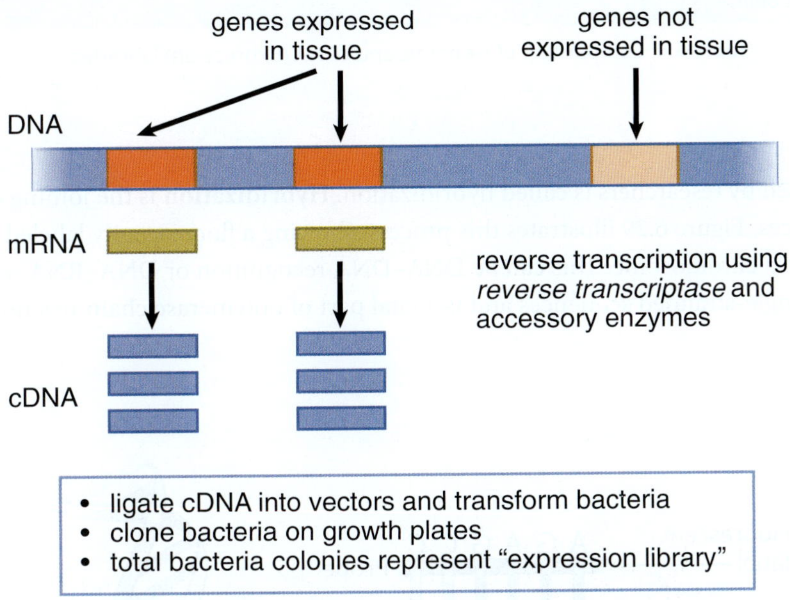

Figure 6.28 Cloning Expressed Genes by Producing cDNA

	Genomic Libraries	cDNA (Expression) Library
Source of DNA	Chromosomal DNA	mRNA (cDNA)
Enzymes to make library	Restriction endonuclease DNA ligase	Reverse transcriptase DNA ligase
Contains nonexpressed sequences of chromosomes	Yes	No
Cloned genes are complete sequences	Not necessarily	Yes
Cloned genes contain introns	Yes	No
Promoter and enhancer sequences present	Yes, but not necessarily in same clone	No
Gene can be expressed in cloning host (recombinant proteins)	No	Yes
Can be used for gene therapy or constructing transgenic animals	No	Yes

Table 6.4 Comparison of Genomic and cDNA (Expression) Libraries

Hybridization

Another tool often used by researchers is called hybridization. **Hybridization** is the joining of complementary base pair sequences. Figure 6.29 illustrates this process, showing a fluorescently labeled probe binding to a specific sequence on a chromosome. This can be DNA–DNA recognition or DNA–RNA recognition. This technique uses two single-stranded sequences and is a vital part of polymerase chain reaction and Southern blotting.

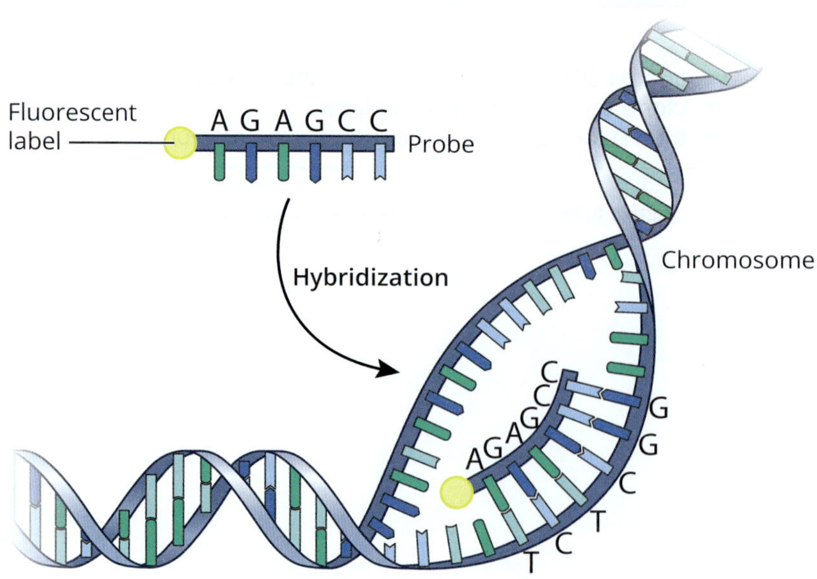

Figure 6.29 DNA Probe Hybridization

Polymerase Chain Reaction

Polymerase chain reaction (PCR) is a powerful and widely-used method of DNA amplification, developed in 1983 by the biochemist Kary Mullis, that can produce millions of copies of a DNA sequence. PCR is fundamental in many research-based assays, and is commonly used as a way to identify criminal suspects, assess familial relationships, and look for the presence of disease-causing organisms in medical samples.

BRIDGE

PCR provides a great example of the temperature dependence of enzymes. While human DNA polymerase denatures at the high temperatures required in PCR, the DNA polymerase from *T. aquaticus* functions optimally at these temperatures. Refer to Chapter 2 of *MCAT Biochemistry Review* for more on the link between temperature and enzyme activity.

To amplify a desired region of DNA, a PCR reaction requires the DNA that contains the region of interest, primers that are complementary to the DNA that flanks the region of interest, nucleotides (dATP, dTTP, dCTP, and dGTP), and DNA polymerase. Once all combined, the reaction mixture will then undergo a thermal cycle to double the amount of initial DNA. A thermal cycle in PCR involves 3 major steps:

1. **Denaturation:** In this step, the PCR reaction mixture is heated to nearly boiling temperatures (around 95°C) to separate the two DNA strands.
2. **Primer annealing:** The solution is cooled enough that the primers are able to bind to the complementary regions that flank the region of interest, while staying warm enough to avoid the two DNA strands from reannealing.
3. **Elongation:** DNA polymerase will synthesize, starting at the primers, a new complementary DNA strand, leading to doubling the amount of DNA that was initially in the mixture.

This process of thermal cycling, with each cycle involving the steps of *denaturation*, *primer annealing*, and *elongation,* is repeated up to 20-40 times, or until there are enough copies of the DNA sequence for further use. Figure 6.30 illustrates an example of this. Unfortunately, the DNA polymerase found in the human body does not work at high temperatures: Thus, heat-resistant DNA polymerases, such as the DNA polymerase Taq Polymerase from *Thermus aquaticus*, a species of bacteria that thrives in the hot springs of Yellowstone National Park at 70°C, are typically used instead.

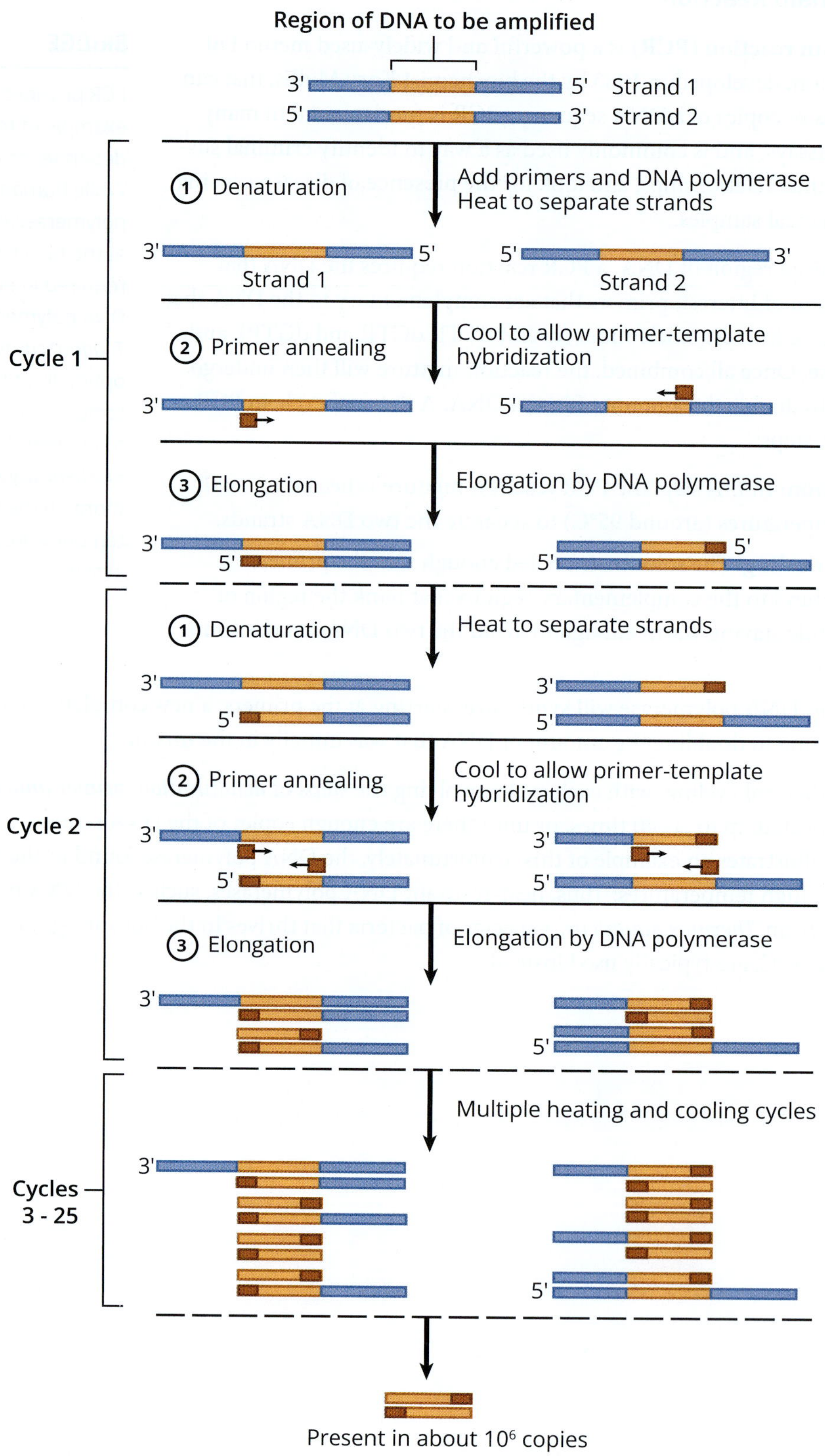

Figure 6.30 Denaturation, Primer Annealing, and Elongation in Each Thermal Cycle in PCR

Reverse Transcription Polymerase Chain Reaction

Reverse transcription polymerase chain reaction (RT-PCR) is a technique used to convert a specific RNA sequence into DNA and then amplify the DNA. This technique can be used for cloning purposes but more commonly is used to measure the transcriptional activity of a gene of interest. In fact, RT-PCR is one of the most commonly used methods for detecting the COVID-19 virus. As seen in Figure 6.31, the RNA from a tissue sample is first extracted. Then, **reverse transcriptase**, an RNA-dependent DNA polymerase derived from retroviruses, is added, along with a primer complementary to the target mRNA, nucleotides, and DNA polymerase. Reverse transcriptase then creates a complementary DNA strand (cDNA) to the RNA, which is followed by amplification of the DNA by PCR with DNA polymerase. This technique allows for the quantification of RNA, even at low levels of expression, as the final amount of DNA produced correlates to how much RNA was in the original sample.

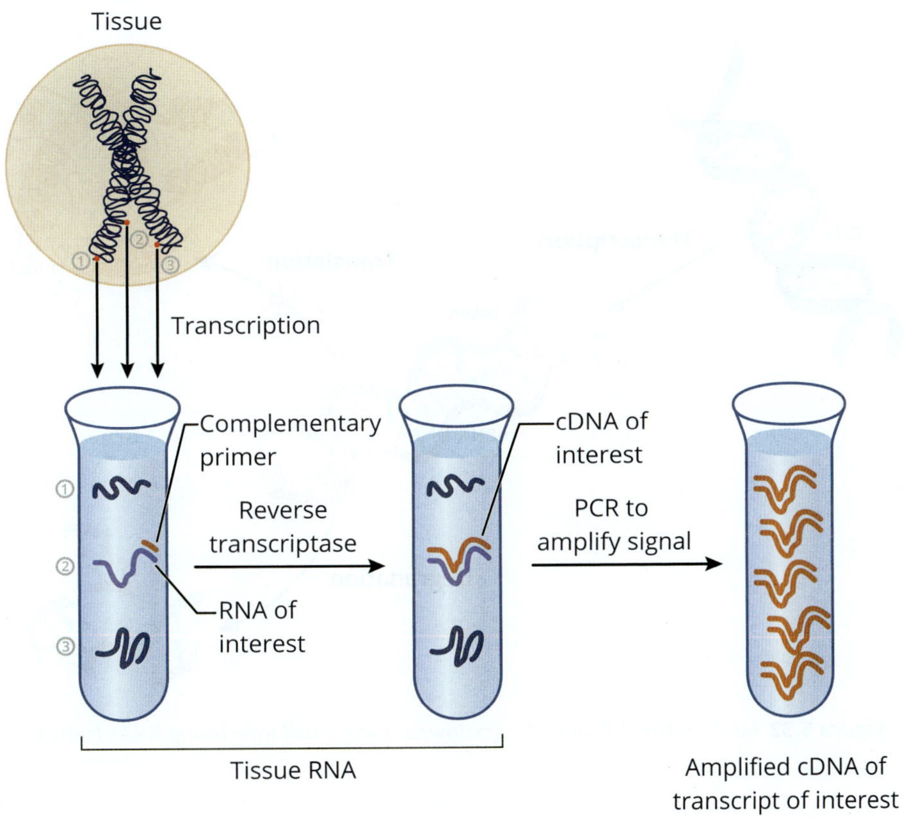

Figure 6.31 Reverse Transcription Polymerase Chain Reaction

Small Interfering RNA

Small interfering RNA (siRNA), also known as **silencing RNA**, are small non-coding RNA molecules that decrease the amount of a particular protein by interfering with the expression of specific mRNA strands before translation. In an experimental technique called a **knockdown**, introduction of siRNA into a cell temporarily represses the levels of a particular protein at the level of translation, in comparison to a **knockout**, which permanently disables gene expression entirely at the level of DNA. Typically, siRNAs are double-stranded RNAs that match the sequence of the mRNA of the target protein. While naturally occurring, they can also be synthetically created to target a specific protein and then transfected into cells, where they are then incorporated into what is known as the **RNA-inducing silencing complex (RISC)**, subsequently binding to the complementary target mRNA sequence. Activated RISC has endonuclease activity, which cleaves the target mRNA, making it unusable for translation and halting new protein creation. Figure 6.32 shows the general process by which siRNAs inhibit translation of proteins.

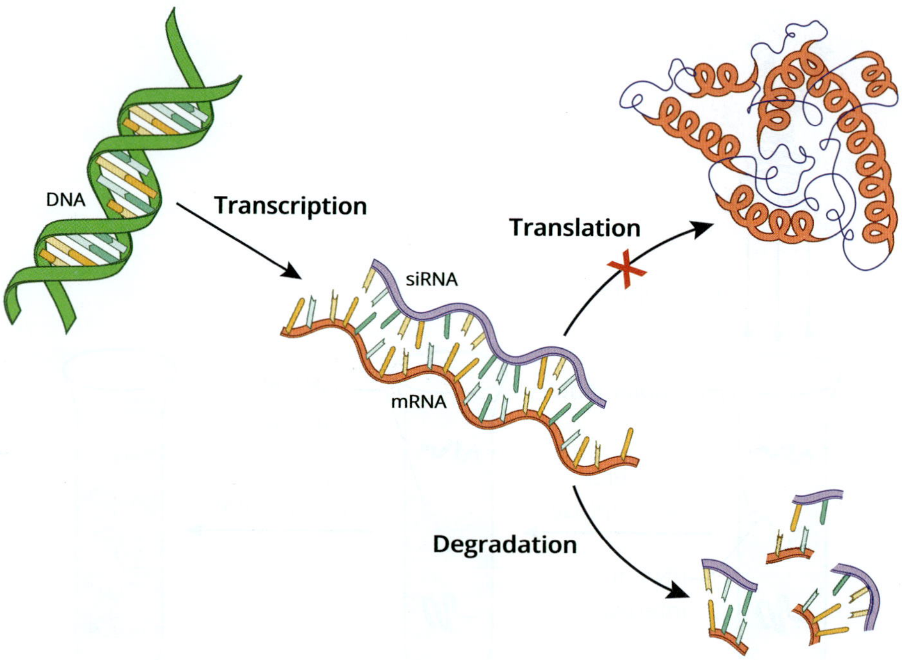

Figure 6.32 Mechanism of Protein Knockdowns Using Small Interfering RNAs (siRNAs)

Blotting and Molecular Labeling

Gel electrophoresis is a technique used to separate macromolecules, such as DNA and proteins, by size and/or charge. Electrophoresis of proteins and the different types of PAGE were discussed in detail in Chapter 3 of *MCAT Biochemistry Review*, but DNA can also be separated using gel electrophoresis. All molecules of DNA are negatively charged because of the phosphate groups in the backbone of the molecule, so all DNA strands will migrate toward the anode of an electrochemical cell. The preferred gel for DNA electrophoresis is **agarose gel**, and—just like proteins in polyacrylamide gel—the longer the DNA strand, the slower it will migrate in the gel.

Gel electrophoresis is often used prior to **blotting**, which is a method of transferring molecules like DNA, RNA, and proteins onto a thin membrane. Once the molecules have transferred onto the membrane, they can then be visualized in a number of different ways, depending on the experimental set-up. On the MCAT, three types of blots are tested on the exam: Southern blots, northern blots, and western blots. In each of these, detection of the molecule of interest creates bands on the membrane. However, it is important to note that blots are semi-quantitative methods of detection. While thicker bands correlate with more of the molecule of interest being present, an exact amount of how much of the molecule of interest is present cannot be determined. Figure 6.33 summarizes Southern, northern, and western blotting, each described in detail below.

MCAT EXPERTISE

The MCAT of course does not test capitalization conventions, but you may have noticed a difference in how the different types of blotting are spelled out. The term "Southern blot" derives its title from its inventor, Edwin Southern. For this reason, Southern is capitalized. However, western and northern blots, which are a play on words of "Southern" and not the name of any individual, are lower case.

Southern Blot

A **Southern blot** is used after gel electrophoresis to detect the presence of specific DNA sequences in a sample, as seen in Figure 6.33. After purification, DNA is cut by restriction enzymes into fragments before being separated by gel electrophoresis. The DNA fragments are then carefully transferred (or blotted) onto a membrane. The membrane is then probed with many copies of a labeled DNA sequence that is complementary to the DNA sequence of interest, which will bind and create double-stranded DNA. The probes are labeled, usually either with radioisotopes or fluorescent proteins, which are used to visualize the presence of the desired DNA sequence after probe binding.

Northern Blot

A **northern blot** is similar to a Southern blot, but instead separates and probes for RNA sequences of interest. Figure 6.33 shows the process of generating a northern blot. After purification, RNA is separated by gel electrophoresis and then transferred onto a membrane that is subsequently washed with labeled nucleotide probes that are complementary to the RNA sequence of interest. Note that unlike DNA, which requires fragmentation due to size, RNA molecules are usually short enough to not need fragmentation with restriction enzymes prior to gel electrophoresis.

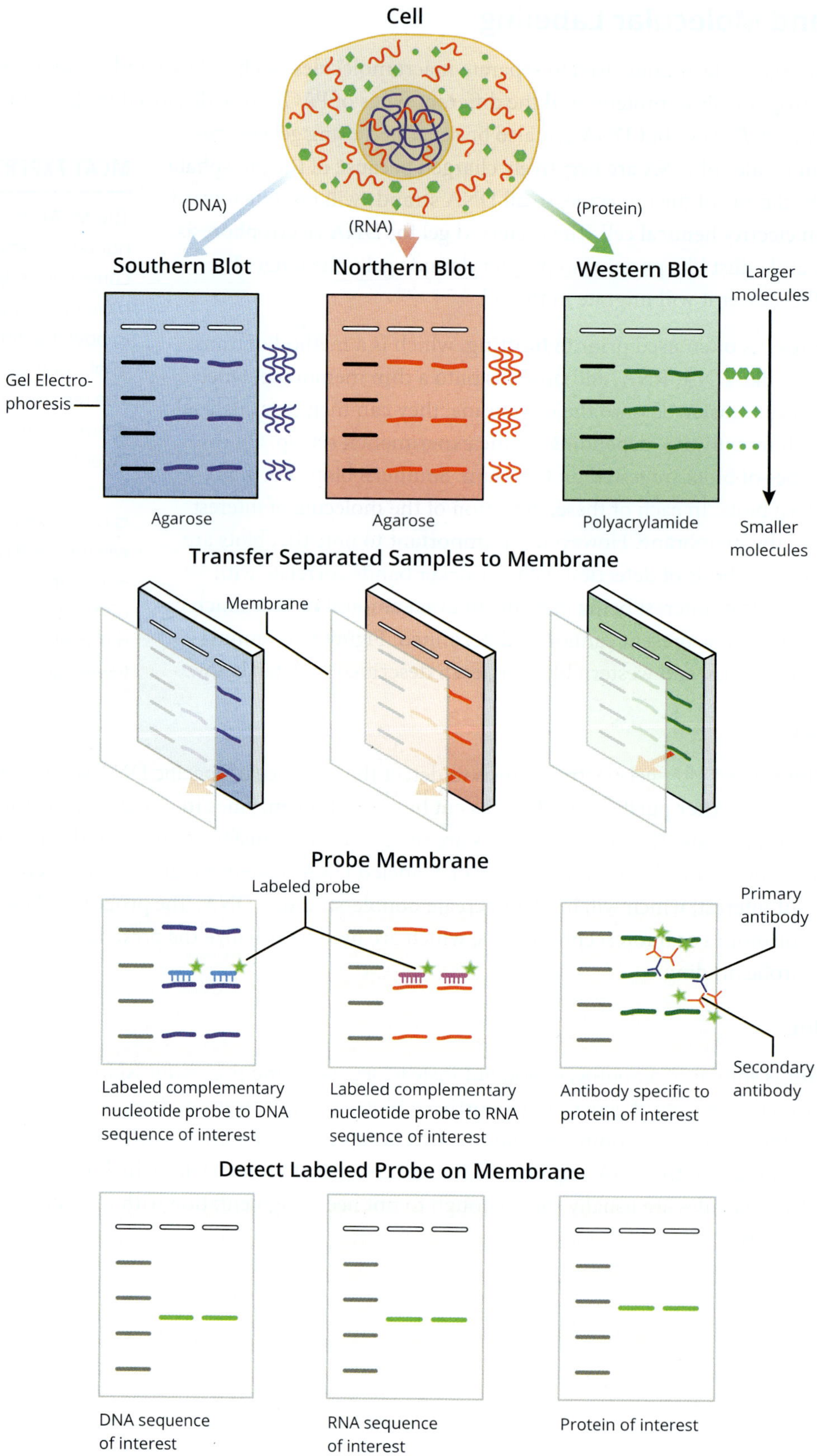

Figure 6.33 Summary of Southern, Western, and Northern Blots

Western Blot

Like northern and Southern blots, **western blots** follow the pattern of separation by gel electrophoresis, transfer to a membrane, and detection through the use of a labeled probe, as shown in Figure 6.33. However, western blots are used to detect specific proteins rather than nucleotides. As discussed in detail in Chapter 3 of *MCAT Biochemistry Review*, after purification, proteins are separated on gels made of polyacrylamide rather than agarose. After transfer to a membrane, proteins are then probed using antibodies specific to that protein. The antibodies that bind directly to the protein of interest are called **primary antibodies**. While primary antibodies can be radiolabeled or bound with a fluorescent protein for detection, it is more common that unlabeled primary antibodies are detected with a labeled **secondary antibody**, which recognizes and binds to the primary antibodies. The use of a secondary antibody amplifies the signal for better detection of proteins on the membrane: for every primary antibody bound to the protein, multiple secondary antibodies can bind to the primary antibody. On a practical level, the use of labeled secondary antibodies is also more widely applicable than using labeled primary antibodies: Primary antibodies bind to very specific molecules and protein sequences, even down to the level of post-translational modifications, meaning detection can only occur if each different primary antibody is labeled. However, secondary antibodies are created to recognize the Fc portion of other antibodies and can therefore bind to multiple different primary antibodies, making for a more generalized method of detection. Antibodies are covered in more depth in Chapter 8 of *MCAT Biology Review*.

Western blots also use **loading controls** to ensure that all the samples loaded onto the gel contain equal amounts of protein. Loading controls in western blots are usually proteins that are known as "house-keeping" genes, which are highly and ubiquitously expressed in cells, and therefore should have consistent levels regardless of experimental conditions. Loading controls are also used in other types of assays, such as Southern and northern blots, but most frequently appear on the MCAT in the context of western blots. The MCAT will not expect memorization or knowledge of specific loading controls, such as β-actin, GAPDH (an enzyme found in glycolysis), or vinculin, but they will expect recognition of loading controls. Without loading controls, it would be impossible to determine if an experimental condition changed the levels of a protein, or if more or less sample was added. Figure 6.34 shows the use of GAPDH as a loading control, where the levels of GAPDH are equal between the three samples, thus ensuring that there was indeed equal loading of all three wells with equal amounts of sample. This means that the levels of BRCA1 and BARD1 truly did decrease in Samples 1 and 2 compared to the control.

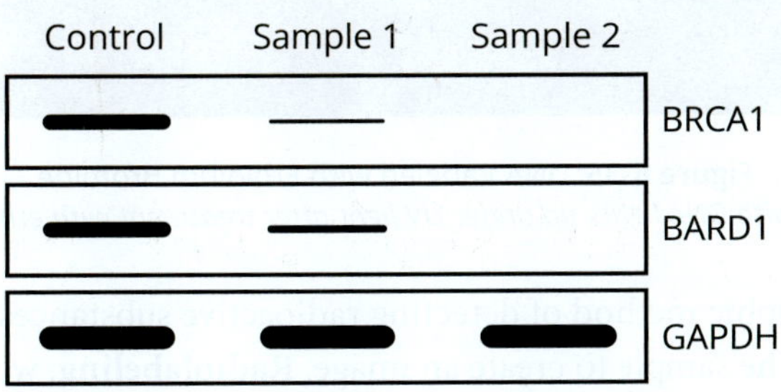

Figure 6.34 GAPDH as a Loading Control
GAPDH levels are equal, indicating BRCA1 and BARD1 levels actually decreased.

Molecular Labeling

Many molecules cannot be directly seen with the human eye. Therefore, methods of detection are crucial for the visualization of what is normally invisible. There are numerous different techniques, many of which are beyond the scope of the MCAT, but a few different types that frequently come up in passages and questions include fluorescence and autoradiography.

A **fluorescent tag**, also called a fluorescent probe, is a fluorescent molecule that is bound or chemically linked to a non-fluorescent molecule, such as a protein, amino acid, or oligonucleotide. The phenomenon of fluorescence is described in detail in Chapter 9 of *MCAT Physics and Math Review*, but in short, the addition of a fluorescent tag allows for the detection of the labeled molecule using light. Fluorescent proteins, such as green fluorescent protein (GFP), can be added to other non-fluorescent proteins for tracking or detection, such as on antibodies during western blot visualization. Ethidium bromide, an **intercalator** that inserts itself between the bases of DNA, is a type of fluorescent dye that allows for the visualization of DNA when exposed to UV light as shown in Figure 6.35.

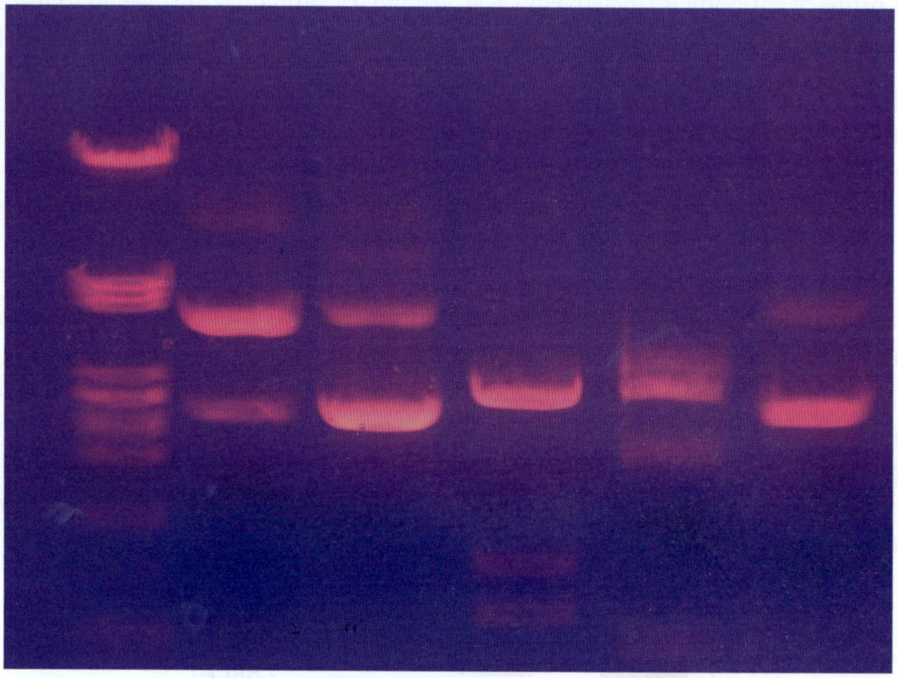

Figure 6.35 DNA Labeled with Ethidium Bromide
An agarose gel with DNA lights up under UV light after treatment with ethidium bromide.

Autoradiography is a photographic method of detecting radioactive substances through the exposure of film or a digital detection device to the sample to create an image. **Radiolabeling**, which is a form of isotopic labeling, is commonly used to label molecules with radioactivity for tracking and detection using autoradiography. This is accomplished by replacing certain atoms with radioactive isotopes. On the MCAT, the most common radioactive isotopes include ^{14}C, ^{35}S, and ^{32}P (note that ^{18}O is not radioactive). The use of radiolabels allows for the tracking and identification of atoms and molecules like proteins and nucleic acids as they go through biochemical reactions. A common method of tagging phosphorylated proteins, as shown in Figure 6.36, is through the use of radiolabeled ATP, where the phosphorous atom in the γ-phosphate group has been tagged with ^{32}P. When the γ-phosphate group is used in protein phosphorylation, the protein gains a radioactive phosphate group, which can then be tracked using autoradiography.

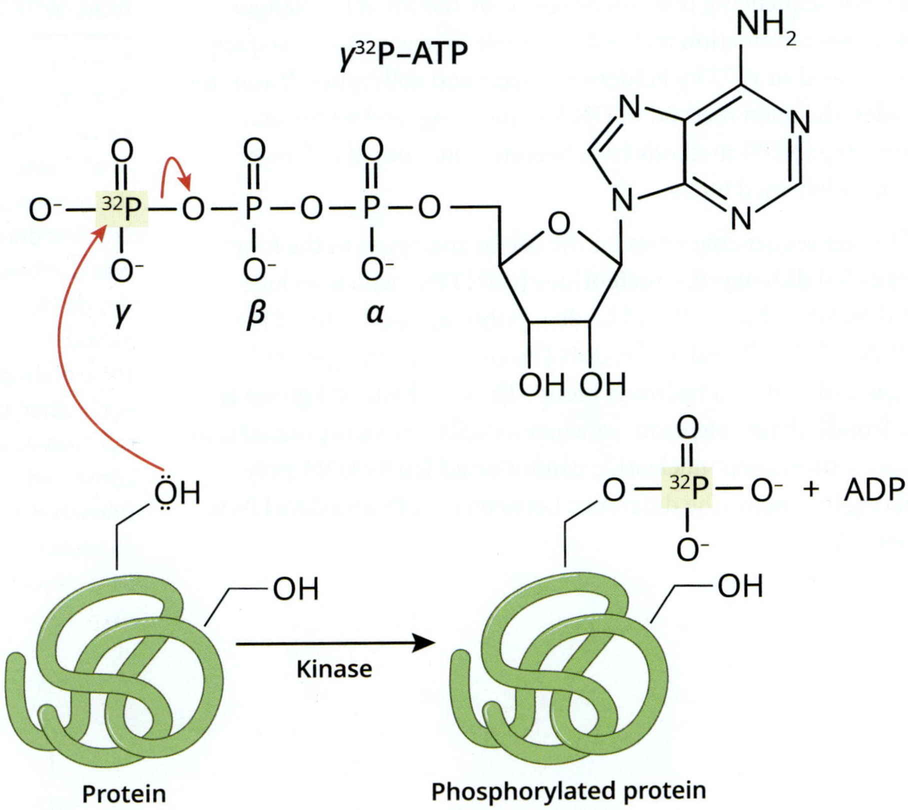

Figure 6.36 Radiolabeling ATP with ^{32}P

Radiolabeling has been used to make many ground-breaking discoveries. In the Hershey-Chase experiments, which helped show that DNA, not protein, was genetic material, bacteriophages were labeled with either radioactive DNA using ^{32}P or with radioactive proteins using ^{35}S. When the bacteriophages were allowed to infect unlabeled bacteria, the viral progenies contained radioactive isotopes only with the bacteriophages labeled with ^{32}P, while the progeny from ^{35}S-labeled bacteriophages remained unlabeled.

DNA Sequencing

DNA sequencing, or the process of determining the nucleic acid sequence of a polynucleotide, has revolutionized the world that we live in. The applications of this technique are far-reaching, from the medical field to the justice system. Since the 1970s when DNA sequencing was first developed, the field has undergone major advancements and is still ever-evolving, with multiple methods of sequencing being used and improved upon in laboratories across the world. As such, the MCAT will not expect detailed knowledge on the many different types of DNA sequencing, but the test will expect a fundamental understanding of the basic principles that underlie many of these techniques.

One method of DNA sequencing that can be tested by the MCAT is **Sanger sequencing** (the chain termination method), an early first-generation sequencing technique developed in 1977 by Frederick Sanger and colleagues. It was, for nearly four decades, the main method of DNA sequencing, and while next-generation sequencing (NGS) methods have become more popular, Sanger sequencing is still widely used today.

The premise of Sanger sequencing relies on the use of analogues to the four nucleotide bases called **dideoxyribonucleotides (ddNTPs)**, which include ddATP, ddCTP, ddGTP, and ddTTP. Unlike deoxyribonucleotides (dNTPs), which are dATP, dCTP, dGTP, and dTTP, ddNTPs contain a hydrogen at C-3′ of the ribose sugar, rather than a hydroxyl group. The C-3′ hydroxyl group is required for nucleotide chain extension, so when a ddNTP is incorporated into the growing chain, a subsequent nucleotide cannot be added by DNA polymerase, terminating the chain. The difference between dNTPs and ddNTPs is shown in Figure 6.37.

REAL WORLD

The Human Genome Project, initiated in 1991, involved the identification of all 3 billion base pairs of the human DNA sequence. The first draft of this project was completed in 2000. This project demonstrated that although humans appear to be quite different from each other, the sequence of our DNA is, in reality, highly conserved. On average, two unrelated individuals still share over 99.9% of their DNA sequences.

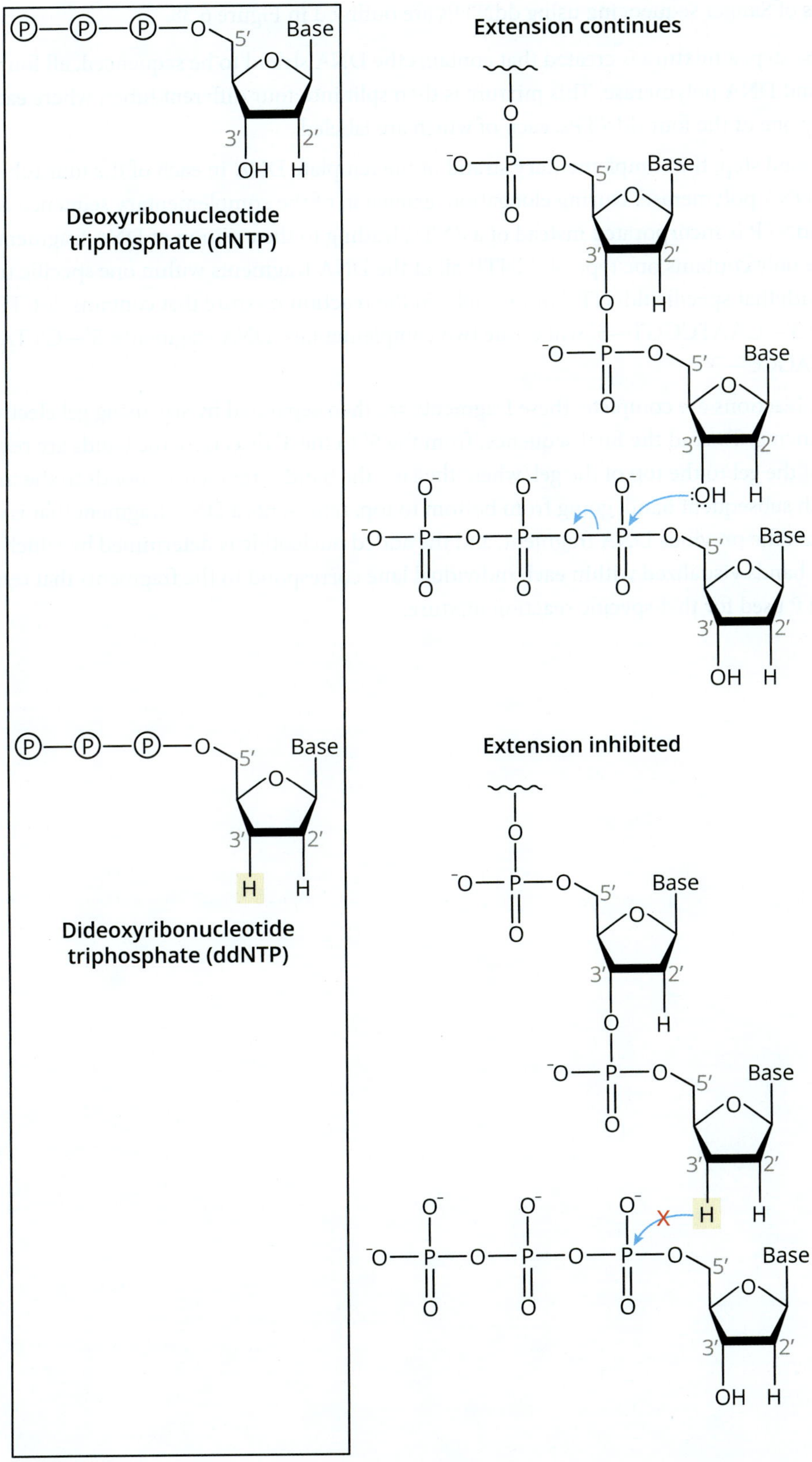

Figure 6.37 Comparison of Deoxynucleotides (dNTPs) and Dideoxynucleotides (ddNTPs)
Once a ddNTP has been incorporated, another nucleotide cannot be added.

The basic steps of Sanger sequencing using ddNTPs are outlined in Figure 6.38.

1. In the first step, a mixture is created that contains the DNA strand to be sequenced, all four dNTPs, a primer, and DNA polymerase. This mixture is then split into four different tubes, where each tube contains only one of the four ddNTPs, each of which are labeled.
2. In the second step, the complementary strand of the template DNA in each of the four tubes is synthesized by DNA polymerase. During elongation, extension of the complementary sequence is terminated when a ddNTP is incorporated instead of a dNTP, leading to the creation of DNA fragments. Because each tube only contains one type of ddNTP, all of the DNA fragments within one specific tube will terminate with that specific ddNTP. For example, in the reaction mixture that contains ddCTP, the template sequence 3′—CAATCGGT—5′ will create two complementary DNA fragments: 5′—GTTAGC—3′ and 5′—GTTAGCC—3′.
3. Once the reactions are complete, these fragments are then separated by size using gel electrophoresis for sequencing. To read the final sequence, from the 5′ to the 3′ direction, the bands are read from the bottom of the gel to the top of the gel, where the lane the bands are in corresponds to the incorporated base. Each subsequent band, going from bottom to top, represents a DNA fragment that is one nucleotide longer than the previous DNA fragment, and the added nucleotide is determined by which lane the band is in. The bands visualized within each individual lane correspond to the fragments that terminate with the ddNTP used for that specific reaction mixture.

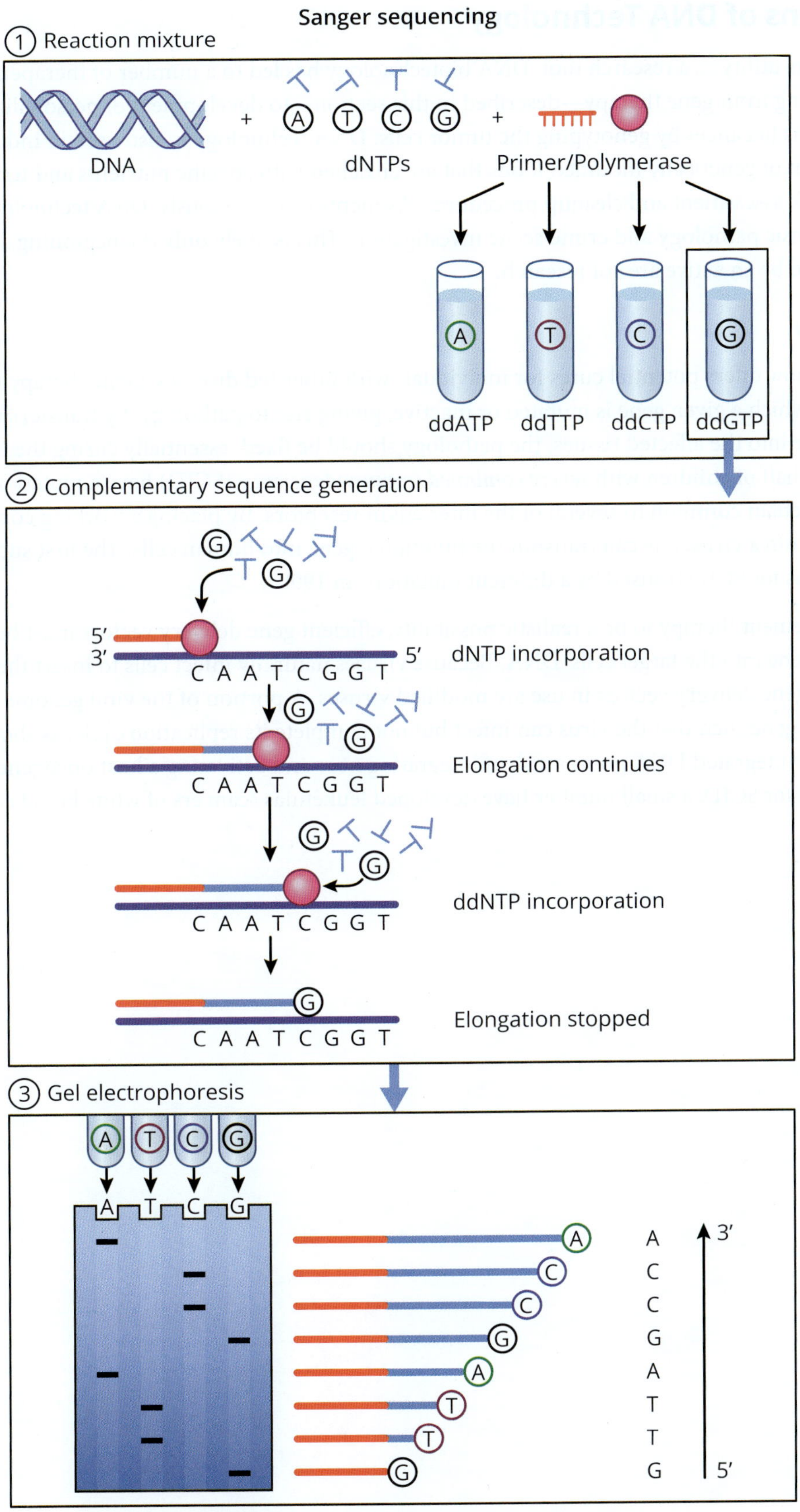

Figure 6.38 The Steps of Sanger Sequencing

Applications of DNA Technology

In addition to its utility as a research tool, DNA biotechnology has led to a number of therapeutic breakthroughs, ranging from gene therapy—described in this section—to development of personalized chemotherapeutic regimens in cancer by genotyping the tumor cells. DNA technology is also used in industry, including the development of genetically modified foods that are enriched with specific nutrients and testing of the environment for risk assessment and cleanup procedures. As mentioned previously, DNA technology also plays a key role in forensic pathology and crime scene investigation. This is likely only the beginning, as biotechnology continues to be an active area of research.

Gene Therapy

Gene therapy now offers potential cures for individuals with inherited diseases. Gene therapy is intended for diseases in which a given gene is mutated or inactive, giving rise to pathology. By transferring a normal copy of the gene into the affected tissues, the pathology should be fixed, essentially curing the individual. For instance, about half of children with *severe combined immunodeficiency* (SCID) have a mutation in the gene encoding the γ chain common to several of the interleukin receptors. By placing a working copy of the gene for the γ chain into a virus, one can transmit the functional gene into human cells. The first successful case of gene therapy was for SCID (caused by a different mutation) in 1990.

For gene replacement therapy to be a realistic possibility, efficient gene delivery vectors must be used to transfer the cloned gene into the target cells' DNA. Because viruses naturally infect cells to insert their own genetic material, most gene delivery vectors in use are modified viruses. A portion of the viral genome is replaced with the cloned gene such that the virus can infect but not complete its replication cycle, as shown in Figure 6.39. Randomly integrated DNA poses a risk of integrating near and activating a host oncogene. Among the children treated for SCID, a small number have developed leukemias (cancers of white blood cells).

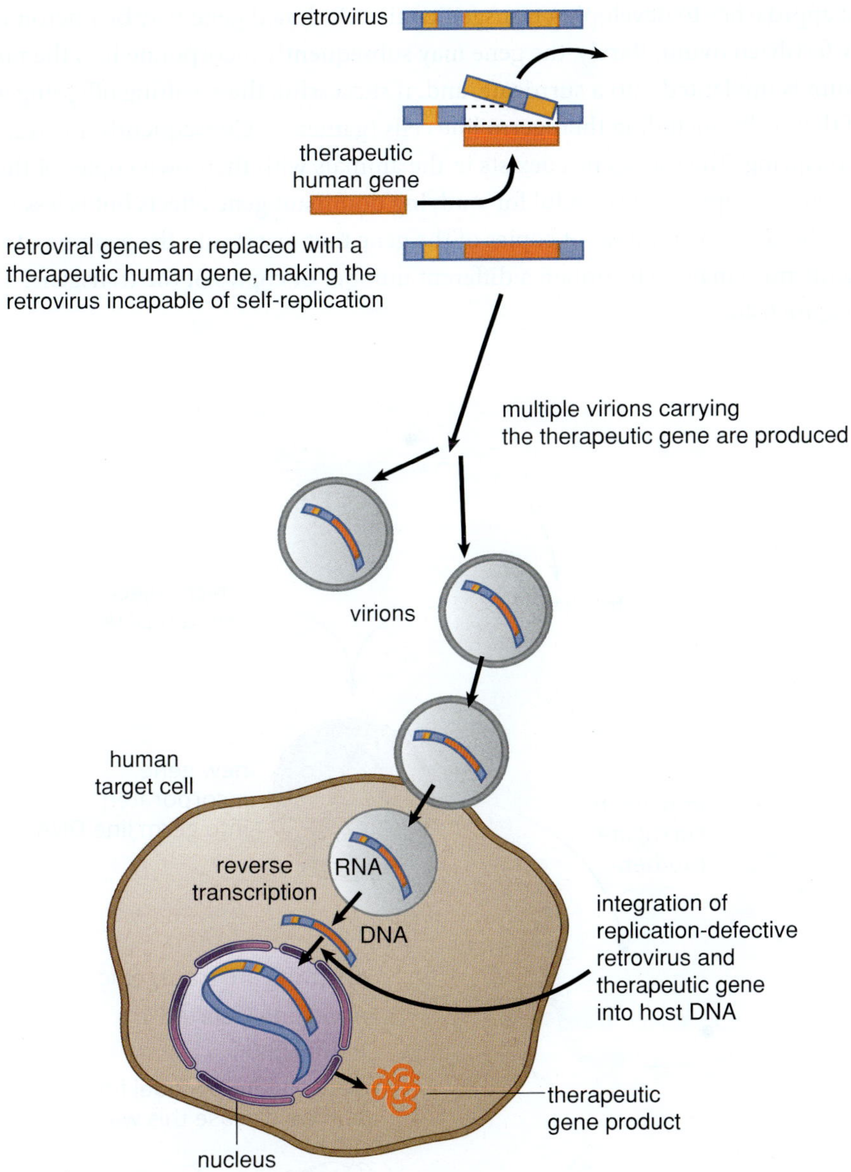

Figure 6.39 Retroviral Gene Therapy
The example given here uses a retrovirus, but other viruses may also be used for gene therapy.

Transgenic and Knockout Mice

Once DNA has been isolated, it can be introduced into eukaryotic cells. **Transgenic mice** are altered at their **germ line** by introducing a cloned gene into fertilized ova or into embryonic stem cells. The cloned gene that is introduced is referred to as a **transgene**. If the transgene is a disease-producing allele, the transgenic mice can be used to study the disease process from early embryonic development through adulthood. A similar approach can be used to produce **knockout mice**, in which a gene has been intentionally deleted (knocked out). These mice provide valuable models in which to study human diseases.

There are different approaches to developing transgenic mice. A cloned gene may be microinjected into the nucleus of a newly fertilized ovum. Rarely, the gene may subsequently incorporate into the nuclear DNA of the zygote. The ovum is implanted into a surrogate, and, if successful, the resulting offspring will contain the transgene in all of their cells, including their germ line cells (gametes). Consequently, the transgene will also be passed to *their* offspring. The transgene coexists in the animals with their own copies of the gene, which have not been deleted. This approach is useful for studying dominant gene effects but is less useful as a model for recessive disease because the number of copies of the gene that insert into the genome cannot be controlled; the transgenic mice may each contain a different number of copies of the transgene. This method is demonstrated in Figure 6.40.

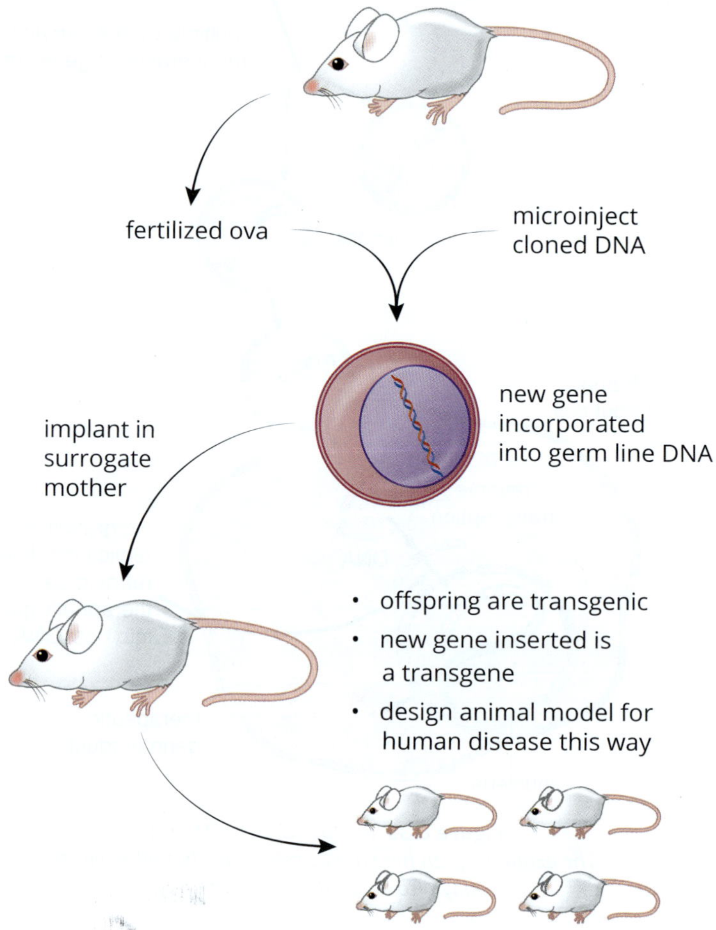

Figure 6.40 Creation of a Transgenic Mouse

Embryonic stem cell lines can also be used for developing transgenic mice. Advantages of using stem cell lines are that the cloned genes can be introduced in cultures, and that one can select for cells with the transgene successfully inserted. The altered stem cells are injected into developing blastocysts and implanted into surrogates. The blastocyst itself is thus composed of two types of stem cells: the ones containing the transgene and the original blastocyst cells that lack the transgene. The resulting offspring is a ***chimera***, meaning that it has patches of cells, including germ cells, derived from each of the two lineages. This is evident if the two cell lineages (transgenic cells and host blastocyst) come from mice with different coat colors. The chimeras will have patchy coats of two colors, allowing them to be easily identified. These chimeras can then be bred to produce mice that are heterozygous for the transgene and mice that are homozygous for the transgene.

Safety and Ethics

The different procedures and techniques that have been reviewed provide great insight for researchers in many different fields of study. However, it is also important to acknowledge the potential risks associated with these technologies. Safety concerns such as increased resistance in viruses and bacteria can impact both humans and the environment in which we live. Ethical dilemmas arise: Is it ethical to test for life-threatening genetic diseases and potentially terminate a pregnancy based on the results? What about testing for eye or hair color? What are the ethical questions around choosing human test subjects? If a disease-causing gene were found in one individual of a family, does this need to be communicated to other relatives at risk, potentially violating principles of privacy? Is it permissible to carry out potentially risky therapies in individuals whose illnesses makes them unable to communicate? The medical community and bioethicists at large continue to wrestle with this question: How much should we meddle with our own genetic makeup?

REAL WORLD

The story of Jesse Gelsinger is one particularly harrowing example of the problems that biotechnology can create. Diagnosed with mild *ornithine transcarbamylase* (OTC) deficiency, a defect of the urea cycle, Gelsinger volunteered for a clinical trial of gene therapy. During the trial (which was also fraught with questionable consent practices), Gelsinger died from a massive immune response to the viral vector, leading to multiple organ failure and brain death. He was 18 years old.

MCAT CONCEPT CHECK 6.5

Before you move on, assess your understanding of the material with these questions.

1. When creating a DNA library, what are some of the advantages of genomic libraries? What about cDNA libraries?
   - Genomic:

   ___

   - cDNA:

   ___

2. What does PCR accomplish for a researcher? What about Southern blotting?
   - PCR:

   ___

   - Southern blotting:

   ___

3. During DNA sequencing, why does the DNA polymer stop growing once a dideoxyribonucleotide is added?

   ___

4. What is the difference between a transgenic and a knockout mouse?

   ___

Conclusion

In this chapter, the DNA molecule was discussed. The importance of this molecule as an archive in the cell was highlighted. The unique structure of the DNA double helix and complementary base-pairing are integral to DNA molecules' ability to replicate and pass information from cell to cell and from generation to generation. Replication of DNA is a complex process involving many enzymes and proteins that are highly coordinated to ensure efficiency. The discoveries of DNA structure and function aid us in understanding how cellular processes take place but also provide us with many tools to exploit in the laboratory.

DNA is one of the most heavily tested concepts on the MCAT. This makes sense because not only has our understanding of the molecule increased exponentially over the last few decades, but also our ability to manipulate DNA. This has led to the creation of an entire industry of biotechnology that will assuredly grow during your career as a medical student and physician. In the next chapter, we turn to DNA's counterpart, RNA. We'll explore how the genes discussed in this chapter can actually turn into functional proteins through the key processes of transcription and translation.

GO ONLINE

You've reviewed the content, now test your knowledge and critical thinking skills by completing a test-like passage set in your online resources!

CONCEPT SUMMARY

DNA Structure

- **Deoxyribonucleic acid** (**DNA**) is a macromolecule that stores genetic information in all living organisms.
- **Nucleosides** contain a five-carbon sugar bonded to a nitrogenous base; **nucleotides** are nucleosides with one to three phosphate groups added.
  - Nucleotides in DNA contain **deoxyribose**; in RNA, they contain **ribose**.
  - Nucleotides are abbreviated by letter: **adenine** (**A**), **cytosine** (**C**), **guanine** (**G**), **thymine** (**T**), and **uracil** (**U**).
- DNA is organized according to the **Watson–Crick model**.
  - The backbone is composed of alternating sugar and phosphate groups, and is always read **5′ to 3′**.
  - There are two strands with **antiparallel** polarity, wound into a **double helix**.
  - **Purines** (A and G) always pair with **pyrimidines** (C, U, and T). In DNA, A pairs with T (via two hydrogen bonds) and C pairs with G (via three hydrogen bonds). RNA does not contain thymine, but contains uracil instead; thus, in RNA, A pairs with U (via two hydrogen bonds).
  - Purines and pyrimidines are biological aromatic heterocycles. **Aromatic** compounds are cyclic, planar, and **conjugated**, and contain $4n + 2$ π electrons (where n is any integer; **Hückel's rule**). Heterocycles are ring structures that contain at least two different elements in the ring.
  - **Chargaff's rules** state that purines and pyrimidines are equal in number in a DNA molecule, and that because of base-pairing, the amount of adenine equals the amount of thymine, and the amount of cytosine equals the amount of guanine.
  - Most DNA is B-DNA, forming a right-handed helix. Low concentrations of Z-DNA, with a zigzag shape, may be seen with high GC-content or high salt concentration.
- DNA strands can be pulled apart (**denatured**) and brought back together (**reannealed**). Heat, alkaline pH, and chemicals like formaldehyde and urea can cause denaturation of DNA; removal of these conditions may result in reannealing of the strands.

Eukaryotic Chromosome Organization

- DNA is organized into 46 chromosomes in human cells.
- In eukaryotes, DNA is wound around **histone proteins** (H2A, H2B, H3, and H4) to form **nucleosomes**, which may be stabilized by another histone protein (H1). As a whole, DNA and its associated histones make up **chromatin** in the nucleus.
  - **Heterochromatin** is dense, transcriptionally silent DNA that appears dark under light microscopy.
  - **Euchromatin** is less dense, transcriptionally active DNA that appears light under light microscopy.
- **Telomeres** are the ends of chromosomes. They contain high GC-content to prevent unraveling of the DNA. During replication, telomeres are slightly shortened, although this can be (partially) reversed by the enzyme telomerase.
- **Centromeres** are located in the middle of chromosomes and hold sister chromatids together until they are separated during anaphase in mitosis. They also contain a high GC-content to maintain a strong bond between chromatids.

DNA Replication

- The **replisome** (**replication complex**) is a set of specialized proteins that assist the DNA polymerases.
- To replicate DNA, it is first unwound at an **origin of replication** by **helicases**. This produces two **replication forks** on either side of the origin.
    - Prokaryotes have a circular chromosome that contains only one origin of replication.
    - Eukaryotes have linear chromosomes that contain many origins of replication.
- Unwound strands are kept from reannealing or being degraded by **single-stranded DNA-binding proteins**.
- **Supercoiling** causes torsional strain on the DNA molecule, which can be released by **DNA topoisomerases**, which create nicks in the DNA molecule.
- DNA replication is **semiconservative**: one old **parent strand** and one new **daughter strand** is incorporated into each of the two new DNA molecules.
- DNA cannot be synthesized without an adjacent nucleotide to hook onto, so a small RNA primer is put down by **primase**.
- **DNA polymerase III** (prokaryotes) or **DNA polymerases** α, δ, and ε (eukaryotes) can then synthesize a new strand of DNA; they read the template DNA $3'$ to $5'$ and synthesize the new strand $5'$ to $3'$.
    - The **leading strand** requires only one primer and can then be synthesized continuously in its entirety.
    - The **lagging strand** requires many primers and is synthesized in discrete sections called **Okazaki fragments**.
- RNA primers can later be removed by **DNA polymerase I** (prokaryotes) or **RNase H** (eukaryotes), and filled in with DNA by DNA polymerase I (prokaryotes) or DNA polymerase δ (eukaryotes). **DNA ligase** can then fuse the DNA strands together to create one complete molecule.

DNA Repair

- **Oncogenes** develop from mutations of **proto-oncogenes**, and promote cell cycling. They may lead to **cancer**, which is defined by unchecked cell proliferation with the ability to spread by local invasion or **metastasize** (migrate to distant sites via the bloodstream or lymphatic system).
- **Tumor suppressor genes** code for proteins that reduce cell cycling or promote DNA repair; mutations of tumor suppressor genes can also lead to cancer.
- During replication, DNA polymerase **proofreads** its work and excises incorrectly matched bases. The daughter strand is identified by its lack of methylation and corrected accordingly.
- **Mismatch repair** also occurs during the G_2 phase of the cell cycle, using the genes *MSH2* and *MLH1*.
- **Nucleotide excision repair** fixes helix-deforming lesions of DNA (such as thymine dimers) via a cut-and-patch process that requires an **excision endonuclease**.
- **Base excision repair** fixes nondeforming lesions of the DNA helix (such as cytosine deamination) by removing the base, leaving an **apurinic/apyrimidinic** (**AP**) **site**. An **AP endonuclease** then removes the damaged sequence, which can be filled in with the correct bases.

Recombinant Biotechnology

- **Recombinant DNA** is DNA composed of nucleotides from two different sources.
- **DNA cloning** introduces a fragment of DNA into a **vector plasmid**. **A restriction enzyme** (**restriction endonuclease**) cuts both the plasmid and the fragment, which are left with **sticky ends**. Once the fragment binds to the plasmid, it can be introduced into a bacterial cell and permitted to replicate, generating many copies of the fragment of interest.
    - Recombinant vectors contain an origin of replication, a polylinker that the fragment of interest is placed into, and at least one type of selection marker (to permit for selection of that colony after replication).
    - Once replicated, the bacterial cells can be used to create a protein of interest, or can be lysed to allow for isolation of the recombinant DNA.
- **DNA libraries** are large collections of known DNA sequences.
    - **Genomic libraries** contain large fragments of DNA, including both coding and noncoding regions of the genome. They cannot be used to make recombinant proteins or for gene therapy.
    - **cDNA libraries** (**expression libraries**) contain smaller fragments of DNA, and only include the exons of genes expressed by the sample tissue. They can be used to make recombinant proteins or for gene therapy.
- **Hybridization** is the joining of complementary base pair sequences.
    - **Polymerase chain reaction** (**PCR**) is an automated process by which millions of copies of a DNA sequence can be created from a very small sample by hybridization.
- **Blotting** is a method of transferring molecules from a gel onto a thin membrane for further analysis.
    - Molecules can be separated by size using **gel electrophoresis**.
    - **Southern blotting** can be used to detect the presence and relative quantity of various DNA strands in a sample. After electrophoresis, the sample is transferred to a membrane that can be probed with single-stranded oligonucleotides to look for a sequence of interest.
    - **Northern blotting** can be used to detect the presence and relative quantity of various RNA strands in a sample. After electrophoresis, the sample is transferred to a membrane that can be probed with single-stranded oligonucleotides to look for a sequence of interest.
    - **Western blotting** can be used to detect the presence and relative quantity of various proteins in a sample. After electrophoresis, the sample is transferred to a membrane that can be probed with primary and secondary antibodies to look for a protein of interest.
- **Sanger sequencing** is a method of DNA sequencing that uses **dideoxyribonucleotides**, which terminate the DNA chain because they lack a 3′ –OH group. The resulting fragments can be separated by gel electrophoresis, and the sequence can be read directly from the gel.
- **Molecular labeling** is used to track molecules.
    - **Fluorescent tags** can be added onto molecules and then imaged using light.
    - **Autoradiography** is a photographic method of detecting radioactive substances.
- **Gene therapy** is a method of curing genetic deficiencies by introducing a functional gene with a viral vector.

- **Transgenic mice** are created by integrating a gene of interest into the germ line or embryonic stem cells of a developing mouse.
    - Organisms that contain cells from two different lineages (such as mice formed by integration of transgenic embryonic stem cells into a normal mouse blastocyst) are called **chimeras**.
    - Transgenic mice can be mated to select for the transgene.
- **Knockout mice** are created by deleting a gene of interest.
- Biotechnology brings up a number of safety and ethical issues, including pathogen resistance and the ethics of choosing individuals for specific traits.

ANSWERS TO CONCEPT CHECKS

6.1

1. Nucleosides contain a five-carbon sugar (pentose) and nitrogenous base. Nucleotides are composed of a nucleoside plus one to three phosphate groups.
2. A pairs with T (in DNA) or U (in RNA), using two hydrogen bonds. C pairs with G, using three hydrogen bonds.
3. DNA contains deoxyribose, while RNA contains ribose. DNA contains thymine, while RNA contains uracil. Usually, DNA is double-stranded, while RNA is single-stranded.
4. The aromaticity of nucleic acids makes these compounds very stable and unreactive. Stability is important for storing genetic information and avoiding spontaneous mutations.
5. This does not violate Chargaff's rules. RNA is single-stranded, and thus the complementarity seen in DNA does not hold true. For single-stranded RNA, %C does not necessarily equal %G; %A does not necessarily equal %U.

6.2

1. The five histone proteins are H1, H2A, H2B, H3, and H4. H1 is the only one not in the histone core.
2.

Characteristic	Heterochromatin	Euchromatin
Density of chromatin packing	Dense	Not dense (uncondensed)
Appearance under light microscopy	Dark	Light
Transcriptional activity	Silent	Active

3. High GC-content increases hydrogen bonding, making the association between DNA strands very strong at telomeres and centromeres.

6.3

1.

Enzyme	Prokaryotes/ Eukaryotes/Both	Function
Helicase	Both	Unwinds DNA double helix
Single-stranded DNA-binding protein	Both	Prevents reannealing of DNA double helix during replication
Primase	Both	Places ~10-nucleotide RNA primer to begin DNA replication
DNA polymerase III	Prokaryotes	Adds nucleotides to growing daughter strand
DNA polymerase α	Eukaryotes	Adds nucleotides to growing daughter strand
DNA polymerase I	Prokaryotes	Fills in gaps left behind after RNA primer excision
RNase H	Eukaryotes	Excises RNA primer
DNA ligase	Both	Joins DNA strands (especially between Okazaki fragments)
DNA topoisomerases	Both	Reduces torsional strain from positive supercoils by introducing nicks in DNA strand

2. The lagging strand is more prone to mutations because it must constantly start and stop the process of DNA replication. Additionally, it contains many more RNA primers, all of which must be removed and filled in with DNA.
3. Telomeres are the ends of eukaryotic chromosomes and contain repetitive sequences of noncoding DNA. These protect the chromosome from losing important genes from the incomplete replication of the 5′ end of the DNA strand.

6.4

1. Oncogenes (or, more properly, proto-oncogenes) code for cell cycle–promoting proteins; when mutated, a proto-oncogene becomes an oncogene, promoting rapid cell cycling. Tumor suppressor genes code for repair or cell cycle–inhibiting proteins; when mutated, the cell cycle is allowed to proceed unchecked. Oncogenes are like stepping on the gas pedal, mutated tumor suppressor genes are like cutting the brakes.
2. The parent strand is more heavily methylated, whereas the daughter strand is barely methylated at all. This allows DNA polymerase to distinguish between the two strands during proofreading.

3.

Repair Mechanism	Phase of Cell Cycle	Key Enzymes/Genes
DNA polymerase (proofreading)	S	DNA polymerase
Mismatch repair	G_2	*MSH2, MLH1*(*MutS* and *MutL* in prokaryotes)
Nucleotide excision repair	G_1, G_2	Excision endonuclease
Base excision repair	G_1, G_2	Glycosylase, AP endonuclease

4. Nucleotide excision repair corrects lesions that are large enough to distort the double helix; base excision repair corrects lesions that are small enough not to distort the double helix.

6.5

1. Genomic libraries include all of the DNA in an organism's genome, including noncoding regions. This may be useful for studying DNA in introns, centromeres, or telomeres. cDNA libraries only include expressed genes from a given tissue, but can be used to express recombinant proteins or to perform gene therapy.
2. PCR increases the number of copies of a given DNA sequence and can be used for a sample containing very few copies of the DNA sequence. Southern blotting is useful when searching for a particular DNA sequence because it separates DNA fragments by length and then probes for a sequence of interest.
3. Dideoxyribonucleotides lack the $3'$ –OH group that is required for DNA strand elongation. Thus, once a dideoxyribonucleotide is added to a growing DNA molecule, no more nucleotides can be added because dideoxyribonucleotides have no $3'$ –OH group with which to form a bond.
4. Transgenic mice have a gene introduced into their germ line or embryonic stem cells to look at the effects of that gene; they are therefore best suited for studying the effects of dominant alleles. Knockout mice are those in which a gene of interest has been removed, rather than added.

SCIENCE MASTERY ASSESSMENT EXPLANATIONS

1. **B**

Nucleotides bond together to form polynucleotides. The 3′ hydroxyl group of one nucleotide's sugar joins the 5′ hydroxyl group of the adjacent nucleotide's sugar by a phosphodiester bond. Hydrogen bonding, **(A)**, is important for holding complementary strands together, but does not play a role in the bonds formed between adjacent nucleotides on a single strand.

2. **D**

Because we are looking for the false statement, we have to read each choice to eliminate those that are true or find one that is overtly false. Let's quickly review the main differences between DNA and RNA. In cells, DNA is double-stranded, with a deoxyribose sugar and the nitrogenous bases A, T, C, and G. RNA, on the other hand, is usually single-stranded, with a ribose sugar and the bases A, U, C, and G. **(D)** is false because both DNA replication and RNA synthesis proceed in a 5′ to 3′ direction.

3. **A**

The melting temperature of DNA is the temperature at which a DNA double helix separates into two single strands (denatures). To do this, the hydrogen bonds linking the base pairs must be broken. Cytosine binds to guanine with three hydrogen bonds, whereas adenine binds to thymine with two hydrogen bonds. The amount of heat needed to disrupt the bonding is proportional to the number of bonds. Thus, the higher the GC-content in a DNA segment, the higher the melting point.

4. **C**

Aromatic rings must contain conjugated π electrons, which require alternating single and multiple bonds, or lone pairs. In carbohydrate ring structures, only single bonds are present, thus preventing aromaticity. Nucleic acids contain aromatic heterocycles, while proteins will generally contain at least one aromatic amino acid (tryptophan, phenylalanine, or tyrosine).

5. **C**

For a compound to be aromatic, it must be cyclic, planar, conjugated, and contain $4n + 2$ π electrons, where n is any integer. Conjugation requires that every atom in the ring have at least one unhybridized p-orbital. While most examples of aromatic compounds have alternating single and double bonds, compounds can be aromatic if they contain triple bonds as well; this would still permit at least one unhybridized p-orbital.

6. **C**

During DNA replication, the strands are separated by DNA helicase. At the replication fork, primase, **(A)**, creates a primer for the initiation of replication, which is followed by DNA polymerase. On the lagging strand, Okazaki fragments form and are joined by DNA ligase, **(B)**. After the chromosome has been processed, the ends, called telomeres, are replicated with the assistance of the enzyme telomerase, **(D)**. RNA polymerase I is located in the nucleolus and synthesizes rRNA.

7. **B**

cDNA (complementary DNA) is formed from a processed mRNA strand by reverse transcription. cDNA is used in DNA libraries and contains only the exons of genes that are transcriptionally active in the sample tissue.

8. **A**

The polymerase chain reaction is used to clone a sequence of DNA using a DNA sample, a primer, free nucleotides, and enzymes. The polymerase from *Thermus aquaticus* is used because the reaction is regulated by thermal cycling, which would denature human enzymes.

9. **D**

Endonucleases are enzymes that cut DNA. They are used by the cell for DNA repair. They are also used by scientists during DNA analysis, as restriction enzymes are endonucleases. Restriction enzymes are used to cleave DNA before electrophoresis and Southern blotting, and to introduce a gene of interest into a viral vector for gene therapy.

10. **D**

Prokaryotic DNA is circular and lacks histone proteins, and thus does not form nucleosomes. Both prokaryotic and eukaryotic DNA are replicated by DNA polymerases, although these polymerases differ in identity. Eukaryotic DNA is organized into chromatin, which can condense to form linear chromosomes; only prokaryotes have circular chromosomes. Only eukaryotic DNA has telomeres.

11. **C**

One common DNA mutation is the transition from cytosine to uracil in the presence of heat. DNA repair enzymes recognize uracil and correct this error by excising the base and inserting cytosine. RNA exists only transiently in the cell, such that cytosine degradation is insignificant. Were uracil to be used in DNA under normal circumstances, it would be impossible to tell if a base *should* be uracil or if it is a damaged cytosine nucleotide.

12. **A**

Oncogenes are most likely to result in cancer through activation, **(B)**, while tumor suppressor genes are most likely to result in cancer through inactivation.

13. **B**

One of the primary ethical concerns related to gene sequencing is the issue of consent and privacy. Because genetic screening provides information on direct relatives, there are potential violations of privacy in communicating this information to family members who may be at risk. There are not significant physical risks, eliminating **(A)**, and gene sequencing is fairly accurate, eliminating **(C)** and **(D)**.

14. **D**

Euchromatin has a classic "beads on a string" appearance that stains lightly, while heterochromatin is tightly packed and stains darkly. Heterochromatin is primarily composed of inactive genes or untranslated regions, while euchromatin is able to be expressed. All chromatin is found in the nucleus, not the cytoplasm.

15. **D**

Mismatch repair mechanisms are active during S phase (proofreading) and G_2 phase (*MSH2* and *MLH1*), eliminating **(B)** and **(C)**. Nucleotide and base excision repair mechanisms are most active during the G_1 and G_2 phases, also eliminating **(A)**. These mechanisms exist during interphase because they are aimed at *preventing* propagation of the error into daughter cells during M phase (mitosis).

▶ **GO ONLINE**

Consult your online resources for additional practice.

SHARED CONCEPTS

Biochemistry Chapter 4
Carbohydrate Structure and Function

Biochemistry Chapter 7
RNA and the Genetic Code

Biology Chapter 1
The Cell

Biology Chapter 2
Reproduction

Biology Chapter 3
Embryogenesis and Development

Biology Chapter 12
Genetics and Evolution

CHAPTER 7

RNA AND THE GENETIC CODE

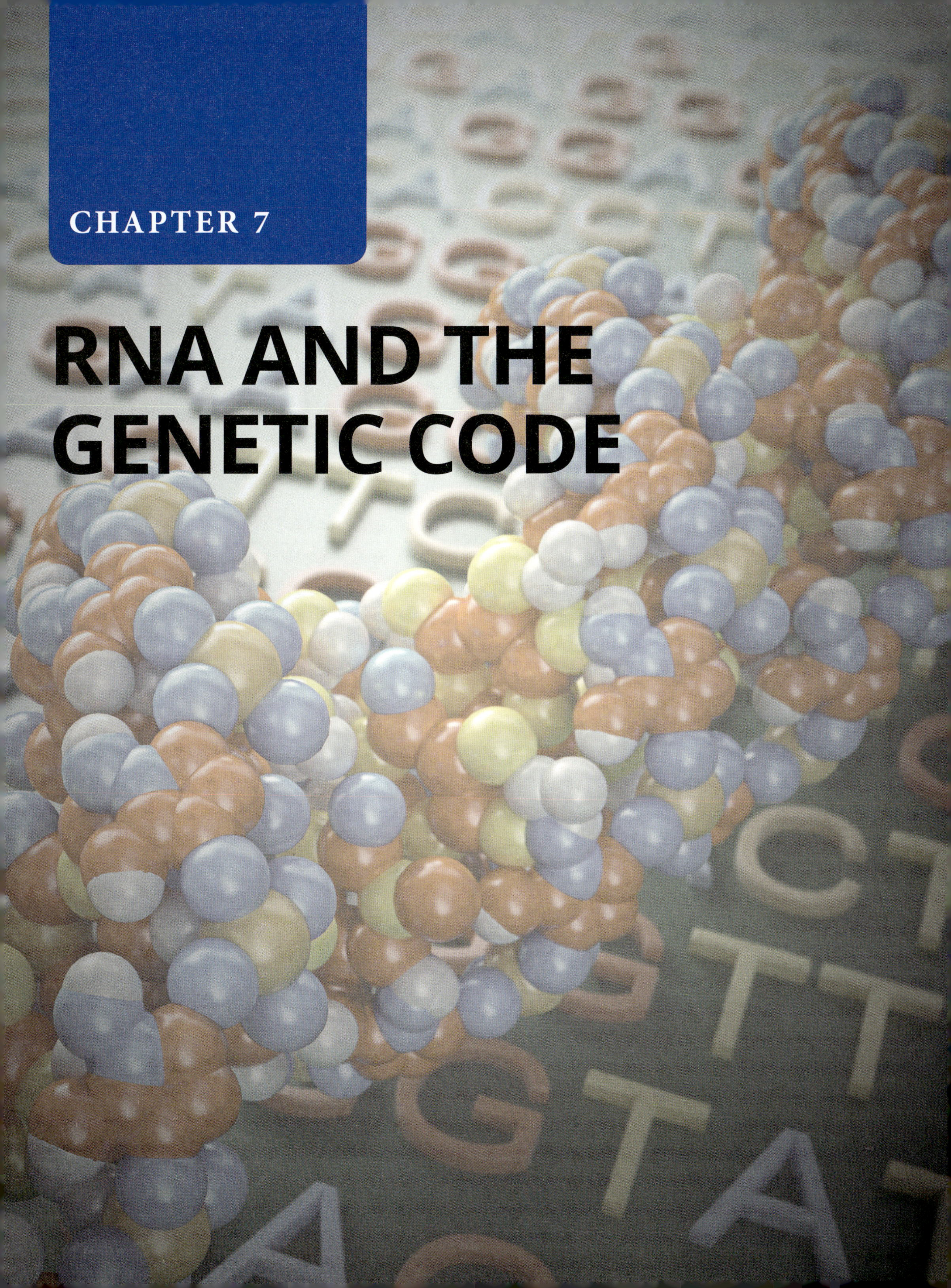

SCIENCE MASTERY ASSESSMENT

Every pre-med knows this feeling: there is so much content I have to know for the MCAT! How do I know what to do first or what's important?

While the high-yield badges throughout this book will help you identify the most important topics, this Science Mastery Assessment is another tool in your MCAT prep arsenal. This quiz (which can also be taken in your online resources) and the guidance below will help ensure that you are spending the appropriate amount of time on this chapter based on your personal strengths and weaknesses. Don't worry though—skipping something now does not mean you'll never study it. Later on in your prep, as you complete full-length tests, you'll uncover specific pieces of content that you need to review and can come back to these chapters as appropriate.

How to Use This Assessment

If you answer 0–7 questions correctly:

Spend about 1 hour to read this chapter in full and take limited notes throughout. Follow up by reviewing **all** quiz questions to ensure that you now understand how to solve each one.

If you answer 8–11 questions correctly:

Spend 20–40 minutes reviewing the quiz questions. Beginning with the questions you missed, read and take notes on the corresponding subchapters. For questions you answered correctly, ensure your thinking matches that of the explanation and you understand why each choice was correct or incorrect.

If you answer 12–15 questions correctly:

Spend less than 20 minutes reviewing all questions from the quiz. If you missed any, then include a quick read-through of the corresponding subchapters, or even just the relevant content within a subchapter, as part of your question review. For questions you got correct, ensure your thinking matches that of the explanation and review the Concept Summary at the end of the chapter.

1. What role does peptidyl transferase play in protein synthesis?
   - **A.** It transports the initiator aminoacyl-tRNA complex.
   - **B.** It helps the ribosome to advance three nucleotides along the mRNA in the 5′ to 3′ direction.
   - **C.** It holds the protein in its tertiary structure.
   - **D.** It catalyzes the formation of a peptide bond.

2. A mutation in which of the following components of the lac operon would lead to a significant reduction in the expression of lactase (one of the structural genes)?
   - **A.** Operator
   - **B.** Regulatory gene
   - **C.** Promoter
   - **D.** Structural genes

3. Topoisomerases are enzymes involved in:
   - **A.** DNA replication and transcription.
   - **B.** posttranscriptional processing.
   - **C.** RNA synthesis and translation.
   - **D.** posttranslational processing.

4. Val-tRNA^{Val} is the tRNA that carries valine to the ribosome during translation. Which of the following sequences gives an appropriate anticodon for this tRNA? (Note: Refer to Figure 7.7 for a genetic code table.)
   - **A.** CAU
   - **B.** AUC
   - **C.** UAC
   - **D.** GUG

5. Enhancers are transcriptional regulatory sequences that function by enhancing the activity of:
   - **A.** RNA polymerase at a single promoter site.
   - **B.** RNA polymerase at multiple promoter sites.
   - **C.** spliceosomes and lariat formation in the ribosome.
   - **D.** transcription factors that bind to the promoter but not to RNA polymerase.

6. In the genetic code of human nuclear DNA, one of the codons specifying the amino acid tyrosine is UAC. If one nucleotide is changed and the codon is mutated to UAG, what type of mutation will occur?
   - **A.** Silent mutation
   - **B.** Missense mutation
   - **C.** Nonsense mutation
   - **D.** Frameshift mutation

7. Which of the following is NOT used by eukaryotes to increase the transcription of a gene?
   - **A.** Gene duplication
   - **B.** Histone acetylation
   - **C.** DNA methylation
   - **D.** Enhancers

8. When trypsin converts chymotrypsinogen to chymotrypsin, some molecules of chymotrypsin bind to a repressor, which in turn binds to an operator region and prevents further transcription of trypsin. This is most similar to which of the following operons?
   - **A.** *trp* operon during lack of tryptophan
   - **B.** *trp* operon during abundance of tryptophan
   - **C.** *lac* operon during lack of lactose
   - **D.** *lac* operon during abundance of lactose

9. Which of the following RNA molecules or proteins is NOT found in the spliceosome during intron excision?
   - **A.** snRNA
   - **B.** hnRNA
   - **C.** shRNA
   - **D.** snRNPs

10. A 4-year-old toddler with cystic fibrosis (CF) is seen by his physician for an upper respiratory infection. Prior genetic testing has shown that there has been a deletion of three base pairs in exon 10 of the *CFTR* gene that affects codons 507 and 508. The nucleotide sequence in this region for normal and mutant alleles is shown below (*X* denotes the missing nucleotide):

Codon Number	**506**	**507**	**508**	**509**	**510**	**511**
Normal gene (coding strand)	ATC	ATC	TTT	GGT	GTT	TCC
Mutant gene (coding strand)	ATC	AT*X*	*XX*T	GGT	GTT	TCC

What effect will this mutation have on the amino acid sequence of the protein encoded by the *CFTR* gene? (Note: Refer to Figure 7.7 for a genetic code table.)

A. Deletion of a phenylalanine residue with no change in the C-terminus sequence
B. Deletion of a leucine residue with no change in the C-terminus sequence
C. Deletion of a phenylalanine residue with a change in the C-terminus sequence
D. Deletion of a leucine residue with a change in the C-terminus sequence

11. A gene encodes a protein with 150 amino acids. There is one intron of 1000 base pairs (bp), a 5′-untranslated region of 100 bp, and a 3′-untranslated region of 200 bp. In the final mRNA, about how many bases lie between the start AUG codon and final termination codon?

A. 150
B. 450
C. 650
D. 1750

12. Peptidyl transferase connects the carboxylate group of one amino acid to the amino group of an incoming amino acid. What type of linkage is created in this peptide bond?

A. Ester
B. Amide
C. Anhydride
D. Ether

13. A eukaryotic cell has been found to exhibit a truncation mutation that creates an inactive RNA polymerase I enzyme. Which type of RNA will be affected by this inactivation?

A. rRNA
B. tRNA
C. snRNA
D. hnRNA

14. You have just sequenced a piece of DNA that reads as follows:

5′—TCTTTGAGACATCC—3′

What would the base sequence of the mRNA transcribed from this DNA be?

A. 5′—AGAAACUCUGUAGG—3′
B. 5′—GGAUGUCUCAAAGA—3′
C. 5′—AGAAACTCTGTAGG—3′
D. 5′—GGATCTCTCAAAGA—3′

15. Double-stranded RNA cannot be translated by the ribosome and is marked for degradation in the cell. Which of the following strands of RNA would prevent mature mRNA in the cytoplasm from being translated?

A. Identical mRNA to the one produced
B. Antisense mRNA to the one produced
C. mRNA with thymine substituted for uracil
D. Sense mRNA to the one produced

Answer Key

1. **D** (See section 7.3)
2. **C** (See section 7.4)
3. **A** (See section 7.2)
4. **C** (See section 7.1)
5. **A** (See section 7.5)
6. **C** (See section 7.1)
7. **C** (See section 7.5)
8. **B** (See section 7.4)
9. **C** (See section 7.2)
10. **A** (See section 7.1)
11. **B** (See section 7.2)
12. **B** (See section 7.3)
13. **A** (See section 7.2)
14. **B** (See section 7.2)
15. **B** (See section 7.2)

The relevant section of the chapter to review for each question is given in parentheses after the correct answer. Detailed explanations can be found at the end of the chapter.

CHAPTER 7

RNA AND THE GENETIC CODE

In This Chapter

CHAPTER PROFILE

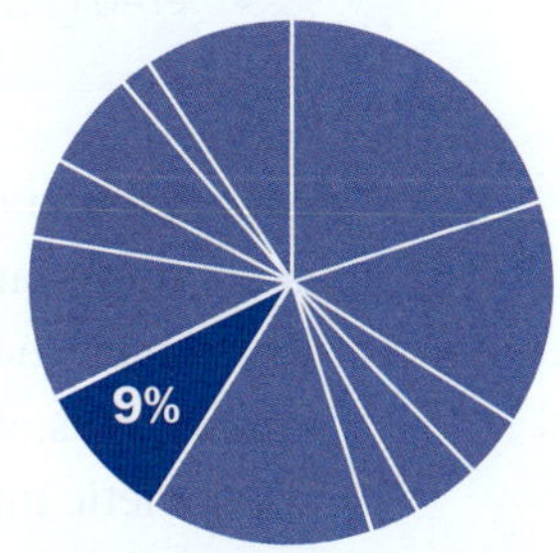

The content in this chapter should be relevant to about 9% of all questions about biochemistry on the MCAT.

This chapter covers material from the following AAMC content categories:

1B: Transmission of genetic information from the gene to the protein

5D: Structure, function, and reactivity of biologically-relevant molecules

Introduction

Hepatitis C virus (HCV) continues to be a major cause of cirrhosis and liver failure in the United States. Usually associated with intravenous drug use, hepatitis C causes ongoing damage and inflammation in the liver, leading to the formation of scar tissue that replaces the normal cells of the organ. Over time, this buildup of scar tissue makes the liver unable to keep up with the metabolic demands of the body, and liver failure ensues. To fight this virus, infected hepatocytes release interferon, a peptide signal that—as the name suggests—interferes with viral replication. Because viruses must hijack the host cell's machinery to replicate, one way the body can limit the spread of the virus is by shutting off the processes of transcription and translation. Interferon not only curtails these processes in virally infected cells, but also induces the production of *RNase L*, which cleaves RNA in cells to further reduce the ability of the virus to replicate. Coupled with other immune defenses, interferon thus serves as an efficient mechanism to protect the body from viral pathogens.

Even in normal, healthy cells, the first step in expressing genetic information is transcription of the information in the base sequence of a double-stranded DNA molecule to form a single-stranded molecule of RNA. The second step is translating that nucleotide sequence into a protein. Not every cell, though, expresses every gene product, and control of gene expression leads to the differentiation of the totipotent zygote into all of the tissues of the body. In this chapter, we will discuss the process through which proteins are produced along with the controls that modulate each step of the path.

7.1 The Genetic Code High Yield

LEARNING OBJECTIVES

After Chapter 7.1, you will be able to:

- Differentiate between three different types of RNA: mRNA, tRNA, and rRNA
- Transcribe a DNA sequence like "GAATTCG" into its mRNA conjugate
- Define the concepts of wobble and degeneracy
- Identify the translation outcomes of key codons, including AUG, UAG, UAA, and UGA
- Predict the likely impact of different mutation types on the resulting peptide

An organism must be able to store and preserve its genetic information, pass that information along to future generations, and express that information as it carries out all the processes of life. We know that DNA and RNA share the same language: they both code using nitrogenous bases. Proteins, however, are composed of amino acids, which constitute a different language altogether. Therefore, we use the genetic code to translate this genetic information into proteins.

While nucleotides play a crucial role in maintaining our genetic identity from generation to generation, it is the proteins they encode that help organisms develop and perform the necessary functions of life. The major steps involved in the transfer of genetic information are illustrated in the **central dogma of molecular biology**, as shown in Figure 7.1.

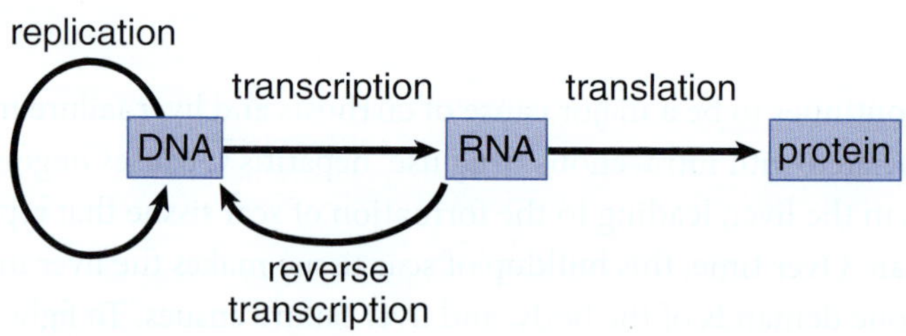

Figure 7.1 The Central Dogma of Molecular Biology

Classically, a **gene** (shown in Figure 7.2) is a unit of DNA that encodes a specific protein or RNA molecule, and through transcription and translation, that gene can be expressed. Although this sequence is now complicated by our increased knowledge of the ways in which genes and nucleic acids may be expressed, it is still useful as a general working definition of the processes of DNA replication, transcription, and translation. We have already discussed DNA synthesis, but will continue learning more about gene expression in the rest of this chapter.

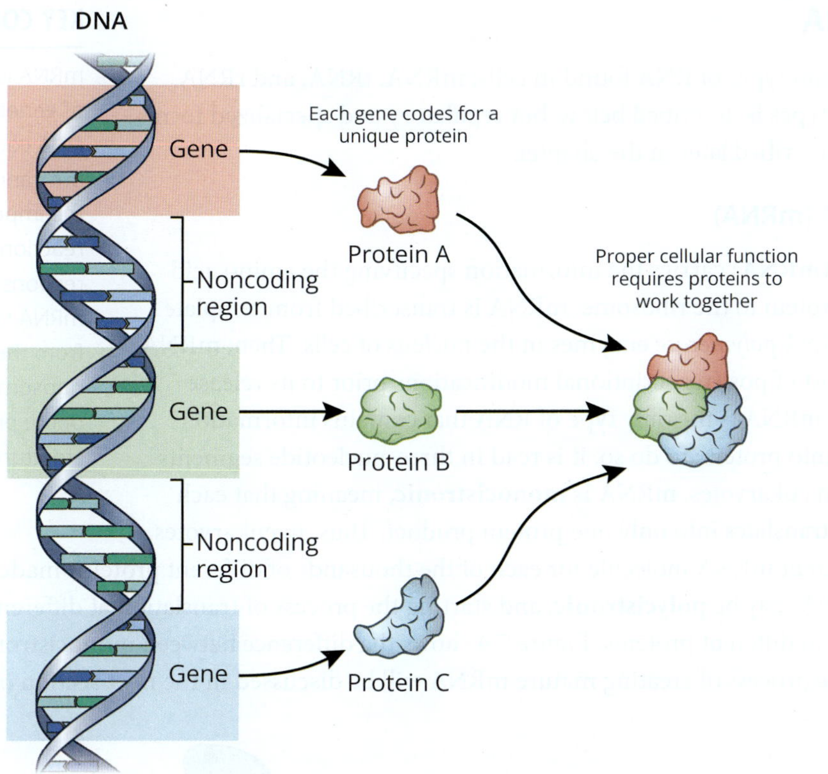

Figure 7.2 Genes to Cellular Function

The relationship between the sequence found in double-stranded DNA, single-stranded RNA, and protein is illustrated in Figure 7.3 for a prototypical gene. Messenger RNA is synthesized in the $5' \rightarrow 3'$ direction and is complementary and antiparallel to the DNA template strand. The ribosome translates the mRNA in the $5' \rightarrow 3'$ direction, as it synthesizes the protein from the amino terminus (N-terminus) to the carboxy terminus (C-terminus).

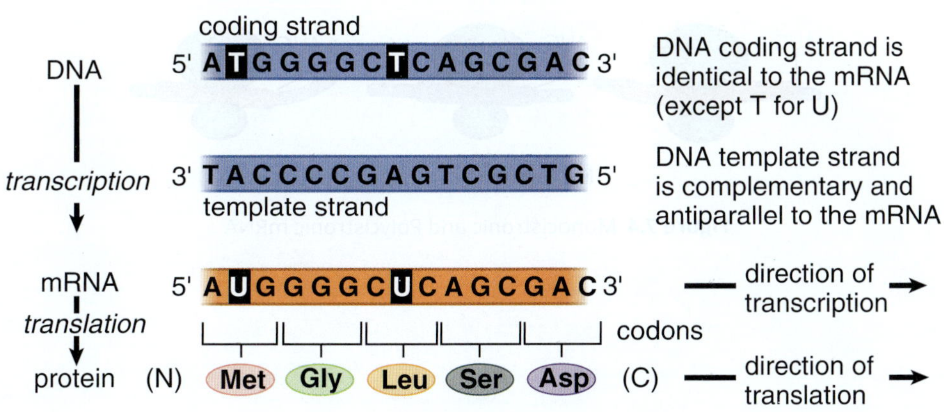

Figure 7.3 Flow of Genetic Information from DNA to Protein

Types of RNA

There are three main types of RNA found in cells: mRNA, tRNA, and rRNA. Each of the main types is described below, but regulatory and specialized forms of RNA are also described later in the chapter.

KEY CONCEPT

mRNA is the messenger of genetic information. DNA codes for proteins but cannot perform any of the important enzymatic reactions that proteins are responsible for in cells. mRNA takes the information from the DNA to the ribosomes, where creation of the primary protein structure occurs.

Messenger RNA (mRNA)

Messenger RNA (mRNA) carries the information specifying the amino acid sequence of the protein to the ribosome. mRNA is transcribed from template DNA strands by *RNA polymerase* enzymes in the nucleus of cells. Then, mRNA may undergo a host of posttranscriptional modifications prior to its release from the nucleus. mRNA is the only type of RNA that contains information that is translated into protein; to do so, it is read in three-nucleotide segments termed **codons**. In eukaryotes, mRNA is **monocistronic**, meaning that each mRNA molecule translates into only one protein product. Thus, in eukaryotes, the cell has a different mRNA molecule for each of the thousands of different proteins made by that cell. In prokaryotes, mRNA may be **polycistronic**, and starting the process of translation at different locations in the mRNA can result in different proteins. Figure 7.4 shows the difference between monocistronic and polycistronic mRNA. The process of creating mature mRNA will be discussed in the next section of this chapter.

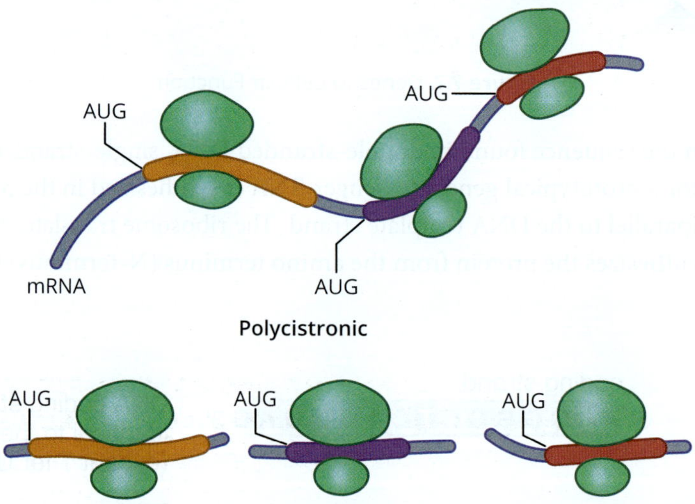

Figure 7.4 Monocistronic and Polycistronic mRNA

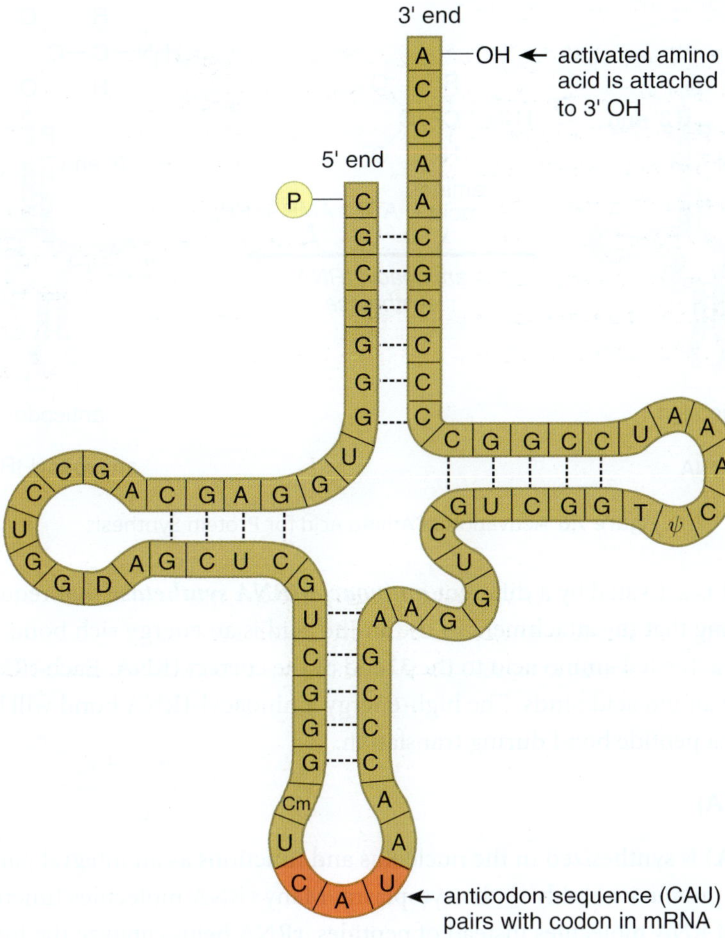

Figure 7.5 The Structure of tRNA

Transfer RNA (tRNA)

Transfer RNA (tRNA) is responsible for converting the language of nucleic acids to the language of amino acids and peptides. Each tRNA molecule contains a folded strand of RNA that includes a three-nucleotide anticodon, as shown in Figure 7.5. This anticodon recognizes and pairs with the appropriate codon on an mRNA molecule while in the ribosome. There are 20 amino acids in eukaryotic proteins, each of which is represented by at least one codon. To become part of a nascent polypeptide in the ribosome, amino acids are connected to a specific tRNA molecule; such tRNA molecules are said to be **charged** or **activated** with an amino acid, as shown in Figure 7.6. Mature tRNA is found in the cytoplasm.

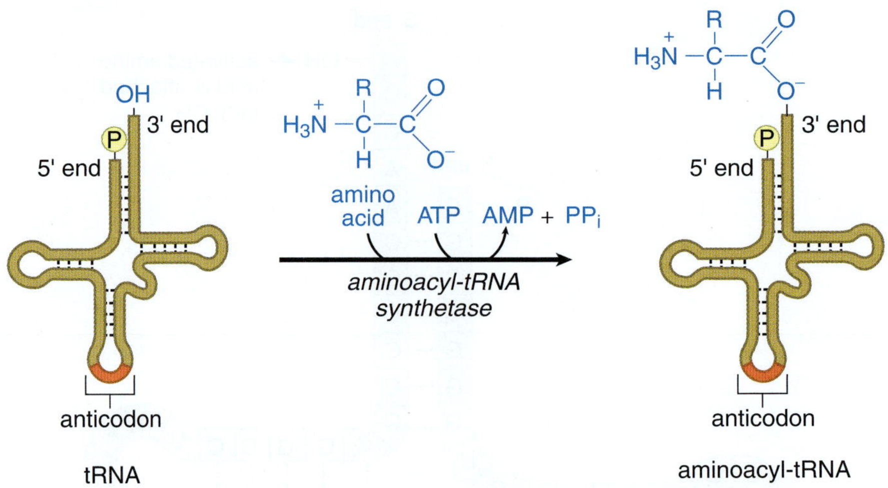

Figure 7.6 Activation of Amino Acid for Protein Synthesis

Each type of amino acid is activated by a different ***aminoacyl-tRNA synthetase*** that requires two high-energy bonds from ATP, implying that the attachment of the amino acid is an energy rich bond. The aminoacyl-tRNA synthetase transfers the activated amino acid to the 3′ end of the correct tRNA. Each tRNA has a CCA nucleotide sequence where the amino acid binds. The high-energy aminoacyl-tRNA bond will be used to supply the energy needed to create a peptide bond during translation.

Ribosomal RNA (rRNA)

Ribosomal RNA (**rRNA**) is synthesized in the nucleolus and functions as an integral part of the ribosomal machinery used during protein assembly in the cytoplasm. Many rRNA molecules function as **ribozymes**; that is, enzymes made of RNA molecules instead of peptides. rRNA helps catalyze the formation of peptide bonds and is also important in splicing out its own introns within the nucleus. The complex structure of the ribosome is described later in this chapter.

Codons

If a gene sequence is a "sentence" describing a protein, then its basic unit is a three-letter "word" known as the **codon**, which is translated into an amino acid. Genetic code tables, such as the one in Figure 7.7, serve as an easy way to determine the amino acid that is translated from each mRNA codon. Each codon consists of three bases; thus, there are 64 codons. Note how all codons are written in the 5′ → 3′ direction, and the code is unambiguous, in that each codon is specific for one and only one amino acid.

First Position (5' End)	Second Position: U	C	A	G	Third Position (3' End)
U	UUU, UUC } Phe UUA, UUG } Leu	UCU, UCC, UCA, UCG } Ser	UAU, UAC } Tyr UAA, UAG } Stop	UGU, UGC } Cys UGA Stop UGG Trp	**U** **C** **A** **G**
C	CUU, CUC, CUA, CUG } Leu	CCU, CCC, CCA, CCG } Pro	CAU, CAC } His CAA, CAG } Gln	CGU, CGC, CGA, CGG } Arg	**U** **C** **A** **G**
A	AUU, AUC, AUA } Ile AUG Met	ACU, ACC, ACA, ACG } Thr	AAU, AAC } Asn AAA, AAG } Lys	AGU, AGC } Ser AGA, AGG } Arg	**U** **C** **A** **G**
G	GUU, GUC, GUA, GUG } Val	GCU, GCC, GCA, GCG } Ala	GAU, GAC } Asp GAA, GAG } Glu	GGU, GGC, GGA, GGG } Gly	**U** **C** **A** **G**

Figure 7.7 The Genetic Code

Note that 61 of the codons code for one of the 20 amino acids, while three codons encode for the termination of translation. This code is universal across species (although there are some exceptions in the mitochondria that are not necessary to know for the MCAT).

KEY CONCEPT

Each codon represents only one amino acid; however, most amino acids are represented by multiple codons.

During translation, the codon of the mRNA is recognized by a complementary **anticodon** on a transfer RNA (tRNA). The anticodon sequence allows the tRNA to pair with the codon in the mRNA. Because base-pairing is involved, the orientation of this interaction will be antiparallel. For example, the aminoacyl tRNA Ile-tRNA^{Ile} has an anticodon sequence 5′—GAU—3′, allowing it to pair with the isoleucine codon 5′—AUC—3′, as seen in Figure 7.8.

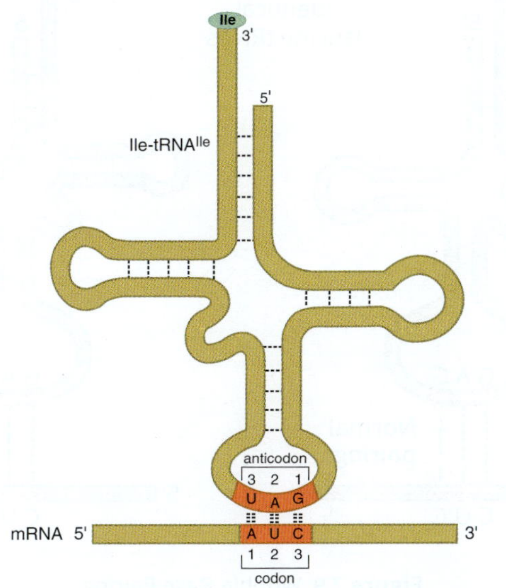

Figure 7.8 Base Pairing of an Aminoacyl-tRNA with a Codon in mRNA

Every preprocessed eukaryotic protein starts with the exact same amino acid: methionine. Because every protein begins with methionine, the codon for methionine (AUG) is considered the **start codon** for translation of the mRNA into protein. There are also three codons that encode for termination of protein translation; there are no charged tRNA molecules that recognize these codons, which leads to the release of the protein from the ribosome. The three **stop codons** are UGA, UAA, and UAG.

MNEMONIC

For Test Day, it is essential to have the one start codon and three stop codons memorized.

Start codon:

- **AUG** (Methionine)—School starts in **AUG**ust

Stop codons:

- **UAA**—**U A**re **A**nnoying
- **UGA**—**U G**o **A**way
- **UAG**—**U A**re **G**one

Mutations

Degeneracy and Wobble

The genetic code is **degenerate** because more than one codon can specify a single amino acid. In fact, all amino acids, except for methionine and tryptophan, are encoded by multiple codons. Referring back to Figure 7.7, we can see that for the amino acids with multiple codons, the first two bases are usually the same, and the third base in the codon is variable. We refer to this variable third base in the codon as the **wobble position**, as illustrated in Figure 7.9. Wobble is an evolutionary development designed to protect against mutations in the coding regions of our DNA. Mutations in the wobble position tend to be called **silent** or **degenerate**, which means there is no effect on the expression of the amino acid and therefore no adverse effects on the polypeptide sequence. The amino acid glycine, for example, requires that only the first two nucleotides of the codon be GG. The third nucleotide could be A, C, G, or U, and the amino acid composition of the protein would remain the same. The sequence that codes for protein can have genetic variance. If the variant is below 1% of allele frequency, it is generally termed a **mutation**. If the variant occurs in greater than 1% of the population, then it is termed as a **polymorphism**.

KEY CONCEPT

The degeneracy of the genetic code allows for mutations in DNA that do not always result in altered protein structure or function. Usually, a mutation within an intron will also not change the protein sequence because introns are cleaved out of the mRNA transcript prior to translation.

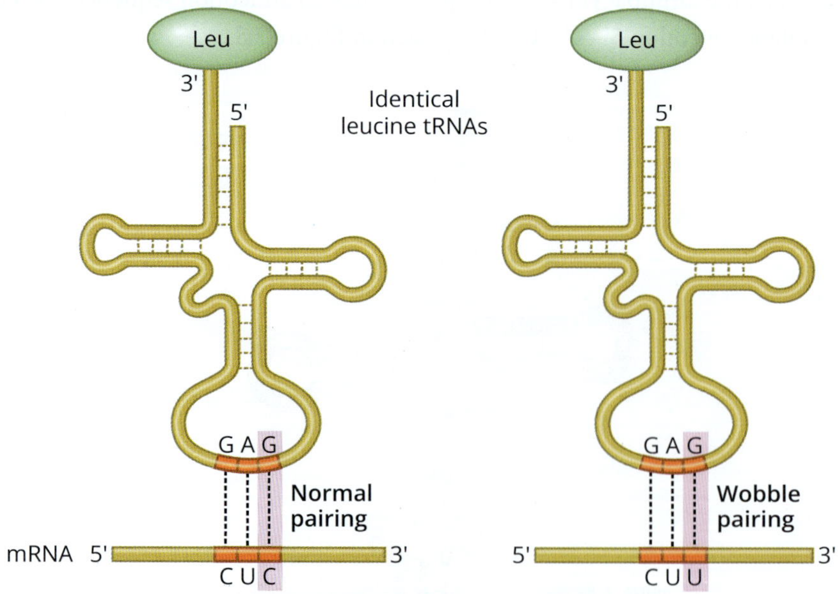

Figure 7.9 Wobble Base Pairing

Missense and Nonsense Mutations

If a mutation occurs and it affects one of the nucleotides in a codon, it is known as a **point mutation**. Although we've already discussed the silent point mutation in the wobble position, other point mutations can have a severe detrimental effect depending on where the mutation occurs in the genome. Because these point mutations can affect the primary amino acid sequence of the protein, they are called **expressed mutations**. Expressed point mutations fall into two categories: missense and nonsense.

- **Missense mutation**—a mutation where one amino acid substitutes for another
- **Nonsense mutation**—a mutation where the codon now encodes for a premature stop codon (also known as a **truncation mutation**)

Frameshift Mutations

The three nucleotides of a codon are referred to as the **reading frame**. Point mutations occur when one nucleotide is changed, but a **frameshift mutation** occurs when some number of nucleotides are added to or deleted from the mRNA sequence. Insertion or deletion of nucleotides will shift the reading frame, usually resulting in changes in the amino acid sequence or premature truncation of the protein. The effects of frameshift mutations are typically more serious than point mutations, although it is heavily dependent on where within the DNA sequence the mutation actually occurred. A synopsis of the different types of mutations can be found in Figure 7.10.

REAL WORLD

Cystic fibrosis is most commonly caused by a frameshift mutation: a deletion at codon 508 in the polypeptide chain of the *CFTR* chloride channel gene. The subsequent loss of a phenylalanine residue at this position results in a defective chloride ion channel. This altered protein never reaches the cell membrane, leading to blocked passage of salt and water into and out of cells. As a result of this blockage, cells that line the passageways of the lungs, pancreas, and other organs produce an abnormally thick, sticky mucus that traps bacteria, increasing the likelihood of infection in patients.

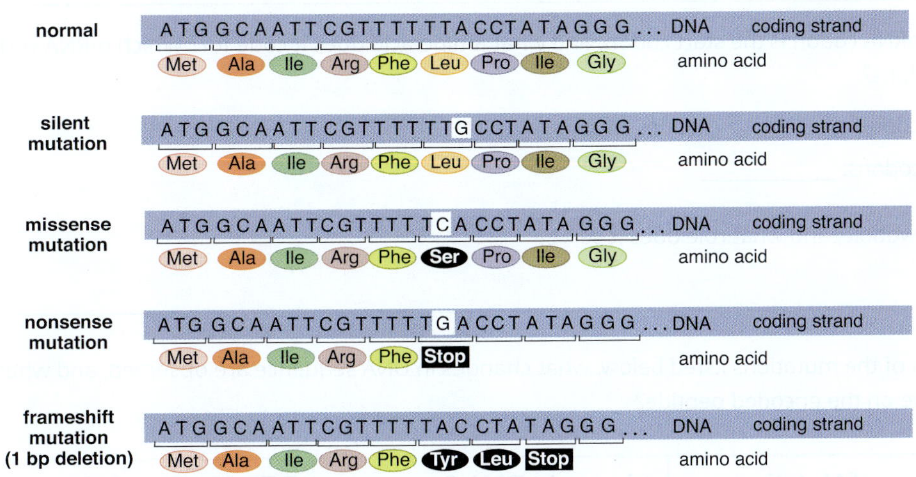

Figure 7.10 Some Common Types of Mutations in DNA

MCAT CONCEPT CHECK 7.1

Before you move on, assess your understanding of the material with these questions.

1. What are the roles of the three main types of RNA?
   - mRNA:
   - tRNA:
   - rRNA:

2. The three-base sequences listed below are DNA sequences from the template (antisense) strand. Using Figure 7.7, which amino acid is encoded by each of these sequences, after transcription and translation?
   - GAT:
   - ATT:
   - CGC:
   - CCA:

3. Which mRNA codon is the start codon, and what amino acid does it code for? Which mRNA codons are the stop codons?
   - Start codon: ____________; codes for: ____________
   - Stop codons: ____________

4. What is wobble, and what role does it serve?

5. For each of the mutations listed below, what changes in DNA sequence are observed, and what effect do they have on the encoded peptide?

Type of Mutation	Change in DNA Sequence	Effect on Encoded Protein
Silent (degenerate)		
Missense		
Nonsense		
Frameshift		

7.2 Transcription High Yield

LEARNING OBJECTIVES

After Chapter 7.2, you will be able to:

- Explain how each of the eukaryotic RNA polymerases (I, II, and III) impacts transcription
- Identify where RNA polymerase would bind to start transcription on a DNA strand
- Determine the mRNA that results from a given hnRNA molecule:

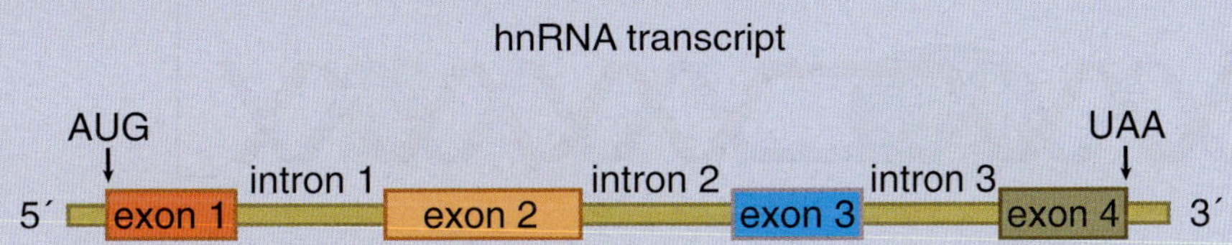

Although DNA contains the actual coding sequence for a protein, the machinery to generate that protein is located in the cytoplasm. DNA cannot leave the nucleus, as it will be quickly degraded, so it must use RNA to transmit genetic information. The creation of mRNA from a DNA template is known as **transcription**, and while mRNA is the only type of RNA that carries information from DNA directly, there are many other types of RNA that exist, two of which will play important roles during protein translation: transfer RNA (tRNA) and ribosomal RNA (rRNA).

Mechanism of Transcription

Transcription proceeds via three general steps:

Initiation: Several enzymes, including *helicase* and *topoisomerase*, are involved in unwinding the double-stranded DNA and preventing formation of super coils, as described in Chapter 6 of *MCAT Biochemistry Review*. This step is important in allowing the transcriptional machinery access to the DNA and the particular gene of interest. RNA is synthesized by a DNA-dependent RNA polymerase; RNA polymerase locates genes by searching for specialized DNA regions known as **promoter regions**, shown in Figure 7.11. In eukaryotes, **RNA polymerase II** is the main player in transcribing mRNA, and one of its major binding sites in the promoter region is known as the **TATA box**, named for its high concentration of thymine and adenine bases. **Transcription factors** help the RNA polymerase locate and bind to this promoter region of the DNA, helping to establish where transcription will start. Unlike DNA polymerase III, which was reviewed during DNA replication, RNA polymerase does not require a primer to start generating a transcript.

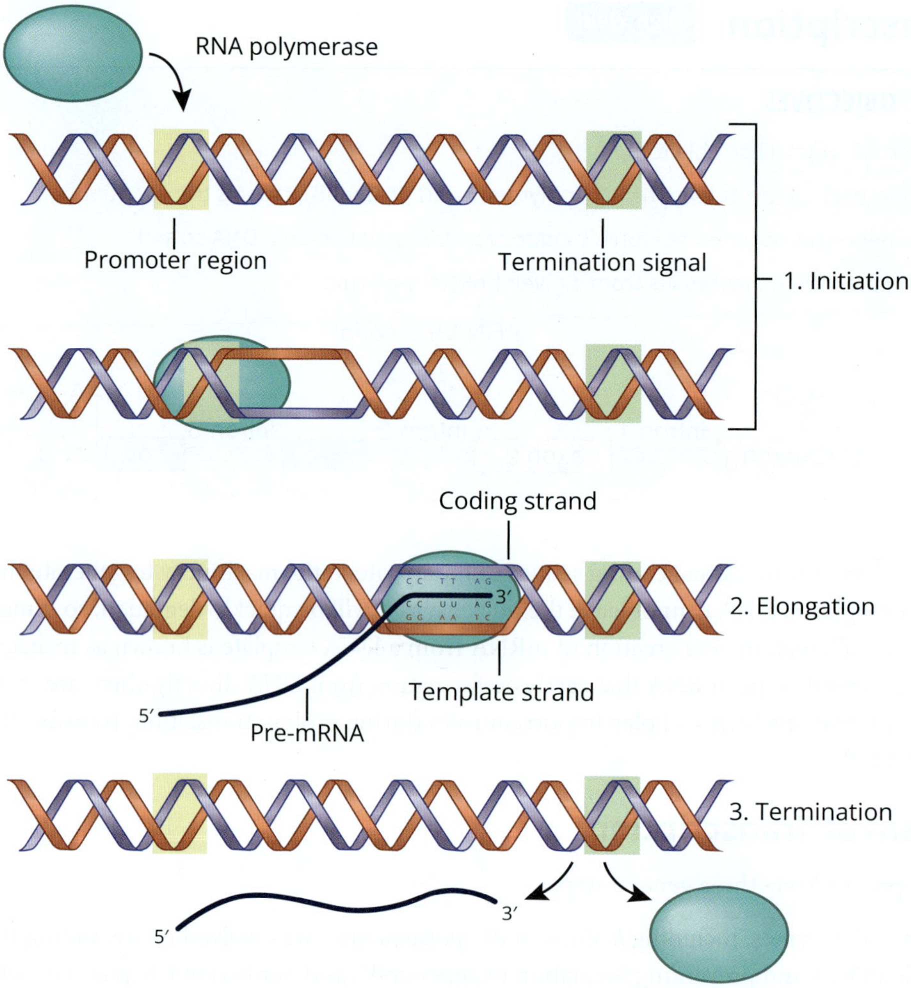

Figure 7.11 Steps in Transcription

Elongation: RNA polymerase travels along the **template strand** (also known as the **antisense strand**) in the 3′ → 5′ direction, which allows for the construction of newly transcribed mRNA in the 5′ → 3′ direction. Unlike DNA polymerase, RNA polymerase does not have proofreading capabilities, so the synthesized transcript will not be edited. The **coding strand** (or **sense strand**) of DNA is not used as a template during transcription. Because the coding strand is also complementary to the template strand, it is identical to the mRNA transcript except that all the thymine nucleotides in DNA have been replaced with uracil in the mRNA molecule.

KEY CONCEPT

Transcription is subject to the 5′ → 3′ rule, just like DNA synthesis. Synthesis of nucleic acids always occurs in the 5′ → 3′ direction.

Termination: Transcription will continue along the DNA coding region until the RNA polymerase reaches a *termination sequence* or *stop signal*, which results in the termination of transcription. The DNA double helix then re-forms, and the primary transcript formed is termed **heterogeneous nuclear RNA (hnRNA)**, sometimes also known as **pre-mRNA**. mRNA is derived from hnRNA via posttranscriptional modifications, as described below.

In eukaryotes, there are three types of RNA polymerases, but only one is involved in the transcription of mRNA:

- *RNA polymerase I* is located in the nucleolus and synthesizes rRNA.
- *RNA polymerase II* is located in the nucleus and synthesizes hnRNA (pre-processed mRNA) and some small nuclear RNA (snRNA).
- *RNA polymerase III* is located in the nucleus and synthesizes tRNA and some rRNA.

In the vicinity of a gene, a numbering system is used to identify the location of important bases in the DNA strand, as shown in Figure 7.12. The first base transcribed from DNA to RNA is defined as the +1 base of that gene region. Bases to the left of this start point (upstream, or toward the 5′ end) are given negative numbers: −1, −2, −3, and so on. Bases to the right (downstream, or toward the 3′ end) are denoted with positive numbers: +2, +3, +4, and so on. Thus, no nucleotide in the gene is numbered 0. The TATA box, where RNA polymerase II binds, usually falls around −25.

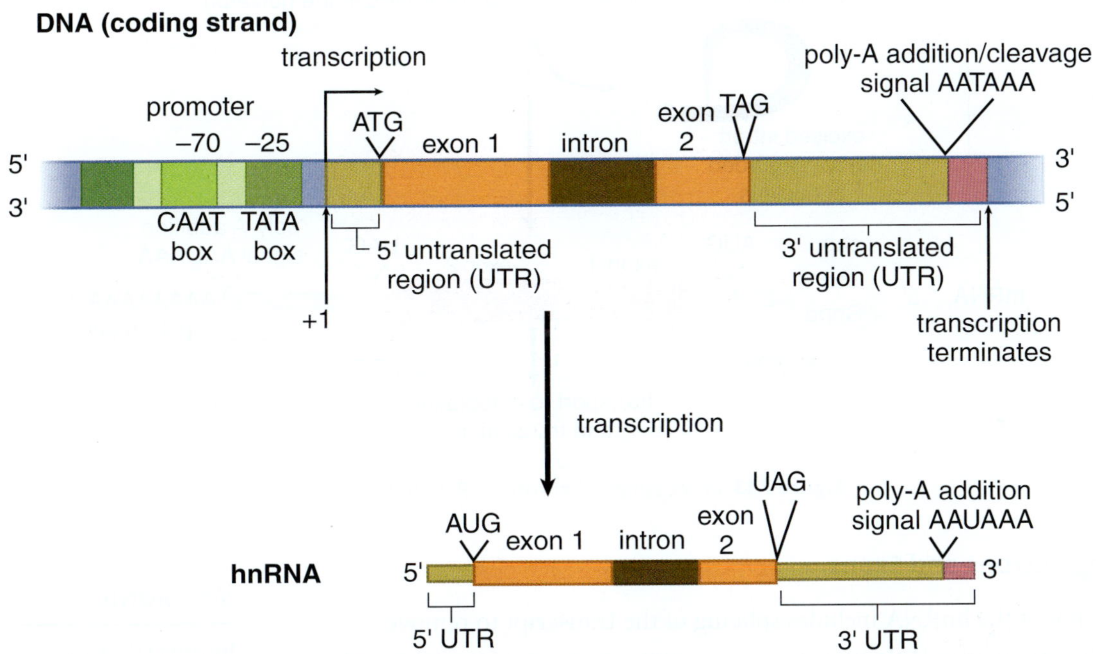

Figure 7.12 Transcription of DNA to hnRNA

Posttranscriptional Processing

Before the hnRNA can leave the nucleus and be translated to protein, it must undergo three specific processes to allow it to interact with the ribosome and survive the conditions of the cytoplasm, as demonstrated in Figure 7.13. You can think of the nucleus as the happy home of the cell; the DNA strands are the caregivers, and the hnRNA is their child. The child must mature in order to survive.

KEY CONCEPT

The MCAT commonly tests post-transcriptional processing:

- Intron/exon splicing
- 5′ cap
- 3′ poly-A tail

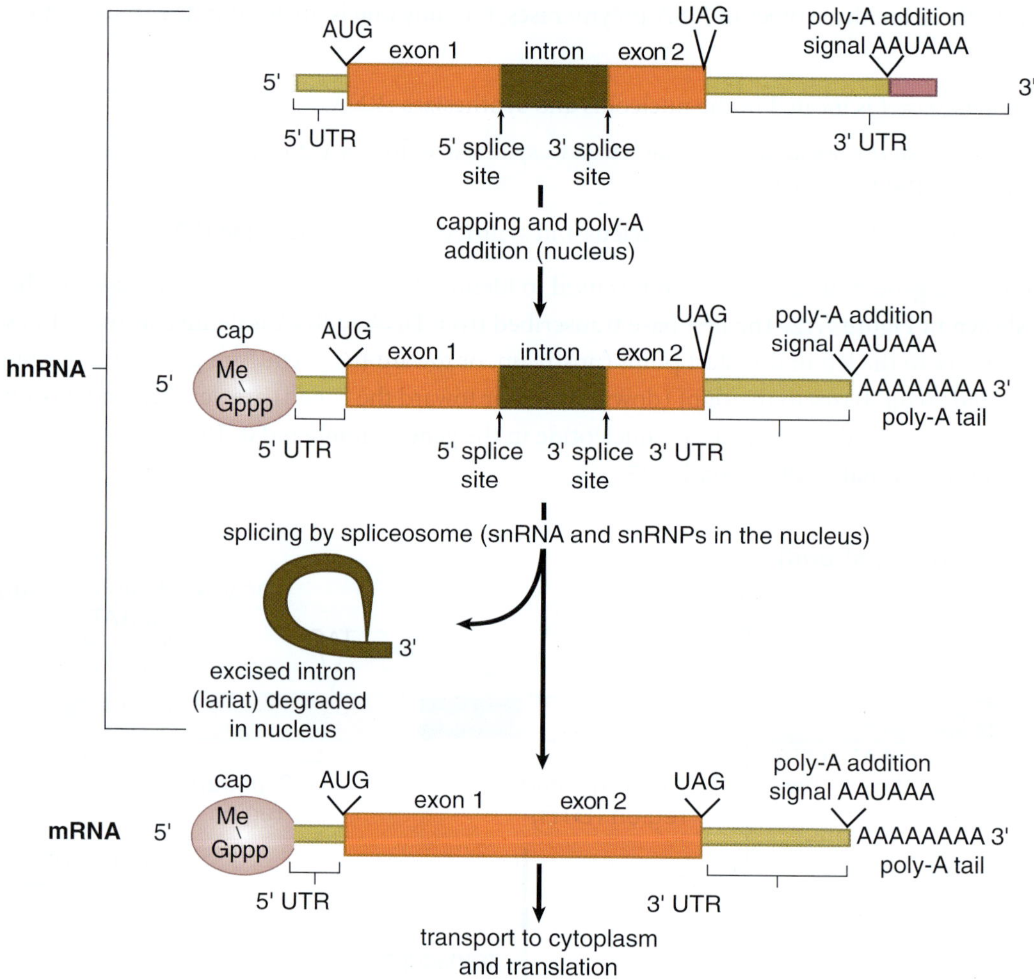

Figure 7.13 Processing Eukaryotic hnRNA to Form mRNA

Splicing: Introns and Exons

> **MNEMONIC**
>
> **In**trons stay **in** the nucleus; **ex**ons will **ex**it the nucleus as part of the mRNA.

Maturation of the hnRNA includes splicing of the transcript to remove noncoding sequences (**introns**) and ligate coding sequences (**exons**) together. Splicing is accomplished by the **spliceosome**. In the spliceosome, **small nuclear RNA (snRNA)** molecules couple with proteins known as **small nuclear ribonucleoproteins** (also known as **snRNPs**, or "snurps"). The snRNP/snRNA complex recognizes both the 5′ and 3′ splice sites of the introns. These noncoding sequences are excised in the form of a **lariat** (lasso-shaped structure) and then degraded.

The evolutionary function of introns in eukaryotic cells is not currently well-understood; however, scientists hypothesize that introns play an important role in the regulation of cellular gene expression levels and in maintaining the size of our genome. The existence of introns has also been hypothesized to allow for rapid protein evolution. Many eukaryotic proteins share peptide sequences in common, suggesting that the genes encoding for these particular peptides may employ a modular function; that is, they contain standard sequences that can be swapped in and out, depending on the needs of the cell.

5′ Cap

At the 5′ end of the hnRNA molecule, a **7-methylguanylate triphosphate cap** is added. The cap is actually added during the process of transcription and is recognized by the ribosome as the binding site. It also protects the mRNA from degradation in the cytoplasm.

3′ Poly-A Tail

A **polyadenosyl (poly-A) tail** is added to the 3′ end of the mRNA transcript and protects the message against rapid degradation. It is composed of adenine bases. Think of the poly-A tail as a fuse for a "time bomb" for the mRNA transcript: as soon as the mRNA leaves the nucleus, it will start to get degraded from its 3′ end. The longer the poly-A tail, the more time the mRNA will be able to survive before being digested in the cytoplasm. The poly-A tail also assists with export of the mature mRNA from the nucleus.

REAL WORLD

Mutations in splice sites can lead to abnormal proteins. For example, mutations that interfere with proper splicing of β-globulin mRNA are responsible for some cases of *β-thalassemia*, a group of blood disorders that hinder the production and efficacy of hemoglobin in the blood. Splice site mutations are one of the few mutations in noncoding DNA that may still have an effect on the translated protein.

At this point, when only the exons remain and the cap and tail have been added, the cell has created the mature mRNA that can now be transported into the cytoplasm for protein translation. Untranslated regions of the mRNA (UTRs) will still exist at the 5′ and 3′ edges of the transcript because the ribosome initiates translation at the start codon (AUG) and will end at a stop codon (UAA, UGA, UAG).

For some genes in eukaryotic cells, however, the primary transcript of hnRNA may be spliced together in different ways to produce multiple variants of proteins encoded by the same original gene. This process is known as **alternative splicing**, and it is illustrated in Figure 7.14. By utilizing alternative splicing, an organism can make many more different proteins from a limited number of genes. For reference, humans are estimated to make at least 100,000 proteins, but the number of human genes is only about 20,000–25,000. Don't worry about memorizing these numbers, though; they are constantly changing with new research. Alternative splicing is also known to function in the regulation of gene expression, in addition to generating protein diversity.

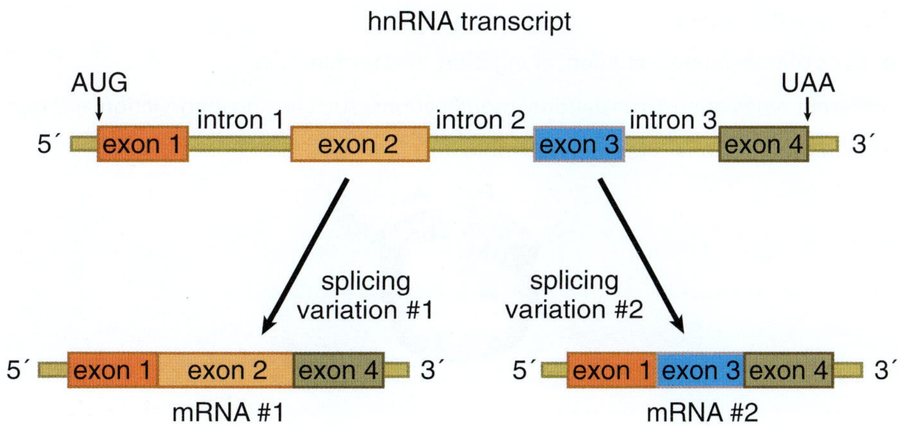

Figure 7.14 Alternative Splicing of Eukaryotic hnRNA to Produce Different Proteins

MCAT CONCEPT CHECK 7.2

Before you move on, assess your understanding of the material with these questions.

1. What is the role of each eukaryotic RNA polymerase?
   - RNA polymerase I:

   ____

   - RNA polymerase II:

   ____

   - RNA polymerase III:

   ____

2. When starting transcription, where does RNA polymerase bind?

   ____

3. What are the three major posttranscriptional modifications that turn hnRNA into mature mRNA?
   1. ______________________________
   2. ______________________________
   3. ______________________________

4. What is alternative splicing, and what does it accomplish?

   ____

7.3 Translation **High Yield**

LEARNING OBJECTIVES

After Chapter 7.3, you will be able to:

- Describe the steps of translation: initiation, elongation, and termination
- Distinguish different types of posttranslational modifications, such as phosphorylation and glycosylation
- Explain the role of the functional sites in a ribosome:

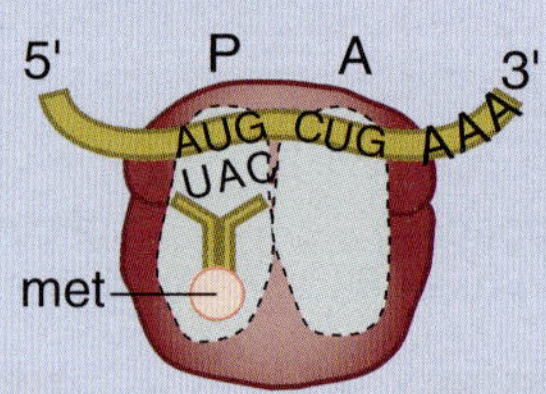

Once the mRNA transcript is created and processed, it can exit the nucleus through **nuclear pores**. Once in the cytoplasm, mRNA finds a ribosome to begin the process of **translation**—converting the mRNA transcript into a functional protein. Translation is a complex process that requires mRNA, tRNA, ribosomes, amino acids, and energy in the form of GTP.

The Ribosome

As mentioned earlier, the anticodon of the tRNA binds to the codon on the mature mRNA in the ribosome. The **ribosome** is composed of proteins and rRNA. In both prokaryotes and eukaryotes, there are large and small subunits; the subunits only bind together during protein synthesis. The structure of the ribosome dictates its main function, which is to bring the mRNA message together with the charged aminoacyl-tRNA complex to generate the protein. There are three binding sites in the ribosome for tRNA: the A site (aminoacyl), P site (peptidyl), and E site (exit). These are described further in the section on translation below.

Eukaryotic ribosomes contain four strands of rRNA, designated the 28S, 18S, 5.8S, and the 5S rRNAs; the "S" values indicate the size of the strand. The genes for some of the rRNAs (28S, 18S, and 5.8S rRNAs) used to construct the ribosome are found in the nucleolus. RNA polymerase I transcribes the 28S, 18S, and 5.8S rRNAs as a single unit within the nucleolus, which results in a 45S ribosomal precursor RNA. This 45S pre-rRNA is processed to become the 18S rRNA of the 40S (small) ribosomal subunit and the 28S and 5.8S rRNAs of the 60S (large) ribosomal subunit. RNA polymerase III transcribes the 5S rRNA, which is also found in the 60S ribosomal subunit; this process takes place outside of the nucleolus. The ribosomal subunits created are the 60S and 40S subunits; these subunits join during protein synthesis to form the whole 80S ribosome.

In comparison with eukaryotes, prokaryotes have 50S and 30S large and small subunits, which assemble to create the complete 70S ribosome. Note that the "S" value is determined experimentally by studying the behavior of particles in an ultracentrifuge; thus, the numbers of each subunit and each rRNA are not additive because they are based on size and shape, not size alone. The structure of eukaryotic and prokaryotic ribosomes are shown in Figure 7.15.

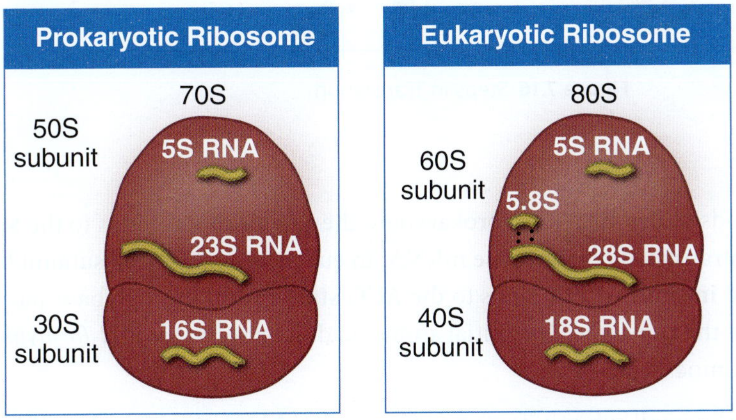

Figure 7.15 The Composition of Prokaryotic and Eukaryotic Ribosomes

Mechanism of Translation

Translation occurs in the cytoplasm in prokaryotes and eukaryotes. In prokaryotes, the ribosomes start translating before the mRNA is complete; in eukaryotes, however, transcription and translation occur at separate times and in separate locations within the cell.

KEY CONCEPT

Terminology and 5′ → 3′

- DNA → DNA = replication: new DNA synthesized in 5′ → 3′ direction
- DNA → RNA = transcription: new RNA synthesized in 5′ → 3′ direction (template is read 3′ → 5′)
- RNA → protein = translation: mRNA read in 5′ → 3′ direction

REAL WORLD

The fact that prokaryotic and eukaryotic ribosomes have slightly different structures is no small fact. This difference allows us to target antibiotics, like macrolides (*azithromycin, erythromycin*), tetracyclines (*doxycycline*), *vancomycin*, and others to bacterial cells with fewer side effects to humans.

The process of translation occurs in three stages, as shown in Figure 7.16: **initiation**, **elongation**, and **termination**. While the names of the three steps are identical to the names of the steps of transcription, the processes involved are quite distinct. In translation, specialized factors for initiation (initiation factors, IF), elongation (elongation factors, EF), and termination (release factors, RF), as well as GTP are required for each step.

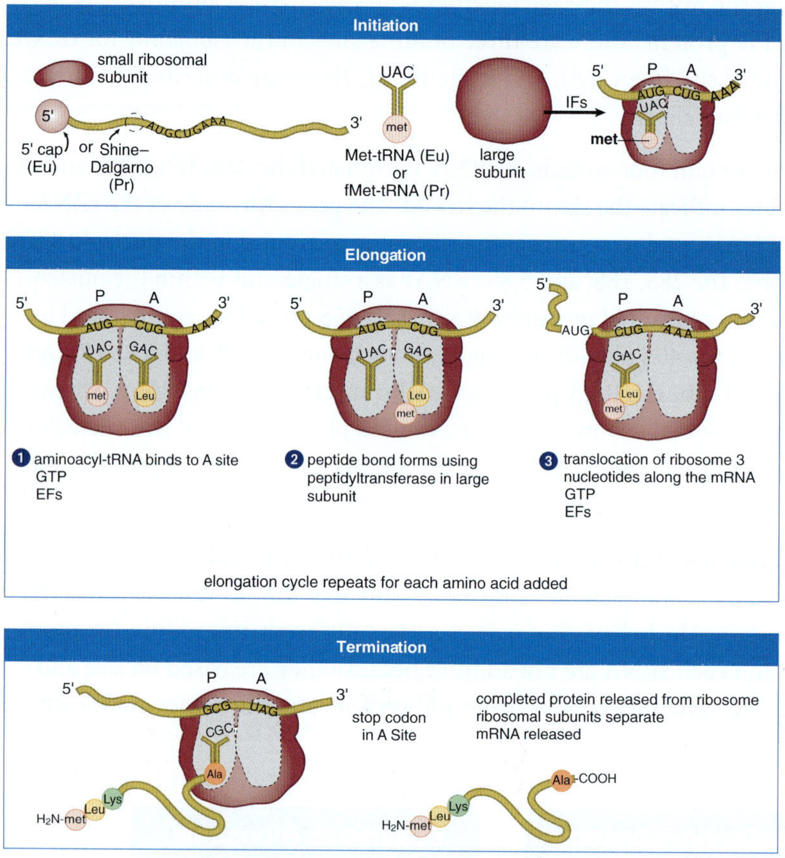

Figure 7.16 Steps in Translation

Initiation

The small ribosomal subunit binds to the mRNA. In prokaryotes, the small subunit binds to the **Shine–Dalgarno sequence** in the 5′ untranslated region of the mRNA. In eukaryotes, the small subunit binds to the 5′ cap structure. The charged **initiator tRNA** binds to the AUG **start codon** through base-pairing with its anticodon within the P site of the ribosome. The initial amino acid in prokaryotes is *N-formylmethionine* (fMet); in eukaryotes, it's methionine.

The large subunit then binds to the small subunit, forming the completed initiation complex. This is assisted by **initiation factors (IF)** that are not permanently associated with the ribosome.

Elongation

Elongation is a three-step cycle that is repeated for each amino acid added to the protein after the initiator methionine. During elongation, the ribosome

MNEMONIC

Order of sites in the ribosome during translation: **APE**.

moves in the 5′ to 3′ direction along the mRNA, synthesizing the protein from its amino (N-) to carboxyl (C-) terminus. The ribosome contains three very important binding sites:

- The **A site** holds the incoming aminoacyl-tRNA complex. This is the next amino acid that is being added to the growing chain, and is determined by the mRNA codon within the A site.
- The **P site** holds the tRNA that carries the growing polypeptide chain. It is also where the first amino acid (methionine) binds because it is starting the polypeptide chain. A **peptide bond** is formed as the polypeptide is passed from the tRNA in the P site to the tRNA in the A site. This requires ***peptidyl transferase***, an enzyme that is part of the large subunit. GTP is used for energy during the formation of this bond.
- The **E site** (not shown in Figure 7.16) is where the now inactivated (uncharged) tRNA pauses transiently before exiting the ribosome. As the now-uncharged tRNA enters the E site, it quickly unbinds from the mRNA and is ready to be recharged.

Elongation factors (**EF**) assist by locating and recruiting aminoacyl-tRNA along with GTP, while helping to remove GDP once the energy has been used.

Some eukaryotic proteins contain signal sequences, which designate a particular destination for the protein, as shown in Figure 7.17. For peptides that will be secreted, such as hormones and digestive enzymes, a signal sequence directs the ribosome to move to the endoplasmic reticulum (ER), so that the protein can be translated directly into the lumen of the rough ER. From there, the protein can be sent to the Golgi apparatus and be secreted from a vesicle via exocytosis. Other signal sequences direct proteins to the nucleus, lysosomes, or cell membrane.

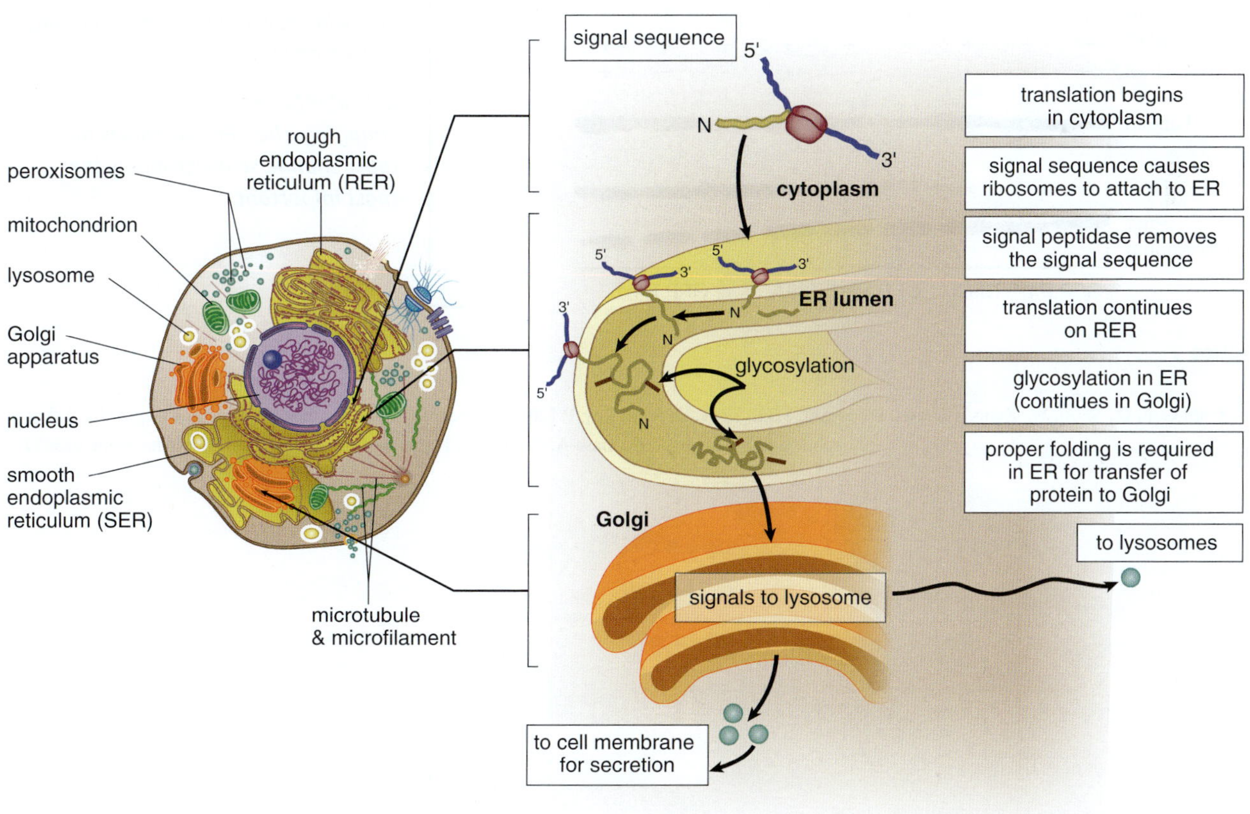

Figure 7.17 Synthesis of Secretory, Membrane, and Lysosomal Proteins

BIOCHEMISTRY GUIDED EXAMPLE WITH EXPERT THINKING

Profilins (Pfn) are a family of actin-monomer binding proteins that strongly inhibit spontaneous elongation of pointed ends of actin filaments, but promote barbed-ended elongation through the addition of ATP-bound monomeric actin. Since actin polymerization is a fundamental component of many physiological properties, the goal of this study is to elucidate the regulation of Pfn1 (the most abundant isoform of Pfn in mammals) by phosphorylation.

Intro to topic: Pfn moderates actin through two mechanisms

Goal: better understand regulation of Pfn1 through phosphorylation

Pfn1 is known to be phosphorylated on tyrosine and serine residues. Using sequence analysis software, threonine-89 was also identified as a possible phosphorylation site by protein kinase A (PKA). To examine the role of threonine-89 in Pfn1 expression, two Pfn1 constructs were created—T89D and T89A. Human embryonic kidney cells (HEK-293) expressing indicated green fluorescent protein-fused Pfn1 (GFP Pfn1) constructs (GFP Pfn1 T89D, T89A, and wild-type) were lysed with either non-denaturing (containing 1% NP-40) or denaturing (containing 1% NP-40, 2% SDS as a mild denaturant for one buffer, and the other with 6 M urea as a strong denaturant in addition) extraction buffers. Misfolded proteins are generally insoluble unless some denaturant is present. HEK-293 lysates were subject to a western blot, where lysates were immunoblotted with anti-tubulin antibody as a loading control, anti-GFP antibody, and anti-Pfn1 antibody specific for endogenous Pfn1.

PKA possibly phosphorylates T89

T89D and T89A mutants made to analyze role of phosphorylation

Cells expressing the 3 constructs were broken apart with one of 3 types of solutions: non-, mild, and strongly denaturing

Ignore the results for tubulin; it's just a control

This will show if any of the constructs are expressed

This will show the Pfn1 that's already expressed in the cells

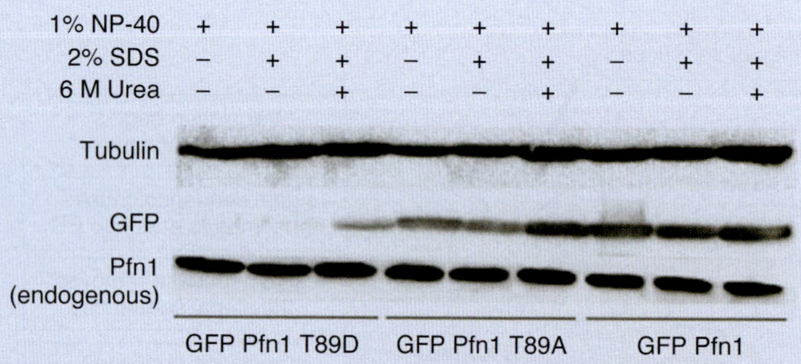

Lots of info here, so focus on what's changing: the GFP row shows the most change so it's probably the most important

Figure 1

Adapted from Gau, D., Veon, W., Zeng, X., Yates, N., Shroff, S. G., Koes, D. R., & Roy, P. (2016). Threonine 89 is an important residue of profilin-1 that is phosphorylatable by protein kinase A. *PLoS One*, 11(5), e0156313. doi:10.1371/journal.pone.0156313.

What is the purpose of mutating the potential phosphorylation site to aspartic acid and alanine, respectively? What is the implication for expression of Pfn1?

Since the question is asking for a reason behind the experimental design, our focus should be on understanding the way the experiment was designed. The passage is focused on clarifying how phosphorylation regulates Pfn1. We know from our content background that phosphorylation of an amino acid (specifically serine, threonine, and tyrosine) will turn a polar amino acid into one that is negatively charged. If we didn't remember that, we could also infer it by thinking about the charge on a phosphate group, which is highly negative. We have enough information to answer the first question. Mutating a threonine phosphorylation site to aspartic acid (which is negatively charged) would mimic the site being constantly phosphorylated, while mutating to alanine would mimic the site being constantly dephosphorylated, since alanine residues cannot be phosphorylated.

One possible phosphorylation site, T89, was identified, and three GFP constructs were made—one mimicking phosphorylation (T89D, lanes 1–3), one eliminating phosphorylation (T89A, lanes 4–6), and one unmodified (lanes 7–9). The GFP tag allows the experimenters to see whether the GFP-fused construct is being expressed (whether the protein is being made). We're told this experimental procedure is a western blot, a technique in which a specific antibody of interest will bind to proteins that were separated on a gel. In western blots, a band appears when the antibody successfully binds to protein. The rows above the gel image display experimental conditions for each of the lanes. All lanes have 1% NP-40, which we're told is non-denaturing. We should recall that the word denaturing means that a substance changes the 3-D structure of a protein. So, non-denaturing means that NP-40 won't change the shape of the protein by itself. The lanes with 2% SDS are in mild denaturing conditions, and the lanes with 2% SDS and 6 M urea are in strong denaturing conditions. Continuing by that same definition, we know that strong denaturing conditions will unfold and solubilize all proteins, greatly changing their 3-D structure. If we look at the row probing for GFP, we see that there is no band for non- and mild denaturing conditions, but there is a faint band under strong denaturing conditions for only the T89D construct. We can see that the lanes for both the wild type and T89A, regardless of condition, are mostly the same. Finally, recall that phosphorylation is a post-translational event, so a change in the phosphorylation state of the protein would occur after Pfn1 has been translated, and wouldn't work to affect its expression.

Therefore, we can conclude that mutating the threonine residue can mimic the effect of constantly phosphorylated or dephosphorylated Pfn. Second, since we only see a GFP band when T89D is in the presence of a strong denaturant, phosphorylation of Pfn1 may cause the protein to fold in a way that makes it insoluble, thereby targeting the protein for degradation. Follow-up studies are required to verify the exact mechanism of action by which this occurs. Therefore, because T89D represents the "always phosphorylated" version of Pfn1, and T89D only appears on the gel in strongly denaturing conditions, we can conclude that Pfn1, when phosphorylated, isn't available/expressed. We can thus conclude that phosphorylation of Pfn1 can potentially be used to down-regulate the availability of Pfn1 for usage with actin polymerization.

Termination

When any of the three stop codons moves into the A site, a protein called **release factor** (**RF**) binds to the termination codon, causing a water molecule to be added to the polypeptide chain. The addition of this water molecule allows peptidyl transferase and **termination factors** to hydrolyze the completed polypeptide chain from the final tRNA. The polypeptide chain will then be released from the tRNA in the P site, and the two ribosomal subunits will dissociate.

Posttranslational Processing

The nascent polypeptide chain is subject to posttranslational modifications before it will become a functioning protein, similar to how hnRNA is modified prior to being released from the nucleus. One essential step for the final synthesis of the protein is proper folding. There is a specialized class of proteins called **chaperones**, the main function of which is to assist in the protein-folding process.

Many proteins are also modified by cleavage events. A common example of this is insulin, which needs to be cleaved from a larger, inactive peptide to achieve its active form. In peptides with signal sequences, the signal sequence must be cleaved if the protein is to enter the organelle and accomplish its function.

In peptides with quaternary structure, subunits come together to form the functional protein. A classic example is hemoglobin, which is composed of two alpha chains and two beta chains.

Other biomolecules may be added to the peptide via the following processes, which are illustrated in Figure 7.18:

- **Phosphorylation**—addition of a phosphate group (PO_4^{2-}) by protein kinases to activate or deactivate proteins; phosphorylation in eukaryotes is most commonly seen with serine, threonine, and tyrosine
- **Carboxylation**—addition of carboxylic acid groups, usually to serve as calcium-binding sites
- **Glycosylation**—addition of oligosaccharides as proteins pass through the ER and Golgi apparatus to determine cellular destination
- **Prenylation**—addition of lipid groups to certain membrane-bound enzymes

REAL WORLD

Posttranslational modifications are often important for proper protein functioning. For example, several clotting factors, including prothrombin, require posttranslational carboxylation of some of their glutamic acid residues in order to function properly. Vitamin K is required as a cofactor for these reactions; thus, vitamin K deficiency may result in a bleeding disorder.

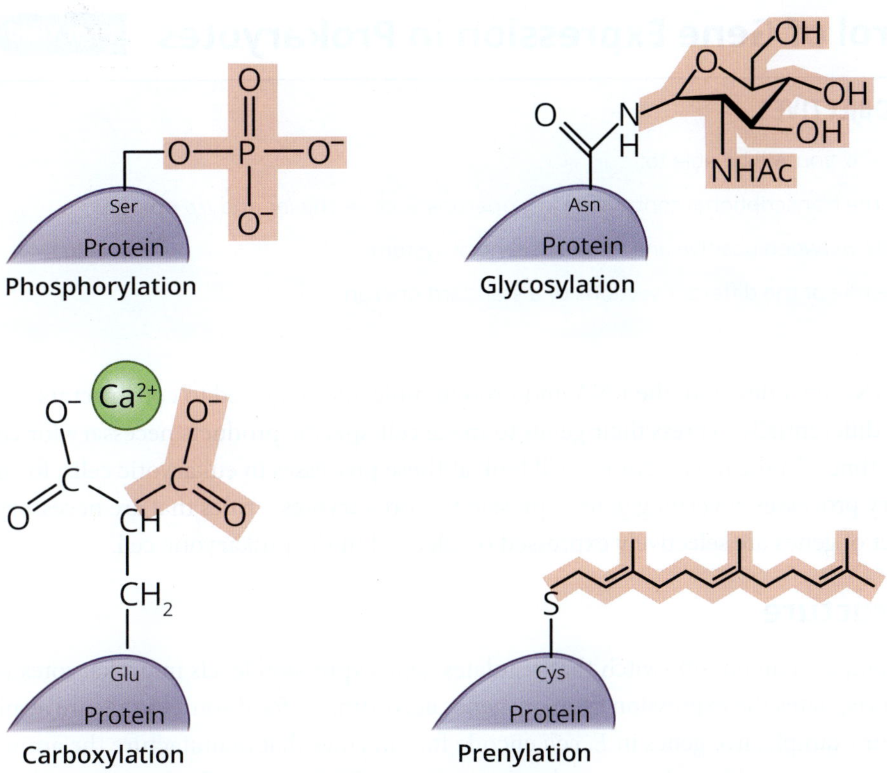

Figure 7.18 Examples of Posttranslational Modifications

MCAT CONCEPT CHECK 7.3

Before you move on, assess your understanding of the material with these questions.

1. What are the three steps of translation?

    1. ______________________________
    2. ______________________________
    3. ______________________________

2. What are the roles of each site in the ribosome?

    - A site:

    ____

    - P site:

    ____

    - E site:

    ____

3. What are the major posttranslational modifications that occur in proteins?

____

7.4 Control of Gene Expression in Prokaryotes High Yield

LEARNING OBJECTIVES

After Chapter 7.4, you will be able to:

- Recognize the transcriptional controls on key operons such as the *lac* and *trp* operons
- Differentiate between positive and negative control systems
- Explain the role of the different sections of a standard operon

An organism's DNA encodes all of the RNA and protein molecules required to construct its cells. Yet organisms are able to differentially express their genes to make cell-specific products necessary for cellular development at specific times. In the next section, we'll look at these processes in eukaryotic cells; for now, we'll focus on the regulatory processes governing gene expression in prokaryotes—rules that are necessary in determining which subset of genes are selectively expressed or silenced in the prokaryotic cell.

Operon Structure

The simplest example of an on–off switch that regulates gene expression levels in prokaryotes was discovered in *E. coli,* which regulates the expression of many genes according to food sources that are available in the environment. For example, five genes in *E. coli* encode for enzymes that manufacture the amino acid tryptophan, and these are arranged in a cluster on the chromosome. By sharing a single common promoter region on the DNA sequence, these genes are transcribed as a group. This type of structure is called an **operon**—a cluster of genes transcribed as a single mRNA; this particular cluster in *E. coli* is known as the *trp* operon. Operons are incredibly common in the prokaryotic cell.

The **Jacob–Monod model** is used to describe the structure and function of operons. In this model, operons contain structural genes, an operator site, a promoter site, and a regulator gene, as shown in Figure 7.19. The **structural gene** codes for the protein of interest. Upstream of the structural gene is the **operator site,** a nontranscribable region of DNA that is capable of binding a repressor protein. Further upstream is the **promoter site**, which is similar in function to promoters in eukaryotes: it provides a place for RNA polymerase to bind. Furthest upstream is the **regulator gene**, which codes for a protein known as the **repressor**. There are two types of operons: inducible systems and repressible systems.

KEY CONCEPT

Operons include both inducible and repressible systems, and offer a simple on–off switch for gene control in prokaryotes.

Inducible Systems

In **inducible systems**, the repressor is bonded tightly to the operator system and thereby acts as a roadblock. RNA polymerase is unable to get from the promoter to the structural gene because the repressor is in the way. Such systems—in which the binding of a protein reduces transcriptional activity—are called **negative control** mechanisms. To remove that block, an inducer must bind the repressor protein so that RNA polymerase can move down the gene, as shown in Figure 7.19. Inducible systems operate on a principle analogous to competitive inhibition for enzyme activity: as the concentration of the inducer increases, it will pull more copies of the repressor off of the operator region, freeing up those genes for transcription. This system is useful because it allows gene products to be produced only when they are needed.

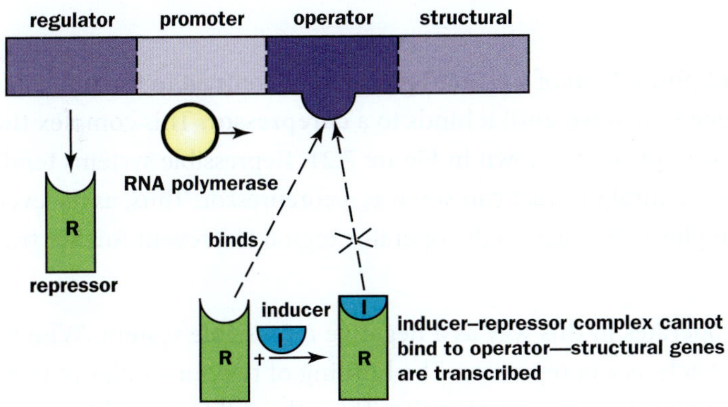

Figure 7.19 Inducible Systems
Allow for gene transcription only when an inducer is present to bind the otherwise present repressor protein

A classic example of an inducible system is the *lac* operon, which contains the gene for *lactase*, as demonstrated in Figure 7.20. Bacteria can digest lactose, but it is more energetically expensive than digesting glucose. Therefore, bacteria only want to use this option if lactose is high and glucose is low. The *lac* operon is induced by the presence of lactose; thus, these genes are only transcribed when it is useful to the cell.

The *lac* operon is assisted by binding of the **catabolite activator protein** (**CAP**). CAP is a transcriptional activator used by *E. coli* when glucose levels are low to signal that alternative carbon sources should be used. Falling levels of glucose cause an increase in the signaling molecule cyclic AMP (cAMP), which binds to CAP. This induces a conformational change in CAP that allows it to bind the promoter region of the operon, further increasing transcription of the lactase gene. Such systems—in which the binding of a molecule increases transcription of a gene—are called **positive control** mechanisms.

KEY CONCEPT

Negative control—The binding of a protein to DNA stops transcription.

Positive control—The binding of a protein to DNA increases transcription.

Inducible system—The system is normally "off" but can be made to turn "on," given a particular signal.

Repressible system—The system is normally "on" but can be made to turn "off," given a particular signal.

Any combination of control and system are possible; the *lac* operon is a negative inducible system whereas the *trp* operon is a negative repressible system.

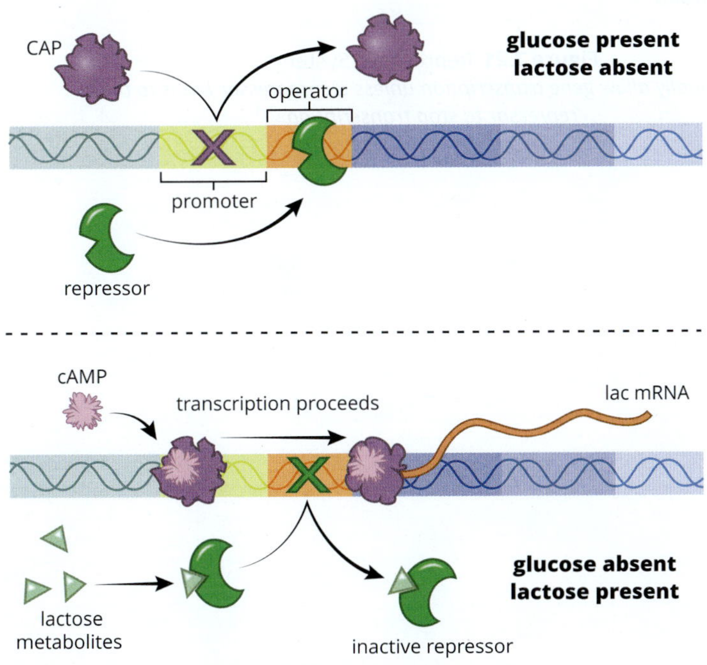

Figure 7.20 The *lac* Operon
An example of an inducible system

Repressible Systems

Repressible systems allow constant production of a protein product. In contrast to the inducible system, the repressor made by the regulator gene is inactive until it binds to a **corepressor**. This complex then binds the operator site to prevent further transcription, as shown in Figure 7.21. Repressible systems tend to serve as negative feedback; often, the final structural product can serve as a corepressor. Thus, as its levels increase, it can bind the repressor, and the complex will attach to the operator region to prevent further transcription of the same gene.

The *trp* operon, described above, operates in this way as a negative repressible system. When tryptophan is high in the local environment, it acts as a corepressor. The binding of two molecules of tryptophan to the repressor causes the repressor to bind to the operator site. Thus, the cell turns off its machinery to synthesize its own tryptophan, which is an energetically expensive process because of its easy availability in the environment.

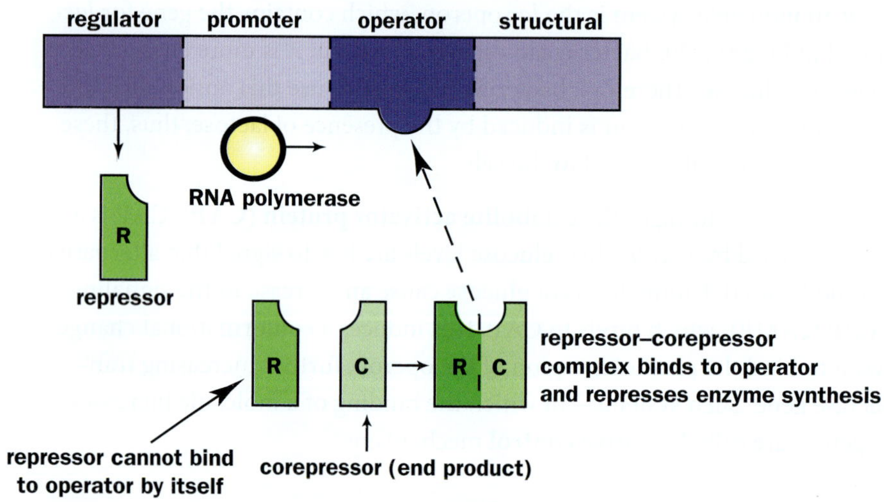

Figure 7.21 Repressible Systems
Continually allow gene transcription unless a corepressor binds to the repressor to stop transcription

MCAT CONCEPT CHECK 7.4

Before you move on, assess your understanding of the material with these questions.

1. What type of operon is the *trp* operon? The *lac* operon?
   - *trp*: ___________________________
   - *lac*: ___________________________

2. From 5′ to 3′, what are the components of the operon, and what are their roles?

Component	Role

3. What is a positive control system? What is a negative control system?
   - Positive control system:

____

   - Negative control system:

____

7.5 Control of Gene Expression in Eukaryotes **High Yield**

LEARNING OBJECTIVES

After Chapter 7.5, you will be able to:

- Identify the different mechanisms that can be used to regulate or amplify the expression of a gene
- Predict how histone and DNA modification will affect the ratio of heterochromatin to euchromatin

Genomic expression in eukaryotes is considerably more complex than in prokaryotes, and you will need to know those differences for Test Day. Regulation of gene expression is an essential feature that helps in maintaining the overall functionality of cells. In addition to basic transcriptional enzymes, however, there are a host of other regulatory proteins that play a prominent role in controlling gene expression levels in the cell.

Transcription Factors

Transcription factors are transcription-activating proteins that search the DNA looking for specific DNA-binding motifs. Transcription factors tend to have two recognizable domains: a DNA-binding domain and an activation domain. The **DNA-binding domain** binds to a specific nucleotide sequence in the promoter region or to a DNA **response element** (a sequence of DNA that binds only to specific transcription factors) to help in the recruitment of transcriptional machinery. The **activation domain** allows for the binding of several transcription factors and other important regulatory proteins, such as RNA polymerase and histone acetylases, which function in the remodeling of the chromatin structure.

Gene Amplification

Once the transcription complex is formed, basal (or low-level) transcription can begin and maintain moderate, but adequate, levels of the protein encoded by this gene in the cell. There are times, however, when the expression must be increased, or **amplified**, in response to specific signals such as hormones, growth factors, and other intracellular conditions. Eukaryotic cells accomplish this through enhancers and gene duplication.

Enhancers

Response elements outside the normal promoter regions can be recognized by specific transcription factors to enhance transcription levels. Several response elements may be grouped together to form an **enhancer**, which allows for the control of one gene's expression by multiple signals. Figure 7.22 demonstrates a eukaryotic example of an enhancer. Signal molecules, such as cyclic AMP (cAMP), cortisol, and estrogen, bind to specific receptors. For the examples given, these receptors are cyclic AMP response element-binding protein (CREB), the glucocorticoid (cortisol) receptor, and the estrogen receptor, respectively; all are transcription factors that bind to their respective response elements within the enhancer. Other proteins are involved in this process, but are outside the scope of the MCAT. Note that the large distance between the enhancer and promoter regions for a given gene means that DNA often must bend into a hairpin loop to bring these elements together spatially.

KEY CONCEPT

The DNA regulatory base sequences (such as promoters, enhancers, and response elements) are known as *cis* regulators because they are in the same vicinity as the gene they control. Transcription factors, however, have to be produced and translocated back to the nucleus; thus they are called *trans* regulators because they travel through the cell to their point of action.

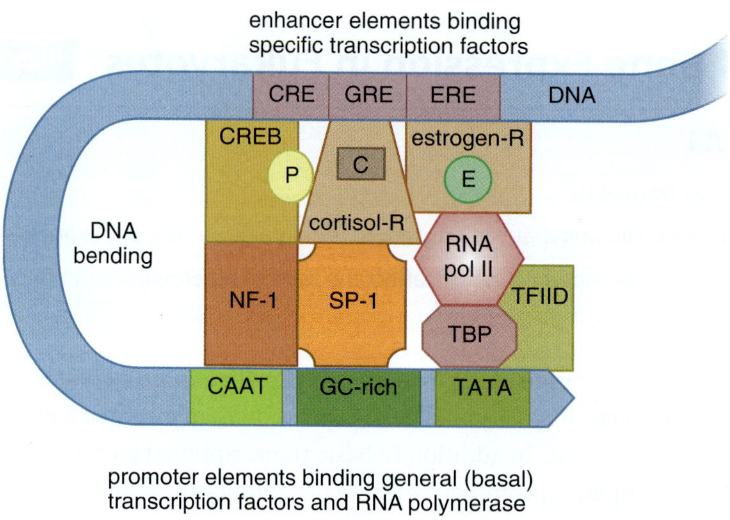

Figure 7.22 Stimulation of Transcription by an Enhancer and Its Associated Transcription Factors

Enhancer regions in the DNA can be up to 1000 base pairs away from the gene they regulate and can even be located within an intron, or noncoding region, of the gene. They differ from upstream promoter elements in their locations because upstream promoter elements must be within 25 bases of the start of a gene. By utilizing enhancer regions, genes have an increased likelihood to be amplified because of the variety of signals that can increase transcription levels.

Gene Duplication

Cells can also increase the expression of a gene product by duplicating the relevant gene. Genes can be duplicated in series on the same chromosome, yielding many copies in a row of the same genetic information. Genes can also be duplicated in parallel by opening the gene with helicases and permitting DNA replication only of that gene; cells can continue replicating the gene until hundreds of copies of the gene exist in parallel on the same chromosome.

Regulation of Chromatin Structure

In eukaryotic cells, DNA is packaged in the nucleus as chromatin, which requires chromatin remodeling to allow transcription factors and the transcriptional machinery easier access to the DNA. **Heterochromatin** is tightly coiled DNA that appears dark under the microscope; its tight coiling makes it inaccessible to the transcription machinery, so these genes are inactive. **Euchromatin**, on the other hand, is looser and appears light under the microscope; the transcription machinery can access the genes of interest, so these genes are active. Remodeling of the chromatin structures regulates gene expression levels in the cell.

Histone Acetylation

Transcription factors that bind to the DNA can recruit other coactivators such as ***histone acetylases***. These proteins are involved in chromatin remodeling, as shown in Figure 7.23, because they acetylate lysine residues found in the amino terminal tail regions of histone proteins. **Acetylation** of histone proteins decreases the positive charge on lysine residues and weakens the interaction of the histone with DNA, resulting in an open chromatin conformation that allows for easier access of the transcriptional machinery to the DNA.

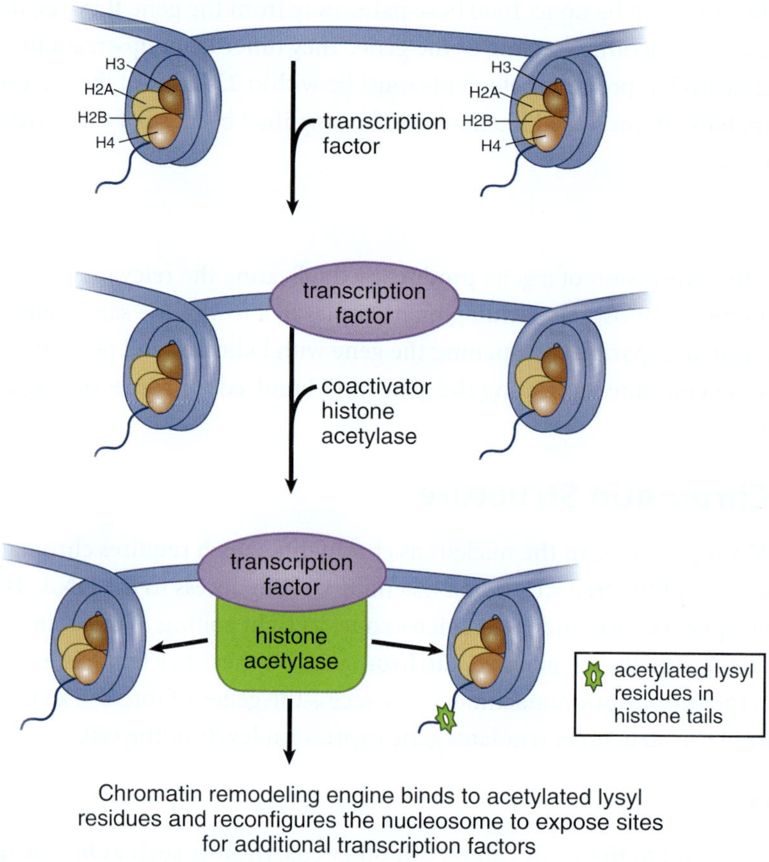

Figure 7.23 Chromatin Remodeling by Acetylation
Increases space between histones, allowing better access to DNA for transcription factors

Specific patterns of histone acetylation can lead to increased gene expression levels. On the other hand, gene silencing can occur just as easily with chromatin remodeling. ***Histone deacetylases*** are proteins that function to remove acetyl groups from histones, which results in a closed chromatin conformation and overall decrease in gene expression levels in the cell.

DNA Methylation

DNA methylation is also involved in chromatin remodeling and regulation of gene expression levels in the cell. ***DNA methylases*** add methyl groups to cytosine and adenine nucleotides, with an example of methylated DNA shown in Figure 7.24; methylation of genes is often linked with the silencing of gene expression. During development, methylation plays an important role in silencing genes that no longer need to be activated. Heterochromatin regions of the DNA are much more heavily methylated, hindering access of the transcriptional machinery to the DNA.

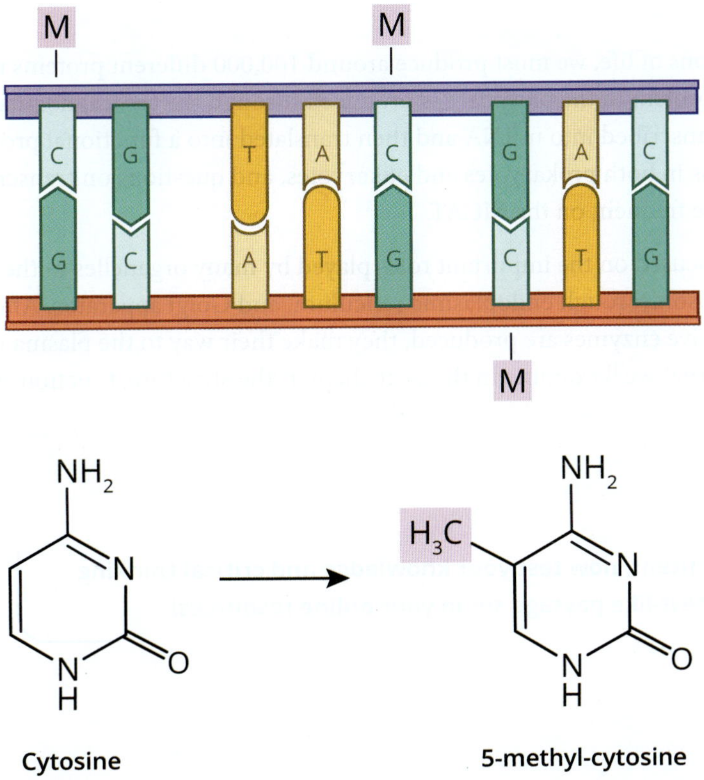

Figure 7.24 DNA Methylation

MCAT CONCEPT CHECK 7.5

Before you move on, assess your understanding of the material with these questions.

1. In an enhancer, what are the differences between signal molecules, transcription factors, and response elements?

____

2. By what histone and DNA modifications can genes be silenced in eukaryotic cells? Would these processes increase the proportion of heterochromatin or euchromatin?

____

Conclusion

To carry out the functions of life, we must produce around 100,000 different proteins using our 20,000–25,000 available genes. Every protein in the biosphere is produced through the central dogma of molecular biology, as genes in DNA are transcribed into mRNA and then translated into a functional protein. This is a complex, highly regulated process in both prokaryotes and eukaryotes, and questions on transcription and translation, and their regulation, are frequent on the MCAT.

The last two chapters focused on the important roles played by many organelles in the cell, including the nucleus, nucleolus, ribosome, rough endoplasmic reticulum, and Golgi apparatus. After secreted proteins such as hormones and digestive enzymes are produced, they make their way to the plasma membrane for exocytosis. It is this last stop that we'll examine in the next chapter: the structure, function, and biochemistry of biological membranes.

GO ONLINE

You've reviewed the content, now test your knowledge and critical thinking skills by completing a test-like passage set in your online resources!

CONCEPT SUMMARY

The Genetic Code

- The **central dogma** states that DNA is transcribed to RNA, which is translated to protein.
- A degenerate code allows multiple codons to encode for the same amino acid.
  - Initiation (start) codon: AUG
  - Termination (stop) codons: UAA, UGA, UAG
- Redundancy and **wobble** (third base in the codon) allows mutations to occur without effects in the protein.
- Point mutations can cause:
  - **Silent** mutations with no effect on protein synthesis.
  - **Nonsense** (**truncation**) mutations that produce a premature stop codon.
  - **Missense** mutations that produce a codon that codes for a different amino acid.
- **Frameshift mutations** result from nucleotide addition or deletion, and change the reading frame of subsequent codons.
- RNA is structurally similar to DNA except:
  - Substitution of a ribose sugar for deoxyribose
  - Substitution of uracil for thymine
  - It is single-stranded instead of double-stranded
- There are three types of RNA with separate jobs in transcription:
  - **Messenger RNA** (**mRNA**) carries the message from DNA in the nucleus via transcription of the gene; it travels into the cytoplasm to be translated.
  - **Transfer RNA** (**tRNA**) brings in amino acids and recognizes the codon on the mRNA using its anticodon.
  - **Ribosomal RNA** (**rRNA**) makes up the ribosome and is enzymatically active.

Transcription

- **Helicase** unwinds the DNA double helix.
- **RNA polymerase II** binds to the **TATA box** within the **promoter** region of the gene (25 base pairs upstream from first transcribed base).
- **hnRNA** is synthesized from the DNA template (antisense) strand.
- Posttranscriptional modifications include:
  - A 7-methylguanylate triphosphate cap is added to the 5′ end.
  - A polyadenosyl (poly-A) tail is added to the 3′ end.
  - Splicing is done by snRNA and snRNPs in the **spliceosome**; introns are removed in a **lariat** structure, and exons are ligated together.
  - Prokaryotic cells can increase the variability of gene products from one transcript through **polycistronic genes** (in which starting transcription in different sites within the gene leads to different gene products).
  - Eukaryotic cells can increase variability of gene products through **alternative splicing** (combining different exons in a modular fashion to acquire different gene products).

Translation

- tRNA translates the codon into the correct amino acid.
- Ribosomes are the factories where translation (protein synthesis) occurs.
- There are three stages of **translation.**
    - **Initiation** in prokaryotes occurs when the 30S ribosome attaches to the **Shine–Dalgarno sequence** and scans for a start codon; it lays down *N*-formylmethionine in the P site of the ribosome.
    - Initiation in eukaryotes occurs when the 40S ribosome attaches to the 5′ cap and scans for a start codon; it lays down methionine in the P site of the ribosome.
    - **Elongation** involves the addition of a new aminoacyl-tRNA into the A site of the ribosome and transfer of the growing polypeptide chain from the tRNA in the P site to the tRNA in the A site. The now uncharged tRNA pauses in the E site before exiting the ribosome.
    - **Termination** occurs when the codon in the A site is a stop codon; a **release factor** places a water molecule on the polypeptide chain and thus releases the protein.
    - Initiation, elongation, and release factors help with each step in recruitment and assembly/disassembly of the ribosome.
- Posttranslational modifications include:
    - Folding by **chaperones**
    - Formation of quaternary structure
    - Cleavage of proteins or signal sequences
    - Covalent addition of other biomolecules (phosphorylation, carboxylation, glycosylation, prenylation)

Control of Gene Expression in Prokaryotes

- The **Jacob–Monod model** of repressors and activators explains how operons work.
    - **Operons** are inducible or repressible clusters of genes transcribed as a single mRNA.
- **Inducible systems** (such as the *lac* operon) are bonded to a **repressor** under normal conditions; they can be turned on by an **inducer** pulling the repressor from the **operator site**.
- **Repressible systems** (such as the *trp* operon) are transcribed under normal conditions; they can be turned off by a corepressor coupling with the repressor and the binding of this complex to the operator site.

Control of Gene Expression in Eukaryotes

- **Transcription factors** search for promoter and enhancer regions in the DNA.
    - **Promoters** are within 25 base pairs of the transcription start site.
    - **Enhancers** are more than 25 base pairs away from the transcription start site.
    - Modification of chromatin structure affects the ability of transcriptional enzymes to access the DNA through histone acetylation (increases accessibility) or DNA methylation (decreases accessibility).

ANSWERS TO CONCEPT CHECKS

7.1

1. mRNA carries information from DNA by traveling from the nucleus (where it is transcribed) to the cytoplasm (where it is translated). tRNA translates nucleic acids to amino acids by pairing its anticodon with mRNA codons; it is charged with an amino acid, which can be added to the growing peptide chain. rRNA forms much of the structural and catalytic component of the ribosome, and acts as a ribozyme to create peptide bonds between amino acids.
2. • GAT: mRNA codon = AUC; Isoleucine (Ile)
   • ATT: mRNA codon = AAU; Asparagine (Asn)
   • CGC: mRNA codon = GCG; Alanine (Ala)
   • CCA: mRNA codon = UGG; Tryptophan (Trp)
3. The start codon is AUG, which codes for methionine; the stop codons are UAA, UGA, and UAG.
4. Wobble refers to the fact that the third base in a codon often plays no role in determining which amino acid is translated from that codon. For example, any codon starting with "CC" codes for proline, regardless of which base is in the third (wobble) position. This is protective because mutations in the wobble position will not have any effect on the protein translated from that gene.
5.

Type of Mutation	Change in DNA Sequence	Effect on Encoded Protein
Silent (degenerate)	Substitution of bases in the wobble position, introns, or noncoding DNA	No change observed
Missense	Substitution of one base, creating an mRNA codon that matches a different amino acid	One amino acid is changed in the protein; variable effects on function depending on specific change
Nonsense	Substitution of one base, creating a stop codon	Early truncation of protein; variable effects on function, but usually more severe than missense mutations
Frameshift	Insertion or deletion of bases, creating a shift in the reading frame of the mRNA	Change in most amino acids after the site of insertion or deletion; usually the most severe of the types listed here

7.2

1. RNA polymerase I synthesizes most rRNA. RNA polymerase II synthesizes mRNA (hnRNA) and snRNA. RNA polymerase III synthesizes tRNA and some rRNA.
2. RNA polymerase II binds to the TATA box, which is located within the promoter region of a relevant gene, at about −25.
3. The major posttranscriptional modifications are:
   - Splicing: removal of introns, joining of exons; uses snRNA and snRNPs in the spliceosome to create a lariat, which is then degraded; exons are ligated together
   - 5′ cap: addition of a 7-methylguanylate triphosphate cap to the 5′ end of the transcript
   - 3′ poly-A tail: addition of adenosine bases to the 3′ end to protect against degradation
4. Alternative splicing is the ability of some genes to use various combinations of exons to create multiple proteins from one hnRNA transcript. This increases protein diversity and allows a species to maximize the number of proteins it can create from a limited number of genes.

7.3

1. Initiation, elongation, and termination
2. A site: binds incoming aminoacyl-tRNA using codon–anticodon pairing

   P site: holds growing polypeptide until peptidyl transferase forms peptide bond and polypeptide is handed to A site

   E site: transiently holds uncharged tRNA as it exits the ribosome
3. Posttranslational modifications include proper folding by chaperones, formation of quaternary structure, cleavage of proteins or signal sequences, and addition of other biomolecules (phosphorylation, carboxylation, glycosylation, prenylation).

7.4

1. The *trp* operon is a negative repressible system; the *lac* operon is a negative inducible system.
2.

Component	Role
Regulator gene	Transcribed to form repressor protein
Promoter site	Site of RNA polymerase binding (similar to promoters in eukaryotes)
Operator site	Binding site for repressor protein
Structural gene	The gene of interest; its transcription is dependent on the repressor being absent from the operator site

3. Positive control systems require the binding of a protein to the operator site to increase transcription. Negative control systems require the binding of a protein to the operator site to decrease transcription.

7.5

1. Signal molecules include steroid hormones and second messengers, which bind to their receptors in the nucleus. These receptors are transcription factors that use their DNA-binding domain to attach to a particular sequence in DNA called a response element. Once bonded to the response element, these transcription factors can then promote increased expression of the relevant gene.
2. Histone deacetylation and DNA methylation will both downregulate the transcription of a gene. These processes allow the relevant DNA to be clumped more tightly, increasing the proportion of heterochromatin.

SCIENCE MASTERY ASSESSMENT EXPLANATIONS

1. **D**

Peptidyl transferase is an enzyme that catalyzes the formation of a peptide bond between the incoming amino acid in the A site and the growing polypeptide chain in the P site. Initiation and elongation factors help transport charged tRNA molecules into the ribosome and advance the ribosome down the mRNA transcript, as in **(A)** and **(B)**. Chaperones maintain a protein's three-dimensional shape as it is formed, as in **(C)**.

2. **C**

The promoter functions as a recruitment site for RNA polymerase and is required for gene expression. A mutation in this region would hinder RNA polymerase recruitment, resulting in a decrease in gene expression. These observations support **(C)** as the correct answer. By contrast, mutations in the operator and regulatory genes would render the repressor less able to block transcription, leading to the opposite effect, i.e. an increase in lactase expression. This result eliminates both **(A)** and **(B)**. Finally, mutations in the structural genes could lead to the production of a nonfunctional enzyme, but are unlikely to affect gene expression, eliminating **(D)**.

3. **A**

Topoisomerases, such as prokaryotic DNA gyrase, are involved in DNA replication and mRNA synthesis (transcription). DNA gyrase is a type of topoisomerase that enhances the action of helicase enzymes by the introduction of negative supercoils into the DNA molecule. These negative supercoils facilitate DNA replication by keeping the strands separated and untangled.

4. **C**

There are four different codons for valine: GUU, GUC, GUA, and GUG. Through base-pairing, we can determine that the proper anticodon must end with "AC." Remember that the codon and anticodon are antiparallel to each other, and that nucleic acids are always written $5' \rightarrow 3'$ on the MCAT. Therefore, we are looking for an answer that ends with "AC" (rather than starting with "CA").

5. **A**

Specific transcription factors bind to a specific DNA sequence, such as an enhancer, and to RNA polymerase at a single promoter sequence. They enable the RNA polymerase to transcribe the specific gene for that enhancer more efficiently.

6. **C**

UAG is one of the three known stop codons, so changing tyrosine to a stop codon must be a nonsense (or truncation) mutation.

7. **C**

In this question, the correct answer is the answer that is *not* associated with increased transcription. DNA methylation, **(C)**, is associated with silencing of gene expression. Regions of DNA with poor gene expression, called heterochromatin, are heavily methylated. These modifications significantly decrease the ability of RNA polymerase to access DNA.

8. **B**

The example given is a sample of repression due to the abundance of a corepressor. In other words, this is a repressible system that is currently blocking transcription. For the *trp* operon, an abundance of tryptophan in the environment allows for the repressor to bind tryptophan and then to the operator site. This blocks transcription of the genes required to synthesize tryptophan within the cell. The system described is a repressible system; the *lac* operon is an inducible system, in which an inducer binds to the repressor, thus permitting transcription.

9. **C**

shRNA (short hairpin RNA) is a useful biotechnology tool used in RNA interference. It is not, however, produced in the nucleus for use in the spliceosome. It targets mRNA to be degraded in the cytoplasm; it is not utilized in splicing of the hnRNA (heterogeneous nuclear RNA). snRNA (small nuclear RNA) and snRNPs (small nuclear ribonucleoproteins), however, do bind to the hnRNA to induce splicing.

10. **A**

In this table, we are given the sequence of the sense (coding) DNA strand. This will be identical to the mRNA transcript, except all thymine nucleotides will be replaced with uracil. With the deletion of these three bases, codon 507 changes from AUC to AUU in the transcript; these both code for isoleucine due to wobble. However, codon 508 (UUU in the transcript) has been lost. UUU codes for phenylalanine. The C-terminus sequence will remain unchanged because the deletion of three bases (exactly one codon) will not throw off the reading frame. For reference, the mutant reading frames would be:

(Note: refer back to Figure 7.7 for a table of the genetic code)

AUC	AUU	GGU	GUU	UCC

11. **B**

The intron will not be a part of the final, processed mRNA, and the untranslated regions of the mRNA will not be turned into amino acids. Translation will begin with codon 1 (which would be AUG). Because there are 150 amino acids, we can surmise that there will be 151 codons. Each codon will use 3 nucleotides, so $150 \times 3 = 450$ because codon 151 will be the stop codon.

12. **B**

Peptidyl transferase connects the incoming amino terminal to the previous carboxyl terminal; the only functional group listed here with a carbonyl and amino group is the amide. Peptide bonds are thus amide linkages, and the correct answer is **(B)**.

13. **A**

RNA polymerase I in eukaryotes is found in the nucleolus and is in charge of transcribing most of the rRNA for use during ribosomal creation. RNA polymerase II is responsible for hnRNA and snRNA. RNA polymerase III is responsible for tRNA and the 5S rRNA.

14. **B**

To answer this question correctly, we must remember that mRNA will be antiparallel to DNA. Our answer should be 5′ to 3′ mRNA, with the 5′ end complementary to the 3′ end of the DNA that is being transcribed. Thus, the mRNA transcribed from this strand will be 5′—GGAUGUCUCAAAGA—3′. mRNA contains uracil, rather than thymine.

15. **B**

The mRNA produced has the same structure as the sense strand of DNA (with uracils instead of thymines). Because bonding of nucleic acids is always complementary but antiparallel, the antisense strand of mRNA would be the one that binds to the produced mRNA, creating double-stranded RNA that is then degraded once found in the cytoplasm.

GO ONLINE

Consult your online resources for additional practice.

SHARED CONCEPTS

Biochemistry Chapter 1
Amino Acids, Peptides, and Proteins

Biochemistry Chapter 2
Enzymes

Biochemistry Chapter 6
DNA and Biotechnology

Biology Chapter 1
The Cell

Biology Chapter 3
Embryogenesis and Development

Biology Chapter 12
Genetics and Evolution

CHAPTER 8

BIOLOGICAL MEMBRANES

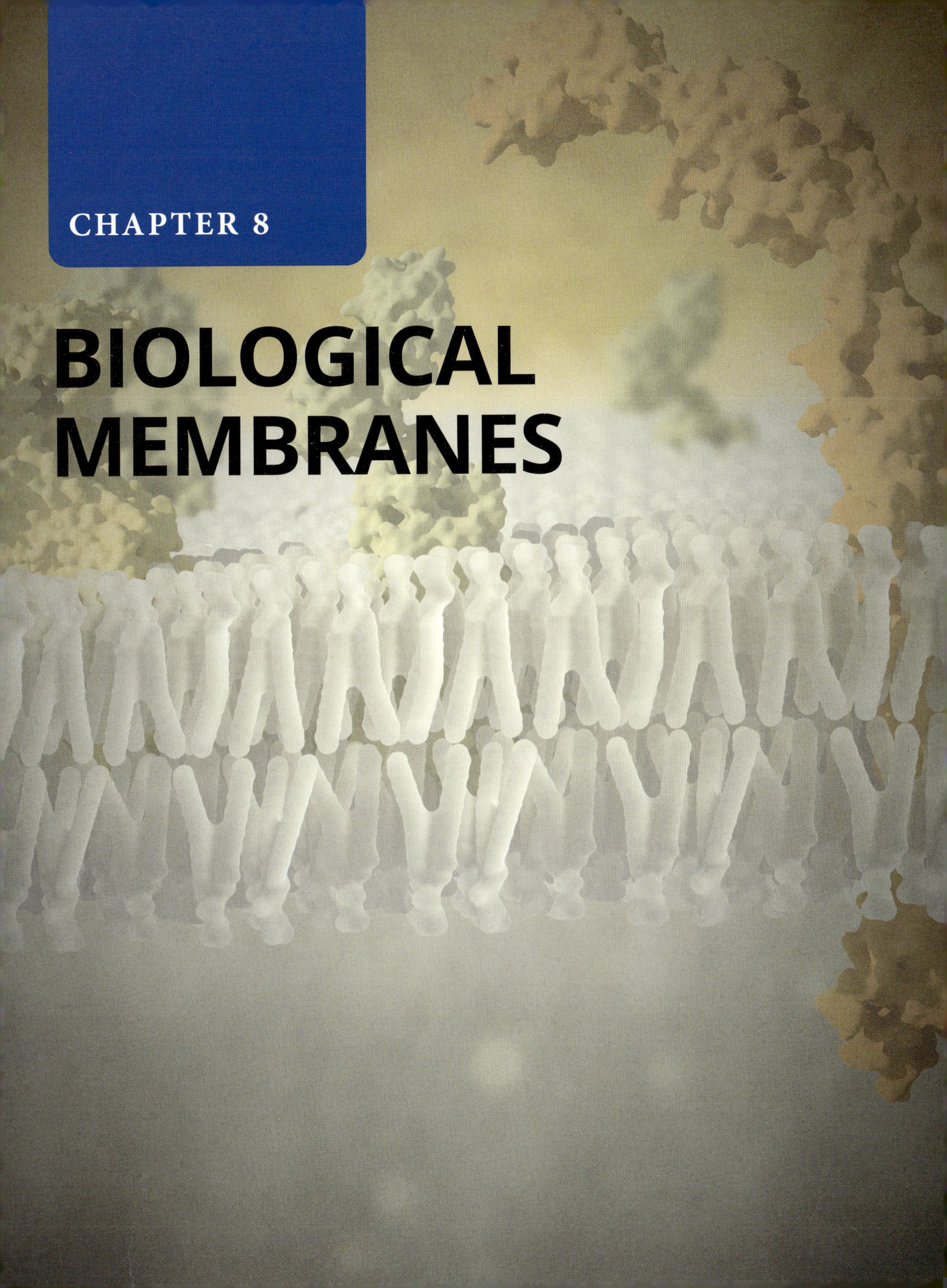

SCIENCE MASTERY ASSESSMENT

Every pre-med knows this feeling: there is so much content I have to know for the MCAT! How do I know what to do first or what's important?

While the high-yield badges throughout this book will help you identify the most important topics, this Science Mastery Assessment is another tool in your MCAT prep arsenal. This quiz (which can also be taken in your online resources) and the guidance below will help ensure that you are spending the appropriate amount of time on this chapter based on your personal strengths and weaknesses. Don't worry though—skipping something now does not mean you'll never study it. Later on in your prep, as you complete full-length tests, you'll uncover specific pieces of content that you need to review and can come back to these chapters as appropriate.

How to Use This Assessment

If you answer 0–7 questions correctly:

Spend about 1 hour to read this chapter in full and take limited notes throughout. Follow up by reviewing **all** quiz questions to ensure that you now understand how to solve each one.

If you answer 8–11 questions correctly:

Spend 20–40 minutes reviewing the quiz questions. Beginning with the questions you missed, read and take notes on the corresponding subchapters. For questions you answered correctly, ensure your thinking matches that of the explanation and you understand why each choice was correct or incorrect.

If you answer 12–15 questions correctly:

Spend less than 20 minutes reviewing all questions from the quiz. If you missed any, then include a quick read-through of the corresponding subchapters, or even just the relevant content within a subchapter, as part of your question review. For questions you got correct, ensure your thinking matches that of the explanation and review the Concept Summary at the end of the chapter.

BIOLOGICAL MEMBRANES

1. A student is trying to determine the type of membrane transport occurring in a cell. The student finds that the molecule to be transported is very large and polar, and when transported across the membrane, no energy is required. Which of the following is the most likely mechanism of transport?
   - **A.** Active transport
   - **B.** Simple diffusion
   - **C.** Facilitated diffusion
   - **D.** Exocytosis

2. A researcher treats a solution containing animal cells with ouabain, a poisonous substance that interferes with the sodium–potassium ATPase embedded in the cell membrane, and the cell lyses as a result. Which of the following statements best describes ouabain's effects?
   - **A.** Treatment with ouabain results in high levels of extracellular calcium.
   - **B.** Treatment with ouabain results in high levels of extracellular potassium and sodium.
   - **C.** Treatment with ouabain increases intracellular concentrations of sodium.
   - **D.** Treatment with ouabain decreases intracellular concentrations of sodium.

3. Resting membrane potential depends on:
   - **I.** the differential distribution of ions across the membrane.
   - **II.** active transport processes.
   - **III.** selective permeability of the phospholipid bilayer.
   - **A.** I only
   - **B.** I and III only
   - **C.** II and III only
   - **D.** I, II, and III

4. Which of the following is NOT a function of the cell membrane?
   - **A.** Cytoskeletal attachment
   - **B.** Protein synthesis
   - **C.** Transport regulation
   - **D.** Second messenger reservoir

5. The dynamic properties of molecules in the cell membrane are most rapid in:
   - **A.** phospholipids moving within the plane of the membrane.
   - **B.** phospholipids moving between the layers of the membrane.
   - **C.** proteins moving within the plane of the membrane.
   - **D.** proteins exiting the cell through exocytosis.

6. Which lipid type is LEAST likely to contribute to membrane fluidity?
   - **A.** Unsaturated glycerophospholipids
   - **B.** *trans* glycerophospholipids
   - **C.** Cholesterol
   - **D.** Unsaturated sphingolipids

7. A membrane receptor is most likely to be a(n):
   - **A.** embedded protein with catalytic activity.
   - **B.** transmembrane protein with sequestration activity.
   - **C.** membrane-associated protein with sequestration activity.
   - **D.** transmembrane protein with catalytic activity.

8. Which of the following is NOT a cell–cell junction in animals?
   - **A.** Desmosomes
   - **B.** Gap junctions
   - **C.** Plasmodesmata
   - **D.** Tight junctions

9. Which of the following is true of diffusion and osmosis?
   - **A.** Diffusion and osmosis rely on the concentration gradient of only the compound of interest.
   - **B.** Diffusion and osmosis rely on the concentration gradient of all compounds in a cell.
   - **C.** Diffusion and osmosis will proceed in the same direction if there is only one solute.
   - **D.** Diffusion and osmosis cannot occur simultaneously.

10. The bulk movement of liquid into a cell through vesicular infoldings is known as:
   - **A.** phagocytosis.
   - **B.** pinocytosis.
   - **C.** exocytosis.
   - **D.** drinking.

11. Which of the following is LEAST likely to be the resting membrane potential of a cell?
   - **A.** −70 mV
   - **B.** −55 mV
   - **C.** 0 mV
   - **D.** +35 mV

12. How does the inner mitochondrial membrane differ from the outer mitochondrial membrane?
   - **A.** The inner mitochondrial membrane is more permeable and lacks cholesterol.
   - **B.** The inner mitochondrial membrane is less permeable and lacks cholesterol.
   - **C.** The inner mitochondrial membrane is more permeable and has cholesterol.
   - **D.** The inner mitochondrial membrane is less permeable and has cholesterol.

13. For most cells, the extracellular calcium concentration is around 10,000 times higher than the intracellular calcium concentration. What is the membrane potential established by this electrochemical gradient?
   - **A.** −123 mV
   - **B.** −61.5 mV
   - **C.** +61.5 mV
   - **D.** +123 mV

14. Which of the following statements conflicts with the fluid mosaic model?
   - **A.** The cell membrane is static in structure.
   - **B.** Membrane components can be derived from multiple biomolecules.
   - **C.** Hydrophobic interactions stabilize the lipid bilayer.
   - **D.** Proteins are asymmetrically distributed within the cell membrane.

15. Which of the following is a sphingolipid?
   - **A.** Lecithin
   - **B.** Phosphatidylinositol
   - **C.** Cholesterol
   - **D.** Ganglioside

Answer Key

1. **C** (See section 8.3)
2. **C** (See section 8.4)
3. **D** (See section 8.4)
4. **B** (See section 8.1)
5. **A** (See section 8.3)
6. **B** (See section 8.2)
7. **D** (See section 8.2)
8. **C** (See section 8.2)
9. **A** (See section 8.3)
10. **B** (See section 8.3)
11. **C** (See section 8.4)
12. **B** (See section 8.4)
13. **D** (See section 8.4)
14. **A** (See section 8.1)
15. **D** (See section 8.2)

The relevant section of the chapter to review for each question is given in parentheses after the correct answer. Detailed explanations can be found at the end of the chapter.

CHAPTER 8

BIOLOGICAL MEMBRANES

In This Chapter

Introduction

Biological membranes are a stunning combination of opposites and contrasts. They are exceptionally thin, structurally bland, and relatively straightforward to describe. Yet, they define the borders of cells, tissues, and organelles; carry out a significant number of the biological functions within cells; and are an unending source of scientific inquiry and discovery. The most commonly tested biological membrane on the MCAT is the plasma membrane. At first, the plasma membrane seems like it's only a shell—just a barrier that defines the cell. But the plasma membrane plays roles in signaling, entry of nutrients and expulsion of waste, cell recognition, transport of materials between tissues, and even electronic functions.

Cell membranes have both a stretchy, flexible component (phospholipids) and an abundance of stabilizing molecules (cholesterol and protein) to make sure that everything remains intact. In this chapter, we will examine the general function, composition, and transport properties of biological membranes. We will conclude by taking a look at a few specialized cell membranes within the body, in addition to specific membrane properties.

CHAPTER PROFILE

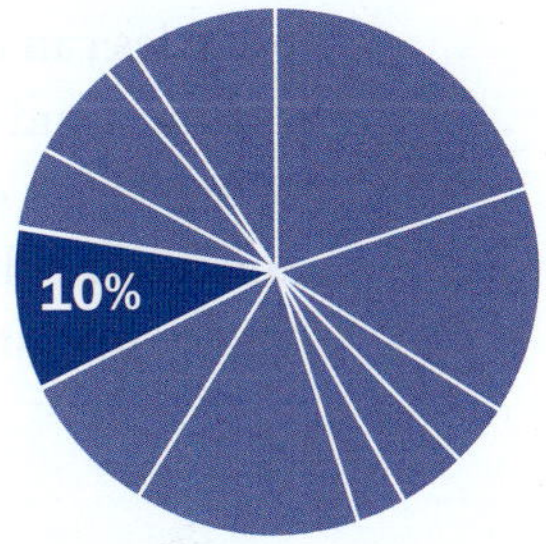

The content in this chapter should be relevant to about 10% of all questions about biochemistry on the MCAT.

This chapter covers material from the following AAMC content categories:

2A: Assemblies of molecules, cells, and groups of cells within single cellular and multicellular organisms

3A: Structure and functions of the nervous and endocrine systems, and ways in which these systems coordinate the organ systems

8.1 Fluid Mosaic Model

LEARNING OBJECTIVES

After Chapter 8.1, you will be able to:

- Describe the functions of flippases and lipid rafts
- Order a given list of membrane components from least to most abundant

The **cell (plasma) membrane** is often described as a semipermeable phospholipid bilayer. This phrase alone describes both the function and structure of the cell membrane: as a semipermeable barrier, it chooses which particles can enter and leave the cell at any point in time. This selectivity is mediated not only by the various channels and carriers that poke holes in the membrane, but also by the membrane itself. Composed primarily of two layers of phospholipids, the cell membrane permits fat-soluble compounds to cross easily, while larger and water-soluble compounds must seek alternative entry. The cell membrane is illustrated in Figure 8.1; the theory that underlies the structure and function of the cell membrane is referred to as the **fluid mosaic model**.

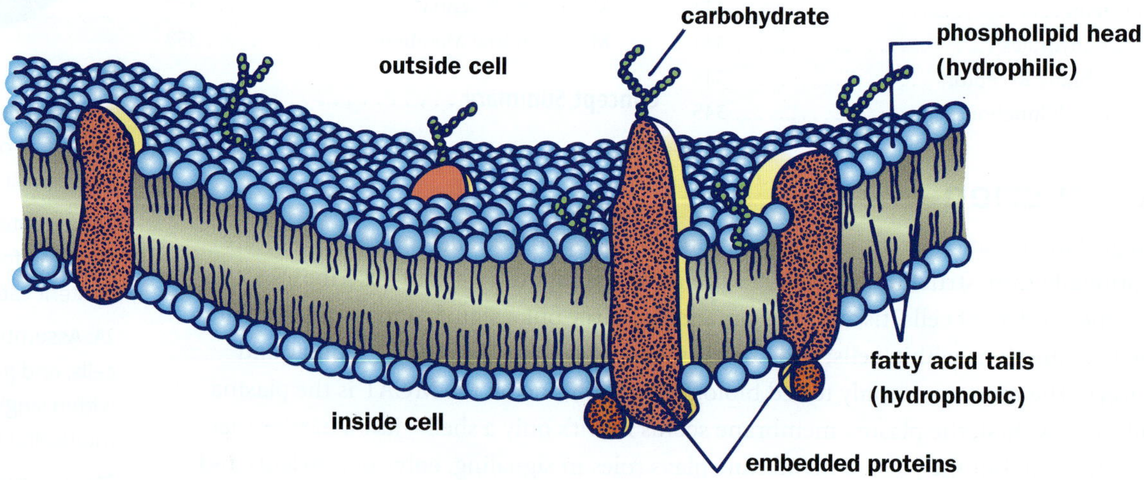

Figure 8.1 Cell Membrane
The cell membrane is a phospholipid bilayer that regulates movement of solutes into and out of the cell.

General Membrane Structure and Function

The phospholipid bilayer also includes proteins and distinct signaling areas within lipid rafts. Carbohydrates associated with membrane-bound proteins create a **glycoprotein coat**. The **cell wall** of plants, bacteria, and fungi contain higher levels of carbohydrates.

The main function of the cell membrane is to protect the interior of the cell from the external environment. Cellular membranes selectively regulate traffic into and out of the cell and are involved in both intracellular and intercellular communication and transport. Cell membranes also contain proteins embedded within the lipid bilayer that act as cellular receptors during signal transduction. These proteins play an important role in regulating and maintaining overall cellular activity.

Membrane Dynamics

The cell membrane functions as a stable semisolid barrier between the cytoplasm and the environment, but it is in a constant state of flux on the molecular level. **Phospholipids** move rapidly in the plane of the membrane through simple diffusion. This can be seen when fusing two membranes that have been tagged with different labels; the tags will migrate with their associated lipids until both types are rapidly intermixed. **Lipid rafts** are collections of similar lipids with or without associated proteins that serve as attachment points for other biomolecules; these rafts often serve roles in signaling. Both lipid rafts and proteins also travel within the plane of the membrane, but more slowly. Lipids can also move between the membrane layers, but this is energetically unfavorable because the polar head group of the phospholipid must be forced through the nonpolar tail region in the interior of the membrane. Specialized enzymes called **flippases** assist in the transition or "flip" between layers. Figure 8.2 illustrates a lipid raft and the role of flippases.

REAL WORLD

Many antidepressants increase levels of neurotransmitters in the brain, but the effects take longer to appear than the changes in neurochemistry. The reason for this delay is that the nervous system must still upregulate its postsynaptic receptors to respond to the new levels of neurotransmitter.

Dynamic changes in the concentrations of various membrane proteins are mediated by gene regulation, endocytic activity, and protein insertion. Many cells, particularly those involved in biosignaling processes, can up- or downregulate the number of specific cellular receptors on their surface in order to meet cellular requirements.

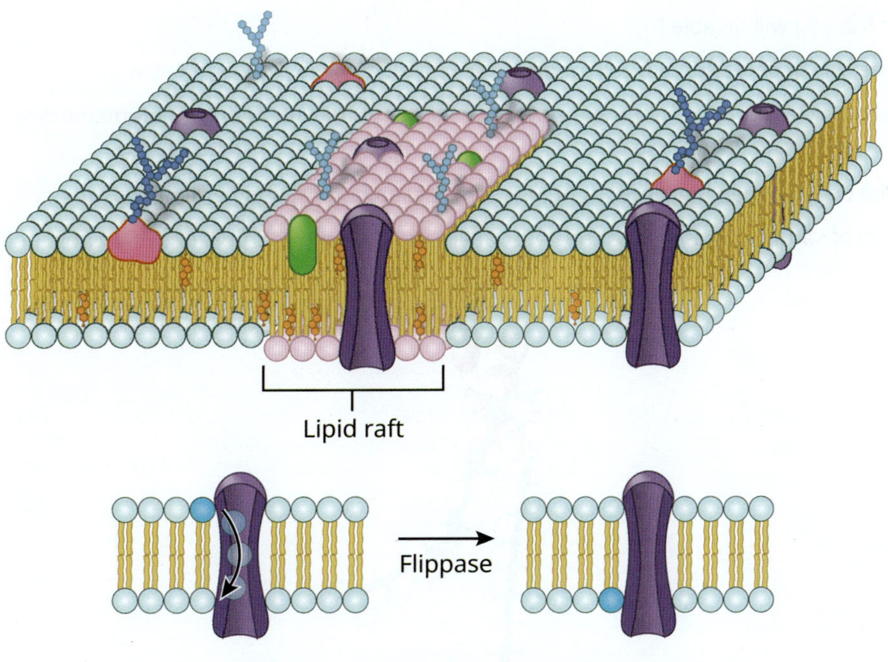

Figure 8.2 Lipid Rafts and Flippases
Lipid rafts and flippases aid in signaling at the cell membrane.

MCAT CONCEPT CHECK 8.1

Before you move on, assess your understanding of the material with these questions.

1. Describe the role of flippases and lipid rafts in biological membranes.
   - Flippases:

   ____

   - Lipid rafts:

   ____

2. List the following membrane components in order from most plentiful to least plentiful: carbohydrates, lipids, proteins, nucleic acids.

   ____________ > ____________ > ____________ > ____________

8.2 Membrane Components High Yield

LEARNING OBJECTIVES

After Chapter 8.2, you will be able to:

- Describe the role of cholesterol in cell membranes
- Define the three classes of membrane proteins: transmembrane, embedded, and membrane-associated proteins
- Differentiate between gap junctions, tight junctions, desmosomes, and hemidesmosomes
- Identify level of saturation, as well as the hydrophilic and hydrophobic portions of a phospholipid:

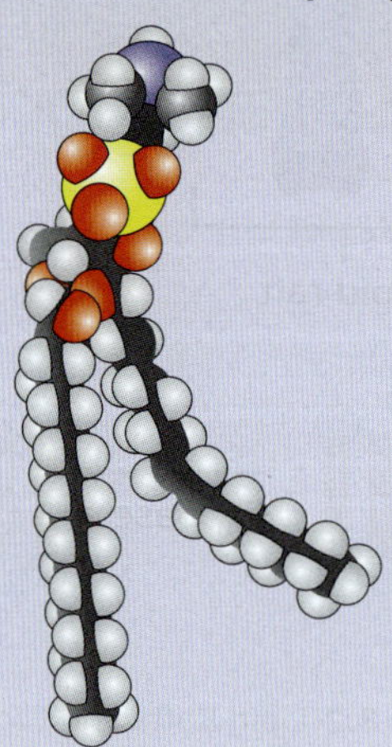

While the fluid mosaic model outlines the general composition of the membrane, the MCAT expects us to have a stronger grasp of the specifics, especially as it pertains to lipids and proteins.

Lipids

The cell membrane is composed predominantly of lipids with some associated proteins and carbohydrates. At times, the cell membrane as a whole will be referred to as a phospholipid bilayer, as it is the primary component of this barrier around the cell. Within the cell membrane, there are a large number of phospholipids with very few free fatty acids. In addition, steroid molecules and cholesterol, which lend fluidity to the membrane, and waxes, which provide membrane stability, help to maintain the structural integrity of the cell. While the structural details of these lipids were discussed in detail in Chapter 5 of *MCAT Biochemistry Review*, we will briefly describe their key points here.

Fatty Acids and Triacylglycerols

Fatty acids are carboxylic acids that contain a hydrocarbon chain and terminal carboxyl group. **Triacylglycerols**, also referred to as **triglycerides**, are storage lipids involved in human metabolic processes. They contain three fatty acid chains esterified to a glycerol molecule. Fatty acid chains can be saturated or unsaturated. **Unsaturated fatty acids** are regarded as "healthier" fats because they tend to have one or more double bonds and exist in liquid form at room temperature; in the plasma membrane, these characteristics impart fluidity to the membrane. Humans can only synthesize a few of the unsaturated fatty acids; the rest come from essential fatty acids in the diet that are transported as triacylglycerols from the intestine inside **chylomicrons**. Two important essential fatty acids for humans are *α-linolenic acid* and *linoleic acid*. **Saturated fatty acids** are the main components of animal fats and tend to exist as solids at room temperature. Saturated fats are found in processed foods and are considered less healthy. As shown in Figure 8.3, when incorporated into phospholipid membranes, saturated fatty acids decrease the overall membrane fluidity.

REAL WORLD

Trans fats, which result from the partial hydrogenation of some unsaturated fatty acids, have been banned from certain stores and cities because of their health risks. Part of the health concern is due to their ability to lower membrane fluidity, in addition to the tendency of *trans* fats to accumulate and form plaques in blood vessels.

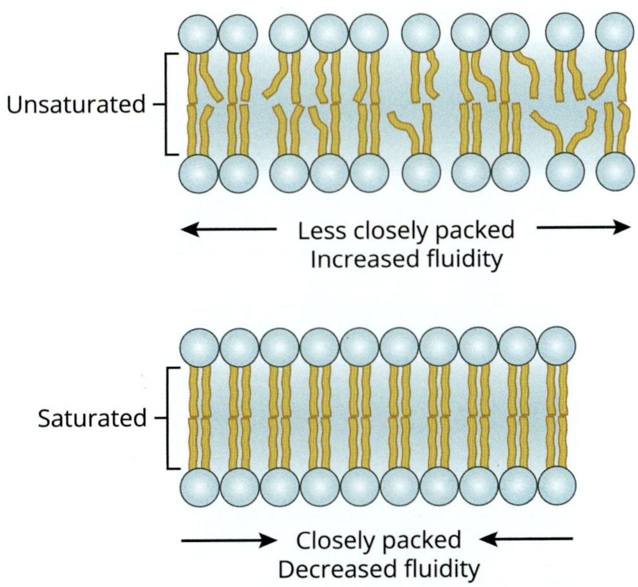

Figure 8.3 Effects of Fatty Acid Saturation on Membrane Fluidity

Phospholipids

By substituting one of the fatty acid chains of triacylglycerol with a phosphate group, a polar head group joins the nonpolar tails, forming a **glycerophospholipid**, commonly called a phospholipid. Phospholipids spontaneously assemble into **micelles** (small monolayer vesicles) or **liposomes** (bilayered vesicles) due to hydrophobic interactions. Glycerophospholipids are used for membrane synthesis and can produce a hydrophilic surface layer on lipoproteins such as *very-low-density lipoprotein* (VLDL), a lipid transporter. In addition, phospholipids are the primary component of cell membranes. Phospholipids serve not only structural roles, but can also serve as second messengers in signal transduction. The phosphate group also provides an attachment point for water-soluble groups, such as *choline* (*phosphatidylcholine*, also known as *lecithin*) or *inositol* (*phosphatidylinositol*). A comparison of triacylglycerols and glycerophospholipids is shown in Figure 8.4.

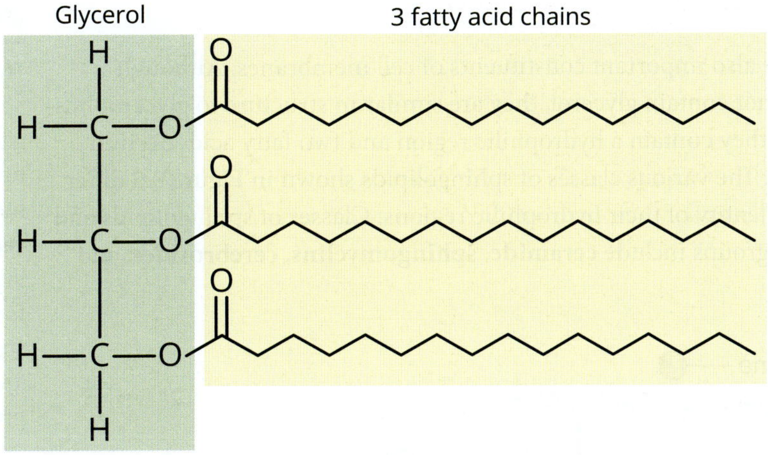

Triglyceride

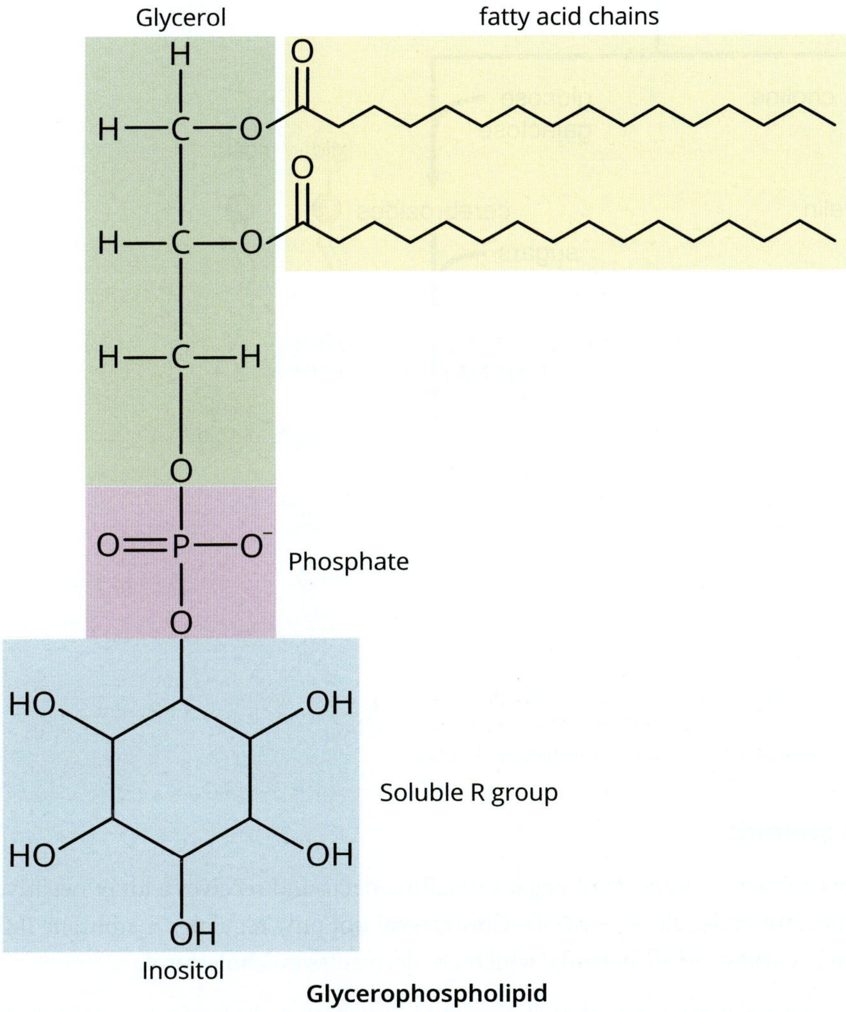

Glycerophospholipid

Figure 8.4 Triacylglycerol and Glycerophospholipid (Phosphatidylinositol)

Sphingolipids

Sphingolipids are also important constituents of cell membranes. Although sphingolipids do not contain glycerol, they are similar in structure to glycerophospholipids, in that they contain a hydrophilic region and two fatty acid–derived hydrophobic tails. The various classes of sphingolipids shown in Figure 8.5 differ primarily in the identity of their hydrophilic regions. Classes of sphingolipids and their hydrophilic groups include **ceramide**, **sphingomyelins**, **cerebrosides**, and **gangliosides**.

MCAT EXPERTISE

The ratio of certain sphingolipids to glycerophospholipids can help to identify particular membranes within the cell, but memorizing this information is unnecessary for Test Day. Where small details like this are important, they will be provided in a passage.

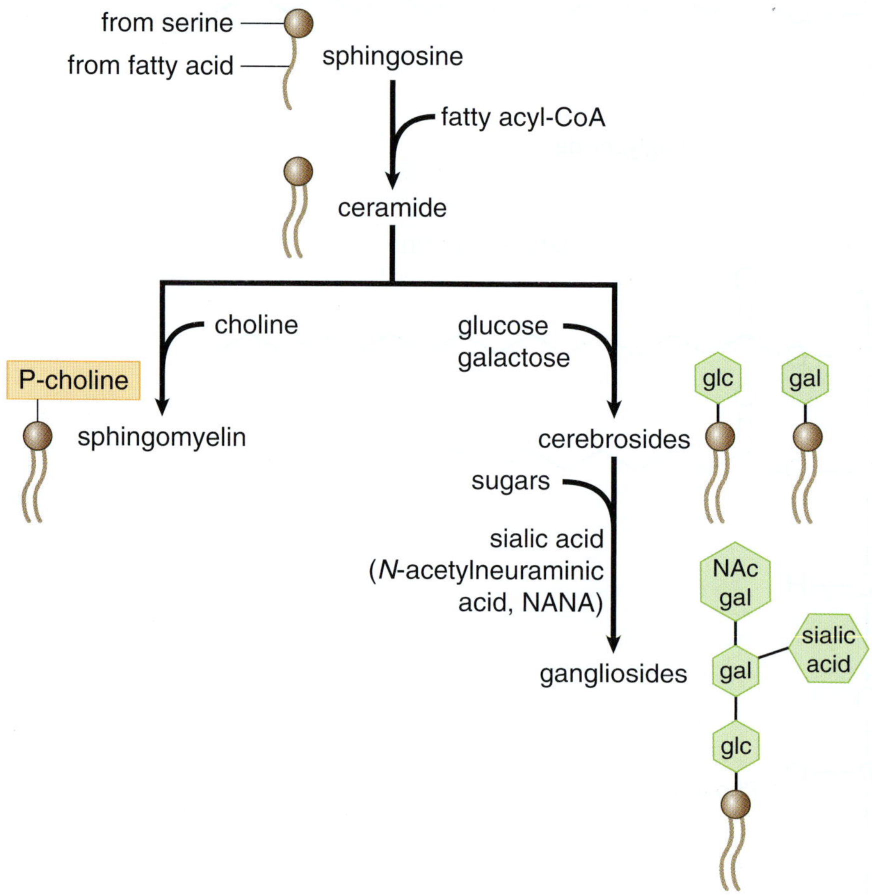

Figure 8.5 Types of Sphingolipids
Sphingolipids are sequentially modified to form each of the biologically necessary molecules in the class.

Cholesterol and Steroids

Cholesterol is associated with a number of negative health effects and receives a lot of negative press; however, it is also a very important molecule in our cells. **Cholesterol** not only regulates membrane fluidity, but it is also necessary in the synthesis of all **steroids**, which are derived from cholesterol.

The structure of cholesterol is similar to that of phospholipids in that cholesterol contains both a hydrophilic and hydrophobic region. Membrane stability is derived from interactions with both the hydrophilic and hydrophobic regions that make up the phospholipid bilayer. While cholesterol stabilizes adjacent phospholipids, it also occupies space between them. This prevents the formation of crystal structures in the membrane, increasing fluidity at lower temperatures. At high temperatures, cholesterol has the opposite effect: by limiting movement of phospholipids within the bilayer, it decreases fluidity and helps hold the membrane intact. The temperature effects of cholesterol on the phospholipid bilayer are shown in Figure 8.6. By mass, cholesterol composes about 20 percent of the cell membrane; by mole fraction, it makes up about half. This large ratio of cholesterol to phospholipid ensures that the membrane remains fluid.

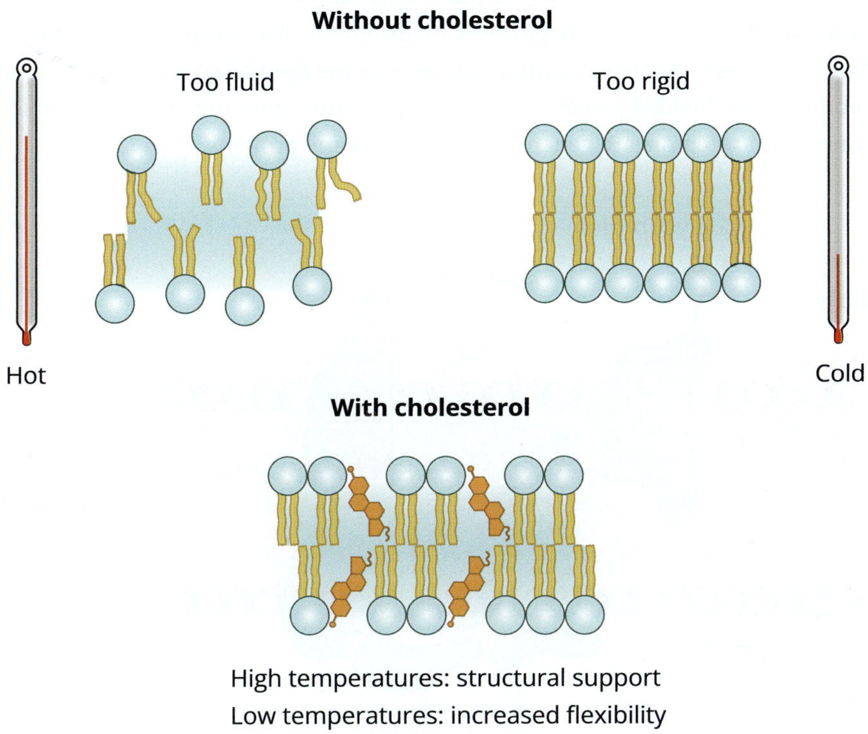

Figure 8.6 Stabilizing Effects of Cholesterol on Membranes

Waxes

Waxes are a class of lipids that are extremely hydrophobic and are rarely found in the cell membranes of animals, but are sometimes found in the cell membranes of plants. A wax, shown in Figure 8.7, is composed of a long-chain fatty acid and a long-chain alcohol, which contribute to the high melting point of these substances. When present within the cell membrane, waxes can provide both stability and rigidity within the nonpolar tail region only. Most waxes serve an extracellular function in protection or waterproofing.

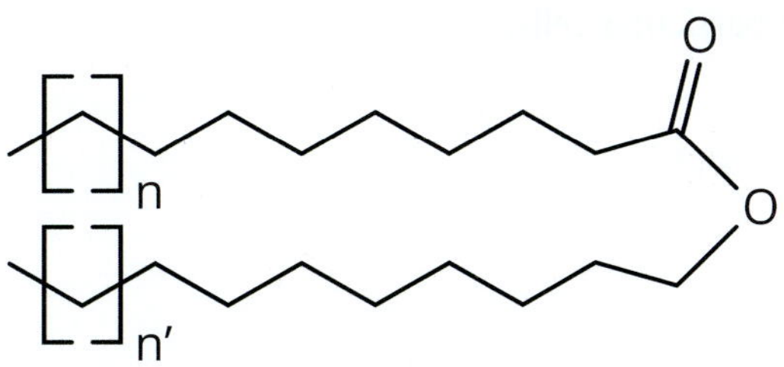

Figure 8.7 General Structure of a Wax

Proteins

The **fluid mosaic model** also accounts for the presence of three types of membrane proteins, as shown in Figure 8.8. **Transmembrane proteins** pass completely through the lipid bilayer. **Embedded proteins**, on the other hand, are associated with only the interior (cytoplasmic) or exterior (extracellular) surface of the cell membrane. Together, transmembrane and embedded proteins are considered **integral proteins** because of their association with the interior of the plasma membrane, which is usually assisted by one or more membrane-associated domains that are partially hydrophobic. **Membrane-associated** (**peripheral**) **proteins** may be bound through electrostatic interactions with the lipid bilayer, especially at lipid rafts, or to other transmembrane or embedded proteins, like the G proteins found in G protein-coupled receptors. Transporters, channels, and receptors are generally transmembrane proteins.

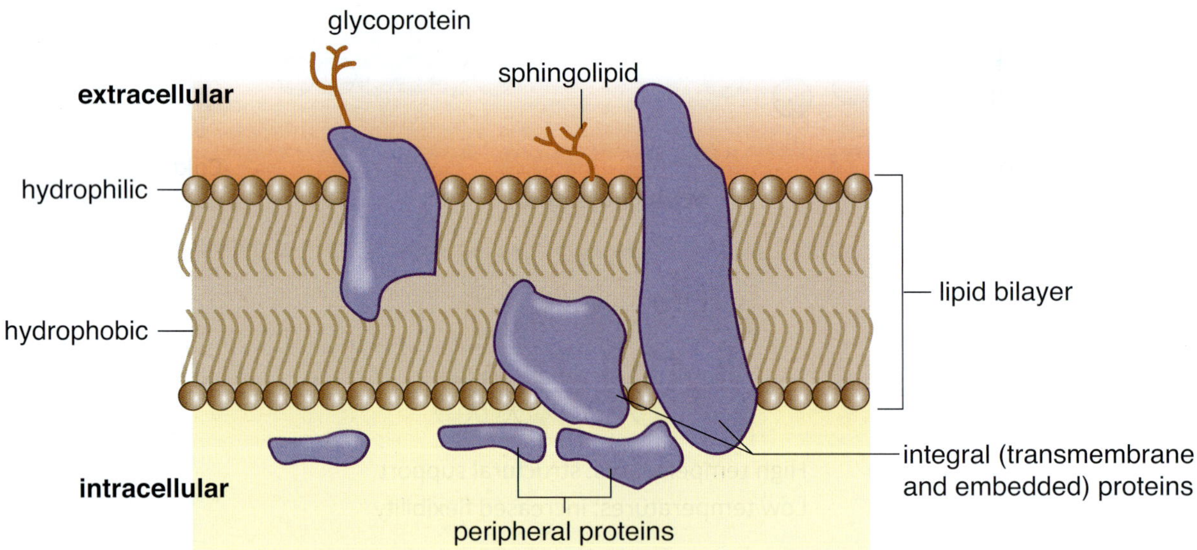

Figure 8.8 Plasma Membrane Proteins

Carbohydrates

Carbohydrates are generally attached to protein molecules on the extracellular surface of cells. Because carbohydrates are generally hydrophilic, interactions between glycoproteins and water can form a coat around the cell, as shown in Figure 8.9. In addition, carbohydrates can act as signaling and recognition molecules. For example, blood group (ABO) antigens on red blood cells are sphingolipids that differ only in their carbohydrate sequence. Our immune systems and some pathogens take advantage of these membrane carbohydrates and membrane proteins to target particular cells.

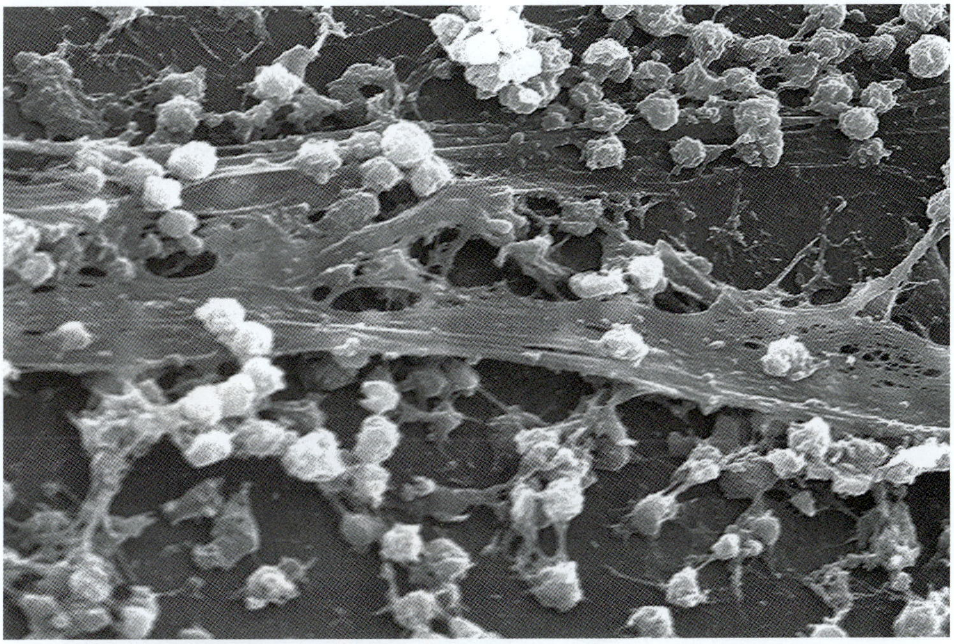

Figure 8.9 Extracellular Membrane-Associated Carbohydrates
Staphylococcus aureus bacteria embedded in bands of extracellular polysaccharides and glycolipids, forming a biofilm.

Membrane Receptors

Some of the transporters for facilitated diffusion and active transport can be activated or deactivated by **membrane receptors**, which tend to be transmembrane proteins. For example, ligand-gated ion channels are membrane receptors that open a channel in response to the binding of a specific ligand. Other membrane receptors participate in biosignaling; for example, G protein-coupled receptors are involved in several different signal transduction cascades. Membrane receptors are generally proteins, although there are some carbohydrate and lipid receptors, especially in viruses.

BRIDGE

Biosignaling is a major function of the cell membrane. Receptors and signal cascades are covered in more detail in Chapter 3 of *MCAT Biochemistry Review.*

Cell–Cell Junctions

Cells within tissues can form a cohesive layer via intercellular junctions. These junctions provide direct pathways of communication between neighboring cells or between cells and the extracellular matrix. Cell–cell junctions are generally comprised of **cell adhesion molecules** (**CAM**), which are proteins that allow cells to recognize each other and contribute to proper cell differentiation and development.

Gap Junctions

Gap junctions allow for direct cell–cell communication and are often found in small bunches together. Gap junctions are also called **connexons** and are formed by the alignment and interaction of pores composed of six molecules of **connexin**, as shown in Figure 8.10. They permit movement of water and some solutes directly between cells. Proteins are generally not transferred through gap junctions.

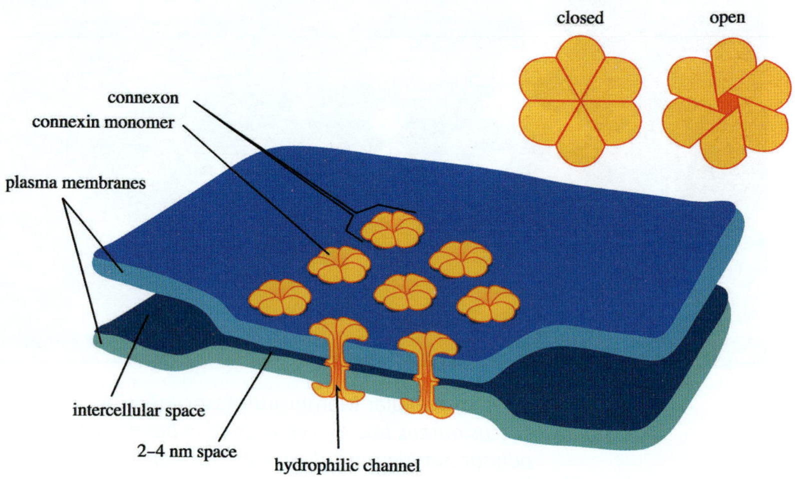

Figure 8.10 Gap Junction
A connexon (gap junction) is composed of six monomers of connexin and permits travel of solutes between cells.

MNEMONIC

Tight junctions form a water**tight** seal, preventing paracellular transport of water and solutes.

BRIDGE

Tight junctions are found in the lining of renal tubules, where they restrict passage of solutes and water without cellular control. Nephrons are discussed in Chapter 10 of *MCAT Biology Review.*

Tight Junctions

Tight junctions prevent solutes from leaking into the space between cells via a **paracellular** route, as shown in Figure 8.11. Tight junctions are found in epithelial cells and function as a physical link between the cells as they form a single layer of tissue. Tight junctions can limit permeability enough to create a transepithelial voltage difference based on differing concentrations of ions on either side of the epithelium. To be effective, tight junctions must form a continuous band around the cell; otherwise, fluid could leak through spaces between tight junctions.

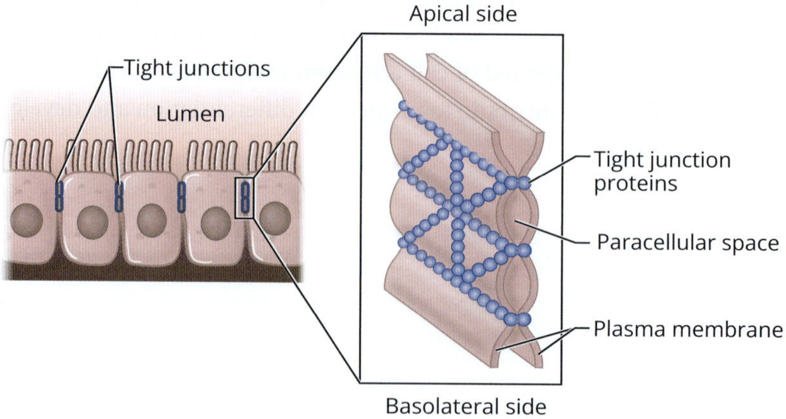

Figure 8.11 Tight Junction Barrier

Desmosomes

Desmosomes bind adjacent cells by anchoring to their cytoskeletons. Desmosomes are formed by interactions between transmembrane proteins associated with intermediate filaments inside adjacent cells, as shown in Figure 8.12. Desmosomes are primarily found at the interface between two layers of epithelial tissue. **Hemidesmosomes** have a similar function, but their main function is to attach epithelial cells to underlying structures, especially the basement membrane.

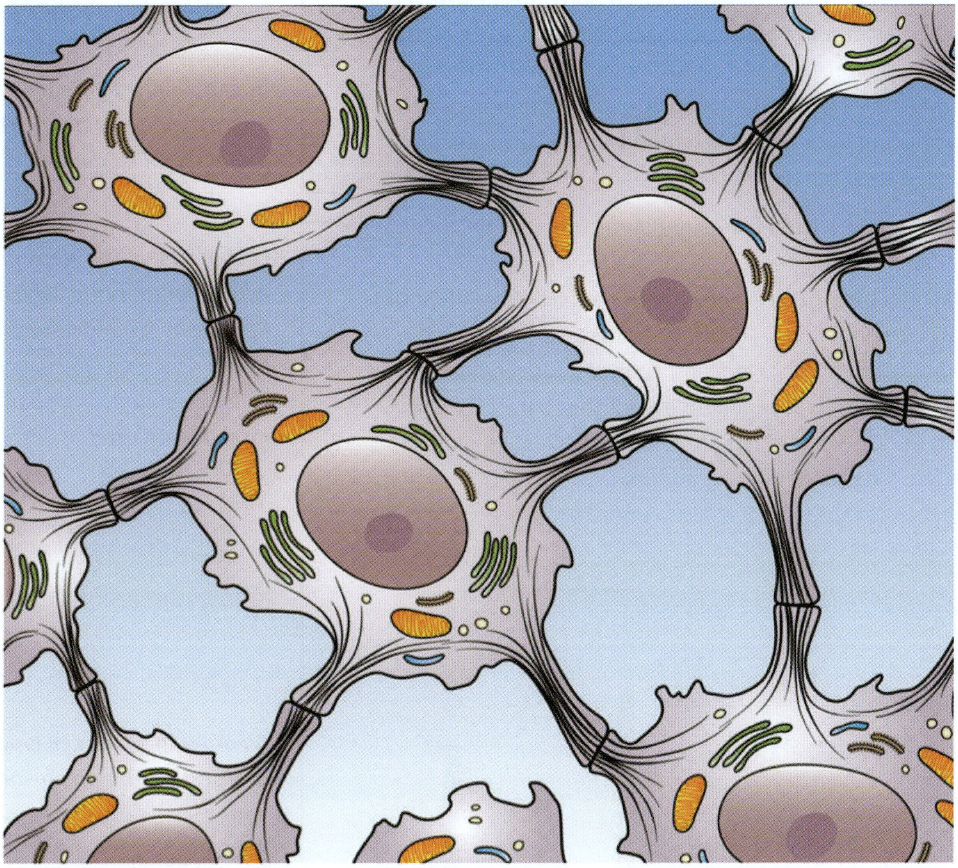

Figure 8.12 Desmosomes Between Adjacent Cells

BIOCHEMISTRY GUIDED EXAMPLE WITH EXPERT THINKING

Transplantation of pancreatic islets into patients who have Type 1 diabetes is hampered by inflammatory reactions at the transplantation site leading to dysfunction and death of insulin producing beta-cells. Recently, it was discovered that co-transplantation of neural crest stem cells (NCSCs) together with islet cells may improve transplantation outcomes. However, it could not be determined whether protection was obtained by the release of soluble factors, or whether direct cell–cell contact was required. Another investigation was conducted to describe the in vitro interaction between NCSCs and insulin-producing beta-TC6 cells that may mediate protection against cytokine-induced beta-cell death.

Problem statement: transplanting insulin producing cells causes inflammation, leading to failure of transplant

Possible solution: using NCSCs with transplant, but not sure how it works

Goal of study: figure out how NCSCs interact with pancreatic cells to protect against death

NCSCs were plated on laminin-coated plates or 0.4 micrometer cell inserts and after three days, beta-TC6 cells were added. The inserts allow for passage of soluble factors, but not direct cell-to-cell contact. After 48 hours, cytokines IL-1β and IFN-β were added. Finally, 48 hours later, cells were labeled with propidium iodide, trypsinized, and analyzed for cell death by flow cytometry. The experiment was repeated except that beta-TC6 cells were plated first, then NCSCs were added after 48 hours. Results plotted below are means for five independent experiments.
** denotes $p < 0.01$

Lots of sequential steps in the experimental setup, which may be important for understanding the figure. There's a specific order in which cells are plated, as well as whether inserts were used.

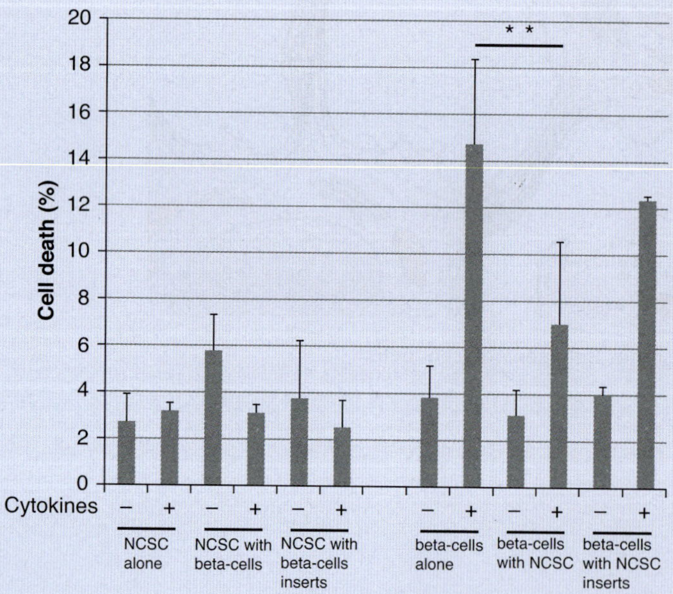

Figure 1

IV: order in which cell type plated, ECM or insert used, cytokine omitted or added

DV: cell death

Trend: significant difference between beta-cell alone and beta-cell with NCSC (no insert)

Adapted from Ngamjariyawat, A., Turpaev, K., Vasylovska, S., Kozlova, E. N., & Welsh, N. (2013). Co-culture of neural crest stem cells (NCSC) and insulin producing beta-TC6 cells results in cadherin junctions and protection against cytokine-induced beta-cell death. *PLoS One*, 8(4), e61828. doi:10.1371/journal.pone.0061828.

Based on this experiment, are NCSCs protecting beta islet cells from cytokine-induced cell death through direct contact, or through indirect contact?

Since the question requires data from the figure, we need to have a solid understanding of the results. The experimental question is asking whether beta-cells require direct contact with NCSCs, or whether the NCSCs are secreting soluble factors that are mediating protection from cytokine-mediated cell death. We'll need to refer to the passage for more information on these phenomena and how they interact. In the introduction to the experiment we can see that we are learning about co-transplantation of NCSCs and beta-cells, and that the experiments are trying to determine why co-transplantation is more effective than transplanting beta-cells alone. The way this was tested in the experimental setup is through the usage of cell inserts, which we are told in paragraph 2 will allow for the passage of factors, but not cell-cell contact.

The results on the left (first 6 bars) correspond to where NCSCs are plated first, then beta-cells are added with and without inserts. All 6 bars are roughly equal and the addition of cytokines do not seem to induce additional cell death, meaning these results cannot be used to make any conclusions since the expected control response (beta-cells inducing cell death in the presence of cytokines) is not shown. Taking a look at the next six columns in the graph, we can see that these are the experiments with the beta-cells being plated first. NCSCs were added 48 hours later, either with or without insert. The graph tells us that in the presence of cytokines, beta-cells alone show a high percentage of cell death (the expected control response), but having the NCSCs without insert shows a significant drop in cell death. This effect goes away when the insert is reintroduced: beta-cells with the NCSC insert have a higher level of cell death, though it's unclear whether that difference is significant.

Because the inserts obstruct cell-to-cell contact, we can conclude that direct contact between beta-cells and NCSCs is required for protection against cytokine-mediated cell death.

MCAT CONCEPT CHECK 8.2

Before you move on, assess your understanding of the material with these questions.

1. In the following phospholipid, determine whether the fatty acids are saturated or unsaturated and label their hydrophobic and hydrophilic regions.

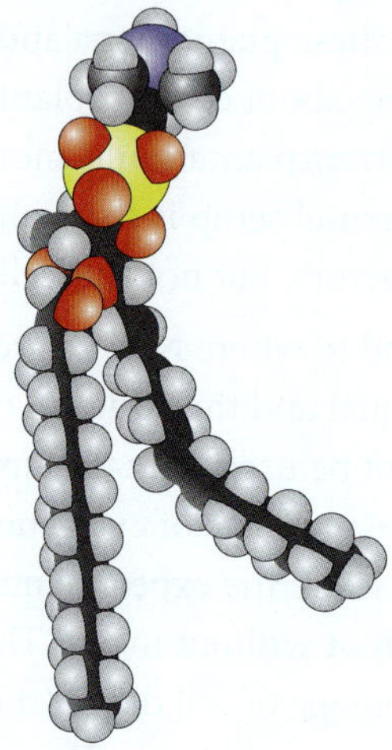

2. How does cholesterol play a role in the fluidity and stability of the plasma membrane?

___

3. What are the three classes of membrane proteins? How are they each most likely to function?

   1. ___
   2. ___
   3. ___

4. Contrast gap junctions and tight junctions.

   - Gap junctions:

   ___

   - Tight junctions:

   ___

8.3 Membrane Transport **High Yield**

LEARNING OBJECTIVES

After Chapter 8.3, you will be able to:

- Explain the driving factors behind passive transport mechanisms
- Contrast symport and antiport mechanisms for active transport
- Relate osmotic pressure to the direction of osmosis:

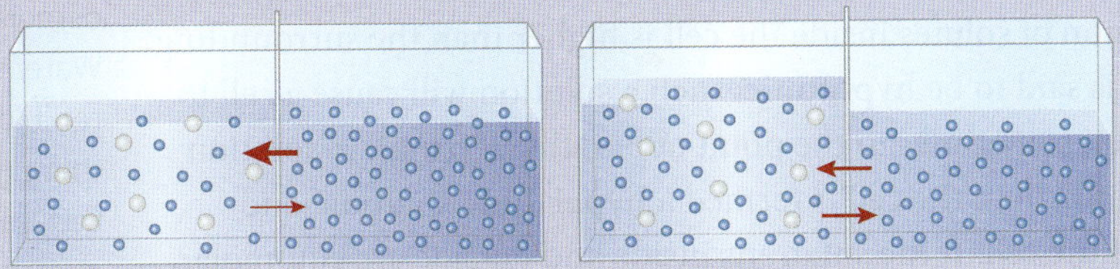

The cell membrane functions to control movement of substances into and out of the cell; however, it varies in its selectivity for different substances. Transport of small nonpolar molecules occurs rapidly through the cell membrane via diffusion, while ions and larger molecules require more specialized transport processes. The different membrane traffic processes are classified as either active or passive, and are driven by concentration gradients or intracellular energy stores.

Concentration Gradients

Transport processes can be classified as active or passive depending on their thermodynamics. Spontaneous processes that do not require energy (negative ΔG) proceed through **passive transport**, while those that are nonspontaneous and require energy (positive ΔG) proceed through **active transport**. Diffusion, facilitated diffusion, and osmosis generally increase in rate as temperature increases, while active transport may or may not be affected by temperature, depending on the enthalpy (ΔH) of the process. The primary thermodynamic motivator in most passive transport is an increase in entropy (ΔS).

MCAT EXPERTISE

An important point to keep in mind is that all transmembrane movement is based on concentration gradients, which are an MCAT favorite; understanding concentration gradients will net you points on Test Day. Remember that the gradient will tell us whether this process will be passive or active.

Passive Transport

Passive transport processes are those that do not require intracellular energy stores but rather utilize the concentration gradient to supply the energy for particles to move.

Simple Diffusion

The most basic of all membrane traffic processes is **simple diffusion**, in which substrates move down their concentration gradient directly across the membrane. Only particles that are freely permeable to the membrane are able to undergo simple diffusion. There is potential energy in a chemical gradient; some of this energy is dissipated as the gradient is utilized during simple diffusion. We can liken this process to a ball rolling down a hill: there is potential energy in the ball when it sits at the top of the hill, and as the ball spontaneously rolls down the hill, some of the energy is dissipated.

Osmosis

Osmosis is a specific kind of simple diffusion that concerns water; water will move from a region of lower solute concentration to one of higher solute concentration. That is, it will move from a region of higher water concentration (more dilute solution) down its gradient to a region of lower water concentration (more concentrated solution). Osmosis is important in several places, most notably when the solute itself is impermeable to the membrane. In such a case, water will move to try to bring solute concentrations to equimolarity, as shown in Figure 8.13. If the concentration of solutes inside the cell is higher than the surrounding solution, the solution is said to be **hypotonic**; such a solution will cause a cell to swell as water rushes in, sometimes to the point of bursting (lysing). A solution that is more concentrated than the cell is termed a **hypertonic** solution, and water will move out of the cell. If the solutions inside and outside are equimolar, they are said to be **isotonic**. A key point here is that isotonicity does not prevent movement; rather, it prevents the *net* movement of particles. Water molecules will continue to move; however, the cell will neither gain nor lose water overall.

REAL WORLD

Osmolarity explains why pure water should never be given intravenously for resuscitation. Red blood cells have an osmolarity around 300 $\frac{\text{mOsm}}{\text{L}}$, while pure water has an osmolarity of 0 $\frac{\text{mOsm}}{\text{L}}$. Water would rush into the red blood cells, causing them to burst. To avoid this, saline or dextrose-containing solutions are used.

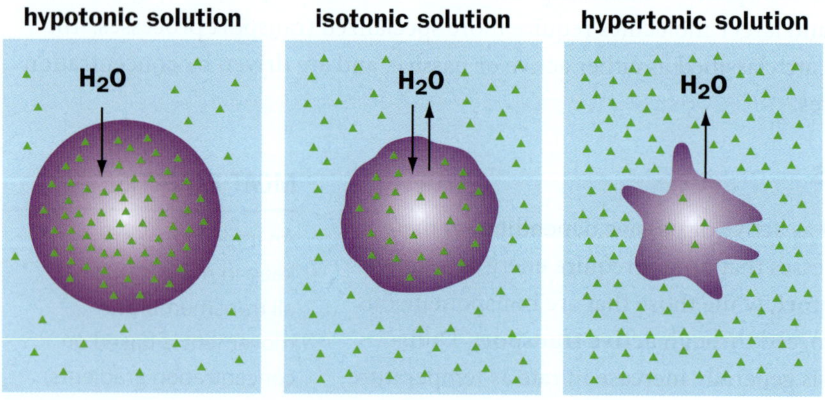

Figure 8.13 Osmosis
Water moves from areas of low solute (high water) concentration to high solute (low water) concentration.

MNEMONIC

To remember that water flows into a cell placed in hyp**O**tonic solution, imagine the cell swelling to form a giant letter **O.**

One method of quantifying the driving force behind osmosis is osmotic pressure. **Osmotic pressure** is a **colligative property**: a physical property of solutions that is dependent on the concentration of dissolved particles but not on the chemical identity of those dissolved particles. Other examples of colligative properties include vapor pressure depression (Raoult's Law), boiling point elevation, and freezing point depression.

To illustrate osmotic pressure, consider a container separated into two compartments by a semipermeable membrane, just like the membranes in our cells. One compartment contains pure water, while the other contains water with dissolved solutes. The membrane allows water but not solutes to pass through. Because substances tend to flow, or diffuse, from higher to lower concentration (which results in an increase in entropy), water will diffuse from the compartment containing pure water into the compartment containing the water–solute mixture. This net flow will cause the water level in the compartment containing the solution to rise above the level in the compartment containing pure water, as shown in Figure 8.14.

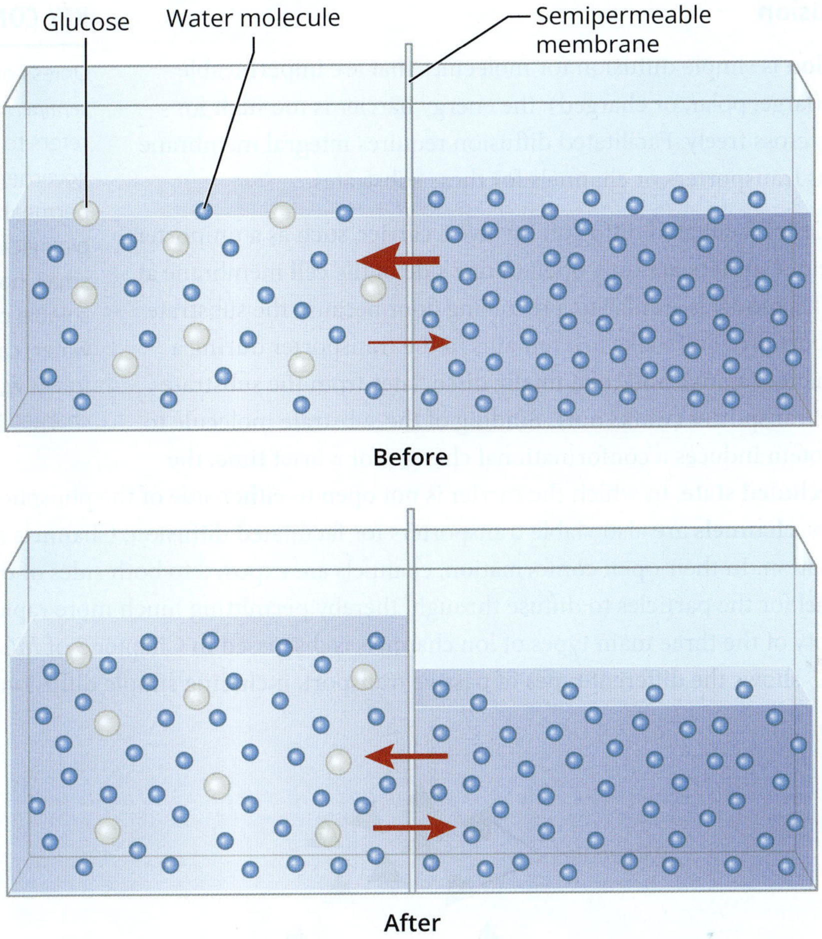

Figure 8.14 Change in Water Level Due to Osmotic Pressure

Because the solute cannot pass through the membrane, the concentrations of solute in the two compartments can never be equal. However, the hydrostatic pressure exerted by the water level in the solute-containing compartment will eventually oppose the influx of water; thus, the water level will only rise to the point at which it exerts a sufficient pressure to counterbalance the tendency of water to flow across the membrane. This pressure, defined as the **osmotic pressure** (Π) of the solution, is given by the formula:

$$\Pi = iMRT$$

Equation 8.1

where M is the molarity of the solution, R is the ideal gas constant, T is the absolute temperature (in kelvins), i is the **van't Hoff factor**, which is simply the number of particles obtained from the molecule when in solution. For example, glucose remains one intact molecule, so $i_{\text{glucose}} = 1$; sodium chloride becomes two ions (Na^+ and Cl^-), so $i_{\text{NaCl}} = 2$. The equation clearly shows that osmotic pressure is directly proportional to the molarity of the solution. Thus, osmotic pressure, like all colligative properties, depends only on the presence and number of particles in solution, but not their actual identity.

In cells, the osmotic pressure is maintained against the cell membrane, rather than the force of gravity. If the osmotic pressure created by the solutes within a cell exceeds the pressure that the cell membrane can withstand, the cell will lyse. Generally, osmotic pressure is best thought of as a "sucking" pressure, drawing water into the cell in proportion to the concentration of the solution.

Facilitated Diffusion

Facilitated diffusion is simple diffusion for molecules that are impermeable to the membrane (large, polar, or charged); the energy barrier is too high for these molecules to cross freely. Facilitated diffusion requires integral membrane proteins to serve as transporters or channels for these substrates.

The classic examples of facilitated diffusion involve a carrier, such as a uniporter, or a channel protein. **Carriers** are only open to one side of the cell membrane at any given point. This model is similar to a revolving door because the substrate binds to the transport protein (walks in), remains in the transporter during a conformational change (spins), and then finally dissociates from the substrate-binding site of the transporter (walks out). Binding of the substrate molecule to the transporter protein induces a conformational change; for a brief time, the carrier is in the **occluded state**, in which the carrier is not open to either side of the phospholipid bilayer. In addition to carriers, **channels** are also viable transporters for facilitated diffusion. Channels may be in an open or closed conformation. In their open conformation, channels are exposed to both sides of the cell membrane and act like a tunnel for the particles to diffuse through, thereby permitting much more rapid transport kinetics. The activity of the three main types of ion channels is discussed in Chapter 3 of *MCAT Biochemistry Review*. Figure 8.15 shows the different types of passive transport, including simple diffusion and facilitated diffusion.

KEY CONCEPT

Unless otherwise specified, *semipermeable membrane* refers to a membrane governed by the same permeability rules as biological membranes: small, nonpolar, lipid-soluble particles (and water) can pass through freely, while large, polar, or charged particles cannot.

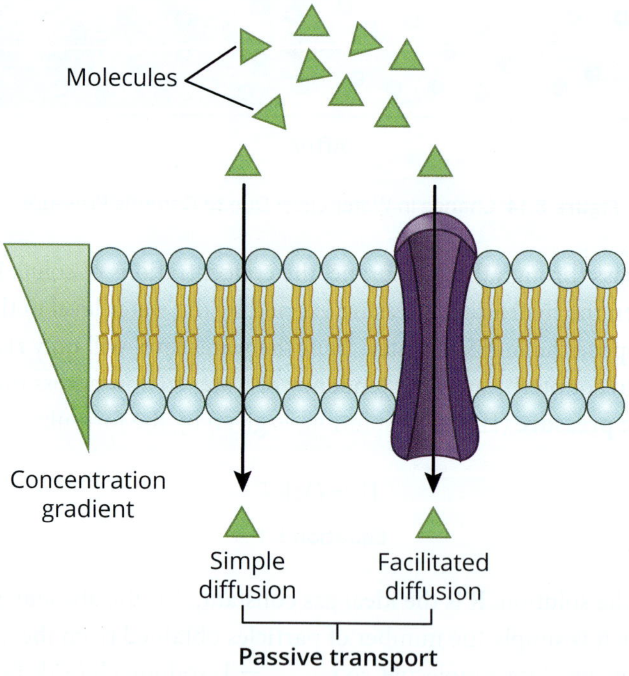

Figure 8.15 Passive Transport Processes
The passive movement of solutes across the cell membrane is mediated by concentration gradients.

Active Transport

Active transport results in the net movement of a solute against its concentration gradient, just like rolling a ball uphill. Active transport always requires energy, but the source of this energy can vary. **Primary active transport** uses ATP or another energy molecule to directly power the transport of molecules across a membrane. Generally, primary active transport involves the use of a *transmembrane ATPase*. **Secondary active transport**, also known as **coupled transport**, also uses energy to transport particles across the membrane; however, in contrast to primary active transport, there is no direct coupling to ATP hydrolysis. Instead, secondary active transport harnesses the energy released by one particle going *down* its electrochemical gradient to drive a different particle *up* its gradient. When both particles flow the same direction across the membrane, it is termed **symport**. When the particles flow in opposite directions, it is called **antiport**. Active transport is important in many tissues. For instance, primary active transport maintains the membrane potential of neurons in the nervous system. The kidneys use secondary active transport, usually driven by sodium, to reabsorb and secrete various solutes into and out of the filtrate. Figure 8.16 shows active transport, while Table 8.1 summarizes how molecules move across membranes.

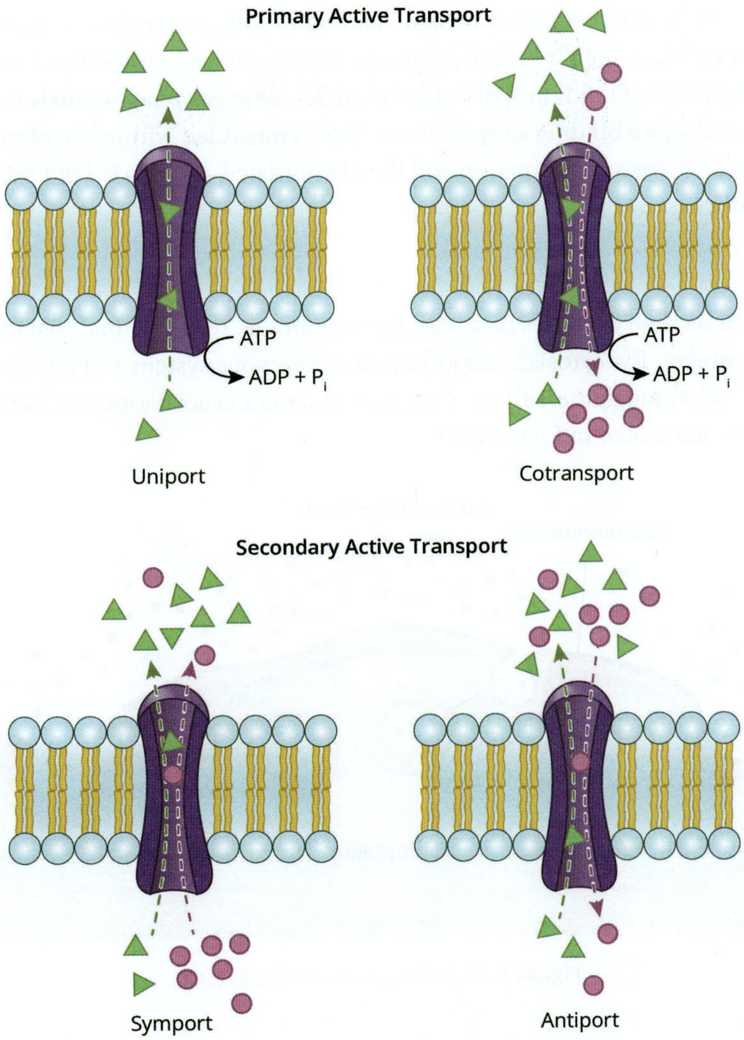

Figure 8.16 Active Transport Processes
The movement of solutes against a gradient requires an input of energy.

	Simple Diffusion	Osmosis	Facilitated Diffusion	Active Transport
Concentration gradient of solute	High → Low	Low → High	High → Low	Low → High
Membrane protein required	No	No	Yes	Yes
Energy required	No—this is a passive process	No—this is a passive process	No—this is a passive process	Yes—this is an active process; requires energy
Example molecule(s) transported	Small, nonpolar (O_2, CO_2)	H_2O	Polar molecules (glucose) or ions (Na^+, Cl^-)	Polar molecules or ions (Na^+, Cl^-, K^+)

Table 8.1 Membrane Transport Processes

Endocytosis and Exocytosis

Endocytosis

Endocytosis occurs when the cell membrane invaginates and engulfs material to bring it into the cell. The material is encased in a vesicle, which is important because cells will sometimes ingest toxic substances. **Pinocytosis** is the endocytosis of fluids and dissolved particles, whereas **phagocytosis** is the ingestion of large solids such as bacteria. Substrate binding to specific receptors embedded within the plasma membrane will initiate the process of endocytosis. Invagination will then be initiated and carried out by **vesicle-coating proteins**, most notably clathrin.

Exocytosis

Exocytosis occurs when secretory vesicles fuse with the membrane, releasing material from inside the cell to the extracellular environment. Exocytosis is important in the nervous system and intercellular signaling. For instance, exocytosis of neurotransmitters from synaptic vesicles is a crucial aspect of neuron physiology. Both endo- and exocytosis are illustrated in Figure 8.17.

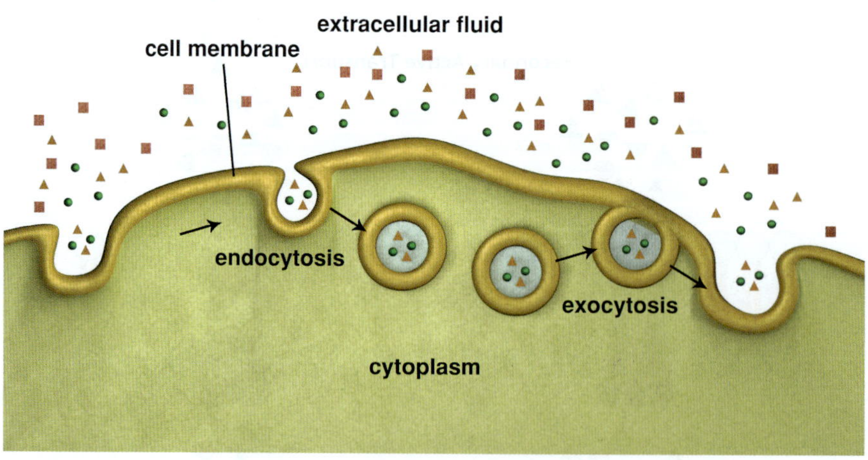

Figure 8.17 Endocytosis and Exocytosis

MCAT CONCEPT CHECK 8.3

Before you move on, assess your understanding of the material with these questions.

1. What is the primary thermodynamic factor responsible for passive transport?

___

2. What is the relationship between osmotic pressure and the direction of osmosis through a semipermeable membrane?

___

3. Compare the two types of active transport. What is the difference between symport and antiport?

___

8.4 Specialized Membranes

LEARNING OBJECTIVES

After Chapter 8.4, you will be able to:

- Identify the channels involved in maintenance of the resting membrane potential
- Calculate resting membrane potential using the Nernst equation
- Distinguish between the different regions of the mitochondrion

The membranes of most organelles are similar to the cell membrane in both composition and general characteristics; however, it is important to note that some membranes are specialized to accomplish specific functions. For instance, the sarcolemma of muscle cells must maintain a membrane potential for muscle contraction to occur. Membrane composition may also be altered slightly, especially in the case of mitochondria.

Membrane Potential

The impermeability of the cell membrane to ions and the selectivity of ion channels both lead to an electrochemical gradient between the exterior and interior of cells. The difference in electrical potential across cell membranes is called the **membrane potential**, V_m. The resting potential for most cells is between -40 and -80 mV, although the potential can rise as high as $+35$ mV during depolarization of the cell. Maintaining membrane potential requires energy because ions may passively diffuse through the cell membrane over time using **leak channels**; therefore, an ion transporter or pump such as the **sodium–potassium pump** (**Na^+/K^+ ATPase**) regulates the concentration of intracellular and extracellular sodium and potassium ions. Chloride ions also participate in establishing membrane potential. The **Nernst equation** can be used to determine the membrane potential from the intra- and extracellular concentrations of the various ions:

$$E = \frac{RT}{zF} \ln \frac{[\text{ion}]_{\text{outside}}}{[\text{ion}]_{\text{inside}}} = \frac{61.5}{z} \log \frac{[\text{ion}]_{\text{outside}}}{[\text{ion}]_{\text{inside}}}$$

Equation 8.2

where R is the ideal gas constant, T is the temperature in kelvins, z is the charge of the ion, and F is the Faraday constant $\left(96{,}485\ \frac{\text{C}}{\text{mol}\ e^-}\right)$. The simplification to 61.5 in the numerator assumes body temperature, 310 K. The **Goldman–Hodgkin–Katz voltage equation** flows from the Nernst equation, taking into account the relative contribution of each major ion to the membrane potential:

$$V_\text{m} = 61.5 \log \left[\frac{P_{\text{Na}^+} \times [\text{Na}^+]_\text{outside} + P_{\text{K}^+} \times [\text{K}^+]_\text{outside} + P_{\text{Cl}^-} \times [\text{Cl}^-]_\text{inside}}{P_{\text{Na}^+} \times [\text{Na}^+]_\text{inside} + P_{\text{K}^+} \times [\text{K}^+]_\text{inside} + P_{\text{Cl}^-} \times [\text{Cl}^-]_\text{outside}}\right]$$

Equation 8.3

where P represents the permeability for the relevant ion. Note that chloride is inverted relative to the other ions because it carries a negative charge.

BRIDGE

The cell membrane is often compared to a capacitor because opposite charges are maintained on either side of the membrane. Capacitance is discussed in Chapter 6 of *MCAT Physics and Math Review.*

Sodium–Potassium Pump

There is a steady-state resting relationship between ion diffusion and the **Na^+/K^+ ATPase**. One of the main functions of the Na^+/K^+ ATPase is to maintain a low concentration of sodium ions and high concentration of potassium ions intracellularly by pumping three sodium ions out for every two potassium ions pumped in. This movement of ions removes one positive charge from the intracellular space of the cell, which maintains the negative resting potential of the cell. As mentioned before, the cell membrane also contains leak channels that allow ions, such as Na^+ and K^+, to passively diffuse into or out of the cell down their concentration gradients. Cell membranes are more permeable to K^+ ions than Na^+ ions at rest because there are more K^+ leak channels than Na^+ leak channels. The combination of Na^+/K^+ ATPase activity and leak channels together maintain a stable resting membrane potential.

Mitochondrial Membranes

Mitochondria are referred to as the "powerhouse" of the cell because of their ability to produce ATP by oxidative respiration. Mitochondria contain two membranes: the inner and outer mitochondrial membranes.

Outer Mitochondrial Membrane

The **outer mitochondrial membrane** is highly permeable due to many large pores that allow the passage of ions and small proteins. The outer membrane completely surrounds the inner mitochondrial membrane, with the presence of a small **intermembrane space** in between the two layers.

Inner Mitochondrial Membrane

The **inner mitochondrial membrane** has a much more restricted permeability compared to the outer mitochondrial membrane. Structurally, the inner mitochondrial membrane contains numerous infoldings, known as **cristae**, which increase the available surface area for the integral proteins associated with the membrane. These proteins, discussed in Chapter 10 of *MCAT Biochemistry Review*, are involved in the electron transport chain and ATP synthesis. The inner membrane also encloses the **mitochondrial matrix**, where the citric acid cycle produces high-energy electron carriers used in the electron transport chain. The inner mitochondrial membrane contains a very high level of *cardiolipin* and does not contain cholesterol.

MCAT CONCEPT CHECK 8.4

Before you move on, assess your understanding of the material with these questions.

1. How is the resting membrane potential maintained?

____

____

____

2. Given the following data, calculate the resting membrane potential of this cell:

Ion	Permeability (Relative)	Intracellular Concentration	Extracellular Concentration
Na^+	0.05	14 mM	140 mM
K^+	1	120 mM	4 mM
Cl^-	0	12 mM	120 mM

____

____

____

3. What distinguishes the inner mitochondrial membrane from other biological membranes? What is the pH gradient between the cytoplasm and the intermembrane space?

____

____

____

Conclusion

Understanding biological membranes becomes increasingly important as you progress in your medical career. At this point, you should have a strong foundation of knowledge about the fluid mosaic model and how membranes exist dynamically. We've also covered the components of cell membranes, with a special emphasis on lipids and the phospholipid bilayer. We reviewed some basic physical properties of the cell, including cell–cell junctions. We also examined membrane transport, such as passive transport (simple diffusion, facilitated diffusion, and osmosis) and active transport, before briefly touching upon endocytosis and exocytosis. Finally, we reviewed specialized membranes within cells. Up to now, you have been exposed to each of the classes of molecules and some of their applications both experimentally and within the cell. This comprehensive review should provide you with a better understanding of what will be expected of you on Test Day and briefly introduce you to topics that you will learn more about in medical school.

The first seven chapters of *MCAT Biochemistry Review* focused on various types of biomolecules, their structures, and their functions. In this chapter, we applied this knowledge of biomolecules to make sense of biological membranes. In the remaining four chapters, we'll turn our attention to the metabolic pathways by which the body builds, stores, and burns these biomolecules.

GO ONLINE

You've reviewed the content, now test your knowledge and critical thinking skills by completing a test-like passage set in your online resources!

CONCEPT SUMMARY

Fluid Mosaic Model

- The **fluid mosaic model** accounts for the presence of lipids, proteins, and carbohydrates in a dynamic, semisolid plasma membrane that surrounds cells.
- The plasma membrane contains proteins embedded within the **phospholipid bilayer**.
- The membrane is not static.
    - Lipids move freely in the plane of the membrane and can assemble into **lipid rafts**.
    - **Flippases** are specific membrane proteins that maintain the bidirectional transport of lipids between the layers of the phospholipid bilayer in cells.
    - Proteins and carbohydrates may also move within the membrane, but are slowed by their relatively large size.

Membrane Components

- Lipids are the primary membrane component, both by mass and mole fraction.
    - **Triacylglycerols** and **free fatty acids** act as phospholipid precursors and are found in low levels in the membrane.
    - **Glycerophospholipids** replace one fatty acid with a phosphate group, which is often linked to other hydrophilic groups.
    - **Cholesterol** is present in large amounts and contributes to membrane fluidity and stability.
    - **Waxes** are present in very small amounts, if at all; they are most prevalent in plants and function in waterproofing and defense.
- Proteins located within the cell membrane act as transporters, cell adhesion molecules, and enzymes.
    - **Transmembrane proteins** can have one or more hydrophobic domains and are most likely to function as receptors or channels.
    - **Embedded proteins** are most likely part of a catalytic complex or involved in cellular communication.
    - **Membrane-associated proteins** may act as recognition molecules or enzymes.
- Carbohydrates can form a protective **glycoprotein coat** and also function in cell recognition.
- Extracellular ligands can bind to membrane receptors, which function as channels or enzymes in second messenger pathways.
- Cell–cell junctions regulate transport intracellularly and intercellularly.
    - **Gap junctions** allow for the rapid exchange of ions and other small molecules between adjacent cells.
    - **Tight junctions** prevent **paracellular** transport, but do not provide intercellular transport.
    - **Desmosomes** and **hemidesmosomes** anchor layers of epithelial tissue together.

Membrane Transport

- **Concentration gradients** help to determine appropriate membrane transport mechanisms in cells.
- **Osmotic pressure**, a **colligative property**, is the pressure applied to a pure solvent to prevent osmosis and is used to express the concentration of the solution.
  - It is often better conceptualized as a "sucking" pressure in which a solution is drawing water in, proportional to its concentration.
- **Passive transport** does not require energy because the molecule is moving down its concentration gradient or from an area with higher concentration to an area with lower concentration.
  - **Simple diffusion** does not require a transporter. Small, nonpolar molecules passively move from an area of high concentration to an area of low concentration until equilibrium is achieved.
  - **Osmosis** describes the diffusion of water across a selectively permeable membrane.
  - **Facilitated diffusion** uses transport proteins to move impermeable solutes across the cell membrane.
- **Active transport** requires energy in the form of ATP or an existing favorable ion gradient.
  - Active transport may be **primary** or **secondary** depending on the energy source. Secondary active transport can be further classified as **symport** or **antiport**.
- **Endocytosis** and **exocytosis** are methods of engulfing material into cells or releasing material to the exterior of cells, both via the cell membrane. **Pinocytosis** is the ingestion of liquid into the cell in vesicles formed from the cell membrane and **phagocytosis** is the ingestion of larger, solid molecules.

Specialized Membranes

- The composition of cell membranes is fairly consistent; however, there are some cells that contain specialized membranes.
- **Membrane potential** is maintained by the sodium–potassium pump and leak channels.
  - The electrical potential created by one ion can be calculated using the **Nernst equation**.
  - The resting potential of a membrane at physiological temperature can be calculated using the **Goldman–Hodgkin–Katz voltage equation**, which is derived from the Nernst equation.
- The mitochondrial membrane differs from the cell membrane:
  - The outer mitochondrial membrane is highly permeable to metabolic molecules and small proteins.
  - The inner mitochondrial membrane surrounds the mitochondrial matrix, where the citric acid cycle produces electrons used in the electron transport chain and where many other enzymes important in cellular respiration are located. The inner mitochondrial membrane also does not contain cholesterol.

ANSWERS TO CONCEPT CHECKS

8.1

1. Flippases are responsible for the movement of phospholipids between the layers of the plasma membrane because it is otherwise energetically unfavorable. Lipid rafts are aggregates of specific lipids in the membrane that function as attachment points for other biomolecules and play roles in signaling.
2. Lipids, including phospholipids, cholesterol, and others, are most plentiful; proteins, including transmembrane proteins (channels and receptors), membrane-associated proteins, and embedded proteins, are next most plentiful; carbohydrates, including the glycoprotein coat and signaling molecules, are next; nucleic acids are essentially absent.

8.2

1. The hydrophilic region is at the top of this diagram. While you need not be able to recognize it, the head group is phosphatidylcholine in this example. The hydrophobic region is at the bottom and is composed of two fatty acid tails. The tail on the left is saturated; the tail on the right is unsaturated, as evidenced by the kink in its chain.
2. Cholesterol moderates membrane fluidity by interfering with the crystal structure of the cell membrane and occupying space between phospholipid molecules at low temperatures, and by restricting excessive movement of phospholipids at high temperatures. Cholesterol also provides stability by cross-linking adjacent phospholipids through interactions at the polar head group and hydrophobic interactions at the nearby fatty acid tail.
3. Transmembrane proteins are most likely to serve as channels or receptors. Embedded membrane proteins are most likely to have catalytic activity linked to nearby enzymes. Membrane-associated (peripheral) proteins are most likely to be involved in signaling or are recognition molecules on the extracellular surface.
4. Gap junctions allow for the intercellular transport of materials and do not prevent paracellular transport of materials. Tight junctions are not used for intercellular transport but do prevent paracellular transport. Gap junctions are in discontinuous bunches around the cell, while tight junctions form bands around the cell.

8.3

1. The primary thermodynamic factor responsible for passive transport is entropy.
2. As osmotic pressure increases, more water will tend to flow into the compartment to decrease solute concentration. Osmotic pressure is often considered a "sucking" pressure because water will move toward the compartment with the highest osmotic pressure.
3. Primary active transport uses ATP as an energy source for the movement of molecules against their concentration gradient, while secondary active transport uses an electrochemical gradient to power the transport. Symport moves both particles in secondary active transport across the membrane in the same direction, while antiport moves particles across the cell membrane in opposite directions.

8.4

1. The membrane potential, which results from a difference in the number of positive and negative charges on either side of the membrane, is maintained primarily by the sodium–potassium pump, which moves three sodium ions out of the cell for every two potassium ions pumped in, and to a minor extent by leak channels that allow the passive transport of ions.

2. $$V_m = 61.5 \log \left[\frac{P_{Na^+} \times [Na^+]_{outside} + P_{K^+} \times [K^+]_{outside} + P_{Cl^-} \times [Cl^-]_{inside}}{P_{Na^+} \times [Na^+]_{inside} + P_{K^+} \times [K^+]_{inside} + P_{Cl^-} \times [Cl^-]_{outside}}\right]$$

$$= 61.5 \log \left[\frac{0.05 \times [140] + 1 \times [4] + 0 \times [12]}{0.05 \times [14] + 1 \times [120] + 0 \times [120]}\right] = 61.5 \log \left[\frac{7+4}{0.7+120}\right]$$

$$= 61.5 \log \left[\frac{11}{120.7}\right] \approx 60 \log \frac{1}{10} = -60 \text{ mV}$$

The exact value is -64.0 mV

3. The inner mitochondrial membrane lacks cholesterol, which differentiates it from most other biological membranes. There is no pH gradient between the cytoplasm and the intermembrane space because the outer mitochondrial membrane has such high permeability to biomolecules (the proton-motive force of the mitochondria is across the inner mitochondrial membrane, not the outer mitochondrial membrane).

SCIENCE MASTERY ASSESSMENT EXPLANATIONS

1. **C**

We are asked to identify the type of transport that would allow a large, polar molecule to cross the membrane without any energy expenditure. This scenario describes facilitated diffusion, which uses a transport protein (or channel) to facilitate the movement of large, polar molecules across the nonpolar, hydrophobic membrane. Facilitated diffusion, like simple diffusion, does not require energy.

2. **C**

This question requires an understanding of osmosis and the action of the sodium–potassium pump. When a cell is placed in a hypertonic solution (a solution having a higher solute concentration than the cell), fluid will diffuse out of the cell and result in cell shrinkage. When a cell is placed in hypotonic solution (a solution having a lower solute concentration than the cell), fluid will diffuse from the solution into the cell, causing the cell to expand and possibly lyse. The sodium–potassium pump moves three sodium ions out of the cell for every two potassium ions it lets into the cell. Therefore, inhibition of the sodium–potassium pump by ouabain will cause a net increase in the sodium concentration inside the cell and water will diffuse in, causing the cell to swell and then lyse.

3. **D**

The polarization of the membrane at rest is the result of an uneven distribution of ions between the inside and outside of the cell. This difference is achieved through active pumping of ions (predominantly sodium and potassium) into and out of the cell and the selective permeability of the membrane, which allows only certain ions to cross.

4. **B**

Ribosomes are the site of protein synthesis within a cell and are not coupled to the cell membrane. The cell membrane functions as a site for cytoskeletal attachment, **(A)**, through proteins and lipid rafts. Transport regulation, **(C)**, is accomplished through channels, transporters, and selective permeability, while the phospholipids act as a reagent for second messenger formation, **(D)**.

5. **A**

Movement of individual molecules in the cell membrane will be affected by size and polarity, just as with diffusion. Lipids are much smaller than proteins in the plasma membrane and will move more quickly. Lipids will move fastest within the plane of the cell membrane because the polar head group does not need to pass through the hydrophobic tail region in the same way that it would if it were moving between the membrane layers.

6. **B**

Compounds that contribute to membrane fluidity will lower the melting point or disrupt the crystal structure. Cholesterol, **(C)**, and unsaturated lipids, **(A)** and **(D)**, are known for these functions. *trans* glycerophospholipids tend to increase the melting point of the membrane and therefore decrease membrane fluidity.

7. **D**

Membrane receptors must have both an extracellular and intracellular domain; therefore, they are considered transmembrane proteins. In order to initiate a second messenger cascade, they typically display enzymatic activity, although some may act strictly as channels.

8. **C**

Plasmodesmata are cell–cell junctions that are found in plants, not animals. Gap junctions, tight junctions, desmosomes, and hemidesmosomes are all found in animals, particularly in epithelia.

9. **A**

The movement of any molecule is dependent on multiple factors, including electric potential, membrane solubility, and concentration gradient. While the electric potential takes into account multiple molecules, the movement of any one solute or water by diffusion or osmosis is dependent only on the concentration gradient of that molecule.

10. **B**

The endocytosis (bulk uptake through vesicle formation) of fluid is known as pinocytosis. Phagocytosis, **(A)**, is the endocytic intake of solids, while exocytosis, **(C)**, is a method of releasing vesicular contents. Drinking, **(D)**, does not apply on a cellular level.

11. **C**

Cell membranes are most likely to have a resting membrane potential that is nonzero because the resting membrane potential creates a state that is capable of responding to stimuli. Signaling molecules and channels would not be as useful with a membrane potential of zero. The values given in the answer choices correspond to different stages of the action potential, but the key information is that a resting potential of 0 mV does not maintain gradients for later activity.

12. **B**

The outer mitochondrial membrane is very permeable while the inner membrane is highly impermeable. The inner mitochondrial membrane is unique within the cell because it lacks cholesterol.

13. **D**

The Nernst equation relates the intra- and extracellular concentrations of an ion to the potential created by that gradient. At physiological temperature, it can be simplified to $E = \frac{61.5}{z} \log \frac{[\text{ion}]_{\text{outside}}}{[\text{ion}]_{\text{inside}}}$. For calcium, $z = +2$ (Ca^{2+}) and the ratio of $[\text{ion}_{\text{outside}}]$ to $[\text{ion}_{\text{inside}}] = 10^4$. Plugging in, we get:

$$E = \frac{61.5}{+2} \log 10^4 = \frac{61.5}{+2} \times 4 = 123 \text{ mV}$$

14. **A**

The fluid mosaic model accounts for a dynamic membrane. In this model, membrane components contain both fatty and carbohydrate-derived components, eliminating **(B)**. Further, the membrane is stabilized by the hydrophobic interactions of both fatty acid tails and membrane proteins, which may be found on the cytosolic or extracellular side of the membrane, or may run directly through the membrane; thus, **(C)** and **(D)** are also eliminated.

15. **D**

Gangliosides, along with ceramide, sphingomyelin, and cerebrosides, are sphingolipids.

GO ONLINE

Consult your online resources for additional practice.

EQUATIONS TO REMEMBER

(8.1) **Osmotic pressure:** $\Pi = iMRT$

(8.2) **Nernst equation:** $E = \frac{RT}{zF}\ln\frac{[\text{ion}]_{\text{outside}}}{[\text{ion}]_{\text{inside}}} = \frac{61.5}{z}\log\frac{[\text{ion}]_{\text{outside}}}{[\text{ion}]_{\text{inside}}}$

(8.3) **Goldman–Hodgkin–Katz voltage equation:**

$$V_{\text{m}} = 61.5\log\left[\frac{P_{\text{Na}^+}\times[\text{Na}^+]_{\text{outside}} + P_{\text{K}^+}\times[\text{K}^+]_{\text{outside}} + P_{\text{Cl}^-}\times[\text{Cl}^-]_{\text{inside}}}{P_{\text{Na}^+}\times[\text{Na}^+]_{\text{inside}} + P_{\text{K}^+}\times[\text{K}^+]_{\text{inside}} + P_{\text{Cl}^-}\times[\text{Cl}^-]_{\text{outside}}}\right]$$

SHARED CONCEPTS

Biochemistry Chapter 3
Nonenzymatic Protein Function and Protein Analysis

Biochemistry Chapter 5
Lipid Structure and Function

Biology Chapter 1
The Cell

Biology Chapter 10
Homeostasis

General Chemistry Chapter 9
Solutions

Physics and Math Chapter 5
Electrostatics

CHAPTER 9

CARBOHYDRATE METABOLISM I: GLYCOLYSIS, GLYCOGEN, GLUCONEOGENESIS, AND THE PENTOSE PHOSPHATE PATHWAY

SCIENCE MASTERY ASSESSMENT

Every pre-med knows this feeling: there is so much content I have to know for the MCAT! How do I know what to do first or what's important?

While the high-yield badges throughout this book will help you identify the most important topics, this Science Mastery Assessment is another tool in your MCAT prep arsenal. This quiz (which can also be taken in your online resources) and the guidance below will help ensure that you are spending the appropriate amount of time on this chapter based on your personal strengths and weaknesses. Don't worry though—skipping something now does not mean you'll never study it. Later on in your prep, as you complete full-length tests, you'll uncover specific pieces of content that you need to review and can come back to these chapters as appropriate.

How to Use This Assessment

If you answer 0–7 questions correctly:

Spend about 1 hour to read this chapter in full and take limited notes throughout. Follow up by reviewing **all** quiz questions to ensure that you now understand how to solve each one.

If you answer 8–11 questions correctly:

Spend 20–40 minutes reviewing the quiz questions. Beginning with the questions you missed, read and take notes on the corresponding subchapters. For questions you answered correctly, ensure your thinking matches that of the explanation and you understand why each choice was correct or incorrect.

If you answer 12–15 questions correctly:

Spend less than 20 minutes reviewing all questions from the quiz. If you missed any, then include a quick read-through of the corresponding subchapters, or even just the relevant content within a subchapter, as part of your question review. For questions you got correct, ensure your thinking matches that of the explanation and review the Concept Summary at the end of the chapter.

1. Which of the following transporters is used by cells in the liver to store excess glucose and by beta cells in the pancreas as a glucose sensor?
   - **A.** GLUT 1
   - **B.** GLUT 2
   - **C.** GLUT 3
   - **D.** GLUT 4

2. Which of the following organs does NOT require a constant supply of glucose from the blood for energy during a fast?
   - **A.** Red blood cells
   - **B.** Brain
   - **C.** Pancreas
   - **D.** Liver

3. When insulin is released, it acts to increase the absorption of glucose into skeletal muscle predominantly through which of the following transporters?
   - **A.** GLUT 1
   - **B.** GLUT 2
   - **C.** GLUT 3
   - **D.** GLUT 4

4. After an overnight fast, which of the following enzymes would be expected to have little, if any, physiological activity?
   - **A.** Malate dehydrogenase
   - **B.** Glucokinase
   - **C.** α-Ketoglutarate dehydrogenase
   - **D.** Phosphofructokinase-1

5. Which of the following enzymes is NOT used to trap sugar in the cell?
   - **A.** Hexokinase
   - **B.** Galactokinase
   - **C.** Phosphofructokinase
   - **D.** Fructokinase

6. When fatty acid β-oxidation predominates in the liver, mitochondrial pyruvate is most likely to be:
   - **A.** carboxylated to phosphoenolpyruvate for entry into gluconeogenesis.
   - **B.** oxidatively decarboxylated to acetyl-CoA for oxidation in the citric acid cycle.
   - **C.** carboxylated to oxaloacetate for entry into gluconeogenesis.
   - **D.** reduced to lactate in the process of fermentation.

7. A biopsy is done on a child with an enlarged liver and shows accumulation of glycogen granules with single glucose residues remaining at the branch points near the periphery of the granule. The most likely genetic defect is in the gene encoding:
   - **A.** α-1,4 phosphorylase (glycogen phosphorylase).
   - **B.** α-1,4:α-1,6 transferase (branching enzyme).
   - **C.** α-1,4:α-1,4 transferase (part of debranching enzyme complex).
   - **D.** α-1,6 glucosidase (part of debranching enzyme complex).

8. An investigator is measuring the activity of various enzymes involved in reactions of intermediary metabolism. One of the enzymes has greatly decreased activity compared to reference values. The buffer of the assay contains citrate. Which of the following enzymes will most likely be directly affected by the use of citrate?
   - **A.** Fructose-2,6-bisphosphatase
   - **B.** Isocitrate dehydrogenase
   - **C.** Phosphofructokinase-1
   - **D.** Pyruvate carboxylase

9. After a brief period of intense exercise, the activity of muscle pyruvate dehydrogenase is greatly increased. This increased activity is most likely due to:
   - **A.** decreased ADP.
   - **B.** increased acetyl-CoA.
   - **C.** increased $NADH/NAD^+$ ratio.
   - **D.** increased pyruvate concentration.

10. The metabolism of which of the following sugars would be LEAST affected by the inhibition of the enzyme phosphofructokinase-1?

- **A.** Lactose
- **B.** Fructose
- **C.** Glucose
- **D.** Galactose

11. A patient is given antibiotics to treat a urinary tract infection and develops an episode of red blood cell lysis. Further studies show weakness of the plasma membrane and Heinz bodies (collections of oxidized hemoglobin). Which of the following enzymes is most likely defective in this patient?

- **A.** Fructose-1,6-bisphosphatase
- **B.** Glucose-6-phosphate dehydrogenase
- **C.** Hexokinase
- **D.** Pyruvate kinase

12. The unique enzymes of gluconeogenesis are used to circumvent specific irreversible steps of glycolysis. Which of the following correctly pairs an enzyme from glycolysis with its corresponding enzyme(s) used in gluconeogenesis?

- **A.** Phosphofructokinase-1/fructose-1,6-bisphosphatase
- **B.** Pyruvate dehydrogenase/pyruvate carboxylase and phosphoenolpyruvate carboxykinase
- **C.** Hexokinase/glucokinase
- **D.** Pyruvate kinase/glucose-6-phosphatase

13. After an overnight fast, which of the following processes would be expected to occur at an elevated rate compared with the well-fed state?

- **A.** Glycolysis
- **B.** Glycogenolysis
- **C.** Glycogenesis
- **D.** Glycerol synthesis

14. Andersen disease is caused by a mutation in branching enzyme and is associated with cirrhosis. Scientists theorize the cause is likely an immune response against abnormal glycogen. Which of the following best describes the ratio of glycogen α-1,4 to α-1,6 linkages in individuals with this disorder?

- **A.** Elevated
- **B.** Decreased
- **C.** No difference
- **D.** Cannot determine

15. Each of the following catalyzes a rate-limiting step of a carbohydrate metabolism pathway EXCEPT:

- **A.** hexokinase.
- **B.** glycogen synthase.
- **C.** glucose-6-phosphate dehydrogenase.
- **D.** fructose-1,6-bisphosphatase.

Answer Key

1. **B** (See section 9.1)
2. **D** (See section 9.6)
3. **D** (See section 9.1)
4. **B** (See section 9.2)
5. **C** (See section 9.3)
6. **C** (See section 9.4)
7. **D** (See section 9.6)
8. **C** (See section 9.2)
9. **D** (See section 9.4)
10. **B** (See section 9.3)
11. **B** (See section 9.7)
12. **A** (See section 9.6)
13. **B** (See section 9.5)
14. **A** (See section 9.5)
15. **A** (See section 9.2)

The relevant section of the chapter to review for each question is given in parentheses after the correct answer. Detailed explanations can be found at the end of the chapter.

CHAPTER 9

CARBOHYDRATE METABOLISM I: GLYCOLYSIS, GLYCOGEN, GLUCONEOGENESIS, AND THE PENTOSE PHOSPHATE PATHWAY

In This Chapter

CHAPTER PROFILE

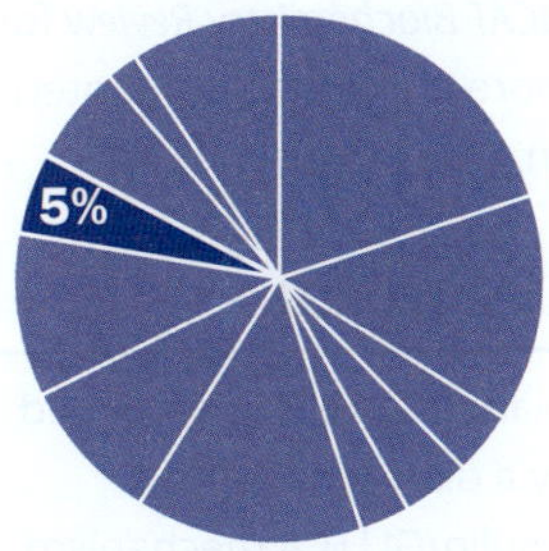

The content in this chapter should be relevant to about 5% of all questions about biochemistry on the MCAT.

This chapter covers material from the following AAMC content categories:

1D: Principles of bioenergetics and fuel molecule metabolism

5D: Structure, function, and reactivity of biologically-relevant molecules

Introduction

Maintaining a constant blood glucose concentration around $100\frac{\text{mg}}{\text{dL}}$ (5.6 mM) is of the utmost importance in the body: high blood sugar causes long-term damage to the retina, kidney, blood vessels, and nerves, while low blood sugar can cause autonomic disturbances, seizures, and even coma. Without the ability to take in glucose constantly, the body must find ways to store and release glucose as it is needed. And given the variety of food we eat on a daily basis, the body must find ways to use all of the various carbohydrates it takes in.

There's a complex interplay between the neurological, endocrine, digestive, and excretory systems to maintain this blood glucose concentration, much of which is discussed in Chapter 12 of *MCAT Biochemistry Review*. In this chapter, we'll take a look at the metabolic pathways that involve glucose: the methods by which our bodies digest glucose and other monosaccharides, store and release glucose for energy, generate glucose from other biomolecules, and use glucose to create some of the coenzymes and substrates needed for biosynthesis.

This chapter is the first of four that focus on metabolism in *MCAT Biochemistry Review*. Here, we focus on metabolic processes of glucose that do not require oxygen; in Chapter 10, we'll turn our focus to the processes that only occur under aerobic conditions. In Chapter 11, we'll explore the metabolism of lipids and amino acids. Finally, in Chapter 12, we'll bring all of metabolism together with a focus on bioenergetics and the regulation of metabolism overall.

9.1 Glucose Transport

LEARNING OBJECTIVES

After Chapter 9.1, you will be able to:

- List the locations and functions of the GLUT 2 and GLUT 4 glucose transport proteins
- Predict how increased blood glucose levels will impact GLUT 2 and GLUT 4 activity

Glucose entry into most cells is driven by concentration and is independent of sodium, unlike absorption from the digestive tract. Normal glucose concentration in peripheral blood is 5.6 mM (normal range: 4–6 mM). There are four glucose transporters, called GLUT 1 through GLUT 4. GLUT 2 and GLUT 4 are the most significant of these because they are located only in specific cells and are highly regulated.

GLUT 2 is a low-affinity transporter in hepatocytes and pancreatic cells. After a meal, blood traveling through the hepatic portal vein from the intestine is rich in glucose. GLUT 2 captures the excess glucose primarily for storage. When the glucose concentration drops below the K_m for the transporter, much of the remainder bypasses the liver and enters the peripheral circulation. The K_m of GLUT 2 is quite high (~15 mM). This means that the liver will pick up glucose in proportion to its concentration in the blood (first-order kinetics). In other words, the liver will pick up excess glucose and store it preferentially after a meal, when blood glucose levels are high. In the β-islet cells of the pancreas, GLUT 2, along with the glycolytic enzyme *glucokinase*, serves as the glucose sensor for insulin release.

GLUT 4 is in adipose tissue and muscle and responds to the glucose concentration in peripheral blood. The rate of glucose transport in these two tissues is increased by insulin, which stimulates the movement of additional GLUT 4 transporters to the membrane by a mechanism involving exocytosis, as shown in Figure 9.1. The K_m of GLUT 4 is close to the normal glucose levels in blood (~5 mM). This means that the transporter is saturated when blood glucose levels are just a bit higher than normal. When a person has high blood sugar concentrations, these transporters will still permit only a constant rate of glucose influx because they will be saturated (zero-order kinetics). Then how can cells with GLUT 4 transporters increase their intake of glucose? By increasing the number of GLUT 4 transporters on their surface.

BRIDGE

The K_m is the concentration of substrate when an enzyme is active at half of its maximum velocity (V_{max}). The lower the K_m, the higher the enzyme's affinity for the substrate. See Chapter 2 of *MCAT Biochemistry Review* for more on Michaelis–Menten enzyme kinetics.

REAL WORLD

Diabetes mellitus is caused by a disruption of the insulin/GLUT 4 mechanism. In type 1 diabetes, insulin is absent and cannot stimulate the insulin receptor. In type 2 diabetes, the receptor becomes insensitive to insulin and fails to bring GLUT 4 transporters to the cell surface. In both cases, blood glucose rises, leading to immediate symptoms (increased urination, increased thirst, ketoacidosis) and long-term symptoms (blindness, heart attacks, strokes, nerve damage).

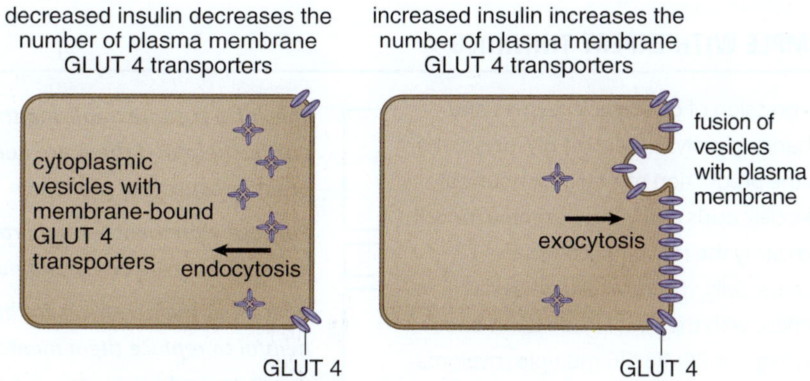

Figure 9.1 Insulin Regulation of Glucose Transport in Muscle and Adipose Cells

Although basal levels of transport occur in all cells independently of insulin, the transport rate increases in adipose tissue and muscle when insulin levels rise. Muscle stores excess glucose as glycogen, and adipose tissue requires glucose to form dihydroxyacetone phosphate (DHAP), which is converted to glycerol phosphate to store incoming fatty acids as *triacylglycerols*.

MCAT CONCEPT CHECK 9.1

Before you move on, assess your understanding of the material with these questions.

1. Compare and contrast GLUT 2 and GLUT 4:

	GLUT 2	GLUT 4
Important tissues		
K_m		
Saturated at normal glucose levels?		
Responsive to insulin?		

2. How does insulin promote glucose entry into cells?

BIOCHEMISTRY GUIDED EXAMPLE WITH EXPERT THINKING

Malignant cells increase their expression of glycolytic enzymes and glucose uptake to markedly enhance glycolysis (aerobic glycolysis; the Warburg effect), which leads to the production of a large amount of ATP and biomolecules such as nucleic acids and lipids essential for cell survival and division. In order to clarify the role of glycolysis in ATP production in malignant and normal cells, the intracellular levels of ATP were measured upon treatment with the hexokinase II inhibitor 3BrPA at 10, 30, and 50 μM, in malignant RPMI8226 multiple myeloma (MM) cells. Data were expressed relative to values for untreated cells (Figure 1). MM cells are known to reside in the bone marrow with normal hematopoietic cells. To compare the effects of inhibiting glycolysis on ATP production between malignant and normal cells, $CD138^+$ primary MM cells and $CD138^-$ non-MM bone marrow mononuclear cells (BMMCs) were cultured for 60 minutes with 50 μM of 3BrPA, and cellular levels of ATP were measured (Figure 2). Finally, to evaluate the effects of 3BrPA on cell viability, RPMI8226 and peripheral blood mononuclear cells (PBMCs), which are non-MM, were cultured for 24 hours with 3BrPA at the indicated concentrations. The cells were stained with propidium iodide (PI), which binds more intensely to non-viable cells, and analyzed by flow cytometry (Figure 3).

This intro is contextualizing the research, so it'll only be helpful if there are questions on the broader context of the study

Purpose statement: explain role of glycolysis to make ATP in cancerous and normal cells

With all of the acronyms in the passage it'll be helpful to replace them mentally with simpler words and add notes to your scratch board: 3BrPA with "glycolytic inhibitor" and RPMI8226 with "cancer"

Fig 2: same as Fig 1, but comparing to normal cells

Replace $CD138^+$ with "cancer", $CD138^-$ with "normal"

This indicates what "new" thing is coming in the next data set

Rephrase: glycolytic inhibitor added to cancer and normal cells

The dye will pick up dead cells!

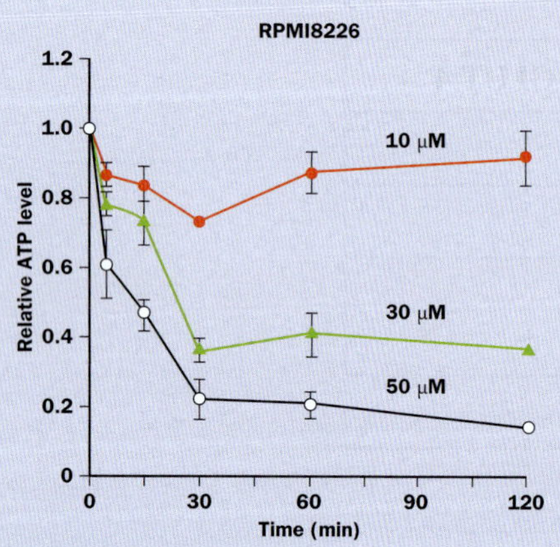

Figure 1

IVs: concentration of glycolytic inhibitor and time

DV: ATP levels

Trend: as glycolysis inhibitor conc goes up, ATP levels decrease in cancer cells

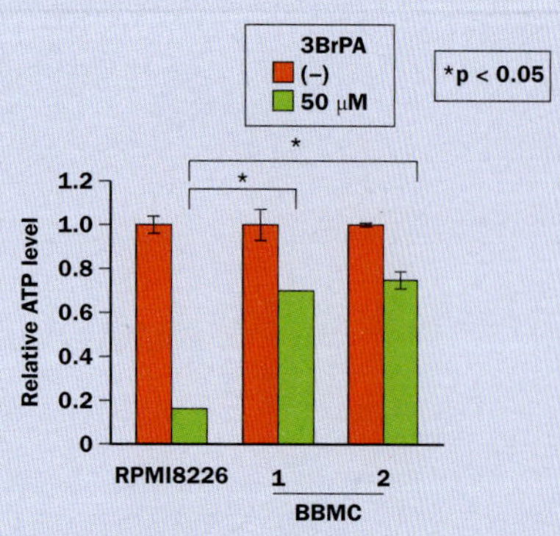

Figure 2

IVs: cancer vs. normal cell type, presence/absence of glycolytic inhibitor

DV: ATP levels

Trend: glycolytic inhibitor lowers ATP levels more in cancer cells compared to normal cells

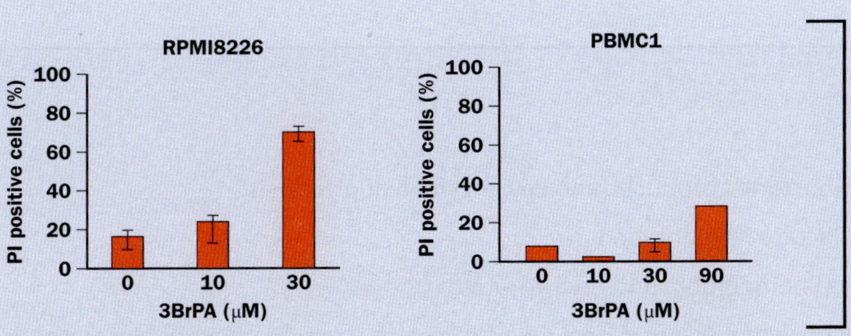

Two sets of graphs, though we can rephrase to essentially make it into one

IVs: normal vs. cancer cells, glycolytic inhibitor concentrations

DVs: levels of dead cells

Trend: the glycolytic inhibitor kills off more cancer cells compared to normal cells

Figure 3

Adapted from Nakano, A., Tsuji, D., Miki, H., Cui, Q., El Sayed, S. M., Ikegame, A., … Abe, M. (2011). Glycolysis inhibition inactivates ABC transporters to restore drug sensitivity in malignant cells. *PLoS One*, 6(11), e27222.

According to the data, do the results support the usage of glycolytic inhibitors like 3BrPA to preferentially target malignant cells? Why or why not?

This question is going to require us to understand what this experiment is testing and how the results are gathered, so let's start by making sure we understand the passage fully. A quick scan of this passage reveals multiple challenges: lots of acronyms, unfamiliar jargon and experimental techniques, and four experimental graphs. While each piece of data will be distinct, they will all be centered around supporting the experiment's purpose. The second sentence states that the overall purpose of this passage is to explore how cancer cells primarily use glycolysis, and how this preference can be used to specifically target tumors.

In Figure 1, we can see what's happening to ATP levels over time in multiple myeloma cells treated with hexokinase inhibitor. Looking at the data, we see that over time, the bigger the dose (written above the lines) of inhibitor, the more the ATP level in the cancer cells drops. If glycolysis is the primary way cancer cells produce ATP, which is what the passage stated in the first sentence, then the results in Figure 1 can be said to support this hypothesis.

Figure 2 shows a comparison of ATP production in the presence and absence of the inhibitor to cancer cells (RPMI8226 and $CD138^{+}$) and normal cells ($CD138^{-}$). While there is a drop in ATP when treated with the inhibitor in all the cell types, there is a statistical difference in the ATP levels of cancer vs. normal cells when the inhibitor is present. The brackets at the top of this figure indicate a statistically significant difference between the cancer cell line with the inhibitor and normal cell lines with the inhibitor. These kinds of statistical significance indications in a graph often point us toward where we should be heading to solve passage-based questions on the MCAT. This is the first piece of evidence that shows how inhibiting glycolysis has a bigger effect on cancer cells compared to normal, because we saw a statistically significant difference between those groups.

However, the most impactful proof comes in Figure 3. The cells have been treated with PI, which the passage tells us will stain non-viable (dead) cells more intensely. The cancer cells have progressively more dead cells (indicated by higher bars) with increasing amounts of the glycolytic inhibitor, which we can see in the first graph of Figure 3, while the normal cells (the second graph of Figure 3) show far fewer dead cells even at the highest dose. To directly compare, one can estimate that ~70% of cancer cells are PI positive with 30 μM 3BrPA, whereas ~10% of nonmalignant cells are PI positive with the same concentration of 3BRPA.

Because the results in Figure 3 tell us that glycolytic inhibitor 3BrPA is far more effective in killing cancerous vs. noncancerous cell lines, the findings are supportive of the idea that 3BrPA could possibly be used to target and treat cancerous cells.

9.2 Glycolysis High Yield

LEARNING OBJECTIVES

After Chapter 9.2, you will be able to:

- Recall the key steps, key intermediates, reactants, products, and key enzymes of glycolysis
- Explain the function and mechanism of lactate fermentation
- Explain the unique effects of glycolysis on hemoglobin and erythrocytes
- Recall function and regulatory mechanisms when given an enzyme of glycolysis, such as phosphoglycerate kinase

All cells can carry out glycolysis. In a few tissues, most importantly red blood cells, glycolysis represents the only energy-yielding pathway available because red blood cells lack mitochondria, which are required for the citric acid cycle, electron transport chain, oxidative phosphorylation, and fatty acid metabolism (β-oxidation). Glucose is the major monosaccharide that enters the pathway, but others such as galactose and fructose can also feed into it.

Glycolysis is a cytoplasmic pathway that converts glucose into two *pyruvate* molecules, releasing a modest amount of energy captured in two substrate-level phosphorylations and one oxidation reaction. If a cell has mitochondria and oxygen, the energy carriers produced in glycolysis (NADH) can feed into the aerobic respiration pathway to generate energy for the cell. If either mitochondria or oxygen is lacking (such as in erythrocytes or exercising skeletal muscle, respectively), glycolysis may occur anaerobically, although some of the available energy is lost.

Glycolysis also provides intermediates for other pathways. In the liver, glycolysis is part of the process by which excess glucose is converted to fatty acids for storage.

BRIDGE

Red blood cells extrude their mitochondria during development, as discussed in Chapter 7 of *MCAT Biology Review*. This helps them carry out their function (carrying oxygen) in two ways:

- Maximizing volume available for hemoglobin, the primary oxygen-carrying protein
- Stopping the red blood cell from utilizing the oxygen it's supposed to be carrying to oxygen-depleted bodily tissues

Important Enzymes of Glycolysis

While glycolysis contains many different steps, as illustrated in Figure 9.2, the MCAT predominantly tests on the enzymes that are highly regulated or that serve an important energetic function. Therefore, we'll focus our attention on five of these enzymes.

REAL WORLD

Because glycolysis is necessary in every cell of the body, there are no known diseases caused by the complete absence of any enzyme in glycolysis; in other words, being unable to carry out glycolysis is incompatible with life. Partial enzyme defects are also rare, but include *pyruvate kinase deficiency*.

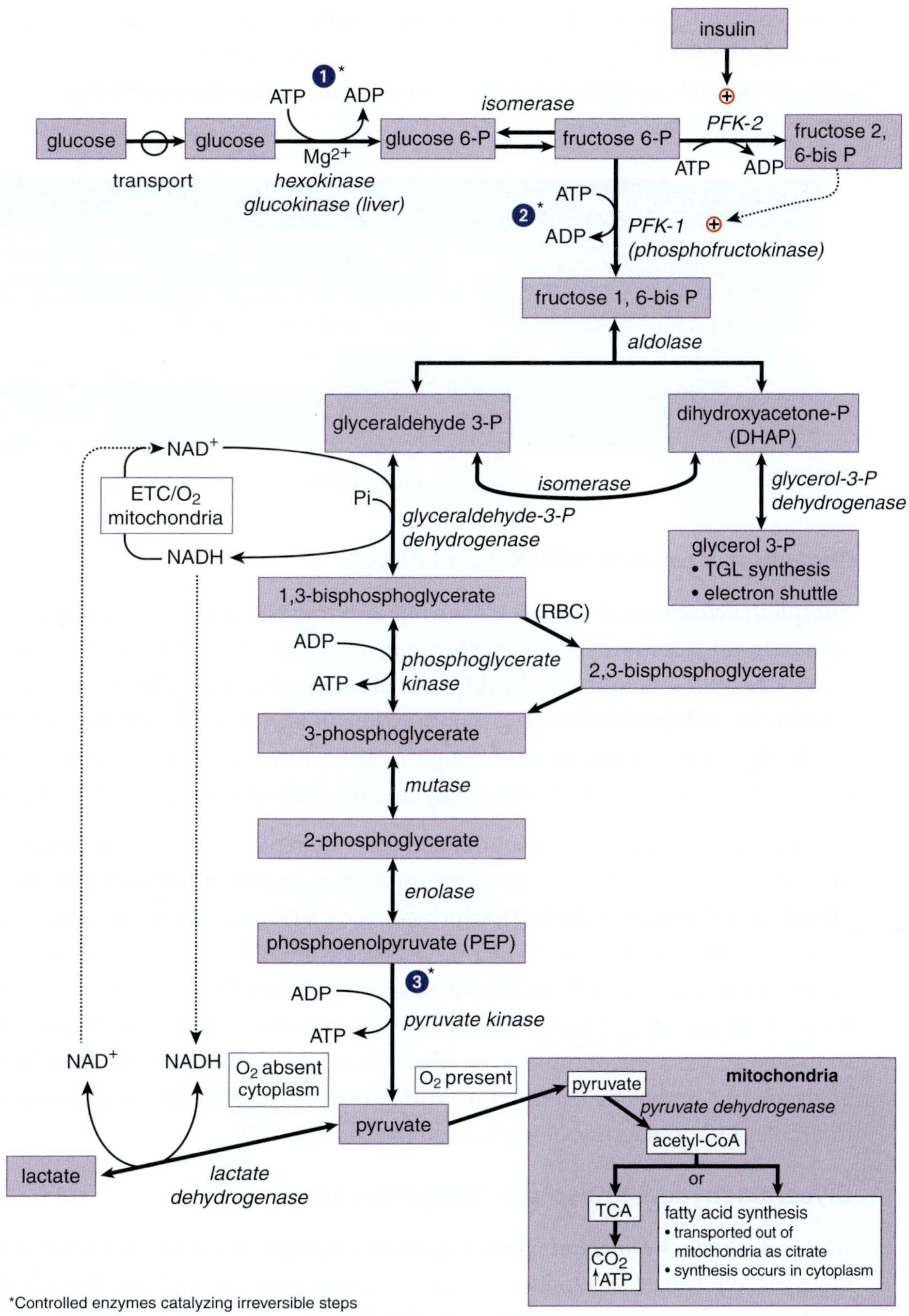

Figure 9.2 Glycolysis

Hexokinase and Glucokinase

The first steps in glucose metabolism in any cell are transport across the membrane and phosphorylation by kinase enzymes inside the cell to prevent glucose from leaving via the transporter. Remember from Chapter 2 of *MCAT Biochemistry Review* that kinases attach a phosphate group from ATP to their substrates. Glucose enters the cell by facilitated diffusion or active transport; in either case, these kinases convert glucose to *glucose 6-phosphate*. Because the GLUT transporters are specific for glucose (not *phosphorylated* glucose), the glucose gets "trapped" inside the cell and cannot leak out. ***Hexokinase*** is widely distributed in tissues and is

KEY CONCEPT

Of all the enzymes the MCAT is most likely to test you on, the rate-limiting enzymes for each process are at the top of the list:

- Glycolysis: *phosphofructokinase-1*
- Fermentation: *lactate dehydrogenase*
- Glycogenesis: *glycogen synthase*
- Glycogenolysis: *glycogen phosphorylase*
- Gluconeogenesis: *fructose-1,6-bisphosphatase*
- Pentose Phosphate Pathway: *glucose-6-phosphate dehydrogenase*

BRIDGE

In Chapter 11 of *MCAT General Chemistry Review*, we learn that oxidation is loss of electrons and reduction is gain of electrons. While this is true with biomolecules, it may be easier to think of oxidation as increasing bonds to oxygen or other heteroatoms (atoms besides C and H) and reduction as increasing bonds to hydrogen, as discussed in Chapter 4 of *MCAT Organic Chemistry Review*. Thus, the conversion of NAD^+ to NADH is a reduction reaction.

inhibited by its product, glucose 6-phosphate. ***Glucokinase*** is found only in liver cells and pancreatic β-islet cells; in the liver, glucokinase is induced by insulin. Table 9.1 identifies the differences between these enzymes. These coincide with the differences between the glucose transporters in these tissues.

Hexokinase	Glucokinase
Present in most tissues	Present in hepatocytes and pancreatic β-islet cells (along with GLUT 2, acts as the glucose sensor)
Low K_m (reaches maximum velocity at low [glucose])	High K_m (acts on glucose proportionally to its concentration)
Inhibited by glucose 6-phosphate	Induced by insulin in hepatocytes

Table 9.1 Comparison of Hexokinase and Glucokinase

Phosphofructokinases (PFK-1 and PFK-2)

Phosphofructokinase-1 **(PFK-1)** is the rate-limiting enzyme and main control point in glycolysis. In this reaction, *fructose 6-phosphate* is phosphorylated to *fructose 1,6-bisphosphate* using ATP. PFK-1 is inhibited by ATP and citrate, and activated by AMP. This makes sense because the cell should turn off glycolysis when it has sufficient energy (high ATP) and turn on glycolysis when it needs energy (high AMP). Citrate is an intermediate of the citric acid cycle, so high levels of citrate also imply that the cell is producing sufficient energy.

Insulin stimulates and glucagon inhibits PFK-1 in hepatocytes by an indirect mechanism involving PFK-2 and fructose 2,6-bisphosphate, as shown in Figure 9.2. Insulin activates ***phosphofructokinase-2*** **(PFK-2)**, which converts a tiny amount of *fructose 6-phosphate* to *fructose 2,6-bisphosphate* (F2,6-BP). F2,6-BP activates PFK-1. On the other hand, glucagon inhibits PFK-2, lowering F2,6-BP and thereby inhibiting PFK-1. PFK-2 is found mostly in the liver. By activating PFK-1, it allows these cells to override the inhibition caused by ATP so that glycolysis can continue, even when the cell is energetically satisfied. The metabolites of glycolysis can thus be fed into the production of glycogen, fatty acids, and other storage molecules rather than just being burned to produce ATP.

Glyceraldehyde-3-Phosphate Dehydrogenase

Glyceraldehyde-3-phosphate dehydrogenase catalyzes an oxidation and addition of inorganic phosphate (P_i) to its substrate, *glyceraldehyde 3-phosphate*. This results in the production of a high-energy intermediate *1,3-bisphosphoglycerate* and the reduction of NAD^+ to NADH. If glycolysis is aerobic, the NADH can be oxidized by the mitochondrial electron transport chain, providing energy for ATP synthesis by oxidative phosphorylation.

3-Phosphoglycerate Kinase

3-Phosphoglycerate kinase transfers the high-energy phosphate from 1,3-bisphosphoglycerate to ADP, forming ATP and *3-phosphoglycerate*. This type of reaction, in which ADP is directly phosphorylated to ATP using a high-energy intermediate, is referred to as **substrate-level phosphorylation**. In contrast to oxidative phosphorylation in mitochondria, substrate-level phosphorylations are not dependent on oxygen, and are the only means of ATP generation in an anaerobic tissue.

Pyruvate Kinase

The last enzyme in aerobic glycolysis, pyruvate kinase catalyzes a substrate-level phosphorylation of ADP using the high-energy substrate *phosphoenolpyruvate* (PEP). ***Pyruvate kinase*** is activated by fructose 1,6-bisphosphate from the PFK-1 reaction. This is referred to as **feed-forward activation**, meaning that the product of an earlier reaction of glycolysis (fructose 1,6-bisphosphate) stimulates, or prepares, a later reaction in glycolysis (by activating pyruvate kinase).

Fermentation

In the absence of oxygen, **fermentation** will occur. The key fermentation enzyme in mammalian cells is ***lactate dehydrogenase***, which converts pyruvate into lactate and concurrently oxidizes NADH to NAD^+. Without oxygen, glycolysis would eventually come to a halt and stop any production of ATP when all the available NAD^+ had been reduced to NADH. Under aerobic conditions, NADH produced by glycolysis donates its electrons to the ETC and is reconverted to NAD^+, replenishing the pool of NAD^+ needed by glyceraldehyde-3-phosphate dehydrogenase (GAPDH) within the glycolysis pathway. However, under anaerobic conditions, the ETC ceases to function and NADH is unable to donate its electrons to regenerate NAD^+. By reducing pyruvate to lactate and oxidizing NADH to NAD^+, lactate dehydrogenase prevents this potential problem from developing and allows glycolysis to continue. There is no net loss of carbon in this process: pyruvate and lactate are both three-carbon molecules. In yeast cells, fermentation is the conversion of pyruvate (three carbons) to ethanol (two carbons) and carbon dioxide (one carbon). While the end products are different, the result of both mammalian and yeast fermentation is the same: replenishing NAD^+.

In aerobic tissues, lactate does not normally form in significant amounts. However, when oxygenation is poor, such as during strenuous exercise, most cellular ATP is generated by anaerobic glycolysis, and lactate production increases. When oxygen once again becomes available, some of this lactate can be converted back into pyruvate. However, most of the lactate will enter into the **Cori cycle,** also called the lactic acid cycle, a metabolic pathway shown in Figure 9.3. In this pathway, lactate produced by muscles during anaerobic respiration is transported to the liver and used in gluconeogenesis to create glucose, which is then returned to the muscles. The muscle cells then break down the glucose, recreating lactate, which can then undergo the same cycle again.

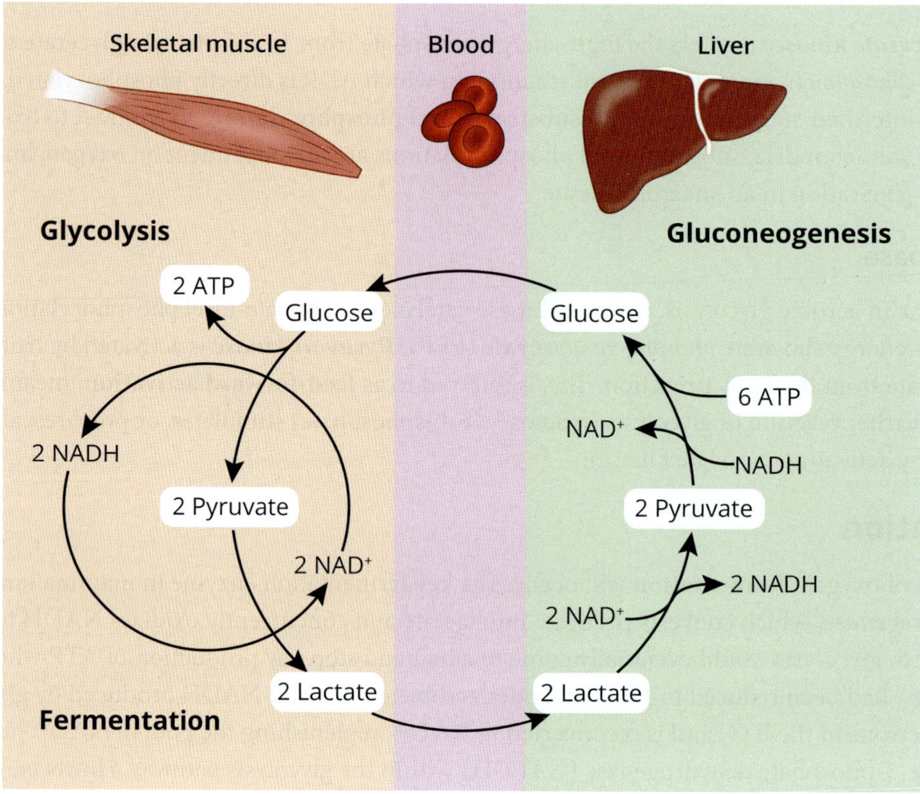

Figure 9.3 The Cori Cycle
Lactate from muscles is used by the liver to create glucose, which is then used and metabolized back into lactate in the muscles.

Important Intermediates of Glycolysis

Glycolysis serves as a crossroads for a number of metabolic processes; the intermediates of glycolysis are often used to link different pathways during both catabolism and anabolism. Three of these intermediates are worth highlighting:

- ***Dihydroxyacetone phosphate*** (**DHAP**) is used in hepatic and adipose tissue for triacylglycerol synthesis. DHAP is formed from fructose 1,6-bisphosphate. It can be isomerized to *glycerol 3-phosphate*, which can then be converted to *glycerol*, the backbone of triacylglycerols.
- 1,3-Bisphosphoglycerate (1,3-BPG) and phosphoenolpyruvate (PEP) are high-energy intermediates used to generate ATP by substrate-level phosphorylation. This is the only ATP gained in anaerobic respiration.

Irreversible Enzymes

Three enzymes in the pathway catalyze reactions that are irreversible. This keeps the pathway moving in only one direction. However, the liver must be able to generate new glucose from other biomolecules through gluconeogenesis, which is essentially the reverse of glycolysis. Because of the irreversible enzymes of

MNEMONIC

Irreversible steps of glycolysis:

How **G**lycolysis **P**ushes **F**orward the **P**rocess: **K**inases.

- **H**exokinase
- **G**lucokinase
- **PF**K-1
- **P**yruvate **K**inase

glycolysis, different reactions, and therefore different enzymes, must be used at these three points:

- Glucokinase or hexokinase
- PFK-1
- Pyruvate kinase

Glycolysis in Erythrocytes

In erythrocytes (red blood cells), anaerobic glycolysis represents the only pathway for ATP production, yielding a net 2 ATP per glucose.

Red blood cells have ***bisphosphoglycerate mutase***, which produces ***2,3-bisphosphoglycerate*** (**2,3-BPG**) from 1,3-BPG in glycolysis. Remember that *mutases* are enzymes that move a functional group from one place in a molecule to another; in this case, the phosphate is moved from the 1-position to the 2-position. 2,3-BPG binds allosterically to the β-chains of hemoglobin A (HbA) and decreases its affinity for oxygen. This effect of 2,3-BPG is seen in the oxygen dissociation curve for HbA, shown in Figure 9.4. The rightward shift in the curve is sufficient to allow unloading of oxygen in tissues, but still allows 100 percent saturation in the lungs. An abnormal increase in erythrocyte 2,3-BPG might shift the curve far enough so that HbA is not fully saturated in the lungs.

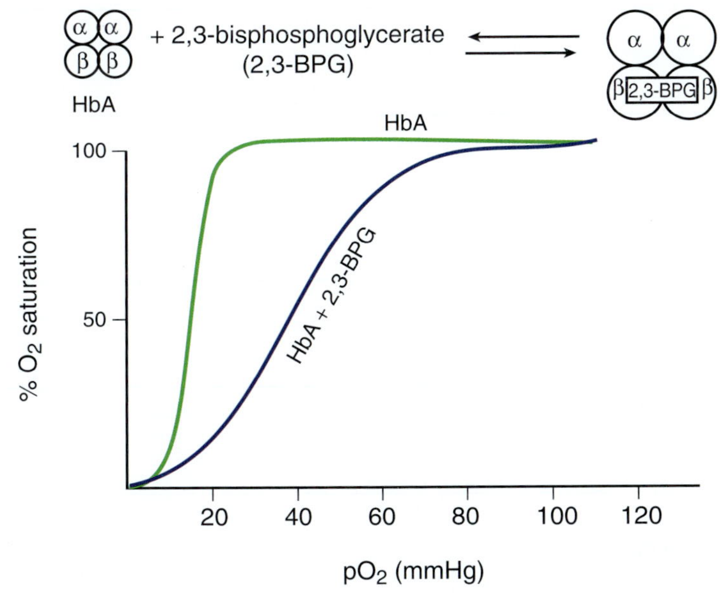

Figure 9.4 Effect of 2,3-Bisphosphoglycerate on Hemoglobin A

Although 2,3-BPG binds to HbA, it does not bind well to fetal hemoglobin (HbF), with the result that HbF has a higher affinity for oxygen than maternal HbA. This allows transplacental passage of oxygen from mother to fetus.

BRIDGE

Adaptation to high altitudes (low pO_2) involves:

- Increased respiration
- Increased oxygen affinity for hemoglobin (initial)
- Increased rate of glycolysis
- Increased [2,3-BPG] in RBC (over a 12–24 hour period)
- Normalized oxygen affinity for hemoglobin restored by the increased level of 2,3-BPG
- Increased hemoglobin (over days to weeks)

Gas exchange is discussed in Chapter 6 of *MCAT Biology Review*, and effects on hemoglobin are discussed in Chapter 7 of *MCAT Biology Review*.

BRIDGE

Remember the other physiological changes that promote a **right** shift of the oxygen dissociation curve (the Bohr effect), discussed in Chapter 7 of *MCAT Biology Review*:

- High 2,3-BPG
- Low pH
- High $[H^+]$
- High pCO_2

These all occur during exercise, giving the mnemonic: "Exercise is the **right** thing to do."

MCAT CONCEPT CHECK 9.2

Before you move on, assess your understanding of the material with these questions.

1. What are the function and key regulators of the following enzymes? Which ones are reversible?

Hexokinase

- Function:

____

- Regulation:

____

- Reversible?

____

Glucokinase

- Function:

____

- Regulation:

____

- Reversible?

____

Phosphofructokinase-1 (PFK-1)

- Function:

____

- Regulation:

____

- Reversible?

____

Glyceraldehyde-3-phosphate dehydrogenase

- Function:

____

- Reversible?

____

3-phosphoglycerate kinase

- Function:

____

- Reversible?

____

Pyruvate kinase

- Function:

____

- Regulation:

____

- Reversible?

____

2. Why must pyruvate undergo fermentation for glycolysis to continue?

____

3. Why is it necessary that fetal hemoglobin does not bind 2,3-BPG?

____

9.3 Other Monosaccharides

LEARNING OBJECTIVES

After Chapter 9.3, you will be able to:

- Explain the importance of trapping a sugar in the cell and linking its metabolism with the glycolysis pathway
- Recognize the key enzymes, reactants, and products of galactose and fructose metabolism

While glucose represents the primary monosaccharide used by cells, other monosaccharides such as *galactose* and *fructose* can also contribute to ATP production by feeding into glycolysis or other metabolic processes. These monosaccharides are tested far less frequently than glucose on the MCAT, but are included here to compare and contrast their metabolism with glycolysis. In particular, notice the similarities between Figure 9.2 (glycolysis) and Figures 9.5 (galactose metabolism) and 9.6 (fructose metabolism).

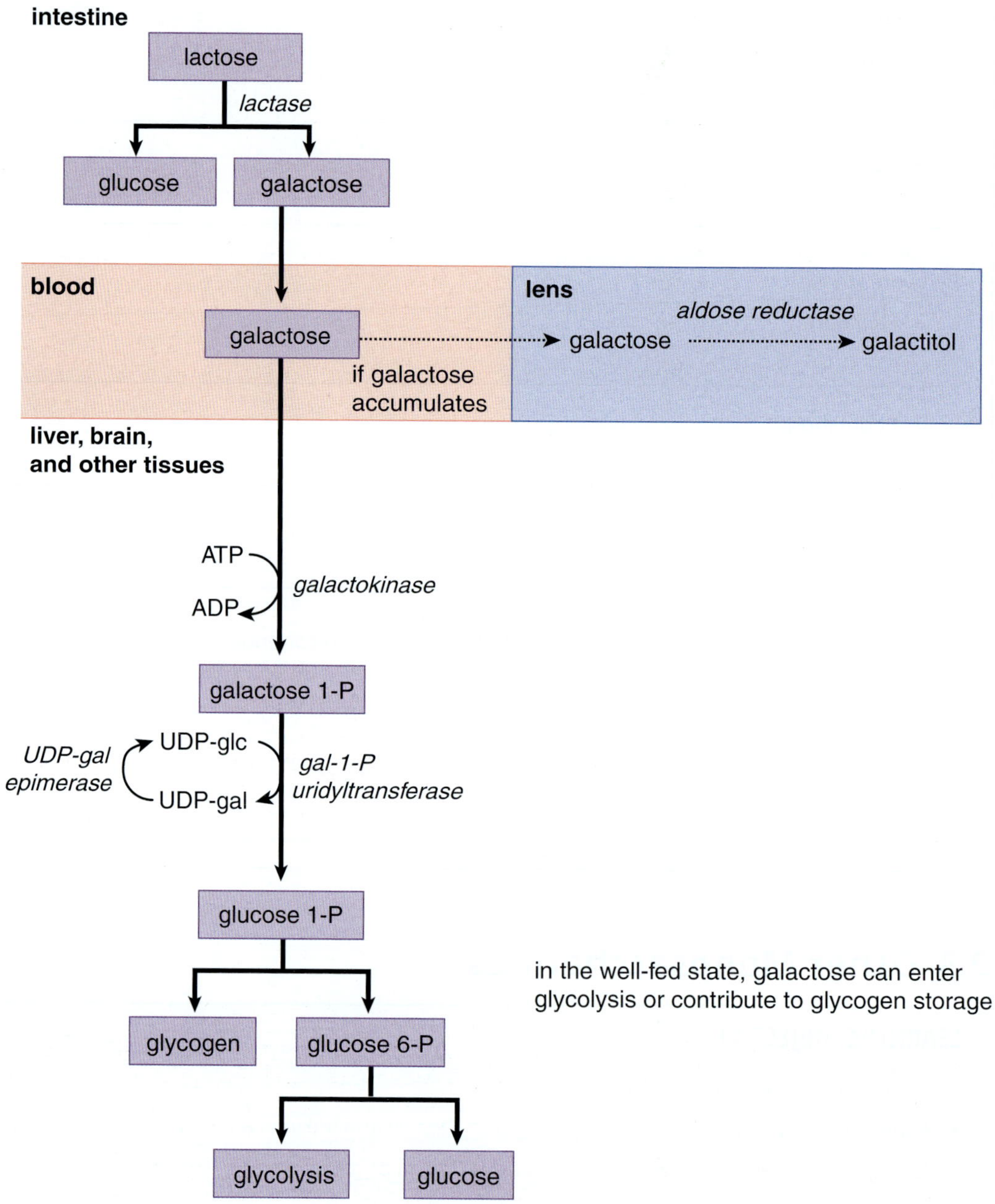

Figure 9.5 Galactose Metabolism

Galactose Metabolism

An important source of **galactose** in the diet is the disaccharide *lactose* present in milk. Lactose is hydrolyzed to galactose and glucose by *lactase,* which is a brush-border enzyme of the duodenum. Along with other monosaccharides, galactose reaches the liver through the hepatic portal vein. Once transported into tissues, galactose is phosphorylated by ***galactokinase***, trapping it in the cell. The resulting *galactose 1-phosphate* is converted to *glucose 1-phosphate* by ***galactose-1-phosphate uridyltransferase*** and an *epimerase.* **Epimerases** are enzymes that catalyze the conversion of one sugar epimer to another;

REAL WORLD

Primary lactose intolerance is caused by a hereditary deficiency of lactase. *Secondary lactose intolerance* can be precipitated at any age by gastrointestinal disturbances that cause damage to the intestinal lining, where lactase is found.

Common symptoms of lactose intolerance include vomiting, bloating, explosive and watery diarrhea, cramps, and dehydration. The symptoms can be attributed to bacterial fermentation of lactose, which produces a mixture of CH_4, H_2, and small organic acids. The acids are osmotically active and result in the movement of water into the intestinal lumen.

remember from Chapter 4 of *MCAT Biochemistry Review* that epimers are diastereomers that differ at exactly one chiral carbon. The pathway is shown in Figure 9.5; important enzymes to remember are:

- Galactokinase
- Galactose-1-phosphate uridyltransferase

Fructose Metabolism

Fructose is found in honey and fruit and as part of the disaccharide *sucrose* (common table sugar). Sucrose is hydrolyzed by the duodenal brush-border enzyme *sucrase*, and the resulting monosaccharides, glucose and fructose, are absorbed into the hepatic portal vein. The liver phosphorylates fructose using ***fructokinase*** to trap it in the cell. The resulting *fructose 1-phosphate* is then cleaved into *glyceraldehyde* and DHAP by *aldolase B*. Smaller amounts are metabolized in renal proximal tubules. The pathway is shown in Figure 9.6.

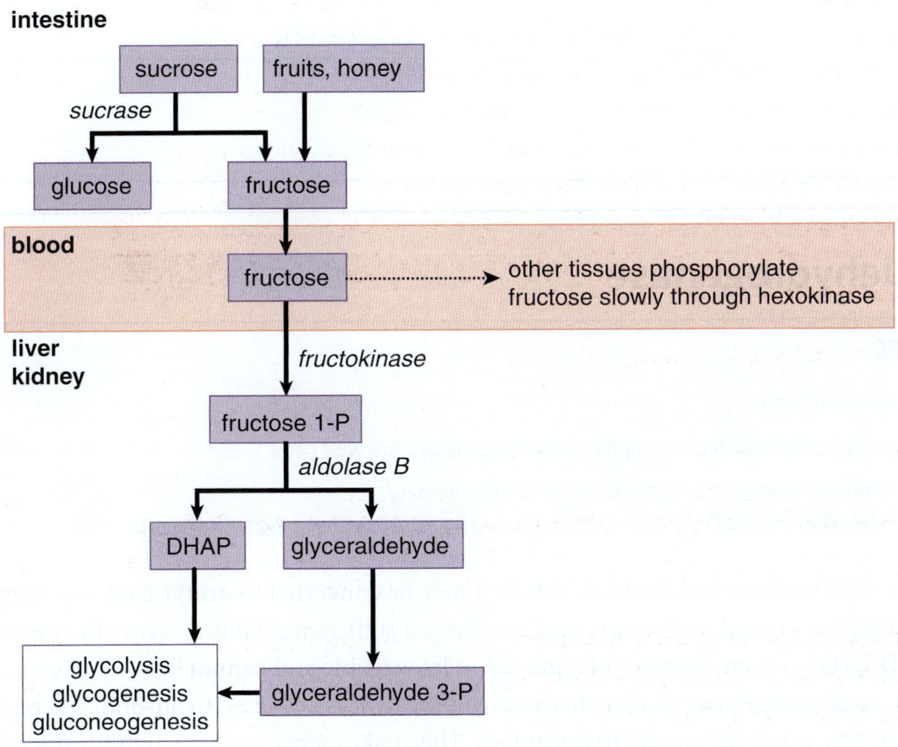

Figure 9.6 Fructose Metabolism

REAL WORLD

Genetic deficiencies of galactokinase or galactose-1-phosphate uridyltransferase lead to galactosemia. Cataracts are a characteristic finding, which result from the conversion of excess galactose in the blood to galactitol in the lens of the eye by aldose reductase. Galactitol is a polyol (a carbon chain with many alcohol groups) and, as such, is hydrophilic. Accumulation of galactitol in the lens causes osmotic damage and cataracts.

Deficiency of galactose-1-phosphate uridyltransferase is more severe because, in addition to causing galactosemia, it leads to galactose 1-phosphate getting stuck intracellularly in the liver, brain, and other tissues and not diffusing out.

KEY CONCEPT

Because dihydroxyacetone phosphate (DHAP) and glyceraldehyde, the products of fructose metabolism, are downstream from the key regulatory and rate-limiting enzyme of glycolysis (PFK-1), a high-fructose drink supplies a quick source of energy in both aerobic and anaerobic cells.

MCAT CONCEPT CHECK 9.3

Before you move on, assess your understanding of the material with these questions.

1. Which enzyme is responsible for trapping galactose in the cell? What enzyme in galactose metabolism results in a product that can feed directly into glycolysis, linking the two pathways?
   - "Trapping" enzyme:
   - "Linking" enzyme:
2. Which enzyme is responsible for trapping fructose in the cell? What enzyme in fructose metabolism results in a product that can feed directly into glycolysis, linking the two pathways?
   - "Trapping" enzyme:
   - "Linking" enzyme:

9.4 Pyruvate Dehydrogenase

LEARNING OBJECTIVES

After Chapter 9.4, you will be able to:

- Recall the reactants and products of the pyruvate dehydrogenase complex
- Describe the relationship between acetyl-CoA levels and PDH activity

Pyruvate from aerobic glycolysis enters mitochondria, where it may be converted to ***acetyl-CoA*** for entry into the citric acid cycle if ATP is needed, or for fatty acid synthesis if sufficient ATP is present. The ***pyruvate dehydrogenase complex*** (**PDH**) reaction, shown in Figure 9.7, is irreversible and cannot be used to convert acetyl-CoA to pyruvate or to glucose. Pyruvate dehydrogenase in the liver is activated by insulin, whereas in the nervous system, the enzyme is not responsive to hormones. This makes sense because high insulin levels signal to the liver that the individual is in a well-fed state; thus, the liver should not only burn glucose for energy, but shift the fatty acid equilibrium toward production and storage, rather than oxidation (fatty acid synthesis, discussed in Chapter 11 of *MCAT Biochemistry Review*, starts from citrate produced in the citric acid cycle).

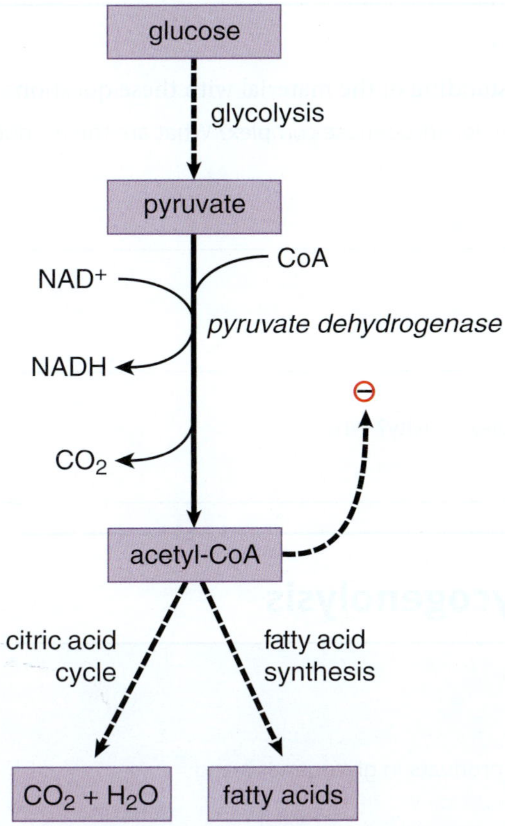

Figure 9.7 Pyruvate Dehydrogenase

Pyruvate dehydrogenase is actually a complex of enzymes carrying out multiple reactions in succession. The details of each of these reactions are covered in Chapter 10 of *MCAT Biochemistry Review*, but an overview of the enzyme is provided here because it represents one of three possible fates of pyruvate: conversion to acetyl-CoA by PDH, conversion to lactate by lactate dehydrogenase, or conversion to *oxaloacetate* by *pyruvate carboxylase*.

This large complex requires multiple cofactors and coenzymes, including *thiamine pyrophosphate*, *lipoic acid*, CoA, FAD, and NAD^+. Insufficient amounts of any of these cofactors or coenzymes can result in metabolic derangements.

Pyruvate dehydrogenase is inhibited by its product acetyl-CoA. This control is important in several contexts and should be considered along with pyruvate carboxylase, the other mitochondrial enzyme that uses pyruvate (introduced in gluconeogenesis, later in this chapter). Essentially, the buildup of acetyl-CoA (which happens during β-oxidation) causes a shift in metabolism: pyruvate is no longer converted into acetyl-CoA (to enter the citric acid cycle), but rather into oxaloacetate (to enter gluconeogenesis).

REAL WORLD

A deficiency in thiamine (vitamin B_1) can result in:

- *Beriberi*, which is characterized by congestive heart failure or nerve damage.
- *Wernicke–Korsakoff syndrome*, which is characterized by difficulty walking, uncoordinated eye movements, confusion, and memory disturbances.

Giving glucose to an individual with thiamine deficiency can lead to severe lactic acidosis and other metabolic derangements because pyruvate cannot be converted into acetyl-CoA without the vitamin. This is why thiamine must be given before an infusion of glucose in individuals suspected to have thiamine deficiency (such as alcoholics).

MCAT CONCEPT CHECK 9.4

Before you move on, assess your understanding of the material with these questions.

1. What are the reactants of the pyruvate dehydrogenase complex? What are the products?
   - Reactants:

   ____

   - Products:

   ____

2. How does acetyl-CoA affect PDH complex activity? Why?

   ____

9.5 Glycogenesis and Glycogenolysis

LEARNING OBJECTIVES

After Chapter 9.5, you will be able to:

- Recall the key enzymes, reactants, and products in glycogenesis and glycogenolysis
- Describe the features of glycogen storage diseases
- Recognize the structural features of glycogen and the major glycosidic links within a glycogen granule:

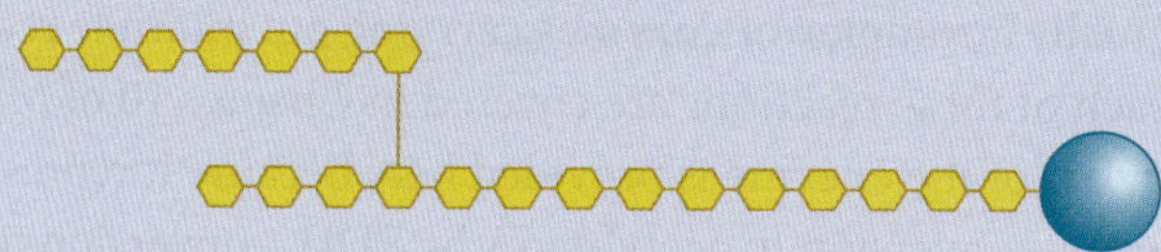

Glycogen, a branched polymer of glucose, represents a storage form of glucose. Glycogen synthesis and degradation occur primarily in liver and skeletal muscle, although other tissues store smaller quantities. Glycogen is stored in the cytoplasm as granules. Each granule has a central protein core with polyglucose chains radiating outward to form a sphere, as shown in Figure 9.8. Glycogen granules composed entirely of linear chains have the highest density of glucose near the core. If the chains are branched, the glucose density is highest at the periphery of the granule, allowing more rapid release of glucose on demand.

KEY CONCEPT

The glycogen in the liver and in skeletal muscle serve two quite different roles. Liver glycogen is broken down to maintain a constant level of glucose in the blood; muscle glycogen is broken down to provide glucose to the muscle during vigorous exercise.

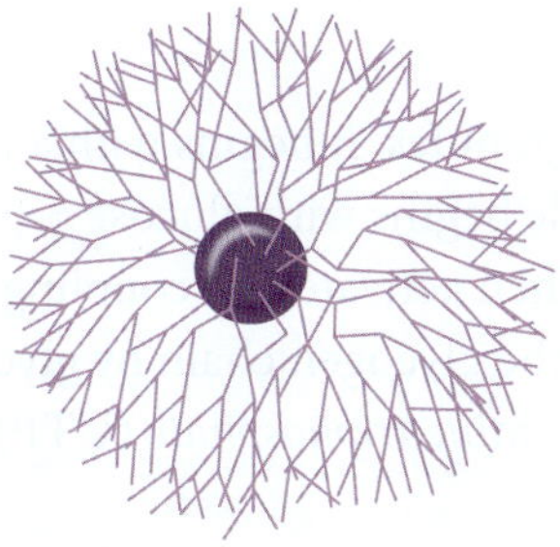

Figure 9.8 A Glycogen Granule

Glycogen stored in the liver is a source of glucose that is mobilized between meals to prevent low blood sugar, whereas muscle glycogen is stored as an energy reserve for muscle contraction.

While our focus is on human metabolism, it is worth mentioning that plants also store excess glucose in long α-linked chains of glucose called **starch**, as seen in Figure 9.9.

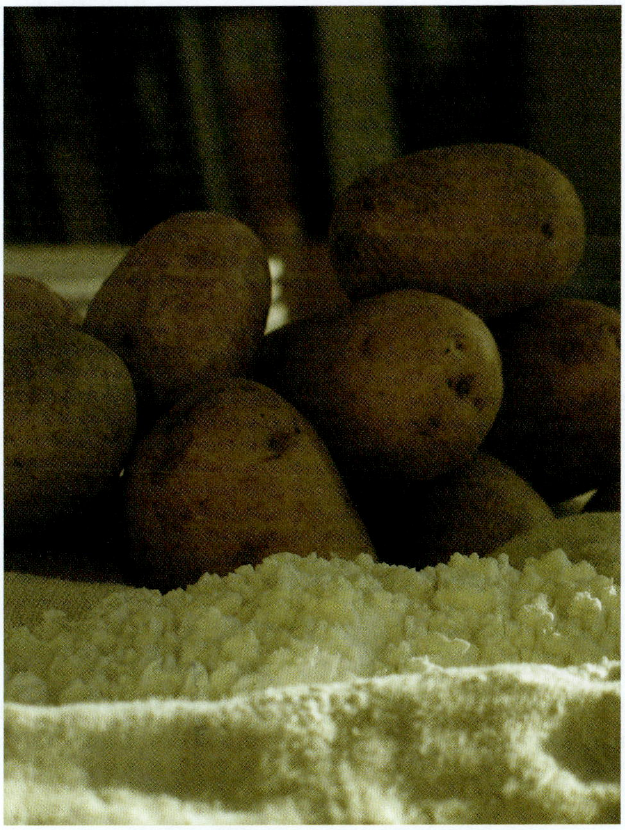

Figure 9.9 Potatoes and Potato Starch

Glycogenesis

Glycogenesis is the synthesis of glycogen granules. It begins with a core protein called *glycogenin*. As shown in Figure 9.10, glucose addition to a granule begins with glucose 6-phosphate, which is converted to glucose 1-phosphate. This glucose 1-phosphate is then activated by coupling to a molecule of *uridine diphosphate* (UDP), which permits its integration into the glycogen chain by glycogen synthase. This activation occurs when glucose 1-phosphate interacts with *uridine triphosphate* (UTP), forming UDP-glucose and a *pyrophosphate* (PP_i).

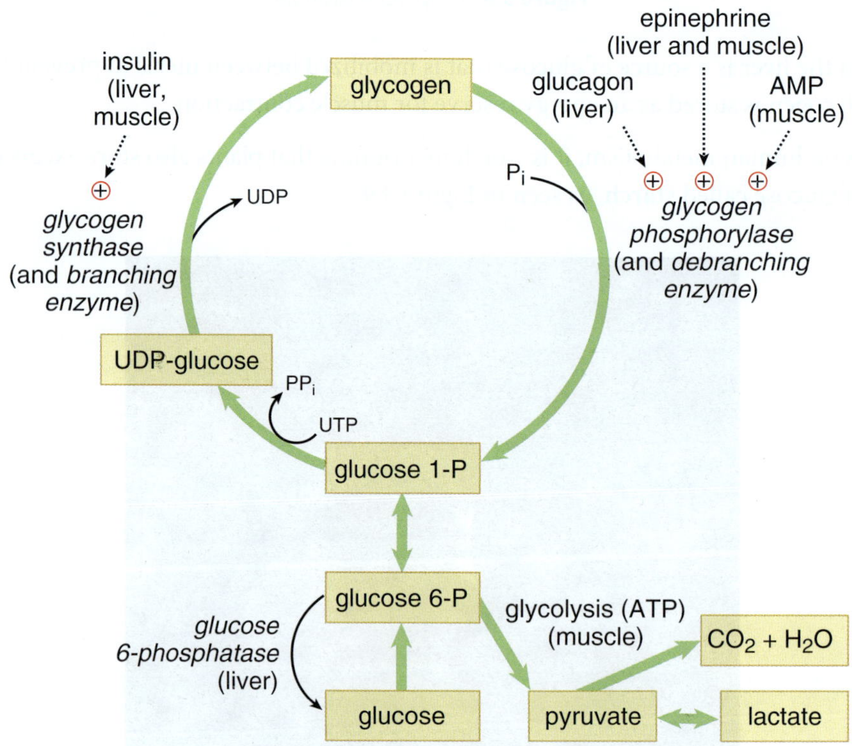

Figure 9.10 Glycogen Metabolism

Glycogen Synthase

Glycogen synthase is the rate-limiting enzyme of glycogen synthesis and forms the α-1,4 glycosidic bond found in the linear glucose chains of the granule. It is stimulated by glucose 6-phosphate and insulin. It is inhibited by epinephrine and glucagon through a protein kinase cascade that phosphorylates and inactivates the enzyme.

Branching Enzyme (Glycosyl α-1,4:α-1,6 Transferase)

Branching enzyme is responsible for introducing α-1,6-linked branches into the granule as it grows. The steps of glycogen synthesis and the process by which branches are introduced are shown schematically in Figure 9.11. Branching enzyme:

- Hydrolyzes one of the α-1,4 bonds to release a block of oligoglucose (a few glucose molecules bonded together in a chain), which is then moved and added in a slightly different location.
- Forms an α-1,6 bond to create a branch.

MNEMONIC

α-1,**4** keeps the same branch moving "**4**ward"; α-1,6 (one-**six**) "puts a branch in the **mix**."

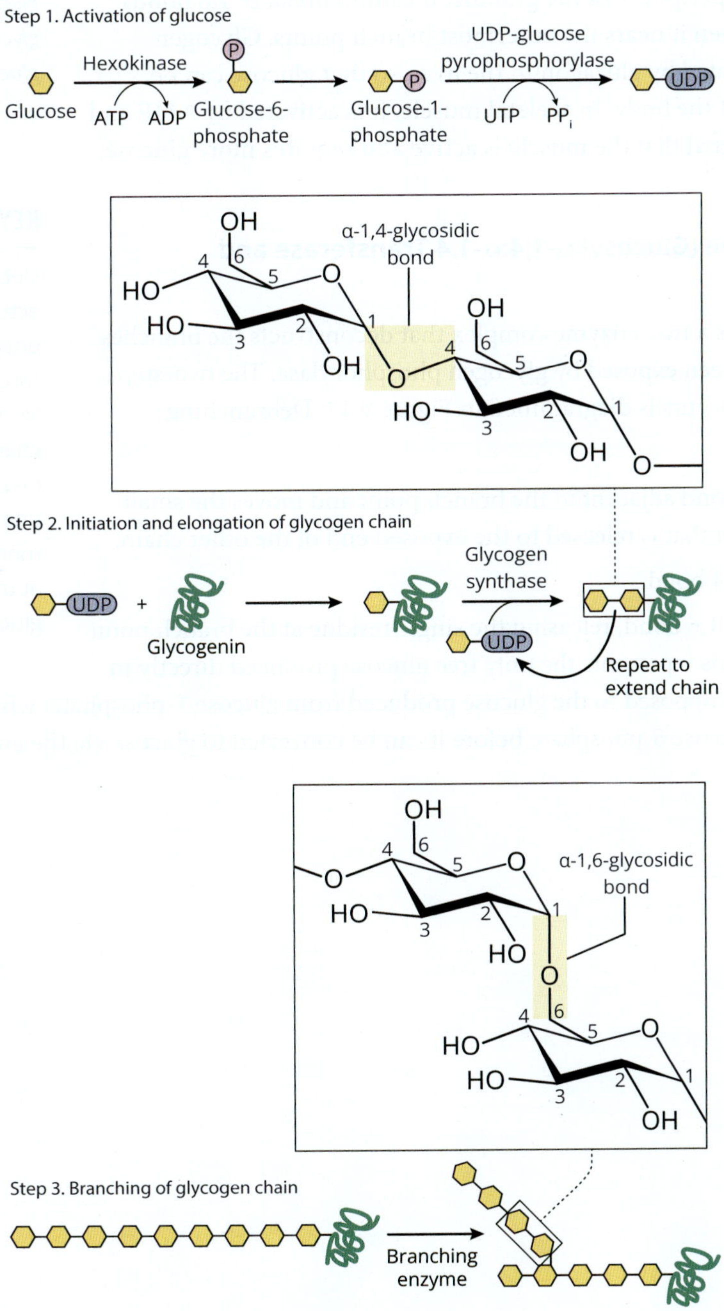

Figure 9.11 Glycogenesis

Glycogenolysis

The rate-limiting enzyme of **glycogenolysis**, the process of breaking down glycogen, is *glycogen phosphorylase*. In contrast to a *hydrolase*, a *phosphorylase* breaks bonds using an inorganic phosphate instead of water. The glucose 1-phosphate formed by glycogen phosphorylase is converted to glucose 6-phosphate by the same mutase used in glycogen synthesis, as shown in Figure 9.10.

MCAT EXPERTISE

Under the pressure of Test Day, it can be easy to misread words. When given a passage or question about carbohydrate metabolism, be sure you focus so you can distinguish between *glycolysis*, *glycogenesis*, *glycogenolysis*, and *gluconeogenesis*.

Glycogen Phosphorylase

Glycogen phosphorylase breaks α-1,4 glycosidic bonds, releasing glucose 1-phosphate from the periphery of the granule. It cannot break α-1,6 bonds and therefore stops when it nears the outermost branch points. Glycogen phosphorylase is activated by glucagon in the liver, so that glucose can be provided for the rest of the body. In skeletal muscle, it is activated by AMP and epinephrine, which signal that the muscle is active and requires more glucose. It is inhibited by ATP.

KEY CONCEPT

Debranching enzyme is actually made up of two enzymes with different functions: one moves the terminal end of a glycogen chain to the branch point (α-1,4:α-1,4 transferase), and one removes the glucose monomer actually present at the branch point (α-1,6 glucosidase).

Debranching Enzyme (Glucosyl α-1,4:α-1,4 Transferase and α-1,6 Glucosidase)

Debranching enzyme is a two-enzyme complex that deconstructs the branches in glycogen that have been exposed by glycogen phosphorylase. The two-step process by which this occurs is diagrammed in Figure 9.12. Debranching enzyme:

- Breaks an α-1,4 bond adjacent to the branch point and moves the small oligoglucose chain that is released to the exposed end of the other chain.
- Forms a new α-1,4 bond.
- Hydrolyzes the α-1,6 bond, releasing the single residue at the branch point as free glucose. This represents the only free glucose produced directly in glycogenolysis (as opposed to the glucose produced from glucose 1-phosphate, which must be converted by a mutase to glucose 6-phosphate before it can be converted to glucose via the enzyme *glucose-6-phosphatase*).

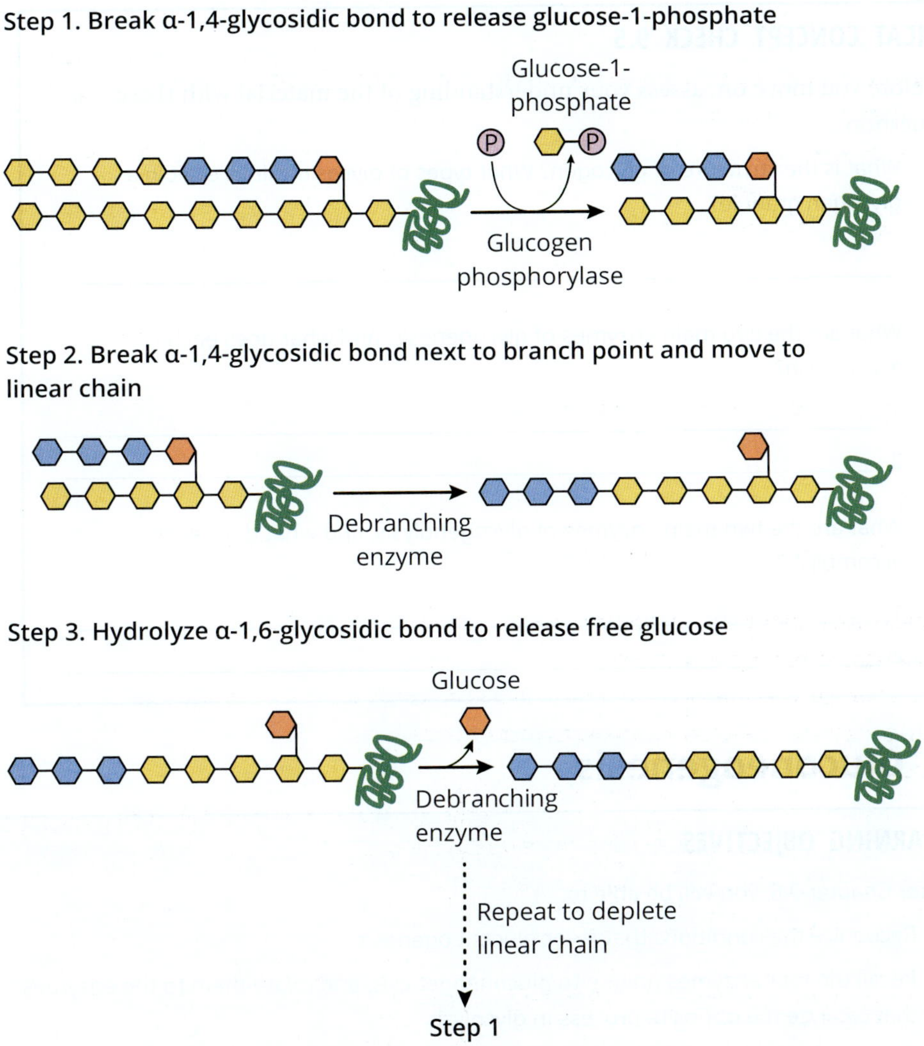

Figure 9.12 Debranching Enzyme

Glycogen Storage Diseases

There are a number of genetic deficiencies that can impact the metabolism of glycogen. The clinical features of a metabolic glycogen defect depend on a few important factors: which enzyme is affected, the degree to which that enzyme's activity is decreased, and which isoform of the enzyme is affected. **Isoforms** are slightly different versions of the same protein; in the case of glycogen enzymes, there are often different isoforms of the enzymes in the liver and muscle. These deficiencies are termed ***glycogen storage diseases*** because all are characterized by accumulation or lack of glycogen in one or more tissues.

REAL WORLD

The most common glycogen storage disease is *von Gierke's disease*, a defect in glucose-6-phosphatase. Because this enzyme is also the last step of gluconeogenesis, this process is also affected, leading to periods of extremely low blood sugar between meals. These patients therefore need continuous feeding with carbohydrates to maintain blood sugar. With the buildup of glucose 6-phosphate in liver cells, the liver enlarges and is damaged over time.

MCAT CONCEPT CHECK 9.5

Before you move on, assess your understanding of the material with these questions.

1. What is the structure of glycogen? What types of glycosidic links exist in a glycogen granule?

____

2. What are the two main enzymes of glycogenesis, and what does each accomplish?

   1. ____
   2. ____

3. What are the two main enzymes of glycogenolysis, and what does each accomplish?

   1. ____
   2. ____

9.6 Gluconeogenesis

KEY CONCEPT

Insulin acts to lower blood sugar levels; the counterregulatory hormones, which include glucagon, epinephrine, cortisol, and growth hormone, act to raise blood sugar levels by stimulating glycogenolysis and gluconeogenesis. The regulation of metabolism is discussed in Chapter 12 of *MCAT Biochemistry Review*.

LEARNING OBJECTIVES

After Chapter 9.6, you will be able to:

- Recognize the conditions that favor gluconeogenesis
- Recall the four enzymes unique to gluconeogenesis, and relate them to the enzymes that catalyze the opposite process in glycolysis
- Detail the regulatory role of acetyl-CoA in the metabolism of pyruvate

The liver maintains glucose levels in blood during fasting through either glycogenolysis or **gluconeogenesis**. The kidney can also carry out gluconeogenesis, although its contribution is much smaller. These pathways are promoted by glucagon and epinephrine, which act to raise blood sugar levels, and are inhibited by insulin, which acts to lower blood sugar levels. During fasting, glycogen reserves drop dramatically in the first 12 hours, during which time gluconeogenesis increases. After 24 hours, it represents the sole source of glucose. Important substrates for gluconeogenesis are:

- Glycerol 3-phosphate (from stored fats, or triacylglycerols, in adipose tissue)
- Lactate (from anaerobic glycolysis)
- Glucogenic amino acids (from muscle proteins)

The last item of this list merits some explaining. Amino acids can be subclassified as glucogenic, ketogenic, or both. **Glucogenic amino acids** (all except leucine and lysine) can be converted into intermediates that feed into gluconeogenesis, while **ketogenic amino acids** can be converted into ketone bodies, which can be used as an alternative fuel, particularly during periods of prolonged starvation. See Chapter 11 of *MCAT Biochemistry Review* for more information on amino acid and protein metabolism.

Dietary fructose and galactose can also be converted to glucose in the liver, as described earlier in this chapter.

BRIDGE

Amino acids and proteins are extremely important topics for the MCAT. Check out Chapter 1 of *MCAT Biochemistry Review* for more information on amino acids, peptides, and proteins.

In humans, while glucose is converted into acetyl-CoA through glycolysis and pyruvate dehydrogenase, it is not possible to convert acetyl-CoA back to glucose. Because most fatty acids are metabolized solely to acetyl-CoA, they are not a major source of glucose either. One minor exception is fatty acids with an odd number of carbon atoms (for example, fatty acid tails containing 17 carbons), which yield a small amount of *propionyl-CoA*, which is glucogenic.

The pathway of gluconeogenesis is diagrammed in Figure 9.13. Each of the important gluconeogenic intermediates—lactate, alanine, and glycerol 3-phosphate—have enzymes that convert them into glycolytic intermediates.

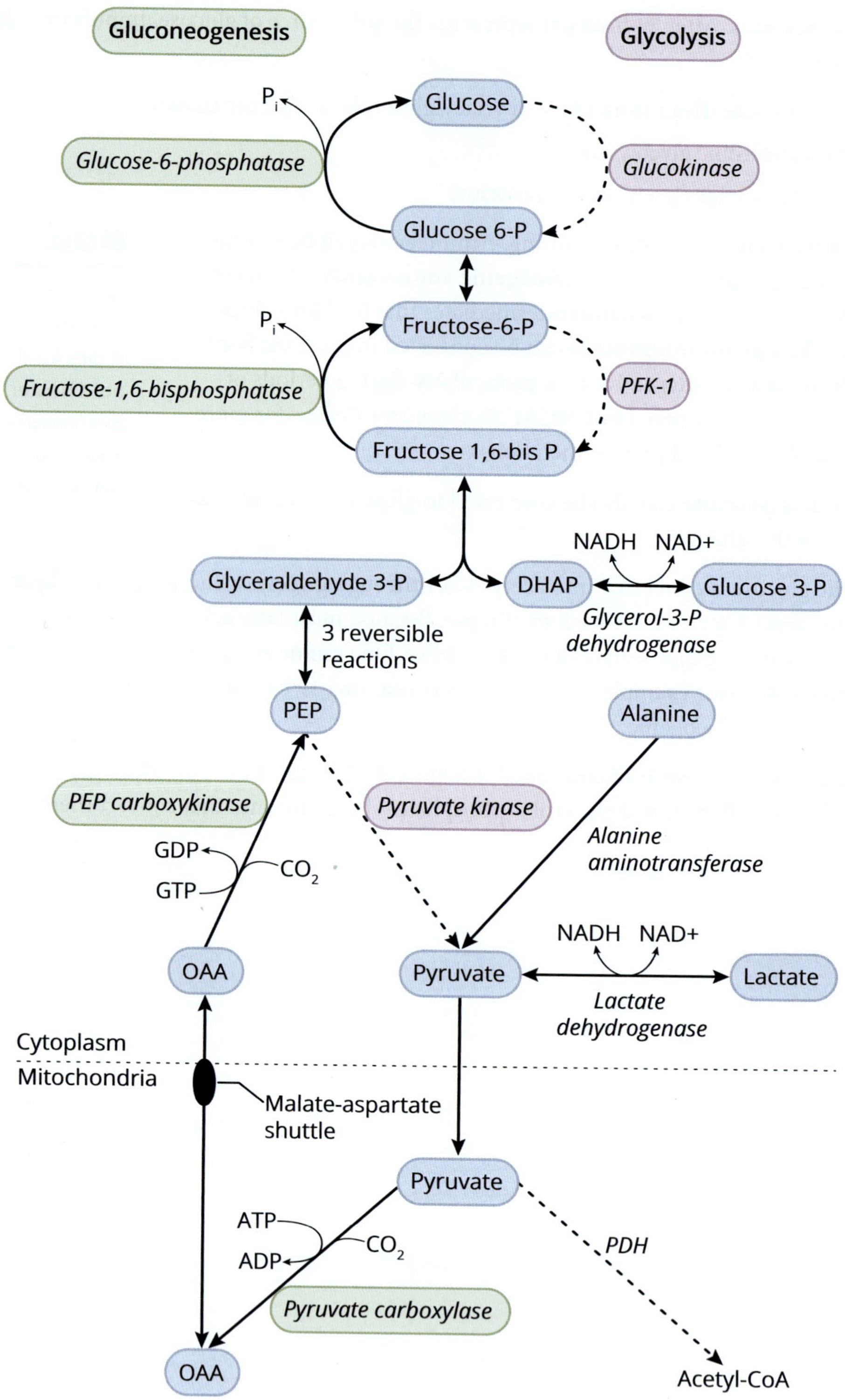

Figure 9.13 Gluconeogenesis

Lactate is converted to pyruvate by *lactate dehydrogenase*. Alanine is converted to pyruvate by *alanine aminotransferase*. Glycerol 3-phosphate is converted to dihydroxyacetone phosphate (DHAP) by *glycerol-3-phosphate dehydrogenase*.

Important Enzymes of Gluconeogenesis

Most steps in gluconeogenesis represent a reversal of glycolysis and have thus been omitted from the diagram. However, the four important enzymes to know are those required to catalyze reactions that circumvent the irreversible steps of glycolysis in the liver (those catalyzed by glucokinase, phosphofructokinase-1, and pyruvate kinase).

Pyruvate Carboxylase

Pyruvate carboxylase is a mitochondrial enzyme that is activated by acetyl-CoA (from β-oxidation). The product, oxaloacetate (OAA), is a citric acid cycle intermediate and cannot leave the mitochondrion. Rather, it is reduced to *malate*, which can leave the mitochondrion via the malate–aspartate shuttle, which is described in Chapter 10 of *MCAT Biochemistry Review*. Once in the cytoplasm, malate is oxidized to OAA. The fact that acetyl-CoA activates pyruvate carboxylase is an important point. Acetyl-CoA inhibits pyruvate dehydrogenase because a high level of acetyl-CoA implies that the cell is energetically satisfied and need not run the citric acid cycle in the forward direction; in other words, the cell should stop burning glucose. Rather, pyruvate will be shunted through pyruvate carboxylase to help generate additional glucose through gluconeogenesis. Note that the source of acetyl-CoA is not from glycolysis and pyruvate dehydrogenase in this case, but from fatty acids. Thus, to produce glucose in the liver during gluconeogenesis, fatty acids must be burned to provide this energy, stop the forward flow of the citric acid cycle, and produce massive amounts of OAA that can eventually lead to glucose production for the rest of the body.

KEY CONCEPT

Because glycolysis contains three irreversible steps (those catalyzed by hexokinase, phosphofructokinase-1, and pyruvate kinase), different enzymes must exist in gluconeogenesis to allow the body to revert pyruvate to glucose.

Phosphoenolpyruvate Carboxykinase (PEPCK)

Phosphoenolpyruvate carboxykinase (**PEPCK**) in the cytoplasm is induced by glucagon and cortisol, which generally act to raise blood sugar levels. It converts OAA to phosphoenolpyruvate (PEP) in a reaction that requires GTP. PEP continues in the pathway to fructose 1,6-bisphosphate. Thus, the combination of pyruvate carboxylase and PEPCK are used to circumvent the action of pyruvate kinase by converting pyruvate back into PEP.

Fructose-1,6-Bisphosphatase

Fructose-1,6-bisphosphatase in the cytoplasm is a key control point of gluconeogenesis and represents the rate-limiting step of the process. It reverses the action of phosphofructokinase-1, the rate-limiting step of glycolysis, by removing phosphate from fructose 1,6-bisphosphate to produce fructose 6-phosphate. A common pattern to note is that *phosphatases* oppose kinases. Fructose-1,6-bisphosphatase is activated by ATP and inhibited by AMP and fructose 2,6-bisphosphate. This should make sense: high levels of ATP imply that a cell is energetically satisfied enough to produce glucose for the rest of the body, whereas high levels of AMP imply that a cell needs energy and cannot afford to produce energy for the rest of the body before satisfying its own requirements. Fructose 2,6-bisphosphate (F2,6-BP) is sometimes thought of as a marker for satisfactory energy levels in liver cells. It helps these cells override the inhibition of phosphofructokinase-1 that occurs when high levels of acetyl-CoA are formed, signaling to the liver cell that it should shift its function from burning to storing fuel. F2,6-BP, produced by PFK-2, controls both gluconeogenesis and glycolysis (in the liver). Recall from the earlier discussion of this enzyme and Figure 9.2 that PFK-2 is activated by insulin and inhibited by glucagon. Thus, glucagon will lower F2,6-BP and stimulate gluconeogenesis, whereas insulin will increase F2,6-BP and inhibit gluconeogenesis.

Glucose-6-Phosphatase

Glucose-6-phosphatase is found only in the lumen of the endoplasmic reticulum in liver cells. Glucose 6-phosphate is transported into the ER, and free glucose is transported back into the cytoplasm, from where it can diffuse out of the cell using GLUT transporters. The absence of glucose-6-phosphatase in skeletal muscle means that muscle glycogen cannot serve as a source of blood glucose and rather is for use only within the muscle. Glucose-6-phosphatase is used to circumvent glucokinase and hexokinase, which convert glucose to glucose 6-phosphate.

Although alanine is the major glucogenic amino acid, almost all amino acids are also glucogenic. Most of these are converted by individual pathways to citric acid cycle intermediates, then to malate, following the same path from there to glucose.

It is important to note that glucose produced by hepatic (liver-based) gluconeogenesis does not represent an energy source for the liver. Gluconeogenesis requires expenditure of ATP that is provided by β-oxidation of fatty acids. Therefore, as mentioned above, hepatic gluconeogenesis is always dependent on β-oxidation of fatty acids in the liver. During periods of low blood sugar, adipose tissue releases these fatty acids by breaking down triacylglycerols to glycerol (which can also be converted to the gluconeogenic intermediate DHAP) and free fatty acids.

Although the acetyl-CoA from fatty acids cannot be converted into glucose, it can be converted into ketone bodies as an alternative fuel for cells, including the brain. Extended periods of low blood sugar are thus usually accompanied by high levels of ketones in the blood. Ketone bodies can be thought of as a transportable form of acetyl-CoA that is primarily utilized in periods of extended starvation.

KEY CONCEPT

Because gluconeogenesis requires acetyl-CoA to occur (to inhibit pyruvate dehydrogenase and stimulate pyruvate carboxylase), gluconeogenesis is inextricably linked to fatty acid oxidation. The source of acetyl-CoA cannot be glycolysis because this would just burn the glucose that is being generated in gluconeogenesis.

REAL WORLD

Because red blood cells lack mitochondria, they cannot carry out aerobic metabolism. Rather, pyruvate is converted to lactic acid to regenerate NAD^+. However, lactate is acidic; it must be removed from the bloodstream to avoid acidifying the blood. Red blood cells deliver this lactate to the liver, where it can be converted back into pyruvate and, through gluconeogenesis, become glucose for the red blood cells to use. This is known as the Cori cycle: glucose is converted to lactate in red blood cells, and lactate is converted to glucose in liver cells.

MCAT CONCEPT CHECK 9.6

Before you move on, assess your understanding of the material with these questions.

1. Under what physiological conditions should the body carry out gluconeogenesis?

____

2. What are the four enzymes unique to gluconeogenesis? Which irreversible glycolytic enzymes do they replace?

Gluconeogenic Enzyme	Replaces

3. How does acetyl-CoA shift the metabolism of pyruvate?

____

4. Given that the glycogen storage disorder von Gierke's disease affects the last enzyme of gluconeogenesis, predict the associated metabolic derangement that occurs.

____

9.7 The Pentose Phosphate Pathway

LEARNING OBJECTIVES

After Chapter 9.7, you will be able to:

- Identify the two major products of the pentose phosphate pathway
- Explain the three primary functions of NADPH in cellular respiration

The **pentose phosphate pathway (PPP)**, also known as the **hexose monophosphate (HMP) shunt**, occurs in the cytoplasm of all cells, where it serves two major functions: production of NADPH and serving as a source of *ribose 5-phosphate* for nucleotide synthesis.

An abbreviated diagram of the pathway is shown in Figure 9.14. The first part of the PPP begins with glucose 6-phosphate, ends with *ribulose 5-phosphate*, and is irreversible. This part produces NADPH and involves the important rate-limiting enzyme ***glucose-6-phosphate dehydrogenase* (G6PD)**. G6PD is induced by insulin because the abundance of sugar entering the cell under insulin stimulation will be shunted into both fuel utilization pathways (glycolysis and aerobic respiration), as well as fuel storage pathways (fatty acid synthesis, glycogenesis, and the PPP). The shunt is also inhibited by its product, NADPH, and is activated by one of its reactants, $NADP^+$.

REAL WORLD

G6PD deficiency is an X-linked disorder and is the most common inherited enzyme defect in the world. Because the PPP is critically important in maintaining levels of glutathione, which helps break down peroxides, these individuals are susceptible to oxidative stress, especially in red blood cells, which carry a large concentration of oxygen. Ingestion of certain oxidizing compounds (especially particular antibiotics and antimalarial medications) or infections can lead to high concentrations of reactive oxygen species, which cause red blood cell lysis. It is hypothesized that the defect evolved because it provides some resistance to malaria infection. G6PD deficiency has also been called *favism* because fava beans are a highly oxidizing food that will also cause hemolysis in these individuals.

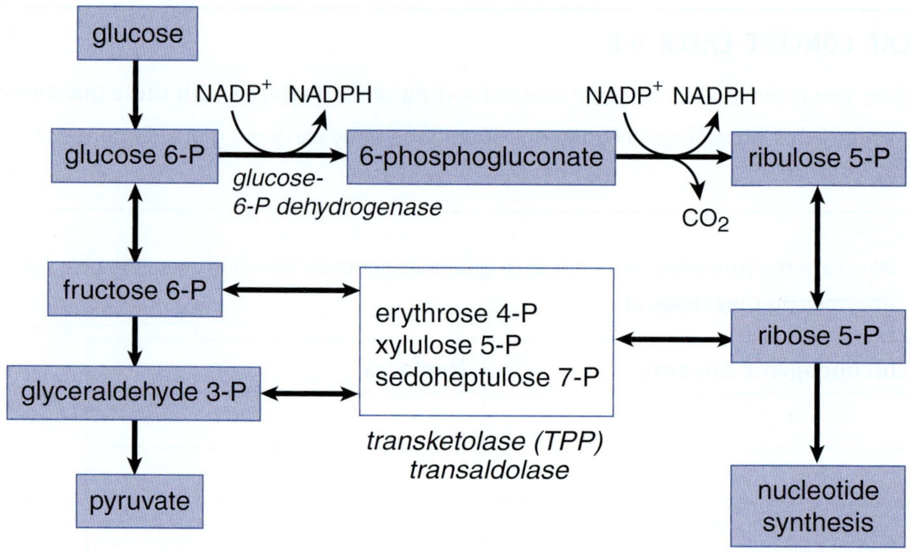

Figure 9.14 The Pentose Phosphate Pathway

The second part of the pathway, beginning with ribulose 5-phosphate, represents a series of reversible reactions that produce an equilibrated pool of sugars for biosynthesis, including ribose 5-phosphate for nucleotide synthesis. Because fructose 6-phosphate and glyceraldehyde 3-phosphate are among the sugars produced, intermediates can feed back into glycolysis; conversely, pentoses can be made from glycolytic intermediates without going through the G6PD reaction. These interconversions are primarily accomplished by the enzymes *transketolase* and *transaldolase*.

Functions of NADPH

While their names appear similar, NADPH and NADH are not the same thing. In the cell, NAD^+ acts as a high-energy electron acceptor from a number of biochemical reactions. It thus can be thought of as a potent oxidizing agent because it helps another molecule be oxidized (and thus is reduced itself during the process). The NADH produced from this reduction of NAD^+ can then feed into the electron transport chain to indirectly produce ATP.

Conversely, **NADPH** primarily acts as an electron donor in a number of biochemical reactions. It thus can be thought of as a potent reducing agent because it helps other molecules be reduced (and thus is oxidized itself during the process). Cells require NADPH for a variety of functions, including:

- Biosynthesis, mainly of fatty acids and cholesterol
- Assisting in cellular bleach production in certain white blood cells, thereby contributing to bactericidal activity
- Maintenance of a supply of reduced *glutathione* to protect against reactive oxygen species (acting as the body's natural antioxidant)

BRIDGE

The ribulose 5-phosphate created in the PPP is isomerized to ribose 5-phosphate, the backbone of nucleic acids. When coupled to a nitrogenous base, it forms a nucleotide that can be integrated into RNA. Make sure to review RNA synthesis (transcription; Chapter 7 of *MCAT Biochemistry Review*), as well as DNA synthesis (Chapter 6 of *MCAT Biochemistry Review*), because these are highly tested topics on the MCAT.

KEY CONCEPT

NADPH and NADH are not the same thing. NAD^+ is an energy carrier; NADPH is used in biosynthesis, in the immune system, and to help prevent oxidative damage.

This last function is important in protecting cells from free radical oxidative damage caused by peroxides. Hydrogen peroxide, H_2O_2, is produced as a byproduct in aerobic metabolism, and can break apart to form hydroxide radicals, $OH^{\bullet}$. Free radicals can attack lipids, including those in the phospholipids of the membrane. When oxidized, these lipids lose their function and can weaken the membrane, causing cell lysis. This is especially true in red blood cells, which contain high levels of oxygen that can be reduced by a single electron to form the superoxide radical $O_2^{\bullet-}$. This radical is neutralized by superoxide dismutase, which catalyzes its conversion into hydrogen peroxide and oxygen ($2O_2^{\bullet-} + 2H^+ \rightarrow H_2O_2 + O_2$). Free radicals can also damage DNA, potentially causing cancer. **Glutathione** is a reducing agent that can help reverse radical formation before damage is done to the cell.

MCAT CONCEPT CHECK 9.7

Before you move on, assess your understanding of the material with these questions.

1. What are the two major metabolic products of the pentose phosphate pathway (PPP)?

   1. ____________________
   2. ____________________

2. What are three primary functions of NADPH?

   1. ____________________
   2. ____________________
   3. ____________________

Conclusion

This chapter is critically important in your studying for the MCAT. The processes of carbohydrate metabolism that do not require oxygen are heavily tested, as is their integration. The body has evolved in such a way that we can use, store, or create fuel 24 hours a day, depending on the demands of the internal and external environment. We can turn on pathways when we need them and turn them off when we don't. And the regulation of these pathways makes sense: for example, acetyl-CoA—a downstream product of glycolysis—can turn off the process of glycolysis and allow us to either store extra sugar as other biomolecules or generate sugar anew if we need it. Return to this chapter repeatedly during your studies to maximize points on metabolism on Test Day. In the next chapter, we'll turn our attention to the oxygen-requiring carbohydrate metabolism processes, including the citric acid cycle, the electron transport chain (ETC), and oxidative phosphorylation.

GO ONLINE

You've reviewed the content, now test your knowledge and critical thinking skills by completing a test-like passage set in your online resources!

CONCEPT SUMMARY

Glucose Transport

- **GLUT 2** is found in the liver (for glucose storage) and pancreatic β-islet cells (as part of the glucose sensor). It has a high K_m.
- **GLUT 4** is found in adipose tissue and muscle and is stimulated by insulin. It has a low K_m.

Glycolysis

- **Glycolysis** occurs in the cytoplasm of all cells and does not require oxygen. It yields 2 ATP per molecule of glucose.
- Important glycolytic enzymes include:
  - **Glucokinase**, which converts glucose to glucose 6-phosphate. It is present in the pancreatic β-islet cells as part of the glucose sensor and is responsive to insulin in the liver.
  - **Hexokinase**, which converts glucose to glucose 6-phosphate in peripheral tissues.
  - **Phosphofructokinase-1** (**PFK-1**), which phosphorylates fructose 6-phosphate to fructose 1,6-bisphosphate in the rate-limiting step of glycolysis. PFK-1 is activated by AMP and fructose 2,6-bisphosphate (F2,6-BP) and is inhibited by ATP and citrate.
  - **Phosphofructokinase-2** (**PFK-2**), which produces the F2,6-BP that activates PFK-1. It is activated by insulin and inhibited by glucagon.
  - **Glyceraldehyde-3-phosphate dehydrogenase** produces NADH, which can feed into the electron transport chain.
  - **3-phosphoglycerate kinase** and **pyruvate kinase** each perform **substrate-level phosphorylation**, placing an inorganic phosphate (P_i) onto ADP to form ATP.
- The enzymes that catalyze irreversible reactions are glucokinase/hexokinase, PFK-1, and pyruvate kinase.
- The NADH produced in glycolysis is oxidized by the mitochondrial electron transport chain when oxygen is present.
- If oxygen or mitochondria are absent, the NADH produced in glycolysis is oxidized by cytoplasmic **lactate dehydrogenase**. Examples include red blood cells, skeletal muscle (during short, intense bursts of exercise), and any cell deprived of oxygen.

Other Monosaccharides

- **Galactose** comes from lactose in milk. It is trapped in the cell by **galactokinase**, and converted to glucose 1-phosphate via **galactose-1-phosphate uridyltransferase** and an epimerase.
- **Fructose** comes from honey, fruit, and sucrose (common table sugar). It is trapped in the cell by **fructokinase**, and then cleaved by **aldolase B** to form glyceraldehyde and DHAP.

Pyruvate Dehydrogenase

- **Pyruvate dehydrogenase** refers to a complex of enzymes that convert pyruvate to acetyl-CoA.
- It is stimulated by insulin and inhibited by acetyl-CoA.

Glycogenesis and Glycogenolysis

- **Glycogenesis** (glycogen synthesis) is the production of glycogen using two main enzymes:
  - **Glycogen synthase**, which creates α-1,4 glycosidic links between glucose molecules. It is activated by insulin in liver and muscle.
  - **Branching enzyme**, which moves a block of oligoglucose from one chain and adds it to the growing glycogen as a new branch using an α-1,6 glycosidic link.
- **Glycogenolysis** is the breakdown of glycogen using two main enzymes:
  - **Glycogen phosphorylase**, which removes single glucose 1-phosphate molecules by breaking α-1,4 glycosidic links. In the liver, it is activated by glucagon to prevent low blood sugar; in exercising skeletal muscle, it is activated by epinephrine and AMP to provide glucose for the muscle itself.
  - **Debranching enzyme**, which moves a block of oligoglucose from one branch and connects it to the chain using an α-1,4 glycosidic link. It also removes the branchpoint, which is connected via an α-1,6 glycosidic link, releasing a free glucose molecule.

Gluconeogenesis

- **Gluconeogenesis** occurs in both the cytoplasm and mitochondria, predominantly in the liver. There is a small contribution from the kidneys.
- Most of gluconeogenesis is simply the reverse of glycolysis, using the same enzymes. The three irreversible steps of glycolysis must be bypassed by different enzymes:
  - **Pyruvate carboxylase** converts pyruvate into oxaloacetate, which is converted to phosphoenolpyruvate by **phosphoenolpyruvate carboxykinase (PEPCK)**. Together, these two enzymes bypass pyruvate kinase. Pyruvate carboxylase is activated by acetyl-CoA from β-oxidation; PEPCK is activated by glucagon and cortisol.
  - **Fructose-1,6-bisphosphatase** converts fructose 1,6-bisphosphate to fructose 6-phosphate, bypassing phosphofructokinase-1. This is the rate-limiting step of gluconeogenesis. It is activated by ATP directly and glucagon indirectly (via decreased levels of fructose 2,6-bisphosphate). It is inhibited by AMP directly and insulin indirectly (via increased levels of fructose 2,6-bisphosphate).
  - **Glucose-6-phosphatase** converts glucose 6-phosphate to free glucose, bypassing glucokinase. It is found only in the endoplasmic reticulum of the liver.

The Pentose Phosphate Pathway

- The **pentose phosphate pathway (PPP)**, also known as the **hexose monophosphate (HMP) shunt**, occurs in the cytoplasm of most cells, generating **NADPH** and sugars for biosynthesis (derived from ribulose 5-phosphate).
- The rate-limiting enzyme is **glucose-6-phosphate dehydrogenase**, which is activated by $NADP^+$ and insulin and inhibited by NADPH.

ANSWERS TO CONCEPT CHECKS

9.1

1.

	GLUT 2	GLUT 4
Important tissues	Liver, pancreas	Adipose tissue, muscle
K_m	High (~15 mM)	Low (~5 mM)
Saturated at normal glucose levels?	No—cannot be saturated under normal physiological conditions	Yes—saturated when glucose levels are only slightly above 5 mM
Responsive to insulin?	No (but serves as glucose sensor to cause release of insulin in pancreatic β-cells)	Yes

2. GLUT 4 is saturated when glucose levels are only slightly above 5 mM, so glucose entry can only be increased by increasing the number of transporters. Insulin promotes the fusion of vesicles containing preformed GLUT 4 with the cell membrane.

9.2

1. • Hexokinase phosphorylates glucose to form glucose 6-phosphate, "trapping" glucose in the cell. It is inhibited by glucose 6-phosphate. It is irreversible.
   - Glucokinase also phosphorylates and "traps" glucose in liver and pancreatic cells, and works with GLUT 2 as part of the glucose sensor in β-islet cells. In liver cells, it is induced by insulin. It is irreversible.
   - PFK-1 catalyzes the rate-limiting step of glycolysis, phosphorylating fructose 6-phosphate to fructose 1,6-bisphosphate using ATP. It is inhibited by ATP, citrate, and glucagon. It is activated by AMP, fructose 2,6-bisphosphate, and insulin. It is irreversible.
   - Glyceraldehyde-3-phosphate dehydrogenase generates NADH while phosphorylating glyceraldehyde 3-phosphate to 1,3-bisphosphoglycerate. It is reversible.
   - 3-Phosphoglycerate kinase performs a substrate-level phosphorylation, transferring a phosphate from 1,3-bisphosphoglycerate to ADP, forming ATP and 3-phosphoglycerate. It is reversible.
   - Pyruvate kinase performs another substrate-level phosphorylation, transferring a phosphate from phosphoenolpyruvate (PEP) to ADP, forming ATP and pyruvate. It is activated by fructose 1,6-bisphosphate. It is irreversible.
2. Fermentation must occur to regenerate NAD^+, which is in limited supply in cells. Fermentation generates no ATP or energy carriers; it merely regenerates the coenzymes needed in glycolysis.
3. The binding of 2,3-BPG decreases hemoglobin's affinity for oxygen. Fetal hemoglobin must be able to "steal" oxygen from maternal hemoglobin at the placental interface; therefore, it would be disadvantageous to lower its affinity for oxygen.

9.3

1. Galactose is phosphorylated by galactokinase, trapping it in the cell. Galactose-1-phosphate uridyltransferase produces glucose 1-phosphate, a glycolytic intermediate, thus linking the pathways.
2. Fructose is phosphorylated by fructokinase, trapping it in the cell (with a small contribution from hexokinase). Aldolase B produces dihydroxyacetone phosphate (DHAP) and glyceraldehyde (which can be phosphorylated to form glyceraldehyde 3-phosphate), which are glycolytic intermediates, thus linking the pathways.

9.4

1. Pyruvate, NAD^+, and CoA are the reactants of the PDH complex. Acetyl-CoA, NADH, and CO_2 are the products.
2. Acetyl-CoA inhibits the PDH complex. As a product of the enzyme complex, a buildup of acetyl-CoA from either the citric acid cycle or fatty acid oxidation signals that the cell is energetically satisfied and that the production of acetyl-CoA should be slowed or stopped. Pyruvate can then be used to form other products, such as oxaloacetate for use in gluconeogenesis.

9.5

1. Glycogen is made up of a core protein of glycogenin with linear chains of glucose emanating out from the center, connected by α-1,4 glycosidic links. Some of these chains are branched, which requires α-1,6 glycosidic links.
2. Glycogen synthase attaches the glucose molecule from UDP-glucose to the growing glycogen chain, forming an α-1,4 link in the process. Branching enzyme creates a branch by breaking an α-1,4 link in the growing chain and moving a block of oligoglucose to another location in the glycogen granule. The oligoglucose is then attached with an α-1,6 link.
3. Glycogen phosphorylase removes a glucose molecule from glycogen using a phosphate, breaking the α-1,4 link and creating glucose 1-phosphate. Debranching enzyme moves all of the glucose from a branch to a longer glycogen chain by breaking an α-1,4 link and forming a new α-1,4 link to the longer chain. The branchpoint is left behind; this is removed by breaking the α-1,6 link to form a free molecule of glucose.

9.6

1. Gluconeogenesis occurs when an individual has been fasting for $>$12 hours. To carry out gluconeogenesis, hepatic (and renal) cells must have enough energy to drive the process of glucose creation, which requires sufficient fat stores to undergo β-oxidation.
2.

Gluconeogenic Enzyme	Replaces
Pyruvate carboxylase	Pyruvate kinase
Phosphoenolpyruvate carboxykinase (PEPCK)	Pyruvate kinase
Fructose-1,6-bisphosphatase	Phosphofructokinase-1
Glucose-6-phosphatase	Glucokinase

3. Acetyl-CoA inhibits pyruvate dehydrogenase complex while activating pyruvate carboxylase. The net effect is to shift from burning pyruvate in the citric acid cycle to creating new glucose molecules for the rest of the body. The acetyl-CoA for this regulation comes predominantly from β-oxidation, not glycolysis.
4. The last enzyme in gluconeogenesis is glucose-6-phosphatase so patients with von Gierke's disease are unable to perform gluconeogenesis in addition to glycogenolysis. This means patients will be unable to produce glucose during periods of fasting (resulting in hypoglycemia). Furthermore, given a blocker in the gluconeogenic pathway, a buildup of intermediates (including lactate resulting in lactic acidosis) would also be expected.

9.7

1. The two major metabolic products of the pentose phosphate pathway are ribose 5-phosphate and NADPH.
2. NADPH is involved in lipid biosynthesis, bactericidal bleach formation in certain white blood cells, and maintenance of glutathione stores to protect against reactive oxygen species.

SCIENCE MASTERY ASSESSMENT EXPLANATIONS

1. **B**

The GLUT 2 receptor, **(B)**, has a high K_m and is expressed in hepatocytes of the liver. When the concentration of glucose in the blood is high, glucose is transported into the liver with first order kinetics. Also, in the pancreas, GLUT 2 and glucokinase serve as a glucose sensor. These observations together support **(B)** as the right answer.

2. **D**

The liver, like all cells, needs a constant supply of glucose; however, it is able to produce its own glucose through gluconeogenesis (cells in the kidney can also complete low levels of gluconeogenesis). The other cells listed here are absolutely dependent on a glucose source from the blood for energy, although they may also use other fuels in addition to glucose. For example, the brain can utilize ketone bodies during lengthy periods of starvation; however, it still requires at least some glucose for proper function.

3. **D**

GLUT is an abbreviation for glucose transporter and describes a family of sugar transporters with varying distributions and activities. GLUT 4 is found in adipose tissue and muscle, and mediates insulin-stimulated glucose uptake; in fact, it is the only insulin-responsive glucose transporter. Insulin acts via its receptor to translocate GLUT 4 to the plasma membrane. GLUT 4 in skeletal muscle is also stimulated by exercise through an insulin-independent pathway.

4. **B**

After an overnight fast, the liver is producing glucose and glucokinase activity would be insignificant. Glucokinase is used to trap extra glucose in liver cells as part of a storage mechanism; with low blood glucose, liver cells would be generating new glucose, not storing it. It is also in the pancreas, where it serves as a glucose sensor; if glucose levels are low, it has little activity in this tissue as well. Malate dehydrogenase, **(A)**, and α-ketoglutarate dehydrogenase, **(C)**, are citric acid cycle enzymes. Phosphofructokinase-1, **(D)**, is a glycolytic enzyme. Other enzymes used in glycolysis, the citric acid cycle, or gluconeogenesis, such as phosphofructokinase-1, would be expected to maintain normal activity after an overnight fast, using glucose derived from glycogen or gluconeogenesis, rather than orally ingested glucose.

5. **C**

This question asks for an enzyme whose role is *not* to trap sugar in the cell. Phosphofructokinase **(C)** is the rate-limiting enzyme of glycolysis. Its role is to phosphorylate fructose-6-phosphate to fructose-1,6-bisphosphate during the third step of glycolysis. Importantly, the substrate of phosphofructokinase, i.e. fructose-6-phosphate, has already been once phosphorylated before reaching phosphofructokinase. Therefore, fructose-6-phosphate is already trapped in the cell before even reaching phosphofructokinase. For this reason, it cannot be said that phosphofructokinase is used to trap sugar in the cell. By contrast, **(A)**, **(B)**, and **(D)**, can be eliminated because hexokinase phosphorylates glucose, galactokinase phosphorylates galactose, and fructokinase phosphorylates fructose, each reaction trapping the previously unphosphorylated sugar in the cell.

6. **C**

Pyruvate is converted primarily into three main intermediates: acetyl-CoA, **(B)**, for the citric acid cycle (via pyruvate dehydrogenase complex); lactate, **(D)**, during fermentation (via lactate dehydrogenase); or oxaloacetate, **(C)**, for gluconeogenesis (via pyruvate carboxylase). High levels of acetyl-CoA, which is produced during β-oxidation, will inhibit pyruvate dehydrogenase and shift the citric acid cycle to run in the reverse direction, producing oxaloacetate for gluconeogenesis. Acetyl-CoA also stimulates pyruvate carboxylase directly.

7. **D**

The pattern described for this child's glycogen demonstrates appropriate production: there are long chains of glucose monomers, implying that glycogen synthase works. There are also branch points, implying that branching enzyme, **(B)** works. During glycogenolysis, it seems that the child is able to remove individual glucose monomers and process glycogen down to the branch point itself, which requires glycogen phosphorylase, **(A)**, and α-1,4:α-1,4 transferase, **(C)**. The metabolic problem here is removing the final glucose at the branch point, which is an α-1,6 (not α-1,4) link. This requires **(D)**, α-1,6 glucosidase.

8. **C**

Citrate is produced by citrate synthase from acetyl-CoA and oxaloacetate. This reaction takes place in the mitochondria. When the citric acid cycle slows down, citrate accumulates. In the cytosol, it acts as a negative allosteric regulator of phosphofructokinase-1, the enzyme that catalyzes the rate-limiting step of glycolysis.

9. **D**

In most biochemical pathways, only a few enzymatic reactions are under regulatory control. These often occur either at the beginning of pathways or at pathway branch points. The pyruvate dehydrogenase (PDH) complex controls the link between glycolysis and the citric acid cycle, and decarboxylates pyruvate (the end product of glycolysis) with production of NADH and acetyl-CoA (the substrate for the citric acid cycle). After intense exercise, one would expect PDH to be highly active to generate ATP. ADP levels, **(A)**, should be high because ATP was just burned by the muscle. Acetyl-CoA, **(B)**, is an inhibitor of PDH, causing a shift of pyruvate into the gluconeogenic pathway. A high NADH/NAD^+ ratio, **(C)**, would imply that the cell is already energetically satisfied and not in need of energy, which would not be expected in intensely exercising muscle.

10. **B**

In this question, the right answer will be the molecule whose metabolism will be the *least* impacted by the inhibition of phosphofructokinase-1 (PFK-1). The enzyme PFK-1 catalyzes the rate-limiting step of glycolysis. So sugars that enter the glycolytic pathway after this rate-limiting step, i.e. downstream of PFK-1, would be least impacted by inhibition of PFK-1. Given this criterion, recall the metabolic pathway of fructose, choice **(B)**, which is phosphorylated and then cleaved into glyceraldehyde and DHAP, both of which enter glycolysis downstream of PFK-1. Therefore the metabolism of fructose does not depend on PFK-1, and would therefore be least impacted by the inhibition of PFK-1, making **(B)** the correct answer. By contrast, glucose, **(C)**, is metabolised using the usual glycolytic pathway, and would therefore be impacted by inhibition of PFK-1. Similarly, galactose, **(D)**, is phosphorylated and subsequently isomerized into glucose-6-phosphate, which then follows the usual pathway and would therefore be impacted by inhibition of PFK-1. And lactose, **(A)**, is cleaved by lactase into glucose and galactose. For these reasons, **(A)**, **(C)**, and **(D)** can be eliminated.

11. **B**

Based on the question stem, we can infer that the antibiotics must have been an oxidative stress on the patient (antibiotics, antimalarial medications, infections, certain foods like fava beans, and other common exposures can induce an oxidative stress). The pentose phosphate pathway is responsible for generating NADPH, which is used to reduce glutathione, one of the natural antioxidants present in the body. In individuals with glucose-6-phosphate dehydrogenase (G6PD) deficiency, NADPH cannot be produced at sufficient levels, and oxidative stresses lead to cell membrane and protein (hemoglobin) damage. Note that you do not need to actually know the disease to answer this question; merely knowing that the enzyme must be from the pentose phosphate pathway, which is involved in mitigating oxidative stress, is sufficient.

12. **A**

The irreversible enzymes in glycolysis are hexokinase (or glucokinase in liver and pancreatic β-cells), phosphofructokinase-1, and pyruvate kinase. Pyruvate dehydrogenase is not considered a glycolytic enzyme because it requires the mitochondria to function. The list below shows the correct pairing of glycolytic enzymes with gluconeogenic enzymes:

- Hexokinase or glucokinase/glucose-6-phosphatase
- Phosphofructokinase-1/fructose-1,6-bisphosphatase
- Pyruvate kinase/pyruvate carboxylase and phosphoenolpyruvate carboxykinase (PEPCK)

13. **B**

After a fast, the liver must contribute glucose into the bloodstream through two main processes: glycogenolysis (early to intermediate fasting) and gluconeogenesis (intermediate to late fasting). The other processes would continue at normal basal levels or have decreased activity after a fast.

14. **A**

A deficiency in branching enzyme would result in chains of unbranched glycogen. Since glycogen synthase is not affected, the chain length would be normal, indicating a normal abundance of α-1,4 linkages. However, a loss of branching would correspond to a decrease in α-1,6, linkages. Thus, the ratio of α-1,4 to α-1,6 would increase as division by a smaller denominator yields a larger value, making **(A)** the correct answer.

15. **A**

Hexokinase catalyzes an important irreversible step of glycolysis, but it is not the rate-limiting step. Phosphofructokinase-1 catalyzes the rate-limiting step of glycolysis. Glycogen synthase, **(B)**, catalyzes the rate-limiting step of glycogenesis; glucose-6-phosphate dehydrogenase, **(C)**, catalyzes the rate-limiting step of the pentose phosphate pathway; and fructose-1,6-bisphosphatase, >**(D)**, catalyzes the rate-limiting step of gluconeogenesis.

GO ONLINE

Consult your online resources for additional practice.

SHARED CONCEPTS

Biochemistry Chapter 4
Carbohydrate Structure and Function

Biochemistry Chapter 10
Carbohydrate Metabolism II

Biochemistry Chapter 12
Bioenergetics and Regulation of Metabolism

Biology Chapter 7
The Cardiovascular System

General Chemistry Chapter 5
Chemical Kinetics

General Chemistry Chapter 11
Oxidation–Reduction Reactions

CHAPTER 10

CARBOHYDRATE METABOLISM II: AEROBIC RESPIRATION

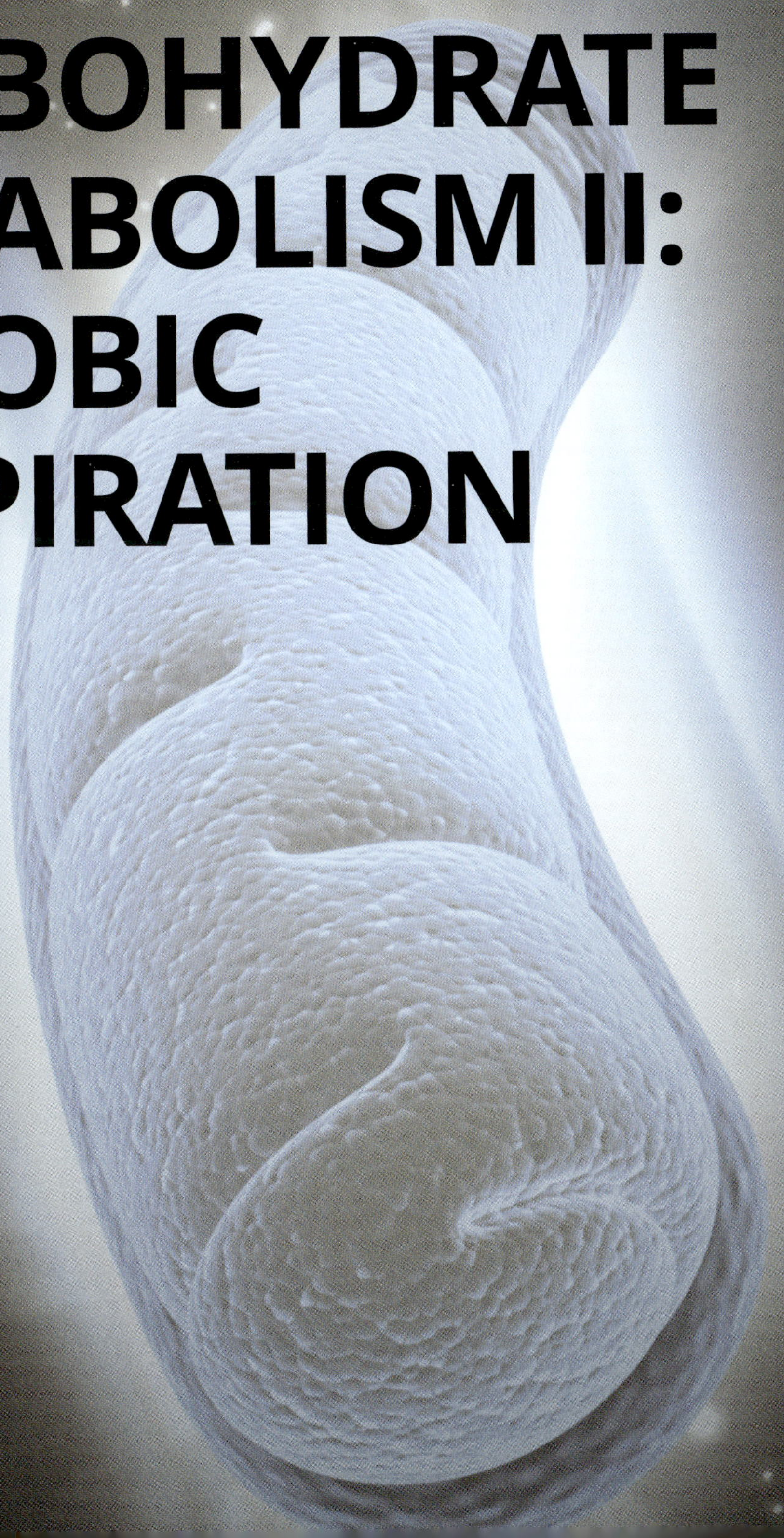

SCIENCE MASTERY ASSESSMENT

Every pre-med knows this feeling: there is so much content I have to know for the MCAT! How do I know what to do first or what's important?

While the high-yield badges throughout this book will help you identify the most important topics, this Science Mastery Assessment is another tool in your MCAT prep arsenal. This quiz (which can also be taken in your online resources) and the guidance below will help ensure that you are spending the appropriate amount of time on this chapter based on your personal strengths and weaknesses. Don't worry though—skipping something now does not mean you'll never study it. Later on in your prep, as you complete full-length tests, you'll uncover specific pieces of content that you need to review and can come back to these chapters as appropriate.

How to Use This Assessment

If you answer 0–7 questions correctly:

Spend about 1 hour to read this chapter in full and take limited notes throughout. Follow up by reviewing **all** quiz questions to ensure that you now understand how to solve each one.

If you answer 8–11 questions correctly:

Spend 20–40 minutes reviewing the quiz questions. Beginning with the questions you missed, read and take notes on the corresponding subchapters. For questions you answered correctly, ensure your thinking matches that of the explanation and you understand why each choice was correct or incorrect.

If you answer 12–15 questions correctly:

Spend less than 20 minutes reviewing all questions from the quiz. If you missed any, then include a quick read-through of the corresponding subchapters, or even just the relevant content within a subchapter, as part of your question review. For questions you got correct, ensure your thinking matches that of the explanation and review the Concept Summary at the end of the chapter.

1. During a myocardial infarction, the oxygen supply to an area of the heart is dramatically reduced, forcing the cardiac myocytes to switch to anaerobic metabolism. Under these conditions, which of the following enzymes would be activated by increased levels of intracellular AMP?
   - **A.** Succinate dehydrogenase
   - **B.** Phosphofructokinase-1
   - **C.** Isocitrate dehydrogenase
   - **D.** Pyruvate dehydrogenase

2. A patient has been exposed to a toxic compound that increases the permeability of mitochondrial membranes to protons. Which of the following metabolic changes would be expected in this patient?
   - **A.** Increased ATP levels
   - **B.** Increased oxygen utilization
   - **C.** Increased ATP synthase activity
   - **D.** Decreased pyruvate dehydrogenase activity

3. Which of the following INCORRECTLY pairs a metabolic process with its site of occurrence?
   - **A.** Glycolysis—cytosol
   - **B.** Citric acid cycle—outer mitochondrial membrane
   - **C.** ATP phosphorylation—cytosol and mitochondria
   - **D.** Electron transport chain—inner mitochondrial membrane

4. Which of the following processes has the following net reaction?

$$2\ \text{acetyl-CoA} + 6\ NAD^+ + 2\ FAD + 2\ GDP + 2\ P_i + 4\ H_2O \rightarrow 4\ CO_2 + 6\ NADH + 2\ FADH_2 + 2\ GTP + 6\ H^+ + 2\ \text{CoA–SH}$$

   - **A.** Pyruvate decarboxylation
   - **B.** Fermentation
   - **C.** Tricarboxylic acid cycle
   - **D.** Electron transport chain

5. In glucose degradation under aerobic conditions:
   - **A.** oxygen is the final electron acceptor.
   - **B.** oxygen is necessary for all ATP synthesis.
   - **C.** net water is consumed.
   - **D.** the proton-motive force is necessary for all ATP synthesis.

6. Fatty acids enter the catabolic pathway in the form of:
   - **A.** glycerol.
   - **B.** adipose tissue.
   - **C.** acetyl-CoA.
   - **D.** ketone bodies.

7. All of the following methods are used to produce acetyl-CoA in cells EXCEPT for one. What is the exception?
   - **A.** Decarboxylation of pyruvate
   - **B.** Catabolism of ketogenic amino acids
   - **C.** Reduction of fatty acids
   - **D.** Metabolism of alcohol

8. In which part of the cell is cytochrome *c* located?
   - **A.** Mitochondrial matrix
   - **B.** Outer mitochondrial membrane
   - **C.** Inner mitochondrial membrane
   - **D.** Cytosol

9. Which of the following correctly shows the amount of ATP produced from the given high-energy carriers?
   - **A.** $FADH_2 \rightarrow 1$ ATP
   - **B.** $FADH_2 \rightarrow 1.5$ ATP
   - **C.** $NADH \rightarrow 3$ ATP
   - **D.** $NADH \rightarrow 3.5$ ATP

10. Why is it preferable to cleave thioester links rather than typical ester links in aerobic metabolism?
    - **A.** Oxygen must be conserved for the electron transport chain.
    - **B.** Thioester hydrolysis has a higher energy yield.
    - **C.** Typical ester hydrolysis cannot occur *in vivo*.
    - **D.** Thioester cleavage requires more energy.

11. Which enzyme converts GDP to GTP?
    - **A.** Nucleosidediphosphate phosphatase
    - **B.** Nucleosidediphosphate kinase
    - **C.** Isocitrate dehydrogenase
    - **D.** Pyruvate dehydrogenase

12. Which of the following best explains why cytosolic NADH can yield potentially less ATP than mitochondrial NADH?
    - **A.** Cytosolic NADH always loses energy when transferring electrons.
    - **B.** Once NADH enters the matrix from the cytosol, it becomes $FADH_2$.
    - **C.** Electron transfer from cytosol to matrix can take more than one pathway.
    - **D.** There is an energy cost for bringing cytosolic NADH into the matrix.

13. In high doses, aspirin functions as a mitochondrial uncoupler. How would this affect glycogen stores?
    - **A.** It causes depletion of glycogen stores.
    - **B.** It has no effect on glycogen stores.
    - **C.** It promotes additional storage of glucose as glycogen.
    - **D.** Its effect on glycogen stores varies from cell to cell.

14. Which complex does NOT contribute to the proton-motive force?
    - **A.** Complex I
    - **B.** Complex II
    - **C.** Complex III
    - **D.** Complex IV

15. Which of the following directly provides the energy needed to form ATP in the mitochondrion?
    - **A.** Electron transfer in the electron transport chain
    - **B.** An electrochemical proton gradient
    - **C.** Oxidation of acetyl-CoA
    - **D.** β-Oxidation of fatty acids

Answer Key

1. **B** (See section 10.2)
2. **B** (See section 10.4)
3. **B** (See section 10.2)
4. **C** (See section 10.2)
5. **A** (See section 10.3)
6. **C** (See section 10.1)
7. **C** (See section 10.1)
8. **C** (See section 10.3)
9. **B** (See section 10.4)
10. **B** (See section 10.4)
11. **B** (See section 10.2)
12. **C** (See section 10.4)
13. **A** (See section 10.4)
14. **B** (See section 10.3)
15. **B** (See section 10.4)

The relevant section of the chapter to review for each question is given in parentheses after the correct answer. Detailed explanations can be found at the end of the chapter.

CHAPTER 10

CARBOHYDRATE METABOLISM II: AEROBIC RESPIRATION

In This Chapter

CHAPTER PROFILE

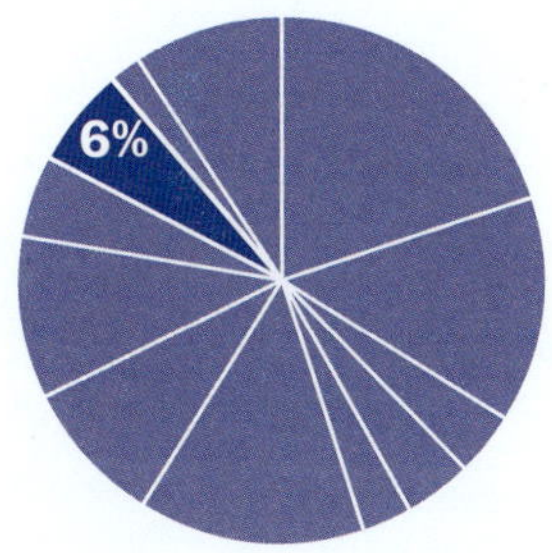

The content in this chapter should be relevant to about 6% of all questions about biochemistry on the MCAT.

This chapter covers material from the following AAMC content category:

1D: Principles of bioenergetics and fuel molecule metabolism

Introduction

Have you ever heard that eating peach pits is deadly? Before you start panicking about the snack you had during your study break, you should know that the accuracy of such a statement is debatable. While it is true that digesting peach pits can result in the formation of trace amounts of cyanide, the concentration is far too low to be clinically worrisome. Cyanide is a poison that binds irreversibly to *cytochrome* a/a_3, a protein located in the electron transport chain of the mitochondria. Why can this be deadly? Blocking the electron transport chain (ETC) inhibits aerobic respiration from yielding the ATP the body requires to function properly. Cyanide poisoning leaves cells unable to utilize oxygen for aerobic respiration because it blocks oxygen from binding to the ETC. Therefore, symptoms resemble those of tissue hypoxia: perceived difficulty breathing, general weakness, and, in higher doses, cardiac arrest followed by death within minutes.

But what about the metabolic pathways described in Chapter 9 of *MCAT Biochemistry Review*—don't they produce energy without oxygen? While glycolysis does not depend on oxygen, it only yields a net 2 ATP per molecule of glucose, which is not nearly enough to maintain the body's energy requirements. This brings us to two of the most tested topics on the MCAT: the citric acid cycle and oxidative phosphorylation (summarized in Figure 10.1).

In this chapter, we'll take a close look at what's gained when the products of glycolysis and other derivatives of metabolic pathways enter the citric acid cycle. We'll also look at how this process is regulated with regard to the substrates, products, and reactions involved. Lastly, we'll observe what happens when this cycle's products undergo oxidative phosphorylation, with particular emphasis on how the electron transport chain facilitates the process and the ATP that is yielded.

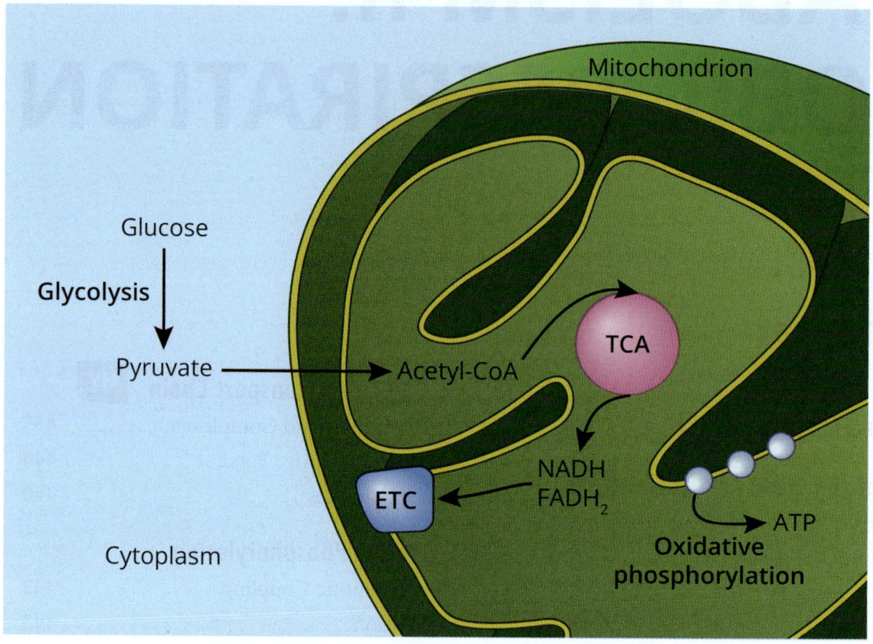

Figure 10.1 Locations of Cellular Respiration

10.1 Acetyl-CoA

LEARNING OBJECTIVES

After Chapter 10.1, you will be able to:

- Detail four potential energy sources for the synthesis of acetyl-CoA
- Identify the major inputs and outputs through the pyruvate dehydrogenase complex

The **citric acid cycle**, also called the **Krebs cycle** or the **tricarboxylic acid (TCA) cycle**, occurs in the mitochondria. The main function of this cycle is the oxidation of acetyl-CoA to CO_2 and H_2O. In addition, the cycle produces the high-energy electron-carrying molecules NADH and $FADH_2$. Acetyl-CoA can be obtained from the metabolism of carbohydrates, fatty acids, and amino acids, making it a key molecule in the crossroads of many metabolic pathways and a highly testable compound.

Methods of Forming Acetyl-CoA

Recall from Chapter 9 of *MCAT Biochemistry Review* that after glucose undergoes glycolysis, its product, *pyruvate*, enters the mitochondrion via active

MCAT EXPERTISE

Similar to the *gluco–/glyco–* terminology in Chapter 9 of *MCAT Biochemistry Review*, it is critical to keep straight the various enzymes containing *pyruvate: pyruvate dehydrogenase* (PDH), its two regulators (*PDH kinase* and *PDH phosphatase*), and *pyruvate carboxylase*, an enzyme in gluconeogenesis.

transport and is oxidized and decarboxylated. These reactions are catalyzed by a multienzyme complex called the ***pyruvate dehydrogenase complex***, which is located in the mitochondrial matrix. As we take a deeper look at the enzymes that make up this complex, as well as the substrates and products of their reactions, it is helpful to follow the carbons in the molecules. For example, the three-carbon pyruvate is cleaved into a two-carbon acetyl group and carbon dioxide. This reaction is irreversible, which explains why glucose cannot be formed directly from acetyl-CoA. In mammals, pyruvate dehydrogenase complex is made up of five enzymes: *pyruvate dehydrogenase* (PDH), *dihydrolipoyl transacetylase*, *dihydrolipoyl dehydrogenase*, *pyruvate dehydrogenase kinase*, and *pyruvate dehydrogenase phosphatase*. While the first three work in concert to convert pyruvate to acetyl-CoA, the latter two regulate the actions of PDH. Figure 10.2 shows the overall reaction for the conversion of pyruvate to acetyl-CoA. The reaction is exergonic $\left(\Delta G^{\circ\prime} = -33.4 \frac{\text{kJ}}{\text{mol}}\right)$. The complex is inhibited by an accumulation of acetyl-CoA and NADH that can occur if the electron transport chain is not properly functioning or is inhibited.

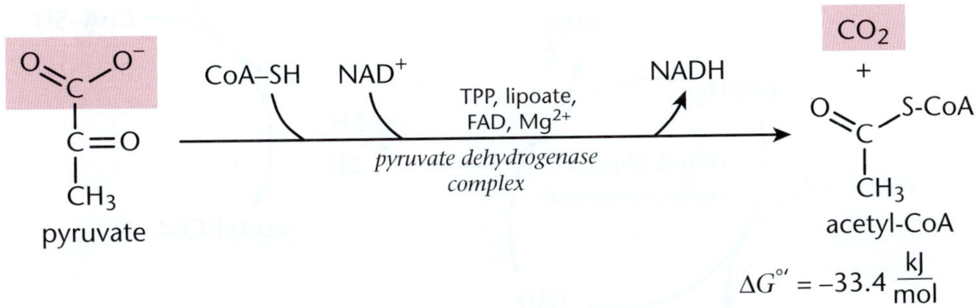

Figure 10.2 Overall Reaction of Pyruvate Dehydrogenase Complex

Note that **coenzyme A (CoA)** is written as CoA–SH in the reaction above. This is because CoA is a thiol, containing an –SH group. When acetyl-CoA forms, it does so via covalent attachment of the acetyl group to the –SH group, resulting in the formation of a thioester, which contains sulfur instead of the typical oxygen ester –OR. The formation of a thioester rather than a typical ester is worth noting because of the high-energy properties of thioesters. That is to say, when a thioester undergoes a reaction such as hydrolysis, a significant amount of energy will be released. This can be enough to drive other reactions forward, like the citric acid cycle. The pyruvate dehydrogenase complex enzymes needed to catalyze acetyl-CoA formation are listed below in sequential order, and the mechanism is shown in Figure 10.3.

- **Pyruvate dehydrogenase (PDH):** Pyruvate is oxidized, yielding CO_2, while the remaining two-carbon molecule binds covalently to *thiamine pyrophosphate* (vitamin B_1, TPP). TPP is a coenzyme held by noncovalent interactions to PDH. Mg^{2+} is also required.
- **Dihydrolipoyl transacetylase:** The two-carbon molecule bonded to TPP is oxidized and transferred to lipoic acid, a coenzyme that is covalently bonded to the enzyme. Lipoic acid's disulfide group acts as an oxidizing agent, creating the acetyl group. The acetyl group is now bonded to lipoic acid via thioester linkage. After this, dihydrolipoyl transacetylase catalyzes the CoA–SH interaction with the newly formed thioester link, causing transfer of an acetyl group to form acetyl-CoA. Lipoic acid is left in its reduced form.

REAL WORLD

In studies of pathologies that affect the central cholinergic system such as Alzheimer's disease, Huntington's disease, and even alcoholism, a decrease in glucose metabolism and oxidative phosphorylation has been observed in the brain. Ongoing research will hopefully determine if the resulting lack of acetyl-CoA could be a cause of the disease or a result of the disease. With decreased amounts of acetyl-CoA, not only is energy production a concern, but also the production of the neurotransmitter acetylcholine.

- **Dihydrolipoyl dehydrogenase:** Flavin adenine dinucleotide (FAD) is used as a coenzyme in order to reoxidize lipoic acid, allowing lipoic acid to facilitate acetyl-CoA formation in future reactions. As lipoic acid is reoxidized, FAD is reduced to $FADH_2$. In subsequent reactions, this $FADH_2$ is reoxidized to FAD, while NAD^+ is reduced to NADH.

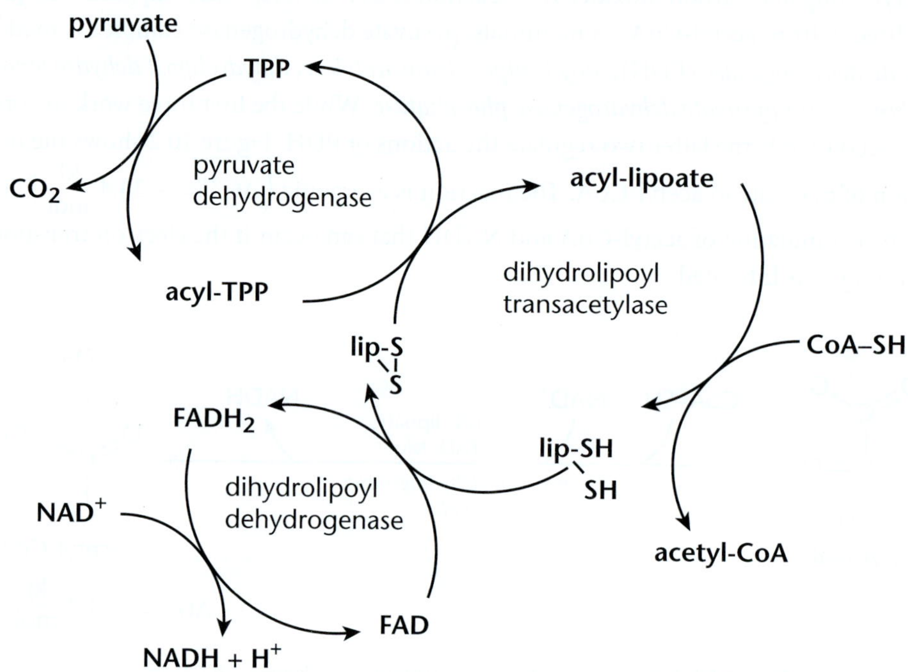

Figure 10.3 Mechanism of Pyruvate Dehydrogenase

While glycolysis is a heavily reviewed and heavily tested contributor to the production of acetyl-CoA, other pathways are capable of forming acetyl-CoA. These pathways act on fatty acids, ketogenic amino acids, ketone bodies, and alcohol. Descriptions of these pathways are provided below. The ultimate production of acetyl-CoA allows all of these pathways to culminate in the final common pathway of the citric acid cycle.

- **Fatty acid oxidation (β-oxidation):** In the cytosol, a process called **activation** causes a thioester bond to form between carboxyl groups of fatty acids and CoA–SH. Because this activated *fatty acyl-CoA* cannot cross the inner mitochondrial membrane, the fatty acyl group is transferred to *carnitine* via a transesterification reaction, as shown in Figure 10.4. Carnitine is a molecule that can cross the inner membrane with a fatty acyl group in tow. Once acyl-carnitine crosses the inner membrane; it transfers the fatty acyl group to a mitochondrial CoA–SH via another transesterification reaction. In other words, carnitine's function is merely to carry the acyl group from a cytosolic CoA–SH to a mitochondrial CoA–SH. Once acyl-CoA is formed in the matrix, β-oxidation can occur, which removes two-carbon fragments from the carboxyl end.

BRIDGE

Once formed, mitochondrial acyl-CoA can undergo β-oxidation. This process is discussed in Chapter 11 of *MCAT Biochemistry Review*.

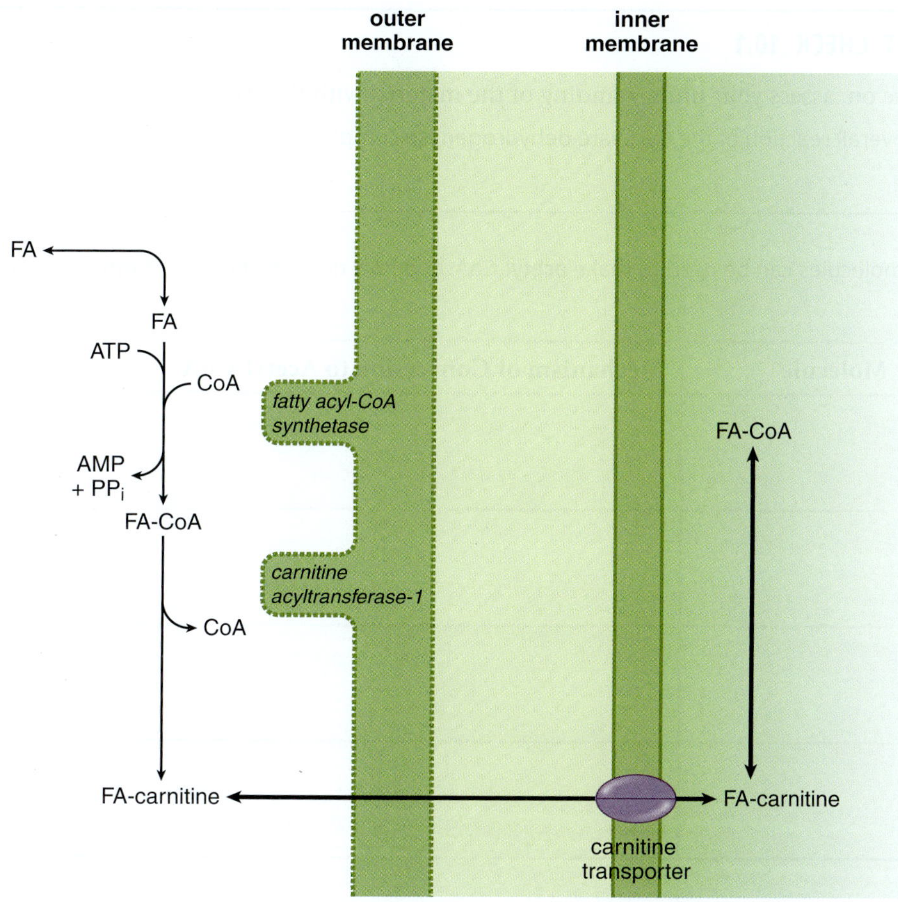

Figure 10.4 Fatty Acid Activation and Transport

- **Amino acid catabolism:** Certain amino acids can be used to form acetyl-CoA. These amino acids must lose their amino group via transamination; their carbon skeletons can then form ketone bodies. These amino acids are termed *ketogenic* for that reason. The conversion of ketone bodies to acetyl-CoA is mentioned below.
- **Ketones:** Although acetyl-CoA is typically used to produce ketones when the pyruvate dehydrogenase complex is inhibited, the reverse reaction can occur as well.
- **Alcohol:** When alcohol is consumed in moderate amounts, the enzymes ***alcohol dehydrogenase*** and ***acetaldehyde dehydrogenase*** convert it to acetyl-CoA. However, this reaction is accompanied by NADH buildup, which inhibits the Krebs cycle. Therefore, the acetyl-CoA formed through this process is used primarily to synthesize fatty acids.

REAL WORLD

While the brain normally uses glucose for energy, under conditions such as starvation, ketone bodies can become the brain's major source of energy.

MCAT CONCEPT CHECK 10.1

Before you move on, assess your understanding of the material with these questions.

1. What is the overall reaction of the pyruvate dehydrogenase complex?

____

2. What other molecules can be used to make acetyl-CoA, and how does the body perform this conversion for each?

Molecule	Mechanism of Conversion to Acetyl-CoA

10.2 Reactions of the Citric Acid Cycle **High Yield**

LEARNING OBJECTIVES

After Chapter 10.2, you will be able to:

- Explain the purpose of the citric acid cycle, including major inputs/outputs
- Identify the importance of key enzymes within the citric acid cycle
- Recall the inhibitors and activators of the enzymes citrate synthase, isocitrate dehydrogenase, and alpha-ketoglutarate dehydrogenase complex

The citric acid cycle takes place in the mitochondrial matrix and begins with the coupling of a molecule of acetyl-CoA to a molecule of *oxaloacetate*. While parts of this molecule are oxidized to carbon dioxide and both energy (GTP) and energy carriers (NADH and $FADH_2$) are produced, the other substrates and products of the cycle are reused over and over again. Although oxygen is not directly required in the cycle, the pathway will not occur anaerobically. This is because NADH and $FADH_2$ will accumulate if oxygen is not available for the electron transport chain and will inhibit the cycle. As we look at the individual reactions that take place during the citric acid cycle, it cannot be overemphasized that this process is exactly what it's called: a *cycle*, not just a series of reactions. An overview of the cycle is provided in Figure 10.5, and we'll take a deeper look at those steps below.

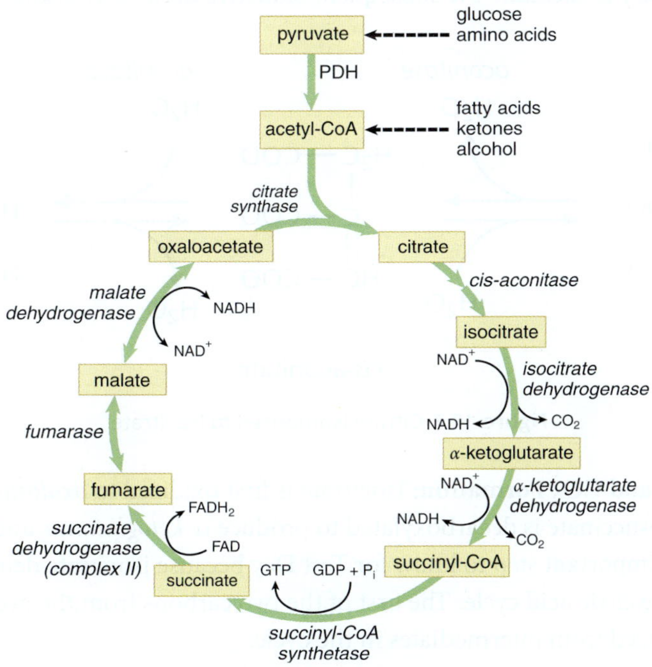

Figure 10.5 The Citric Acid Cycle

Key Reactions

Step 1—Citrate Formation: First, acetyl-CoA and *oxaloacetate* undergo a condensation reaction to form *citryl-CoA*, an intermediate. Then, the hydrolysis of citryl-CoA yields citrate and CoA–SH. This reaction is catalyzed by *citrate synthase.* As discussed in Chapter 2 of *MCAT Biochemistry Review*, *synthases* are enzymes that form new covalent bonds without needing significant energy. This second part of this step energetically favors the formation of citrate and helps the cycle revolve in the forward direction. This reaction can be seen in Figure 10.6.

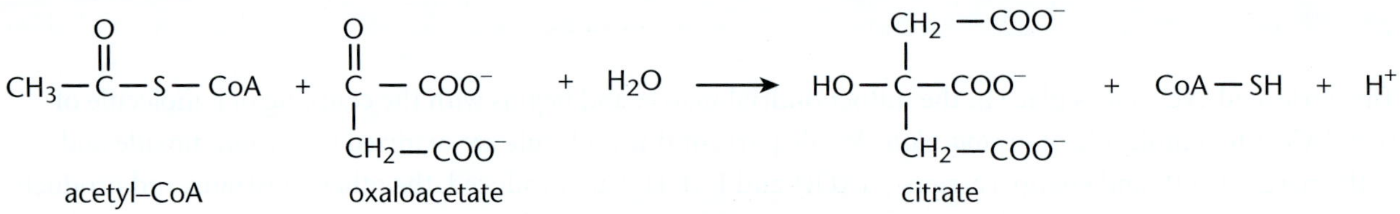

Figure 10.6 Citrate Formation

Step 2—Citrate Isomerized to Isocitrate: Achiral citrate is isomerized to one of four possible isomers of *isocitrate*. First, citrate binds at three points to the enzyme *aconitase*. Then water is lost from citrate, yielding cis-*aconitate*. Finally, water is added back to form isocitrate. The enzyme is a metalloprotein that requires Fe^{2+}. In Figure 10.7, you can see that this results in a switching of a hydrogen and a hydroxyl group. Overall, this step is necessary to facilitate the subsequent oxidative decarboxylation.

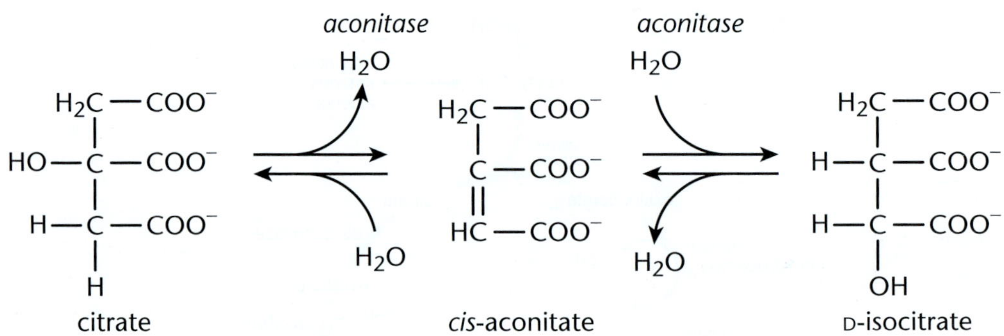

Figure 10.7 Citrate Isomerized to Isocitrate

Step 3—α-Ketoglutarate and CO_2 Formation: Isocitrate is first oxidized to *oxalosuccinate* by *isocitrate dehydrogenase*. Then oxalosuccinate is decarboxylated to produce *α-ketoglutarate* and CO_2, as shown in Figure 10.8. This is a very important step to know for Test Day because isocitrate dehydrogenase is the rate-limiting enzyme of the citric acid cycle. The first of the two carbons from the cycle is lost here. This is also the first NADH produced from intermediates in the cycle.

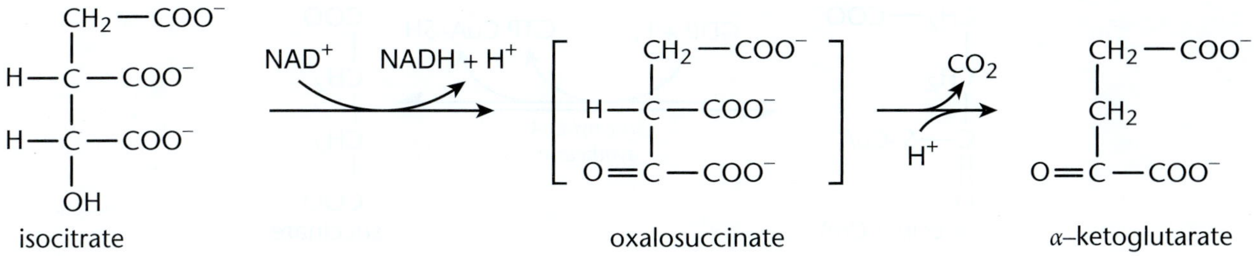

Figure 10.8 α-Ketoglutarate and CO_2 Formation

Step 4—Succinyl-CoA and CO_2 Formation: These reactions are carried out by the *α-ketoglutarate dehydrogenase complex*, which is similar in mechanism, cofactors, and coenzymes to the pyruvate dehydrogenase (PDH) complex. In the formation of succinyl-CoA, α-ketoglutarate and CoA come together and produce a molecule of carbon dioxide, as shown in Figure 10.9. This carbon dioxide represents the second and last carbon lost from the cycle. Reducing NAD^+ produces another NADH.

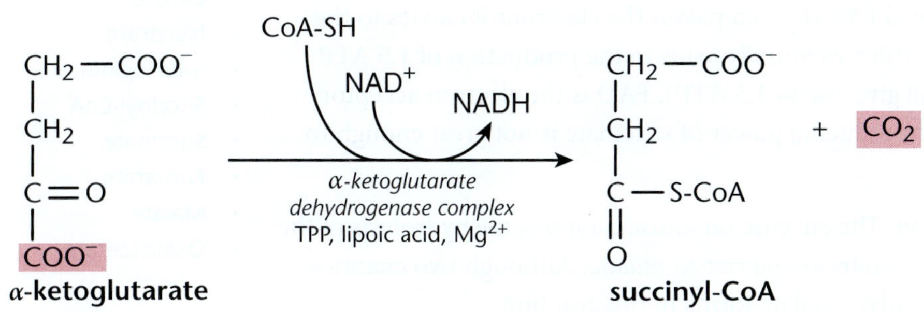

Figure 10.9 Succinyl-CoA and CO_2 Formation

Step 5—Succinate Formation: Hydrolysis of the thioester bond on succinyl-CoA yields *succinate* and CoA–SH, and is coupled to the phosphorylation of GDP to GTP. This reaction is catalyzed by *succinyl-CoA synthetase*, as shown in Figure 10.10. *Synthetases*, unlike *synthases*, create new covalent bonds *with* energy input. Recall the earlier discussion about thioester bonds with regard to acetyl-CoA: they're unique in that their hydrolysis is accompanied by a significant release of energy. Therefore, phosphorylation of GDP to GTP is driven by the energy released by thioester hydrolysis. Once GTP is formed, an enzyme called *nucleosidediphosphate kinase* catalyzes phosphate transfer from GTP to ADP, thus producing ATP. Note that this is the only time in the entire citric acid cycle that ATP is produced directly; ATP production occurs predominantly within the electron transport chain.

KEY CONCEPT

Dehydrogenases are a subtype of *oxidoreductases* (enzymes that catalyze an oxidation–reduction reaction). Dehydrogenases transfer a hydride ion (H^-) to an electron acceptor, usually NAD^+ or FAD. Therefore, whenever you see *dehydrogenase* in aerobic metabolism, be on the lookout for a high-energy electron carrier being formed!

KEY CONCEPT

Citrate *synthase* doesn't require energy input in order to form covalent bonds, but succinyl-CoA *synthetase* certainly does. Pay careful attention to enzyme names: little things can add up to careless mistakes on Test Day otherwise!

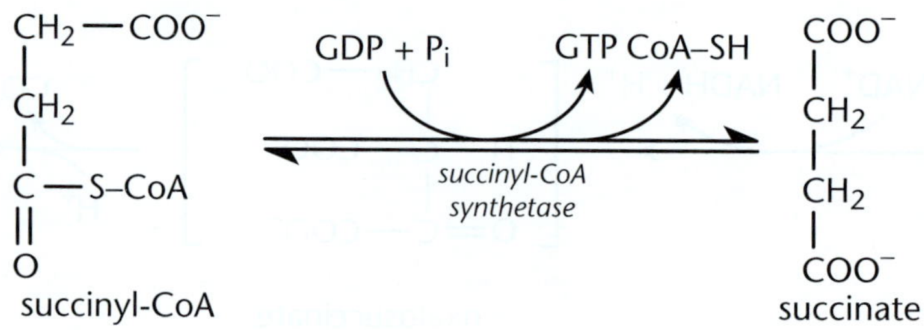

Figure 10.10 Succinate Formation

Step 6—Fumarate Formation: This is the only step of the citric acid cycle that doesn't take place in the mitochondrial matrix; instead, it occurs on the inner membrane. Let's look at why: succinate undergoes oxidation to yield *fumarate*. This reaction is catalyzed by *succinate dehydrogenase*. Succinate dehydrogenase is considered a **flavoprotein** because it is covalently bonded to FAD, the electron acceptor in this reaction. This enzyme is an integral protein on the inner mitochondrial membrane. As succinate is oxidized to fumarate, FAD is reduced to $FADH_2$. Each molecule of $FADH_2$ then passes the electrons it carries to the electron transport chain, which eventually leads to the production of 1.5 ATP (unlike NADH, which will give rise to 2.5 ATP). FAD is the electron acceptor in this reaction because the reducing power of succinate is not great enough to reduce NAD^+.

Step 7—Malate Formation: The enzyme *fumarase* catalyzes the hydrolysis of the alkene bond in fumarate, thereby giving rise to *malate*. Although two enantiomeric forms are possible, only L-malate forms in this reaction.

MNEMONIC

Substrates of Citric Acid Cycle: **P**lease, **Can I K**eep **S**elling **S**eashells **F**or **M**oney, **O**fficer?

- **P**yruvate
- **C**itrate
- **I**socitrate
- α-**K**etoglutarate
- **S**uccinyl-CoA
- **S**uccinate
- **F**umarate
- **M**alate
- **O**xaloacetate

Step 8—Oxaloacetate Formed Anew: The enzyme *malate dehydrogenase* catalyzes the oxidation of malate to *oxaloacetate*. A third and final molecule of NAD^+ is reduced to NADH. The newly formed oxaloacetate is ready to take part in another turn of the citric acid cycle, and we've gained all of the high-energy electron carriers possible from one turn of the cycle. The last steps of the citric acid cycle—from succinate to oxaloacetate—are shown in Figure 10.11.

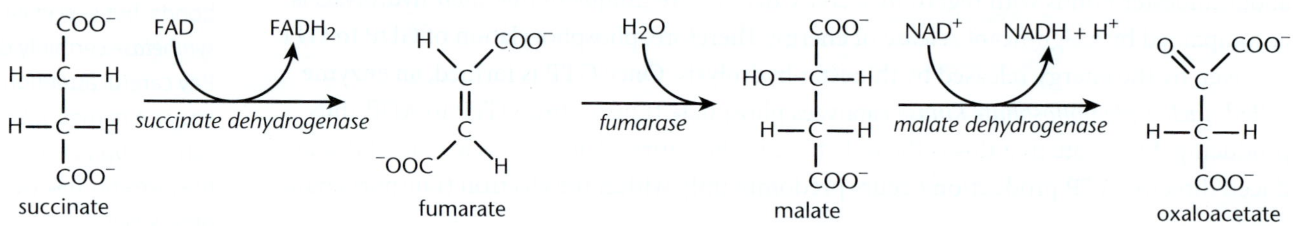

Figure 10.11 The Final Steps of the Citric Acid Cycle

Net Results and ATP Yield

Now let's take a step back and see what our net yield is from the steps we just took. Starting with the pyruvate dehydrogenase complex, recall that the products of this reaction include one acetyl-CoA and one NADH. In the citric acid cycle, steps 3, 4, and 8 each produce one NADH, while step 6 forms one $FADH_2$. Step 5 yields one GTP, which can be converted to ATP. Two carbons leave the cycle in the form of CO_2. Each NADH can be converted to approximately 2.5 ATP, while each $FADH_2$ molecule can yield about 1.5 ATP. The total amount of chemical energy harvested per pyruvate is listed below.

Pyruvate Dehydrogenase Complex:

pyruvate + CoA–SH + NAD^+ → acetyl-CoA + **NADH** + CO_2 + H^+

Citric Acid Cycle:

acetyl-CoA + 3 NAD^+ + FAD + GDP + P_i + 2 H_2O →
2 CO_2 + CoA–SH + **3 NADH** + 3 H^+ + **$FADH_2$** + **GTP**

ATP Production:

- 4 NADH → 10 ATP (2.5 ATP per NADH)
- 1 $FADH_2$ → 1.5 ATP (1.5 ATP per $FADH_2$)
- 1 GTP → 1 ATP
- Total: 12.5 ATP per pyruvate = 25 ATP per glucose

Glycolysis yields two ATP and two NADH, providing another seven molecules of ATP; thus, the net yield of ATP for one glucose molecule from glycolysis through oxidative phosphorylation is 30–32 ATP. Note that the efficiency of glycolysis varies slightly from cell to cell, so there is a range of ATP yield from one molecule of glucose.

Regulation

Let's say it's Test Day, and you see the following question: *Which of the following is an inhibitor of isocitrate dehydrogenase?* Before you start to panic, take a step back and use critical thinking. Where have we heard of isocitrate dehydrogenase—or merely isocitrate—before? The Krebs cycle. By knowing this, you can already make a fair attempt at such a question. Because energy (ATP) and energy carriers (NADH and $FADH_2$) are products of this process, it makes sense that these molecules would have a negative feedback effect on the citric acid cycle. Always consider the big picture when faced with questions like these. For now, we'll outline how regulation occurs throughout the citric acid cycle; look for the recurring theme that energy products inhibit energy production processes.

Pyruvate Dehydrogenase Complex Regulation

Even upstream from its actual starting point, the citric acid cycle can be regulated. The mechanism by which this happens is phosphorylation of PDH, which is facilitated by the enzyme ***pyruvate dehydrogenase kinase***. Thus, whenever levels of ATP rise, phosphorylating PDH inhibits acetyl-CoA production. Conversely, the pyruvate dehydrogenase complex is reactivated by the enzyme ***pyruvate dehydrogenase phosphatase*** in response to high levels of ADP. By removing a phosphate from PDH, pyruvate dehydrogenase phosphatase is able to reactivate acetyl-CoA production. Acetyl-CoA also has a negative feedback effect on its own production. When using alternative fuel sources such as fats, the acetyl-CoA production is sufficient to make it redundant to continue producing acetyl-CoA from carbohydrate metabolism—that's part of why eating a high-fat meal fills you up so quickly! ATP and NADH, as markers of the cell being satisfied energetically, also inhibit PDH.

Control Points of the Citric Acid Cycle

There are three essential checkpoints that regulate the citric acid cycle from within, and allosteric activators and inhibitors regulate all of them. The details of these mechanisms are outlined below and in Figure 10.12.

- **Citrate synthase:** ATP and NADH function as allosteric inhibitors of citrate synthase, which makes sense because both are products (indirect and direct, respectively) of the enzyme. Citrate also allosterically inhibits citrate synthase directly, as does succinyl-CoA.
- **Isocitrate dehydrogenase:** As we discussed in the beginning of this section, this enzyme that catalyzes the citric acid cycle is likely to be inhibited by energy products: ATP and NADH. Conversely, ADP and NAD^+ function as allosteric activators for the enzyme and enhance its affinity for substrates.
- **α-Ketoglutarate dehydrogenase complex:** Once again, the reaction products of succinyl-CoA and NADH function as inhibitors of this enzyme complex. ATP is also inhibitory and slows the rate of the cycle when the cell has high levels of ATP. The complex is stimulated by ADP and calcium ions.

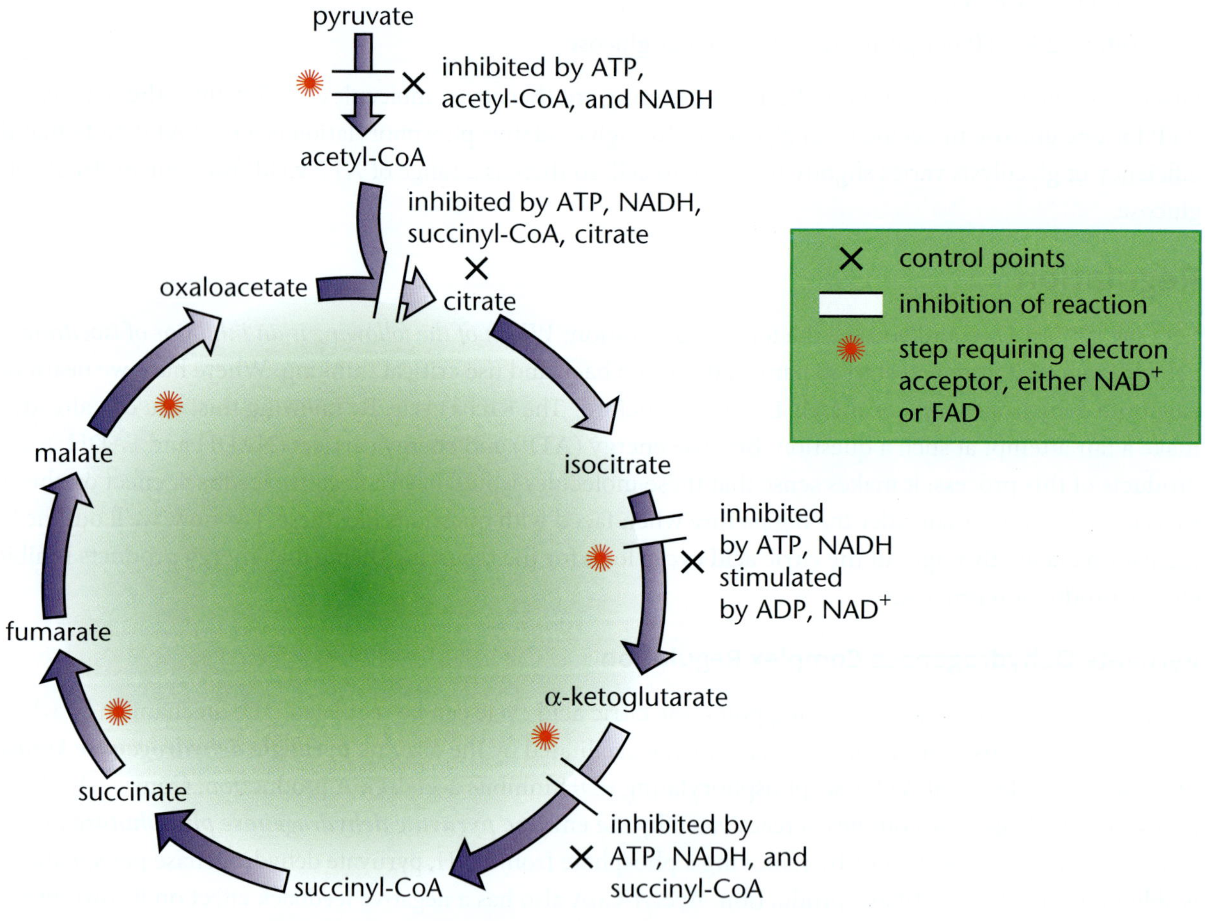

Figure 10.12 Checkpoints and Regulation of the Citric Acid Cycle

Note that high levels of ATP and NADH inhibit the citric acid cycle, while high levels of ADP and NAD^+ promote it. This isn't a coincidence! When energy is being consumed in large amounts, more and more ATP is converted to ADP and NADH is converted to NAD^+. It is therefore the ATP/ADP ratio and NADH/NAD^+ ratio that help determine whether the citric acid cycle will be inhibited or activated. During a metabolically active state, ADP and NAD^+ levels should rise as ATP and NADH levels decline, thus inducing activation at all the various checkpoints described above, replacing the energy used up by active tissues.

MCAT CONCEPT CHECK 10.2

Before you move on, assess your understanding of the material with these questions.

1. What is the purpose of all the reactions that collectively make up the citric acid cycle?

___

2. What enzyme catalyzes the rate-limiting step of the citric acid cycle?

___

3. What are the three main sites of regulation within the citric acid cycle? What molecules inhibit and activate the three main checkpoints?

Checkpoints	Inhibitors	Activators

10.3 The Electron Transport Chain High Yield

LEARNING OBJECTIVES

After Chapter 10.3, you will be able to:

- Connect the reactions of the electron transport chain to the generation of ATP
- Distinguish between the two shuttle mechanisms for NADH transport into the mitochondrion
- Recall the inputs, outputs, and major components of the four complexes of the electron transport chain:

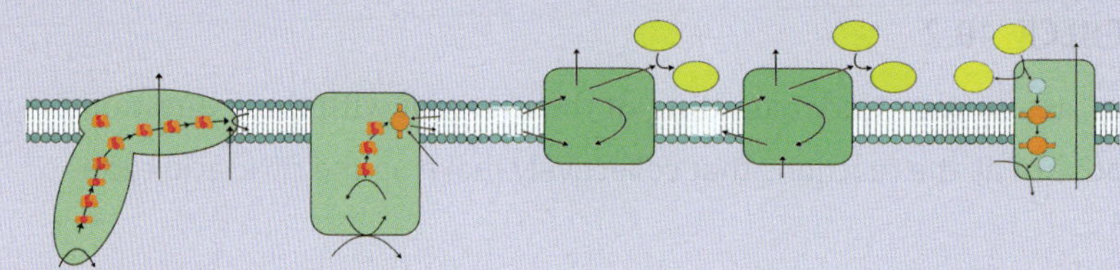

The electron transport chain is the final common pathway that utilizes the harvested electrons from different fuels in the body. It is important to make the distinction that it is not the flow of electrons but the proton gradient it generates that ultimately produces ATP. Aerobic metabolism is the most efficient way of generating energy in living systems, and the mitochondrion is the reason why. In eukaryotes, the aerobic components of respiration are executed in mitochondria, while anaerobic processes such as glycolysis and fermentation occur in the cytosol. Looking at Figure 10.13, notice how the components of the mitochondria are critical in the harvesting of energy. The citric acid cycle takes place in the mitochondrial matrix. The assemblies needed to complete oxidative phosphorylation are housed adjacent to the matrix in the inner membrane of the mitochondria. The inner mitochondrial membrane is assembled into folds called ***cristae***, which maximize surface area. It is the inner mitochondrial membrane that will be essential for generating ATP using the **proton-motive force**, an electrochemical proton gradient generated by the complexes of the electron transport chain.

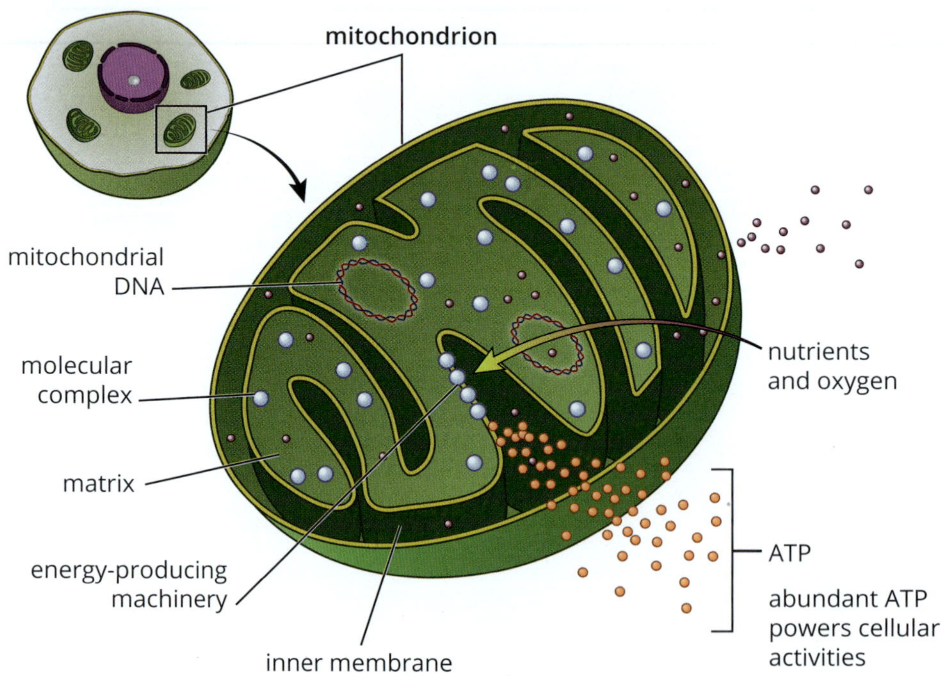

Figure 10.13 Mitochondrial Structure

The final step in aerobic respiration is actually two steps: electron transport along the inner mitochondrial membrane and the generation of ATP via ADP phosphorylation. While these two processes are actually separate entities, they are very much coupled, so explaining these steps together makes a great deal of sense. The electron-rich molecules NADH and $FADH_2$ are formed as byproducts at earlier steps in respiration. They transfer their electrons to carrier proteins located along the inner mitochondrial membrane. Finally, these electrons are given to oxygen in the form of hydride ions (H^-) and water is formed. While this is happening, energy released from transporting electrons facilitates proton transport at three specific locations in the chain. Protons are moved from the mitochondrial matrix into the intermembrane space of the mitochondria, thereby creating a greater concentration gradient of hydrogen ions that can be used to drive ATP production.

Electron Flow and Complexes

The formation of ATP is endergonic and electron transport is an exergonic pathway. By coupling these reactions, the energy yielded by one reaction can fuel the other. In order for energy to be harnessed via electron transport reactions, the proteins along the inner membrane must transfer the electrons donated by NADH and $FADH_2$ in a specific order and direction. The physical property that determines the direction of electron flow is reduction potential. Recall from Chapter 12 of *MCAT General Chemistry Review* that if you pair two molecules with different reduction potentials, the molecule with the higher potential will be reduced, while the other molecule will become oxidized. The electron transport chain is therefore nothing more than a series of oxidations and reductions that occur via the same mechanism. NADH is a good electron donor, and the high reduction potential of oxygen makes it a great final acceptor in the electron transport chain. The organizational structure of the membrane-bound complexes that make up the transport chain is diagrammed in Figure 10.14 and further detailed below.

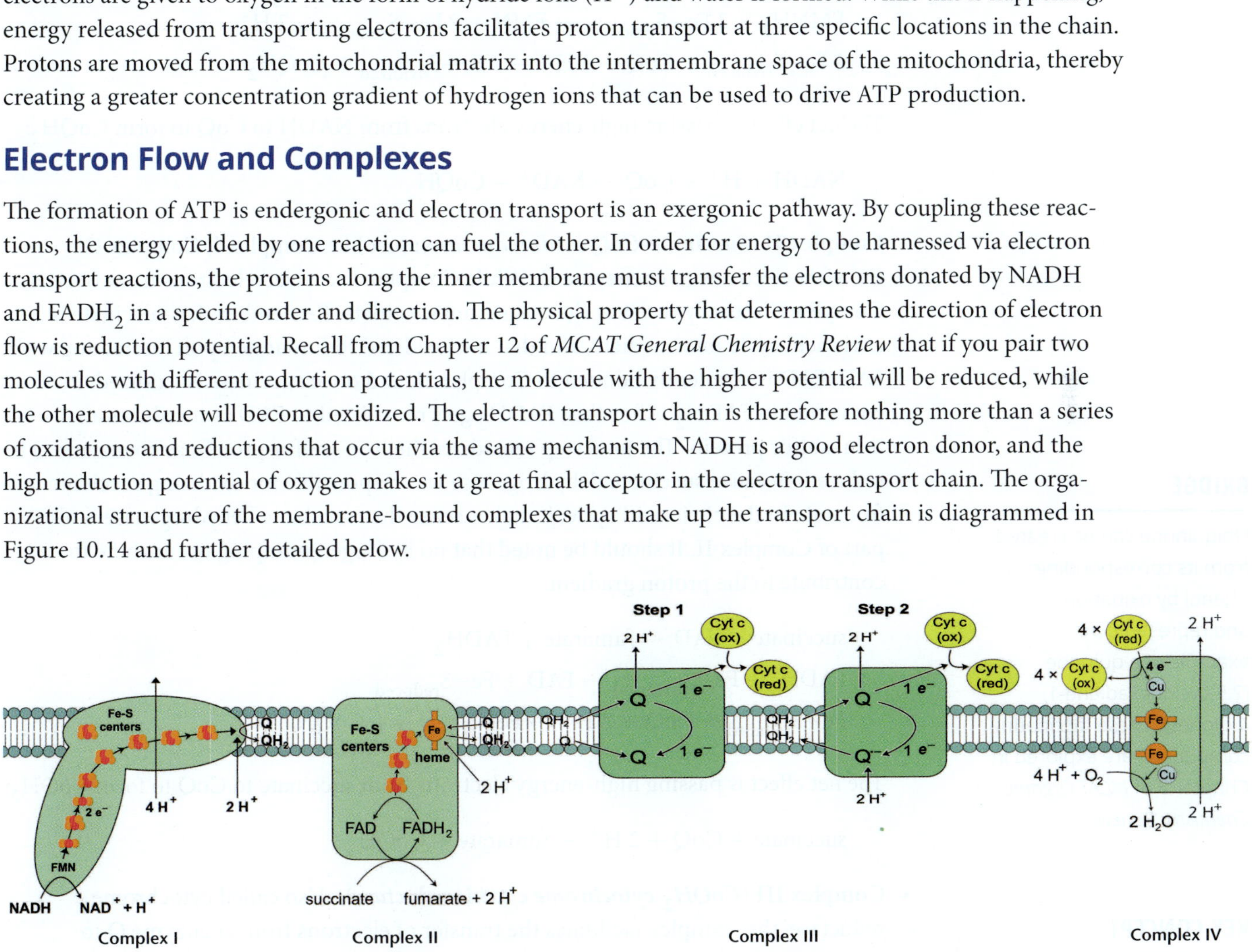

Figure 10.14 Respiratory Complexes on the Inner Mitochondrial Membrane
Steps 1 and 2 of Complex III are drawn as two separate steps here for clarity; however, the same ***$CoQH_2$-cytochrome c oxidoreductase*** *complex is used for both steps.*

- **Complex I (*NADH-CoQ oxidoreductase*):** The transfer of electrons from NADH to coenzyme Q (CoQ) is catalyzed in this first complex. This complex has over 20 subunits, but the two highlighted here include a protein that has an iron–sulfur cluster and a flavoprotein that oxidizes NADH. The flavoprotein has a coenzyme called *flavin mononucleotide* (FMN) covalently bonded to it. FMN is quite similar in structure to FAD, flavin adenine dinucleotide. The first step in the reaction involves NADH transferring its electrons over to FMN, thereby becoming oxidized to NAD^+ as FMN is reduced to $FMNH_2$. Next, the flavoprotein becomes reoxidized while the iron–sulfur subunit is reduced. Finally, the reduced iron–sulfur subunit donates the electrons it received from $FMNH_2$ to coenzyme Q (also called *ubiquinone*). Coenzyme Q becomes $CoQH_2$. This first complex is one of three sites where proton pumping occurs, as four protons are moved to the intermembrane space.

$$NADH + H^+ + FMN \rightarrow NAD^+ + FMNH_2$$
$$FMNH_2 + 2\ Fe{-}S_{oxidized} \rightarrow FMN + 2\ Fe{-}S_{reduced} + 2\ H^+$$
$$2\ Fe{-}S_{reduced} + CoQ + 2\ H^+ \rightarrow 2\ Fe{-}S_{oxidized} + CoQH_2$$

The net effect is passing high-energy electrons from NADH to CoQ to form $CoQH_2$:

$$NADH + H^+ + CoQ \rightarrow NAD^+ + CoQH_2$$

- **Complex II (*Succinate-CoQ oxidoreductase*):** Just like Complex I, Complex II transfers electrons to coenzyme Q. While Complex I received electrons from NADH, Complex II actually receives electrons from succinate. Remember that succinate is a citric acid cycle intermediate, and that it is oxidized to fumarate upon interacting with FAD. FAD is covalently bonded to Complex II, and once succinate is oxidized, it's converted to $FADH_2$. After this, $FADH_2$ gets reoxidized to FAD as it reduces an iron–sulfur protein. The final step reoxidizes the iron–sulfur protein as coenzyme Q is reduced. Because succinate dehydrogenase was responsible for oxidizing succinate to fumarate in the citric acid cycle, it makes sense that succinate dehydrogenase is also a part of Complex II. It should be noted that no hydrogen pumping occurs here to contribute to the proton gradient.

$$\text{succinate} + FAD \rightarrow \text{fumarate} + FADH_2$$
$$FADH_2 + Fe{-}S_{oxidized} \rightarrow FAD + Fe{-}S_{reduced}$$
$$Fe{-}S_{reduced} + CoQ + 2\ H^+ \rightarrow Fe{-}S_{oxidized} + CoQH_2$$

The net effect is passing high-energy electrons from succinate to CoQ to form $CoQH_2$:

$$\text{succinate} + CoQ + 2\ H^+ \rightarrow \text{fumarate} + CoQH_2$$

- **Complex III (*$CoQH_2$-cytochrome* c *oxidoreductase*):** Also called cytochrome reductase, this complex facilitates the transfer of electrons from coenzyme Q to cytochrome *c* in a few steps. Though Complex III is drawn as two separate complexes in Figure 10.14 to illustrate the sequential reactions that occur within the complex, both of these steps are occurring within the same complex, using the same coenzyme Q. The overall reaction is written below. The following steps involve the oxidation and reduction of ***cytochromes***: proteins with heme groups in which iron is reduced to Fe^{2+} and reoxidized to Fe^{3+}.

$$CoQH_2 + 2\ \text{cytochrome } c\ [\text{with } Fe^{3+}] \rightarrow$$
$$CoQ + 2\ \text{cytochrome } c\ [\text{with } Fe^{2+}] + 2\ H^+$$

In the transfer of electrons from iron, only one electron is transferred per reaction, but because coenzyme Q has two electrons to transfer, two cytochrome *c* molecules will be needed. Complex III's main contribution to the proton-motive force is via

BRIDGE

Ubiquinone can be created from its corresponding phenol by oxidation and represents an example of a quinone (2,5-cyclohexadiene-1, 4-diones). These fascinating compounds are explored in Chapter 5 of *MCAT Organic Chemistry Review*.

KEY CONCEPT

Both coenzyme Q and cytochrome *c* aren't technically part of the complexes we're describing. However, because both are able to move freely in the inner mitochondrial membrane, this degree of mobility allows these carriers to transfer electrons by physically interacting with the next component of the transport chain.

the **Q cycle**. In the Q cycle, two electrons are shuttled from a molecule of *ubiquinol* ($CoQH_2$) near the intermembrane space to a molecule of *ubiquinone* (CoQ) near the mitochondrial matrix. Another two electrons are attached to heme moieties, reducing two molecules of cytochrome *c*. A carrier containing iron and sulfur assists this process. In shuttling these electrons, four protons are also displaced to the intermembrane space; therefore, the Q cycle continues to increase the gradient of the proton-motive force across the inner mitochondrial membrane.

- **Complex IV (*cytochrome* c *oxidase*):** This complex facilitates the culminating step of the electron transport chain: transfer of electrons from cytochrome *c* to oxygen, the final electron acceptor. This complex includes subunits of cytochrome *a*, cytochrome a_3, and Cu^{2+} ions. Together, cytochromes *a* and a_3 make up *cytochrome oxidase*. Through a series of redox reactions, cytochrome oxidase gets oxidized as oxygen, becomes reduced, and forms water. This is the final location on the transport chain where proton pumping occurs, as two protons are moved across the membrane. The role proton pumping plays in ATP synthesis is an essential one that we will describe in detail next. The overall reaction is:

$$4 \text{ cytochrome } c \text{ [with } Fe^{2+}] + 4\,H^+ + O_2 \rightarrow 4 \text{ cytochrome } c \text{ [with } Fe^{3+}] + 2\,H_2O$$

KEY CONCEPT

Cyanide, mentioned in the introduction to this chapter, is an inhibitor of cytochrome subunits *a* and a_3. The cyanide anion is able to attach to the iron group and prevent the transfer of electrons. Tissues that rely heavily on aerobic respiration such as the heart and the central nervous system can be greatly impacted.

BIOCHEMISTRY GUIDED EXAMPLE WITH EXPERT THINKING

Mitochondrial disorders are genetically and clinically heterogeneous, mainly affecting energy-demanding organs due to impaired oxidative phosphorylation. Complex I deficiency (NADH:ubiquinone oxidoreductase) in the electron transport chain is the most prevalent oxidative phosphorylation disorder; treatment options are currently limited and successes are often anecdotal. There have been reports of increased muscle endurance by diet modification, and, following these reports, this study seeks to examine dietary treatment options for Complex I deficiency.

Focus on the big idea: there is a disease where Complex I of the ETC is broken

Possible treatment and goal of study: see if diet helps with symptoms

A Dutch female patient with known Complex I deficiency was subjected to HPLC-based metabolite profiling on blood plasma and urine to reveal metabolic abnormalities. The patient's muscle endurance was examined by performing a bicycle test, with dietary intake for this assessment based on the patient's usual diet, in which 34.5% of the energy was derived from fat. A dietary intervention study was then performed where the patient was instructed to consume a high-carbohydrate diet for 3 weeks with 25% of the energy derived from fat, and subsequently a high-fat diet for 3 weeks with 55% of the energy derived from fat. The same bicycle endurance test was performed after each diet. Differences in muscle endurance during the bicycle test were examined with direct substrate infusion, comparing intra-lipid infusion to glucose infusion. In each of the conditions, the mean oxygen consumption ($VO_{2\ mean}$) was also measured during the bicycle test. The results are plotted below.

Assessing how long the patient biked as a measure of muscle endurance

Five different conditions: normal diet, high-carb diet, high fat diet, glucose infused, fat infused

Also assessed oxygen consumed during the bike test

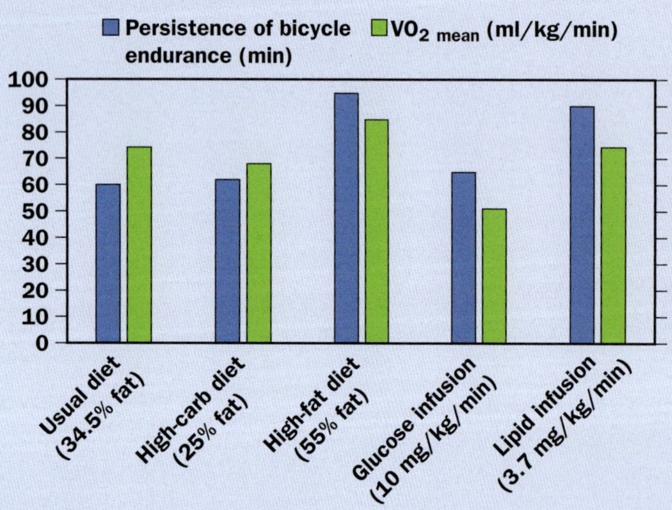

Figure 1

IVs: five diet conditions

DVs: time spent biking and how much oxygen consumed

Trend: longest bike endurance and highest oxygen consumption with high-fat diet, lowest with glucose infusion

Adapted from Theunissen, T., Gerards, M., Hellebrekers, D., van Tienen, F. H., Kamps, R., Sallevelt, S., … Smeets, H. (2017). Selection and characterization of palmitic acid responsive patients with an OXPHOS Complex I defect. *Frontiers in Molecular Neuroscience*, 10, 336. doi:10.3389/fnmol.2017.00336.

According to the data, what is the best treatment option for the patient's Complex I deficiency and why?

The question stem starts with "according to the data", so we need to ensure that we have a firm understanding of the passage presenting the context for that data. The experimental context introduced in paragraph 1 is a malfunction of Complex I in the ETC, and the hypothesis centers on dietary treatment that can help increase muscle endurance. We can recall from our content background that the ETC functions to transfer electrons from NADH and $FADH_2$ to electron acceptors, thereby creating a proton gradient to fuel the production of ATP. The coupling of the ETC to ATP synthase is termed oxidative phosphorylation and requires the availability of oxygen, as oxygen is the final electron acceptor in the ETC. Since ATP is required for muscle contraction, and oxygen is an essential component of the ETC, both high endurance and high oxygen consumption would indicate a high level of aerobic respiration.

The question asks us about the mechanism behind the best treatment option, so we must now analyze the data to see which treatment was best. According to the graph, the high-fat diet allowed the patient to endure the bicycle test the longest, and have the highest level of oxygen consumption. Therefore, the best treatment option is a diet with a high proportion of fat. This conclusion is supported by the fact that lipid infusion also gave higher values compared to glucose infusion, though not as much as the high-fat diet. The next aspect of the question to address is to examine the "why?"—why does ingesting high-fat work this way? Again, using prior knowledge, recall that metabolism of fats generates acetyl-CoA, and acetyl-CoA can then enter the citric acid cycle to produce NADH and $FADH_2$. Complex I receives electrons from NADH, and Complex II receives electrons from $FADH_2$, so in this patient with a Complex I disorder, only the production of $FADH_2$ is fueling aerobic respiration. So, why is there such a large difference between the high-fat and high-carbohydrate diets, especially considering the fact that metabolism of glucose will also eventually generate acetyl-CoA? Glycolysis (break down of glucose into pyruvate) only generates NADH, so the ratio of $FADH_2$/NADH is higher in fat metabolism vs. carbohydrate metabolism, leading to more efficient generation of energy by funneling more electron carriers to Complex II.

In summary, the best treatment for the patient's Complex I deficiency is the high-fat diet, due to increased funneling of electron carriers to Complex II.

The Proton-Motive Force

Let's take a step back and look at the proton gradient that formed as electrons were passed along the ETC. As $[H^+]$ increases in the intermembrane space, two things happen simultaneously: pH drops in the intermembrane space, and the voltage difference between the intermembrane space and matrix increases due to proton pumping. Together, these two changes contribute to what is referred to as an **electrochemical gradient**: a gradient that has both chemical and electrostatic properties. Because it is based on protons, we often refer to the electrochemical gradient across the inner mitochondrial membrane as the proton-motive force. Any electrochemical gradient stores energy, and it will be the responsibility of ***ATP synthase*** to harness this energy to form ATP from ADP and an inorganic phosphate.

NADH Shuttles

As we look at the net ATP yield per glucose, note that a range exists between 30 and 32. This is because efficiency of aerobic respiration varies between cells. This variable efficiency is caused by the fact that cytosolic NADH formed through glycolysis cannot directly cross into the mitochondrial matrix. Because it cannot contribute its electrons to the transport chain directly, it must find alternate means of transportation referred to as **shuttle mechanisms**. A shuttle mechanism transfers the high-energy electrons of NADH to a carrier that can cross the inner mitochondrial membrane. Depending on which of the two shuttle mechanisms NADH participates in, either 1.5 or 2.5 ATP will end up being produced. Let's take a look at the two mechanisms:

BRIDGE

Glycerol 3-phosphate is an important link between lipid metabolism, discussed in Chapter 11 of *MCAT Biochemistry Review*, and glycolysis, discussed in Chapter 9. Its ability to be converted to DHAP, an intermediate of glycolysis, means that the glycerol of triacylglycerols can be shunted into glycolysis for energy.

- **Glycerol 3-phosphate shuttle:** The cytosol contains one isoform of *glycerol-3-phosphate dehydrogenase*, which oxidizes cytosolic NADH to NAD^+ while forming glycerol 3-phosphate from dihydroxyacetone phosphate (DHAP). On the outer face of the inner mitochondrial membrane, there exists another isoform of glycerol-3-phosphate dehydrogenase that is FAD-dependent. This mitochondrial FAD is the oxidizing agent, and ends up being reduced to $FADH_2$. Once reduced, $FADH_2$ proceeds to transfer its electrons to the ETC via Complex II, thus generating 1.5 ATP for every molecule of cytosolic NADH that participates in this pathway, which is shown in Figure 10.15.
- **Malate–aspartate shuttle:** Cytosolic oxaloacetate, which cannot pass through the inner mitochondrial membrane, is reduced to malate, which can. This is accomplished by cytosolic *malate dehydrogenase*. Accompanying this reduction is the oxidation of cytosolic NADH to NAD^+. Once malate crosses into the matrix, mitochondrial malate dehydrogenase reverses the reaction to form mitochondrial NADH. Now that NADH is in the matrix, it can pass along its electrons to the ETC via Complex I and generate 2.5 ATP per molecule of NADH. Recycling the malate requires oxidation to oxaloacetate, which can be transaminated to form aspartate. Aspartate crosses into the cytosol, and can be reconverted to oxaloacetate to restart the cycle, as shown in Figure 10.16.

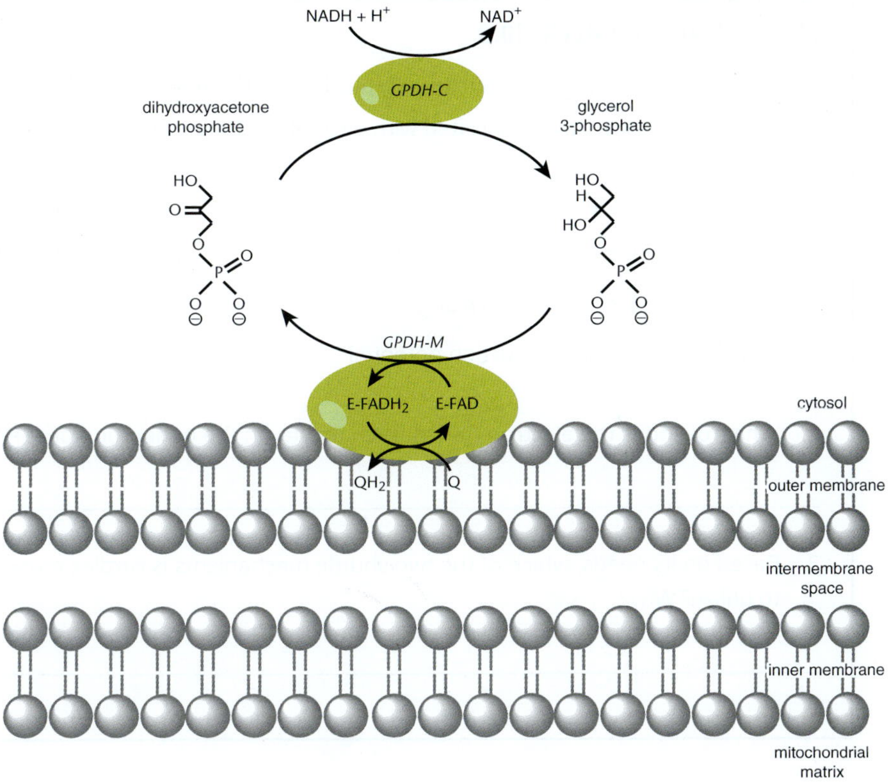

Figure 10.15 Glycerol-3-Phosphate Shuttle

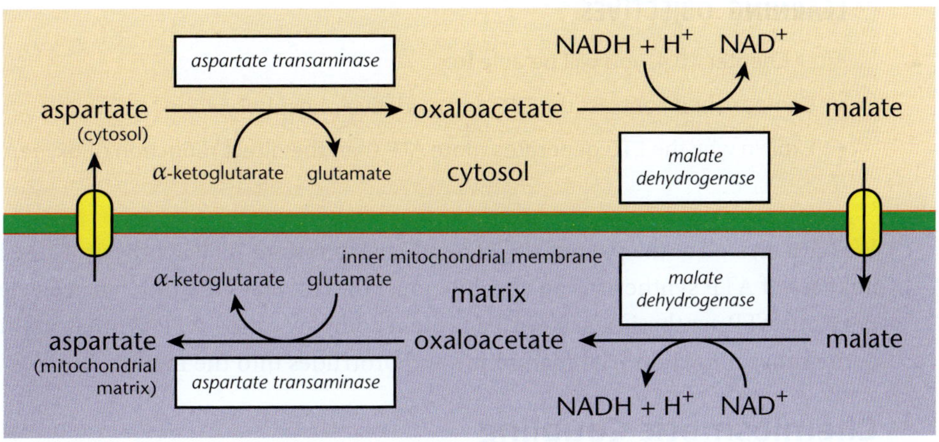

Figure 10.16 Malate–Aspartate Shuttle

MCAT CONCEPT CHECK 10.3

Before you move on, assess your understanding of the material with these questions.

1. Which complex(es) are associated with each of the following? (circle all that apply)

• Pumping a proton into the intermembrane space	I	II	III	IV
• Acquiring electrons from NADH	I	II	III	IV
• Acquiring electrons from $FADH_2$	I	II	III	IV
• Having the highest reduction potential	I	II	III	IV

2. What role does the electron transport chain play in the generation of ATP?

____

3. Based on its needs, which of the two shuttle mechanisms is cardiac muscle most likely to utilize? Why?

____

10.4 Oxidative Phosphorylation

LEARNING OBJECTIVES

After Chapter 10.4, you will be able to:

- Compare and contrast the ETC and oxidative phosphorylation
- Explain why the ETC generates more ATP than the direct reduction of oxygen by NADH

REAL WORLD

A small fraction—only 13 of approximately 100 polypeptides–that are necessary for oxidative phosphorylation are encoded by mitochondrial DNA. The significance of this fact is that mitochondrial DNA has a mutation rate nearly ten times higher than that of nuclear DNA.

We have arrived at the payout site of aerobic respiration: ATP synthesis. Knowing the nuances of ATP synthesis is an absolute must by Test Day. The link between electron transport and ATP synthesis starts with a protein complex called ATP synthase, which spans the entire inner mitochondrial membrane and protrudes into the matrix.

Chemiosmotic Coupling

The proton-motive force interacts with the portion of ATP synthase that spans the membrane, which is called the F_0 portion. $\mathbf{F_0}$ functions as an ion channel, so protons travel through F_0 along their gradient back into the matrix. As this happens, a process called **chemiosmotic coupling** allows the chemical energy of the gradient to be harnessed as a means of phosphorylating ADP, thus forming ATP. In other words, the ETC generates a high concentration of protons in the intermembrane space; the protons then flow through the F_0 ion channel of ATP synthase back into the matrix. As this happens, the other portion of ATP synthase, which is called the $\mathbf{F_1}$ **portion**, utilizes the energy released from this electrochemical gradient to phosphorylate ADP to ATP, as demonstrated in Figure 10.17. The specific mechanism by which ADP is actually phosphorylated is still a matter of debate.

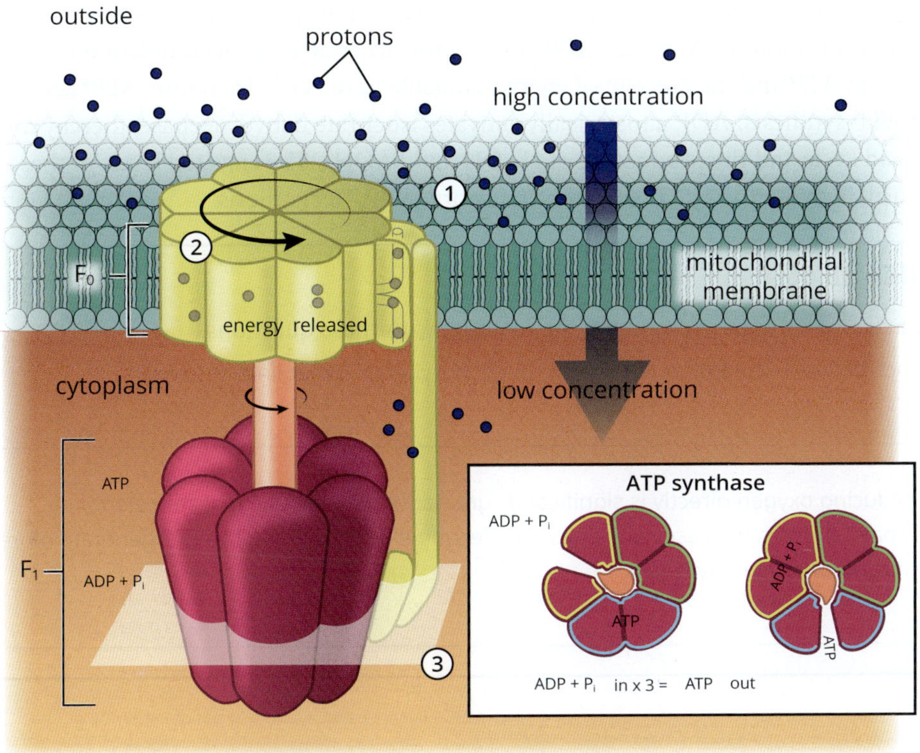

Figure 10.17 ATP Synthase Reaction
ATP synthase generates ATP from ADP and inorganic phosphate by allowing high-energy protons to move down the concentration gradient created by the electron transport chain.

Chemiosmotic coupling describes a direct relationship between the proton gradient and ATP synthesis. It is the predominant mechanism accepted in the scientific community when describing oxidative phosphorylation. However, another mechanism called **conformational coupling** suggests that the relationship between the proton gradient and ATP synthesis is indirect. Instead, ATP is released by the synthase as a result of conformational change caused by the gradient. In this mechanism, the F_1 portion of ATP synthase is reminiscent of a turbine, spinning within a stationary compartment to facilitate the harnessing of gradient energy for chemical bonding.

So we now know how we generate ATP, but how much energy was required to do so? When the proton-motive force is dissipated through the F_0 portion of ATP synthase, the free energy change of the reaction, $\Delta G^{\circ\prime}$, is $-220\ \frac{\text{kJ}}{\text{mol}}$, a highly exergonic reaction. This makes sense because phosphorylating ADP to form ATP is an endergonic process. So, by coupling these reactions, the energy harnessed from one reaction can drive another.

Regulation

Because the citric acid cycle provides the electron-rich molecules that feed into the ETC, it should come as no surprise that the rates of oxidative phosphorylation and the citric acid cycle are closely coordinated. Always think of O_2 and ADP as the key regulators of oxidative phosphorylation. If O_2 is limited, the rate of oxidative phosphorylation decreases, and the concentrations of NADH and $FADH_2$ increase. The accumulation of NADH, in turn, inhibits the citric acid cycle. The coordinated regulation of these pathways is known as

MCAT EXPERTISE

When tackling complex mechanisms such as chemiosmotic coupling on Test Day, it's easy to make mistakes such as interpreting *a pH drop* to be *a [H^+] drop* instead of a rise in proton concentration. Always read actively to avoid such mistakes.

REAL WORLD

Uncouplers are compounds that prevent ATP synthesis without affecting the ETC, thus greatly decreasing the efficiency of the ETC/oxidative phosphorylation pathway. Because ADP builds up and ATP synthesis decreases, the body responds to this perceived lack of energy by increasing O_2 consumption and NADH oxidation. The energy produced from the transport of electrons is released as heat. An example would be the fever experienced with toxic levels of salicylates, including aspirin.

respiratory control. In the presence of adequate O_2, the rate of oxidative phosphorylation is dependent on the availability of ADP. The concentrations of ADP and ATP are reciprocally related; an accumulation of ADP is accompanied by a decrease in ATP and the amount of energy available to the cell. Therefore, ADP accumulation signals the need for ATP synthesis. ADP allosterically activates isocitrate dehydrogenase, thereby increasing the rate of the citric acid cycle and the production of NADH and $FADH_2$. The elevated levels of these reduced coenzymes, in turn, increase the rate of electron transport and ATP synthesis.

MCAT CONCEPT CHECK 10.4

Before you move on, assess your understanding of the material with these questions.

1. What is the difference between the ETC and oxidative phosphorylation? What links the two?

____

2. The $\Delta G°$ of NADH reducing oxygen directly is significantly greater than any individual step along the electron transport chain. If this is the case, why does transferring electrons along the ETC generate more ATP than direct reduction of oxygen by NADH?

____

Conclusion

Both topics discussed in this chapter—the citric acid cycle and oxidative phosphorylation—take place in the mitochondria. In the mitochondrial matrix, the citric acid cycle completely oxidizes acetyl-CoA to carbon dioxide. While this happens, energy is conserved via reduction reactions, forming high-energy electron carriers such as $FADH_2$ and NADH. ATP is also indirectly formed via GTP synthesis. These electron-rich carriers then transfer their electrons to the electron transport chain, which is located along the inner mitochondrial membrane. A series of oxidation–reduction reactions occurs in specific complexes until oxygen, the final electron acceptor, gets reduced and forms H_2O. This electrical pathway generates an electrochemical proton gradient that is harnessed by ATP synthase to generate ATP. The link between these two processes is highlighted by the fact that control of the citric acid cycle is NADH-dependent. When NADH accumulates, isocitrate dehydrogenase inhibition occurs, thus stopping both the citric acid cycle and electron transport chain.

It is worth noting that, while glycolysis is a major source of acetyl-CoA for the citric acid cycle, fatty acids also serve as an important source. In the next chapter, we turn our attention to the metabolism of two other types of biomolecules: lipids and amino acids.

GO ONLINE

You've reviewed the content, now test your knowledge and critical thinking skills by completing a test-like passage set in your online resources!

CONCEPT SUMMARY

Acetyl-CoA

- **Acetyl-CoA** contains a high-energy thioester bond that can be used to drive other reactions when hydrolysis occurs.
- It can be formed from pyruvate via **pyruvate dehydrogenase complex**, a five-enzyme complex in the mitochondrial matrix that forms—and is also inhibited by—acetyl-CoA and NADH.
  - **Pyruvate dehydrogenase** (PDH) oxidizes pyruvate, creating CO_2; it requires thiamine pyrophosphate (vitamin B_1, TPP) and Mg^{2+}.
  - **Dihydrolipoyl transacetylase** oxidizes the remaining two-carbon molecule using lipoic acid, and transfers the resulting acetyl group to CoA, forming acetyl-CoA.
  - **Dihydrolipoyl dehydrogenase** uses FAD to reoxidize lipoic acid, forming $FADH_2$. This $FADH_2$ can later transfer electrons to NAD^+, forming NADH that can feed into the electron transport chain.
  - **Pyruvate dehydrogenase kinase** phosphorylates PDH when ATP or acetyl-CoA levels are high, turning it off.
  - **Pyruvate dehydrogenase phosphatase** dephosphorylates PDH when ADP levels are high, turning it on.
- Acetyl-CoA can be formed from fatty acids, which enter the mitochondria using carriers.
  - The fatty acid couples with CoA in the cytosol to form fatty acyl-CoA, which moves to the intermembrane space.
  - The acyl (fatty acid) group is transferred to carnitine to form acyl-carnitine, which crosses the inner membrane.
  - The acyl group is transferred to a mitochondrial CoA to re-form fatty acyl-CoA, which can undergo β-oxidation to form acetyl-CoA.
- Acetyl-CoA can be formed from the carbon skeletons of ketogenic amino acids, ketone bodies, and alcohol.

Reactions of the Citric Acid Cycle

- The **citric acid cycle** takes place in the mitochondrial matrix.
- Its main purpose is to oxidize carbons in intermediates to CO_2 and generate high-energy electron carriers (NADH and $FADH_2$) and GTP.
- Key enzymes and reactions:
  - **Citrate synthase** couples acetyl-CoA to oxaloacetate and then hydrolyzes the resulting product, forming **citrate** and CoA–SH. This enzyme is regulated by negative feedback from ATP, NADH, succinyl-CoA, and citrate.
  - **Aconitase** isomerizes citrate to **isocitrate.**
  - **Isocitrate dehydrogenase** oxidizes and decarboxylates isocitrate to form **α-ketoglutarate.** This enzyme generates the first CO_2 and first NADH of the cycle. As the rate-limiting step of the citric acid cycle, it is heavily regulated: ATP and NADH are inhibitors; ADP and NAD^+ are activators.
  - **α-Ketoglutarate dehydrogenase complex** acts similarly to PDH complex, metabolizing **α-ketoglutarate** to form **succinyl-CoA.** This enzyme generates the second CO_2 and second NADH of the cycle. It is inhibited by ATP, NADH, and succinyl-CoA; it is activated by ADP and Ca^{2+}.

- **Succinyl-CoA synthetase** hydrolyzes the thioester bond in succinyl-CoA to form **succinate** and CoA–SH. This enzyme generates the one GTP generated in the cycle.
- **Succinate dehydrogenase** oxidizes succinate to form **fumarate**. This **flavoprotein** is anchored to the inner mitochondrial membrane because it requires FAD, which is reduced to form the one $FADH_2$ generated in the cycle.
- **Fumarase** hydrolyzes the alkene bond of fumarate, forming **malate**.
- **Malate dehydrogenase** oxidizes malate to **oxaloacetate**. This enzyme generates the third and final NADH of the cycle.

The Electron Transport Chain

- The **electron transport chain** takes place on the matrix-facing surface of the inner mitochondrial membrane.
- NADH donates electrons to the chain, which are passed from one complex to the next. As the ETC progresses, reduction potentials increase until oxygen, which has the highest reduction potential, receives the electrons.
  - **Complex I** (**NADH-CoQ oxidoreductase**) uses an iron–sulfur cluster to transfer electrons from NADH to flavin mononucleotide (FMN), and then to **coenzyme Q** (**CoQ**), forming $CoQH_2$. Four protons are translocated by Complex I.
  - **Complex II** (**Succinate-CoQ oxidoreductase**) uses an iron–sulfur cluster to transfer electrons from succinate to FAD, and then to CoQ, forming $CoQH_2$. No proton pumping occurs at Complex II.
  - **Complex III** (**$CoQH_2$-cytochrome *c* oxidoreductase**) uses an iron–sulfur cluster to transfer electrons from $CoQH_2$ to heme, forming cytochrome *c* as part of the **Q cycle**. Four protons are translocated by Complex III.
  - **Complex IV** (**cytochrome *c* oxidase**) uses cytochromes and Cu^{2+} to transfer electrons in the form of hydride ions (H^-) from cytochrome *c* to oxygen, forming water. Two protons are translocated by Complex IV.
- NADH cannot cross the inner mitochondrial membrane. Therefore, one of two available shuttle mechanisms to transfer electrons in the mitochondrial matrix must be used.
  - In the **glycerol 3-phosphate shuttle**, electrons are transferred from NADH to dihydroxyacetone phosphate (DHAP), forming glycerol 3-phosphate. These electrons can then be transferred to mitochondrial FAD, forming $FADH_2$.
  - In the **malate–aspartate shuttle**, electrons are transferred from NADH to oxaloacetate, forming malate. Malate can then cross the inner mitochondrial membrane and transfer the electrons to mitochondrial NAD^+, forming NADH.

Oxidative Phosphorylation

- The **proton-motive force** is the electrochemical gradient generated by the electron transport chain across the inner mitochondrial membrane. The intermembrane space has a higher concentration of protons than the matrix; this gradient stores energy, which can be used to form ATP via **chemiosmotic coupling**.
- **ATP synthase** is the enzyme responsible for generating ATP from ADP and an inorganic phosphate (P_i).
  - The **F_0 portion** is an ion channel, allowing protons to flow down the gradient from the intermembrane space to the matrix.
  - The **F_1 portion** uses the energy released by the gradient to phosphorylate ADP into ATP.

- The following is a summary of the energy yield of the various carbohydrate metabolism processes:
  - Glycolysis generates 2 NADH and 2 ATP.
  - Pyruvate dehydrogenase generates 1 NADH per molecule of pyruvate. Because each glucose forms two molecules of pyruvate, this complex produces a net of 2 NADH.
  - The citric acid cycle generates 3 NADH, 1 $FADH_2$, and 1 GTP (6 NADH, 2 $FADH_2$, and 2 GTP per molecule of glucose).
  - Each NADH yields 2.5 ATP; 10 NADH form 25 ATP.
  - Each $FADH_2$ yields 1.5 ATP; 2 $FADH_2$ form 3 ATP.
  - GTP are converted to ATP.
  - 2 ATP from glycolysis + 2 ATP (GTP) the citric acid cycle + 25 ATP from NADH + 3 ATP from $FADH_2$ = 32 ATP per molecule of glucose (optimal). Inefficiencies of the system and variability between cells make 30–32 ATP/glucose the commonly accepted range for energy yield.

ANSWERS TO CONCEPT CHECKS

10.1

1. Pyruvate + CoA–SH + $NAD^+ \rightarrow$ acetyl-CoA + CO_2 + NADH + H^+
2.

Molecule	Mechanism of Conversion to Acetyl-CoA
Fatty acids	Shuttle acyl group from cytosolic CoA–SH to mitochondrial CoA–SH via carnitine; then undergo β-oxidation
Ketogenic amino acids	Transaminate to lose nitrogen; convert carbon skeleton into ketone body, which can be converted into acetyl-CoA
Ketones	Reverse of ketone body formation
Alcohol	Alcohol dehydrogenase and acetaldehyde dehydrogenase convert alcohol into acetyl-CoA

10.2

1. Complete oxidation of carbons in intermediates to CO_2 so that reduction reactions can be coupled with CO_2 formation, thus forming energy carriers such as NADH and $FADH_2$ for the electron transport chain.
2. Isocitrate dehydrogenase
3.

Checkpoints	Inhibitors	Activators
Citrate synthase	ATP, NADH, succinyl-CoA, citrate	None
Isocitrate dehydrogenase	ATP, NADH	ADP, NAD^+
α-Ketoglutarate complex	ATP, NADH, succinyl-CoA	ADP, Ca^{2+}

10.3

1. - Pumping a proton into the intermembrane space: I, III, and IV
   - Acquiring electrons from NADH: I
   - Acquiring electrons from $FADH_2$: II
   - Having the highest reduction potential: IV (reduction potentials increase along the ETC)
2. The electron transport chain generates the proton-motive force, an electrochemical gradient across the inner mitochondrial membrane, which provides the energy for ATP synthase to function.
3. The malate–aspartate shuttle. Because this mechanism is the more efficient one, it makes sense for a highly aerobic organ such as the heart to utilize it in order to maximize its ATP yield.

10.4

1. The ETC is made up of the physical set of intermembrane proteins located on the inner mitochondrial matrix, and they undergo oxidation–reduction reactions as they transfer electrons to oxygen, the final electron acceptor. As electrons are transferred, a proton-motive force is generated in the intermembrane space. Oxidative phosphorylation is the process by which ATP is generated via harnessing the proton gradient, and it utilizes ATP synthase to do so.
2. By splitting up electron transfer into several complexes, enough energy is released to facilitate the creation of a proton gradient at many locations, rather than just one. The greater the proton gradient is, the greater the ATP generation will be. Direct reduction of oxygen by NADH would release a significant amount of energy to the environment, resulting in inefficient electron transport.

SCIENCE MASTERY ASSESSMENT EXPLANATIONS

1. **B**

Phosphofructokinase-1 (PFK-1), which catalyzes the rate-limiting step of glycolysis, is the only enzyme listed here that functions under anaerobic conditions. The other enzymes are all involved in the oxygen-requiring processes discussed in this chapter. Succinate dehydrogenase, **(A)**, appears in both the citric acid cycle and as part of Complex II of the electron transport chain. Isocitrate dehydrogenase, **(C)**, catalyzes the rate-limiting step of the citric acid cycle. Pyruvate dehydrogenase, **(D)**, is one of the five enzymes that make up the pyruvate dehydrogenase complex.

2. **B**

The increased permeability of the inner mitochondrial membrane allows the proton-motive force to be dissipated through locations besides the F_0 portion of ATP synthase. Therefore, ATP synthase is less active and is forming less ATP, invalidating **(A)** and **(C)**. The body will attempt to regenerate the proton-motive force by increasing fuel catabolism, eliminating **(D)**. This increase in fuel use requires more oxygen utilization in the electron transport chain.

3. **B**

The citric acid cycle takes place in the mitochondrial matrix, not the outer mitochondrial membrane. While most citric acid cycle enzymes are located within the matrix, succinate dehydrogenase is located on the inner mitochondrial membrane.

4. **C**

It is not necessary to have all the net reactions memorized for each metabolic process to answer this question; all we need is to identify a few key reactants and products. In this case, we start with acetyl-CoA and end with CoA–SH. We also notice that in this reaction, NAD^+ and FAD are reduced to NADH and $FADH_2$, and that CO_2 is formed. The only metabolic process in which all of the above reactions would occur is the citric acid cycle, also called the tricarboxylic acid (TCA) or Krebs cycle.

5. **A**

This question is testing our general knowledge of cellular respiration. Notice that all types of cellular respiration (aerobic and anaerobic) start with the degradation of glucose by glycolysis. In aerobic respiration, oxygen is the final electron acceptor, and water is therefore produced at the end of the electron transport chain. While oxygen is needed for aerobic respiration in order to produce the optimal 32 molecules of ATP per glucose, it is not the only method by which ATP is produced. Glycolysis still provides 2 ATP per glucose without the need for oxygen, thus making **(B)** and **(D)** incorrect. Water, mentioned in **(C)**, is produced in aerobic metabolism, not consumed.

6. **C**

Fat molecules stored in adipose tissue can be hydrolyzed by lipases to fatty acids and glycerol. While glycerol can be converted into glyceraldehyde 3-phosphate, a glycolytic intermediate, a fatty acid must first be activated in the cytoplasm by coupling the fatty acid to CoA–SH, forming fatty acyl-CoA. The fatty acid is then transferred to a molecule of carnitine, which can carry it across the inner mitochondrial membrane. Once inside, the fatty acid is transferred to a mitochondrial CoA–SH, re-forming fatty acyl-CoA. Through fatty acid oxidation, this fatty acyl-CoA can become acetyl-CoA, which enters the citric acid cycle.

7. **C**

Based on the wording of this question, three choices are used to produce acetyl-CoA and one is not. As part of aerobic metabolism, decarboxylation of pyruvate by the pyruvate dehydrogenase complex yields acetyl-CoA, NADH, and CO_2. Other sources of acetyl-CoA include amino acid catabolism, beta oxidation of fatty acids, and alcohol metabolism. Fatty acids are produced via reduction of acetyl-CoA and cannot be further reduced, making **(C)** correct.

8. **C**

Cytochrome *c* carries electrons from $CoQH_2$-cytochrome *c* oxidoreductase (Complex III) to cytochrome *c* oxidase (Complex IV) as part of the electron transport chain. The ETC takes place on the inner mitochondrial membrane.

9. **B**

During oxidative phosphorylation, energy is harvested from the energy carriers $FADH_2$ and NADH in order to form ATP. One molecule of mitochondrial $FADH_2$ is oxidized to produce 1.5 molecules of ATP. Similarly, one molecule of mitochondrial NADH is oxidized to produce 2.5 molecules of ATP in the electron transport chain.

10. **B**

Thioester links release a great deal of energy when hydrolyzed, making them well-suited as respiration reaction drivers. They are particularly useful because they release more energy than typical ester cleavage. It is thioester formation, not hydrolysis, that requires a great deal of energy, making **(D)** incorrect.

11. **B**

The conversion of GDP to GTP is a phosphorylation reaction, in which a phosphate group is added to a molecule. Such reactions are catalyzed by kinases. Nomenclature is helpful here, as nucleosidediphosphate kinase is the only enzyme that contains *kinase* in its name.

12. **C**

The wording of these answer choices is critical. The electrons from cytosolic NADH can enter the mitochondrion through one of two shuttle mechanisms: the glycerol 3-phosphate shuttle, which ultimately moves these electrons to mitochondrial FAD, and the malate–aspartate shuttle, which ultimately moves these electrons to mitochondrial NAD^+. If the electrons are transferred using the malate–aspartate shuttle, then no energy is lost, making **(A)** and **(D)** incorrect. NADH cannot enter the matrix directly, making **(B)** incorrect. It is the fact that electrons can use more than one pathway—one of which loses energy that could be used for ATP synthesis—that accounts for the potentially decreased yield of ATP from cytosolic NADH.

13. **A**

Uncouplers inhibit ATP synthesis without affecting the electron transport chain. Because the body must burn more fuel to maintain the proton-motive force, glycogen stores will be mobilized to feed into glycolysis, then the TCA, and finally oxidative phosphorylation.

14. **B**

Complex II is the only complex of the ETC that does not contribute to the proton gradient. Complexes I and III each add four protons to the gradient; Complex IV adds two protons to the gradient.

15. **B**

While all of the other answers contribute to energy production, it is the electrochemical gradient (proton-motive force) that directly drives the phosphorylation of ATP by the F_1 portion of ATP synthase.

GO ONLINE

Consult your online resources for additional practice.

SHARED CONCEPTS

Biochemistry Chapter 2
Enzymes

Biochemistry Chapter 4
Carbohydrate Structure and Function

Biochemistry Chapter 9
Carbohydrate Metabolism I

Biochemistry Chapter 11
Lipid and Amino Acid Metabolism

Biochemistry Chapter 12
Bioenergetics and Regulation of Metabolism

General Chemistry Chapter 12
Electrochemistry

CHAPTER 11

LIPID AND AMINO ACID METABOLISM

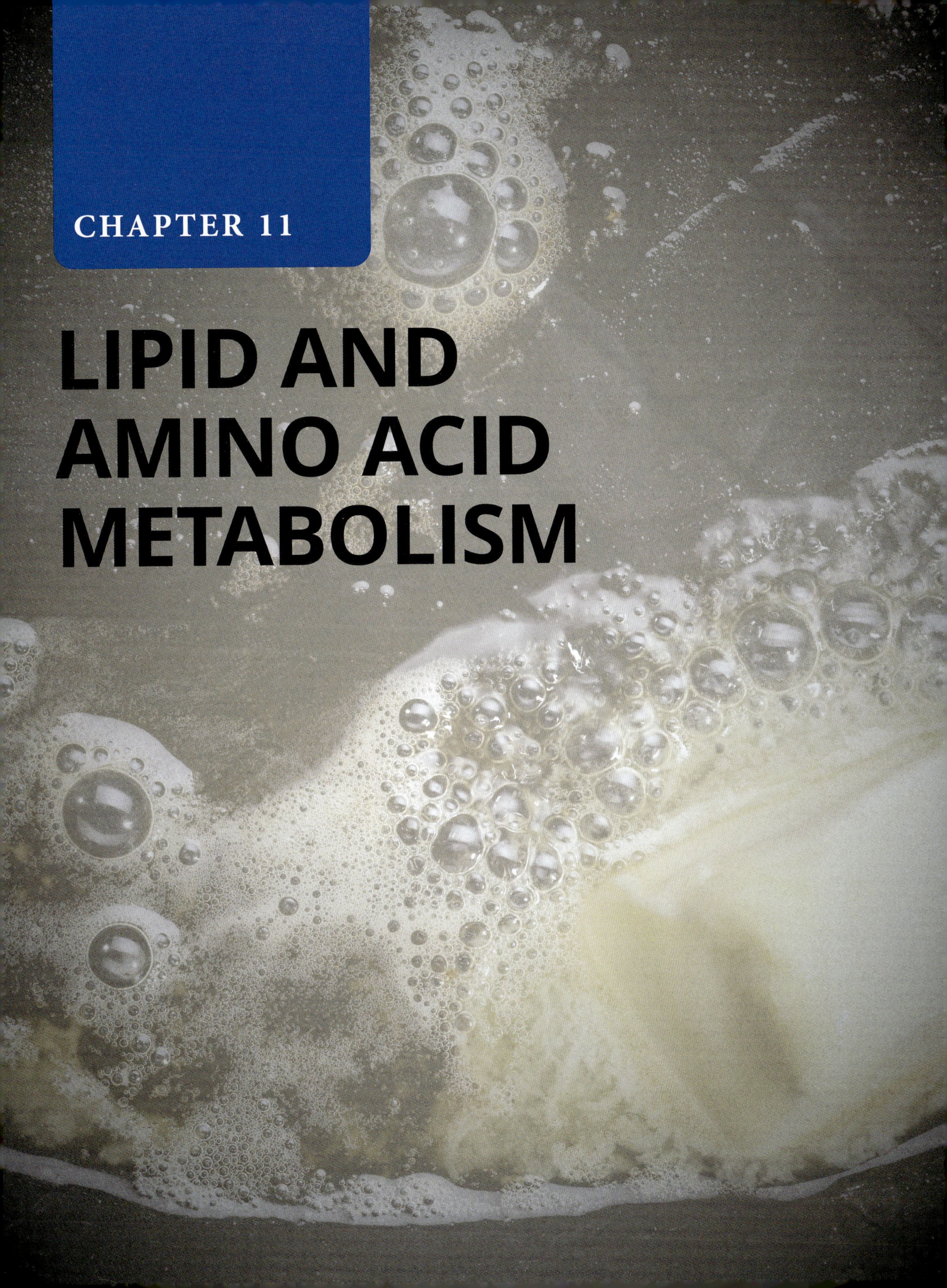

SCIENCE MASTERY ASSESSMENT

Every pre-med knows this feeling: there is so much content I have to know for the MCAT! How do I know what to do first or what's important?

While the high-yield badges throughout this book will help you identify the most important topics, this Science Mastery Assessment is another tool in your MCAT prep arsenal. This quiz (which can also be taken in your online resources) and the guidance below will help ensure that you are spending the appropriate amount of time on this chapter based on your personal strengths and weaknesses. Don't worry though—skipping something now does not mean you'll never study it. Later on in your prep, as you complete full-length tests, you'll uncover specific pieces of content that you need to review and can come back to these chapters as appropriate.

How to Use This Assessment

If you answer 0–7 questions correctly:

Spend about 1 hour to read this chapter in full and take limited notes throughout. Follow up by reviewing **all** quiz questions to ensure that you now understand how to solve each one.

If you answer 8–11 questions correctly:

Spend 20–40 minutes reviewing the quiz questions. Beginning with the questions you missed, read and take notes on the corresponding subchapters. For questions you answered correctly, ensure your thinking matches that of the explanation and you understand why each choice was correct or incorrect.

If you answer 12–15 questions correctly:

Spend less than 20 minutes reviewing all questions from the quiz. If you missed any, then include a quick read-through of the corresponding subchapters, or even just the relevant content within a subchapter, as part of your question review. For questions you got correct, ensure your thinking matches that of the explanation and review the Concept Summary at the end of the chapter.

1. Which of the following hormones does NOT directly regulate the activity of hormone-sensitive lipase in adipose tissue?
   - **A.** Insulin
   - **B.** Glucogen
   - **C.** Epinephrine
   - **D.** Cortisol

2. What is the fate of long-chain fatty acids that are contained within micelles?
   - **A.** Transport into chylomicrons released into the lymphatic system
   - **B.** Transport into chylomicrons released into the circulatory system
   - **C.** Direct diffusion across the intestine into the lymphatic system
   - **D.** Direct diffusion across the intestine into the circulatory system

3. During fatty acid mobilization, which of the following occur(s)?
   - **I.** HSL is activated.
   - **II.** Free fatty acids are released.
   - **III.** Gluconeogenesis proceeds in adipocytes.
   - **A.** I only
   - **B.** III only
   - **C.** I and II only
   - **D.** II and III only

4. How do chylomicrons and VLDL differ?
   - **A.** Chylomicrons contain apoproteins, VLDL do not.
   - **B.** Chylomicrons are synthesized in the intestine, VLDL are synthesized in the liver.
   - **C.** Chylomicrons transport triacylglycerol, VLDL transport cholesterol.
   - **D.** VLDL are another term for chylomicron remnants; they differ in age.

5. Which of the following could result from an absence of apolipoproteins?
   - **I.** An inability to secrete lipid transport lipoproteins
   - **II.** An inability to endocytose lipoproteins
   - **III.** A decreased ability to remove excess cholesterol from blood vessels
   - **A.** I only
   - **B.** III only
   - **C.** I and II only
   - **D.** I, II, and III

6. Statin drugs inhibit HMG-CoA reductase. As such, they are likely prescribed for:
   - **A.** hypercholesterolemia (high cholesterol).
   - **B.** hypertriglyceridemia (high triacylglycerol).
   - **C.** hypocholesterolemia (low cholesterol).
   - **D.** visceral adiposity (obesity).

7. What is the function of LCAT?
   - **A.** LCAT catalyzes the production of cholesteryl esters.
   - **B.** LCAT catalyzes the production of cholesterol.
   - **C.** LCAT catalyzes the transfer of cholesteryl esters.
   - **D.** LCAT catalyzes the transfer of cholesterol.

8. Which fatty acid can be synthesized by humans?
   - **A.** 12:0
   - **B.** 16:0
   - **C.** 16:1
   - **D.** 18:3

9. Which of the following best characterizes the process of fatty acid synthesis?
   - **A.** Two reductions followed by a dehydration and bond formation
   - **B.** Reduction followed by activation, bond formation, dehydration, and reduction
   - **C.** Activation followed by bond formation, reduction, dehydration, and reduction
   - **D.** Activation followed by bond formation, oxidation, dehydration, and reduction

10. Which of the following best describes how the body creates or processes ketone bodies?
    - **A.** Ketone bodies are produced in the peroxisomes of liver cells during periods of fasting.
    - **B.** Acetyl-CoA is converted into acetoacetate, 3-hydroxybutyrate, or acetone, all of which are utilized for energy.
    - **C.** Ketone bodies are produced in the mitochondria of liver cells after prolonged fasting.
    - **D.** The brain is the first organ to use ketone bodies.

11. The majority of triacylglycerols stored in adipocytes originate from:
    - **A.** synthesis in the adipocyte.
    - **B.** dietary intake.
    - **C.** ketone bodies.
    - **D.** synthesis in the liver.

12. 2,4-Dienoyl-CoA reductase is used in the oxidation of:
    - **A.** saturated fatty acids.
    - **B.** monounsaturated fatty acids.
    - **C.** polyunsaturated fatty acids.
    - **D.** cholesterol.

13. Which of the following is true regarding ketolysis?
    - **A.** Ketolysis occurs only in the brain.
    - **B.** Ketolysis occurs in the liver.
    - **C.** Ketolysis generates acetyl-CoA.
    - **D.** Ketolysis increases glucose metabolism.

14. Which of the following amino acids will provide the most energy when degraded?
    - **A.** Glycine
    - **B.** Alanine
    - **C.** Valine
    - **D.** Isoleucine

15. Which of the following is LEAST likely to result from protein degradation and processing by the liver?
    - **A.** Fatty acids
    - **B.** Glucose
    - **C.** Acetoacetate
    - **D.** 3-Hydroxybutyrate

Answer Key

1. **B** (See section 11.2)
2. **A** (See section 11.1)
3. **C** (See section 11.2)
4. **B** (See section 11.3)
5. **D** (See section 11.3)
6. **A** (See section 11.4)
7. **A** (See section 11.4)
8. **B** (See section 11.5)
9. **C** (See section 11.5)
10. **C** (See section 11.6)
11. **D** (See section 11.5)
12. **C** (See section 11.5)
13. **C** (See section 11.6)
14. **D** (See section 11.7)
15. **A** (See section 11.7)

The relevant section of the chapter to review for each question is given in parentheses after the correct answer. Detailed explanations can be found at the end of the chapter.

CHAPTER 11

LIPID AND AMINO ACID METABOLISM

In This Chapter

CHAPTER PROFILE

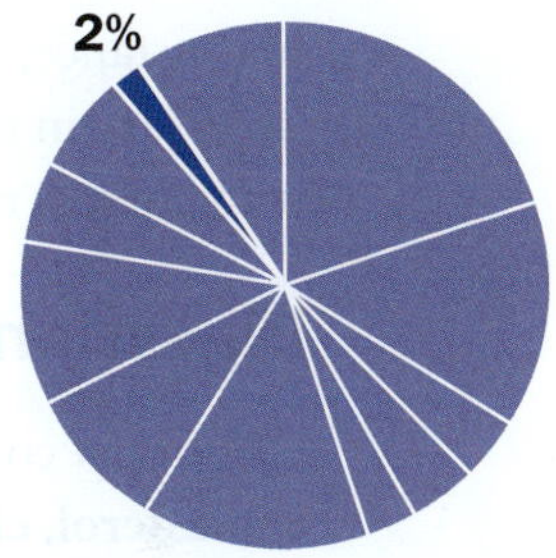

The content in this chapter should be relevant to about 2% of all questions about Biochemistry on the MCAT.

This chapter covers material from the following AAMC content category:

1D: Principles of bioenergetics and fuel molecule metabolism

MCAT EXPERTISE

Chapter 11 contains some of the most complex and difficult material in this book. However, the content within this chapter is not particularly high-yield on Test Day, as can be seen in the chapter profile above. This chapter is still worth reviewing, but its content will be most relevant to students seeking full mastery of all testable content for an extremely competitive score.

Introduction

For weeks before the winter season begins, bears and certain mammals increase their food intake to prepare for hibernation. During this time, they increase their weight by storing energy. Different organisms store fuel and supplies in different ways. Hamsters store extra food in pouches in their cheeks. Cacti absorb and conserve water in preparation for dry seasons. But hibernating animals store extra calories as fat. Over the course of the winter, fat stores are mobilized and metabolized for basic bodily functions, which are minimal during hibernation. Come spring and summer, these reserves will be replenished in preparation for the next winter season. Humans also store extra energy as fat. While we may not hibernate through the winter, fat stores allow us to store energy to use during prolonged periods without food.

As discussed in Chapter 8 of *MCAT Biochemistry Review*, lipids play a major role in maintaining the structure and function of cells; however, they also have important roles as storage molecules for energy and in biological signaling. In this chapter, we'll examine the metabolism of lipids, starting with ingestion of food particles and continuing through absorption, transport, and energy catabolism. We will also cover energy storage via lipid synthesis, as well as the metabolism of cholesterol and ketone bodies. In addition, we will learn about how protein degradation feeds into lipid and carbohydrate pathways and the urea cycle.

11.1 Lipid Digestion and Absorption

LEARNING OBJECTIVES

After Chapter 11.1, you will be able to:

- Differentiate between lipid digestion in the stomach and lipid digestion in the intestines
- Identify the methods by which lipids can enter circulation
- Describe the structure of a micelle

In addition to being a major source of energy in the body, lipids serve a variety of other functions in the body. For instance, some fat-soluble vitamins play roles as coenzymes; prostaglandins and steroid hormones are necessary in the control and maintenance of homeostasis. Aberrant lipid metabolism may also be associated with clinical manifestations such as atherosclerosis and obesity.

Digestion

Dietary fat consists mainly of **triacylglycerols**, with the remainder comprised of **cholesterol**, **cholesteryl esters**, **phospholipids**, and free **fatty acids**. Lipid digestion is minimal in the mouth and stomach; lipids are transported to the small intestine essentially intact. Upon entry into the duodenum, **emulsification** occurs, which is the mixing of two normally immiscible liquids (in this case, fat and water). Formation of an emulsion increases the surface area of the lipid, which permits greater enzymatic interaction and processing. Emulsification is aided by bile, which contains **bile salts**, **pigments**, and **cholesterol**; bile is secreted by the liver and stored in the gallbladder. Finally, the pancreas secretes ***pancreatic lipase***, ***colipase***, and ***cholesterol esterase*** into the small intestine; together, these enzymes hydrolyze the lipid components to *2-monoacylglycerol*, free fatty acids, and cholesterol. Figure 11.1 summarizes the digestion and absorption of dietary lipid components.

BRIDGE

Digestion is covered in Chapter 9 of *MCAT Biology Review*

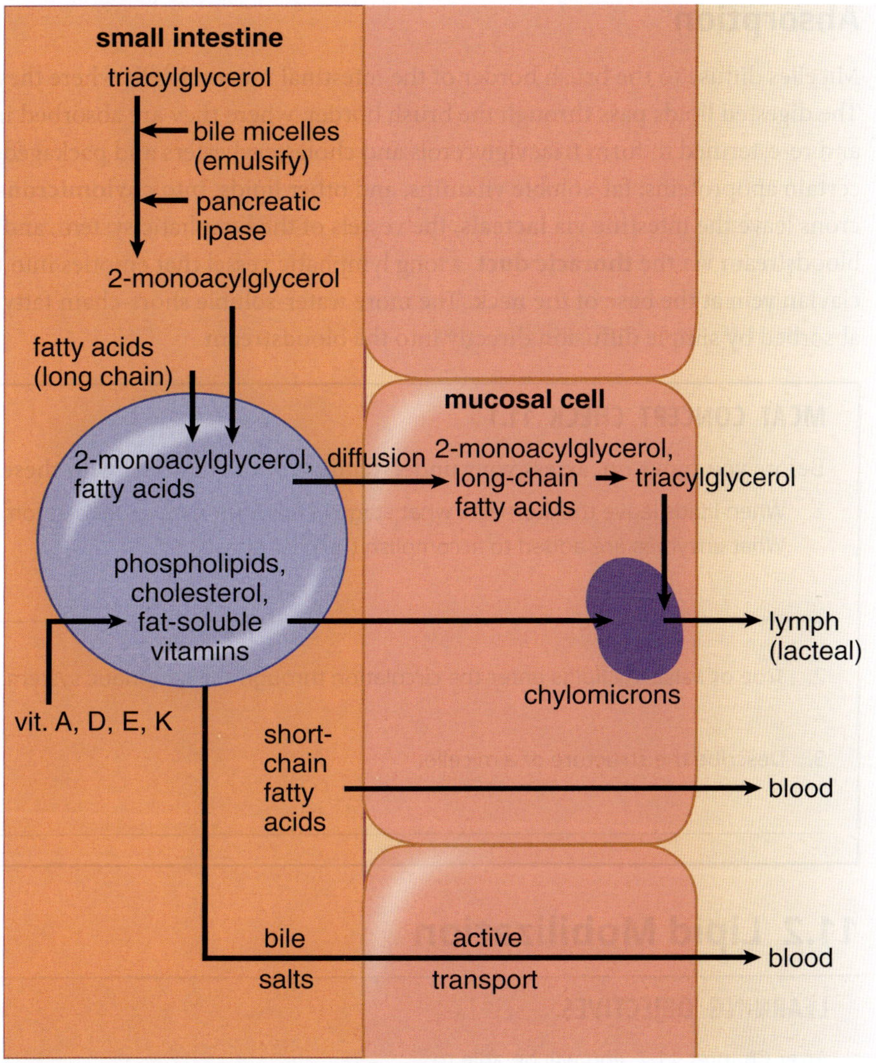

Figure 11.1 Absorption of Lipids

Micelle Formation

Emulsification is followed by absorption of fats by intestinal cells. Free fatty acids, cholesterol, 2-monoacylglycerol, and bile salts contribute to the formation of **micelles**, which are clusters of amphipathic lipids that are soluble in the aqueous environment of the intestinal lumen. Essentially, micelles are water-soluble spheres with a lipid-soluble interior. Micelles are vital in digestion, transport, and absorption of lipid-soluble substances starting from the duodenum all the way to the end of the ileum. At the end of the ileum, bile salts are actively reabsorbed and recycled; any fat that remains in the intestine will pass into the colon, and ultimately ends up in the stool.

BRIDGE

Absorption in the small intestine and colon follows a characteristic pattern. This is a good time to review digestion, discussed in Chapter 9 of *MCAT Biology Review*, to create a complete schema for the absorption and metabolism of all the macronutrients.

Absorption

Micelles diffuse to the brush border of the intestinal mucosal cells where they are absorbed. The digested lipids pass through the brush border, where they are absorbed into the mucosa and re-esterified to form triacylglycerols and cholesteryl esters and packaged, along with certain apoproteins, fat-soluble vitamins, and other lipids, into **chylomicrons**. Chylomicrons leave the intestine via **lacteals**, the vessels of the lymphatic system, and re-enter the bloodstream via the **thoracic duct**, a long lymphatic vessel that empties into the left subclavian vein at the base of the neck. The more water-soluble short-chain fatty acids can be absorbed by simple diffusion directly into the bloodstream.

MCAT CONCEPT CHECK 11.1

Before you move on, assess your understanding of the material with these questions.

1. When lipids leave the stomach, what stages of digestion have been accomplished? What enzymes are added to accomplish the next phase?

___

2. True or False: All lipids enter the circulation through the lymphatic system.

3. Describe the structure of a micelle.

___

11.2 Lipid Mobilization

LEARNING OBJECTIVES

After Chapter 11.2, you will be able to:

- Identify the conditions and hormones that promote lipid mobilization
- Predict the ratio of free fatty acids per glycerol molecule broken down via lipid mobilization

At night, the body is in the postabsorptive state, utilizing energy stores instead of food for fuel. In the postabsorptive state, fatty acids are released from adipose tissue and used for energy. Although human adipose tissue does not respond directly to glucagon, a fall in insulin levels activates a ***hormone-sensitive lipase*** (**HSL**) that hydrolyzes triacylglycerols, yielding fatty acids and glycerol. Epinephrine and cortisol can also activate HSL, as shown in Figure 11.2; we will discuss the effects of these hormones on metabolism in more detail in the next chapter. Released glycerol from fat may be transported to the liver for glycolysis or gluconeogenesis. HSL is effective within adipose cells, but ***lipoprotein lipase*** (**LPL**) is necessary for the metabolism of chylomicrons and very-low-density lipoproteins (VLDL). LPL is an enzyme that can release free fatty acids from triacylglycerols in these lipoproteins.

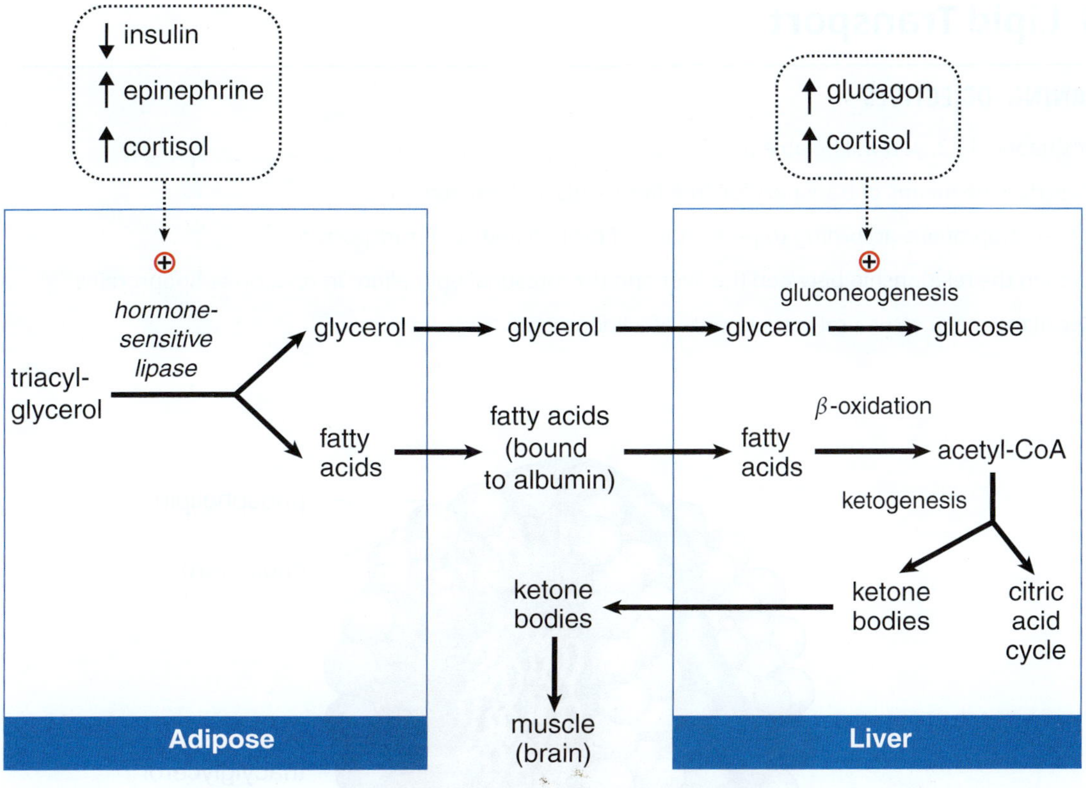

Figure 11.2 Mobilization of Triacylglycerols and Metabolism by the Liver

MCAT CONCEPT CHECK 11.2

Before you move on, assess your understanding of the material with these questions.

1. A patient who has diabetes begins insulin injections for management of blood glucose levels. What is the expected impact on the patient's weight?

____

2. What is the ratio of free fatty acids to glycerol produced through lipid mobilization?

____

11.3 Lipid Transport

LEARNING OBJECTIVES

After Chapter 11.3, you will be able to:

- Describe the means of transport for free fatty acids in the blood
- Order lipoproteins according to percentage of protein and lipid transported
- Explain the relationship between the liver and the intestinal epithelium in relation to lipoproteins
- Recall the major structural components of a lipoprotein

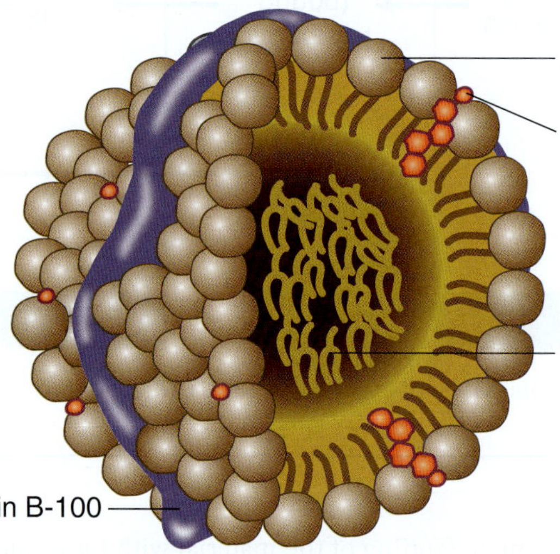

Figure 11.3 Lipoprotein Structure

While free fatty acids are transported through the blood in association with albumin, a carrier protein, triacylglycerol and cholesterol are transported in the blood as **lipoproteins**: aggregates of **apolipoproteins** and lipids, as shown in Figure 11.3. Lipoproteins are named according to their density, which increases in direct proportion to the percentage of protein in the particle. Chylomicrons are the least dense, with the highest fat-to-protein ratio. VLDL (very-low-density lipoprotein) is slightly more dense, followed by IDL (intermediate-density), LDL (low-density), and HDL (high-density). The main functions of each lipoprotein are shown in Table 11.1. Note that chylomicrons and VLDL primarily carry triacylglycerols, but also contain small quantities of cholesteryl esters. LDL and HDL are primarily cholesterol transport molecules.

Lipoprotein	Functions
Chylomicrons	Transport dietary triacylglycerols, cholesterol, and cholesteryl esters from intestine to tissues
VLDL	Transports triacylglycerols and fatty acids from liver to tissues
IDL (VLDL remnants)	Picks up cholesteryl esters from HDL to become LDL Picked up by the liver
LDL	Delivers cholesterol into cells
HDL	Picks up cholesterol accumulating in blood vessels Delivers cholesterol to liver and steroidogenic tissues Transfers apolipoproteins to other lipoproteins

Table 11.1 Classes of Lipoproteins

Chylomicrons

Chylomicrons are highly soluble in both lymphatic fluid and blood and function in the transport of dietary triacylglycerols, cholesterol, and cholesteryl esters to other tissues. Assembly of chylomicrons occurs in the intestinal lining and results in a nascent chylomicron that contains lipids and apolipoproteins.

VLDL (Very-Low-Density Lipoprotein)

VLDL metabolism is similar to that of chylomicrons; however, VLDL is produced and assembled in liver cells. Like chylomicrons, the main function of VLDL is the transport of triacylglycerols to other tissues. VLDLs also contain fatty acids that are synthesized from excess glucose or retrieved from chylomicron remnants.

KEY CONCEPT

Chylomicrons and VLDL primarily carry triacylglycerols. LDL and HDL primarily carry cholesterol. IDL is intermediate; it is a transition state between VLDL and LDL, occurring as the primary lipid within the lipoprotein changes from triacylglycerol to cholesterol.

IDL (Intermediate-Density Lipoprotein)

Once triacylglycerol is removed from VLDL, the resulting particle is referred to as either a **VLDL remnant** or **IDL**. Some IDL is reabsorbed by the liver by apolipoproteins on its exterior, and some is further processed in the bloodstream. For example, some IDL picks up cholesteryl esters from HDL to become LDL. IDL thus exists as a transition particle between triacylglycerol transport (associated with chylomicrons and VLDL) and cholesterol transport (associated with LDL and HDL). This process is shown in Figure 11.4.

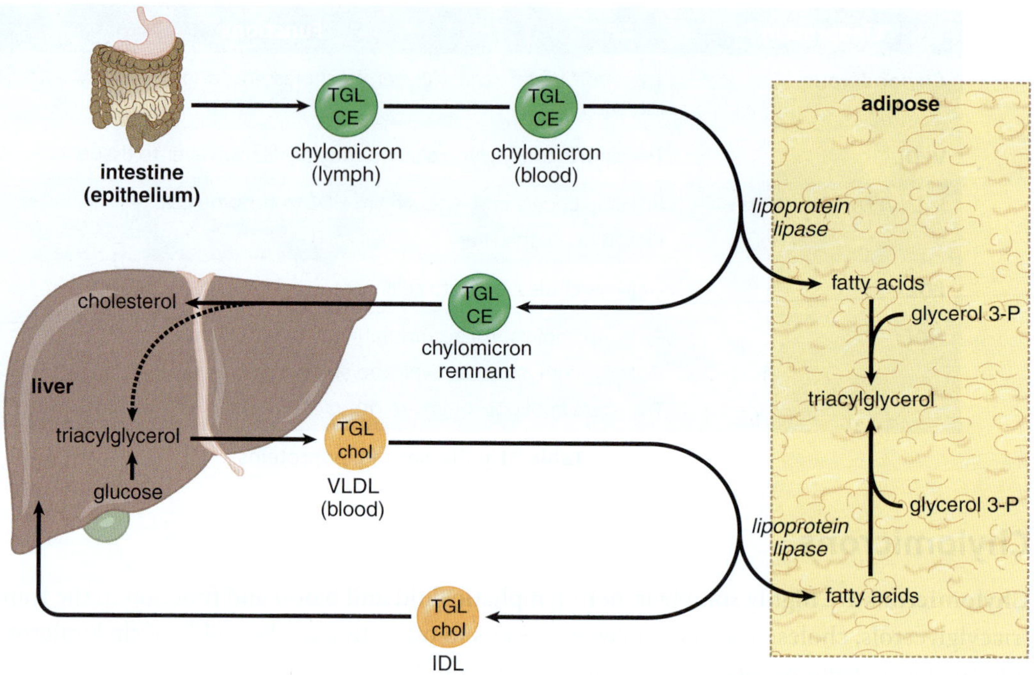

Figure 11.4 Lipid Transport in Lipoproteins
TGL = triacylglycerol; CE = cholesteryl esters; chol = cholesterol

LDL (Low-Density Lipoprotein)

Although both LDL and HDL are primarily cholesterol particles, the majority of the cholesterol measured in blood is associated with **LDL**. The normal role of LDL is to deliver cholesterol to tissues for biosynthesis. However, cholesterol also plays an important role in cell membranes. In addition, bile acids and salts are made from cholesterol in the liver, and many other tissues require cholesterol for steroid hormone synthesis (steroidogenesis).

HDL (High-Density Lipoprotein)

HDL is synthesized in the liver and intestines and released as dense, protein-rich particles into the blood. HDL contains apolipoproteins used for cholesterol recovery—that is, the cleaning up of excess cholesterol from blood vessels for excretion. HDL also delivers some cholesterol to steroidogenic tissues and transfers necessary apolipoproteins to some of the other lipoproteins.

REAL WORLD

When a physician orders a blood test for cholesterol, they are actually measuring levels of LDL and HDL in the blood. HDL is often considered "good" cholesterol because it picks up excess cholesterol from blood vessels for excretion.

Apolipoproteins

Apolipoproteins, also referred to as **apoproteins**, form the protein component of the lipoproteins described above. Apolipoproteins are receptor molecules and are involved in signaling. While it is highly unlikely that specific functions of each apolipoprotein will be tested on the MCAT, they are briefly summarized below to illustrate their diverse purposes:

- **apoA-I:** activates LCAT, an enzyme that catalyzes cholesterol esterification
- **apoB-48:** mediates chylomicron secretion
- **apoB-100:** permits uptake of LDL by the liver
- **apoC-II:** activates lipoprotein lipase
- **apoE:** permits uptake of chylomicron remnants and VLDL by the liver

MCAT CONCEPT CHECK 11.3

Before you move on, assess your understanding of the material with these questions.

1. What is the primary method of transporting free fatty acids in the blood?

____

2. Order the lipoproteins from greatest percentage of protein to least percentage of protein. Circle the molecules that are primarily involved in triacylglycerol transport.

____

3. Lipoproteins are synthesized primarily by which two organs?

____

4. When physicians order a lipid panel to evaluate a patient, which value do they prefer to see over a minimum threshold rather than below a maximum?

____

11.4 Cholesterol Metabolism

LEARNING OBJECTIVES

After Chapter 11.4, you will be able to:

- Predict optimal conditions for HMG-CoA reductase activity
- Recall the functions of the citrate shuttle, HMG-CoA reductase, LCAT, and CETP

Cholesterol is a ubiquitous component of all cells in the human body and plays a major role in the synthesis of cell membranes, steroid hormones, bile acids, and vitamin D.

Sources

Most cells derive their cholesterol from LDL or HDL, but some cholesterol may be synthesized *de novo*. *De novo* synthesis of cholesterol occurs in the liver and is driven by acetyl-CoA and ATP. The **citrate shuttle** carries mitochondrial acetyl-CoA into the cytoplasm, where synthesis occurs. NADPH (from the pentose phosphate pathway) supplies reducing equivalents. Synthesis of ***mevalonic acid*** in the smooth endoplasmic reticulum (SER) is the rate-limiting step in cholesterol biosynthesis and is catalyzed by ***3-hydroxy-3-methylglutaryl* (HMG) *CoA reductase***. Cholesterol synthesis is regulated in several ways. First, increased levels of cholesterol can inhibit further synthesis by a feedback inhibition mechanism. Next, insulin promotes cholesterol synthesis. Control over *de novo* cholesterol synthesis is also dependent on regulation of HMG-CoA reductase gene expression in the cell.

Specific Enzymes

Specialized enzymes involved in the transport of cholesterol include LCAT and CETP. ***Lecithin–cholesterol acyltransferase* (LCAT)** is an enzyme found in the bloodstream that is activated by HDL apoproteins. LCAT adds a fatty acid to cholesterol, which produces soluble cholesteryl esters such as those in HDL. HDL cholesteryl esters can be distributed to other lipoproteins like IDL, which becomes LDL by acquiring these cholesteryl esters. The **cholesteryl ester transfer protein (CETP)** facilitates this transfer process.

MCAT CONCEPT CHECK 11.4

Before you move on, assess your understanding of the material with these questions.

1. Under what conditions is HMG-CoA reductase most active? In what cellular region does it exist?

____

____

____

2. What proteins are specific to the formation and transmission of cholesteryl esters, and what are their functions?

____

____

11.5 Fatty Acids and Triacylglycerols

LEARNING OBJECTIVES

After Chapter 11.5, you will be able to:

- Recall and sequence the five steps in the addition of acetyl-CoA to a growing fatty acid chain
- Differentiate β-oxidation of unsaturated fatty acids from that of saturated fatty acids
- Identify the cellular locations involved in fatty acid synthesis and modification
- Name fatty acids and predict their structure based on their nomenclature:

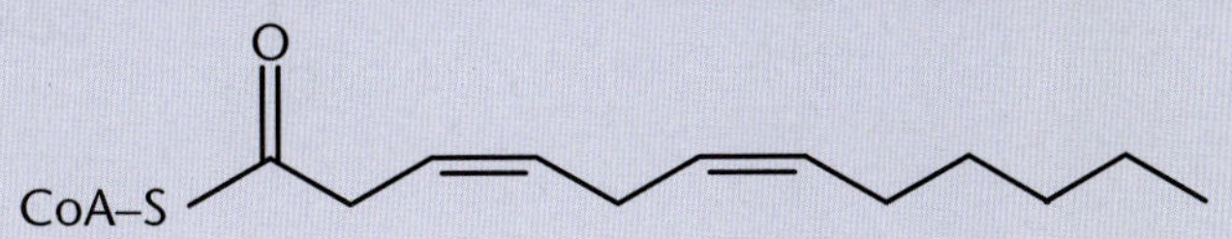

Fatty acids are long-chain carboxylic acids. The carboxyl carbon is carbon 1, and carbon 2 is referred to as the ***α-carbon***. Fatty acids found within the body occur as salts that are capable of forming micelles or are esterified to other compounds, such as the membrane lipids discussed in Chapter 8 of *MCAT Biochemistry Review*.

Nomenclature

When describing a fatty acid, the total number of carbons is given along with the number of double bonds, written as *carbons:double bonds*. Further description can be given by indicating the position and isomerism of the double bonds in an unsaturated fatty acid. **Saturated fatty acids** have no double bonds while **unsaturated fatty acids** have one or more double bonds. Humans can synthesize only a few of the unsaturated fatty acids; the rest come from essential fatty acids found in the diet that are transported in chylomicrons as triacylglycerols from the intestine. Two important essential fatty acids are ***α-linolenic acid*** and ***linoleic acid***. These polyunsaturated fatty acids, as well as other acids formed from them, are important in maintaining cell membrane fluidity, which is critical for proper functioning of the cell. The **omega (ω) numbering system** is also used for unsaturated fatty acids. The ω designation describes the position of the last double bond relative to the end of the chain and identifies the major precursor fatty acid. For example, linoleic acid (18:2 *cis*,*cis*-9,12) is the precursor of the ω-6 family, which includes *arachidonic acid*. α-Linolenic acid (18:3 all-*cis*-9,12,15) is the primary precursor of the ω-3 family. Double bonds in natural fatty acids are generally in the *cis* configuration.

REAL WORLD

Trans double bonds are uncommon in natural fatty acids; they predominate in fatty acids found in margarine and other foods that use partial hydrogenation of vegetable oils in their preparation. Compared with liquid oils, these partially hydrogenated fatty acids are solids at room temperature. These fatty acids contribute to arterial diseases and decreased membrane fluidity.

Synthesis

Fatty acids used by the body for fuel are supplied primarily by the diet. In addition, excess carbohydrate and protein acquired from the diet can be converted to fatty acids and stored as energy reserves in the form of triacylglycerols. Lipid and carbohydrate synthesis are often called **nontemplate synthesis** processes because they do not rely directly on the coding of a nucleic acid, unlike protein and nucleic acid synthesis.

Fatty Acid Biosynthesis

Fatty acid biosynthesis, shown in Figure 11.5, occurs in the liver and its products are subsequently transported to adipose tissue for storage. Adipose tissue can also synthesize smaller quantities of fatty acids. Both of the major enzymes of fatty acid synthesis, *acetyl-CoA carboxylase* and *fatty acid synthase*, are also stimulated by insulin. ***Palmitic acid*** (***palmitate***) is the primary end product of fatty acid synthesis.

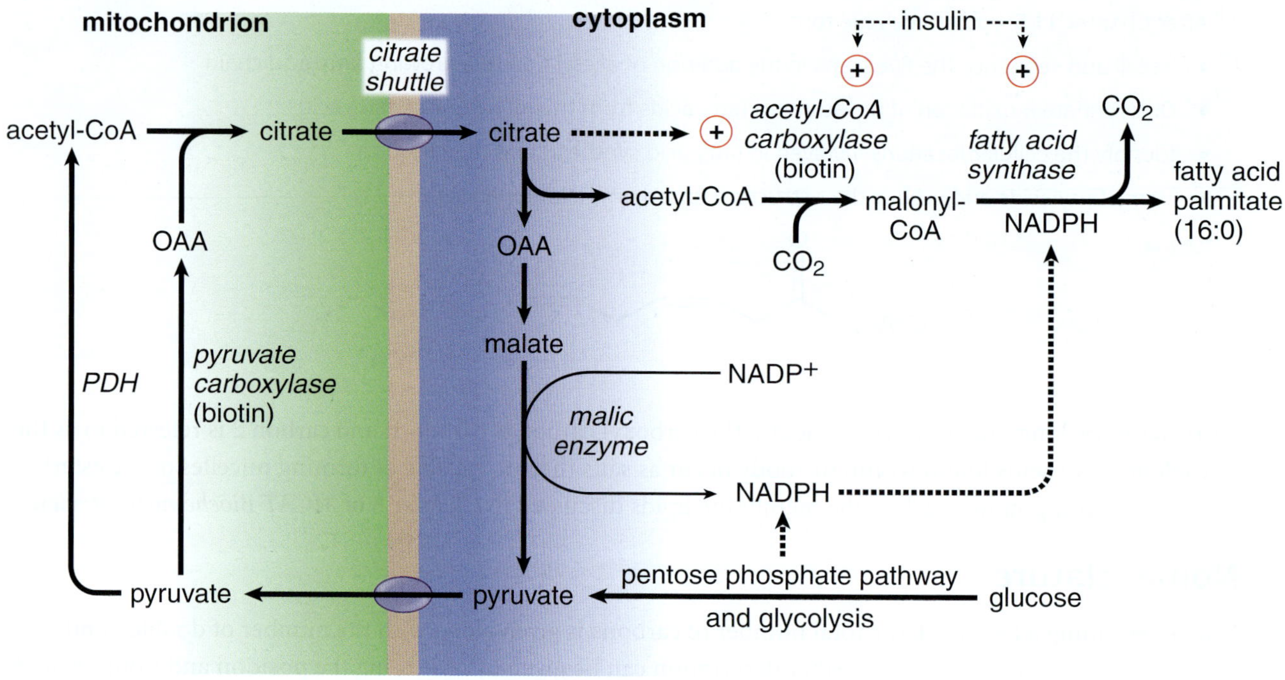

Figure 11.5 Fatty Acid Synthesis from Glucose

Acetyl-CoA Shuttling

Following a large meal, acetyl-CoA accumulates in the mitochondrial matrix and needs to be moved to the cytosol for fatty acid biosynthesis. Acetyl-CoA is the product of the ***pyruvate dehydrogenase complex***, and it couples with *oxaloacetate* to form *citrate* at the beginning of the citric acid cycle. Remember that *isocitrate dehydrogenase* is the rate-limiting enzyme of citric acid cycle; as the cell becomes energetically satisfied, it slows the citric acid cycle, which causes citrate accumulation. Citrate can then diffuse across the mitochondrial membrane. In the cytosol, ***citrate lyase*** splits citrate back into acetyl-CoA and oxaloacetate. The oxaloacetate can then return to the mitochondrion to continue moving acetyl-CoA.

Acetyl-CoA Carboxylase

Acetyl-CoA is activated in the cytoplasm for incorporation into fatty acids by acetyl-CoA carboxylase, the rate-limiting enzyme of fatty acid biosynthesis. **Acetyl-CoA carboxylase** requires biotin and ATP to function, and adds CO_2 to acetyl-CoA to form *malonyl-CoA*. The enzyme is activated by insulin and citrate. The CO_2 added to form malonyl-CoA is never actually incorporated into the fatty acid because it is removed by fatty acid synthase during addition of the activated acetyl group to the fatty acid.

Fatty Acid Synthase

Fatty acid synthase is more appropriately called ***palmitate synthase*** because palmitate is the only fatty acid that humans can synthesize *de novo*. Fatty acid synthase is a large multienzyme complex found in the cytosol that is rapidly induced in the liver following a meal high in carbohydrates because of elevated insulin levels. The enzyme complex contains an acyl carrier protein (ACP) that requires *pantothenic acid* (vitamin B_5). NADPH is also required to reduce the acetyl groups added to the fatty acid. Eight acetyl-CoA groups are required to produce palmitate (16:0). Fatty acyl-CoA may be elongated and desaturated, to a limited extent, using enzymes associated with the smooth endoplasmic reticulum (SER). The steps involved in fatty acid biosynthesis are shown in Figure 11.6 and include attachment to an acyl carrier protein, bond formation between activated malonyl-CoA (malonyl-ACP) and the growing chain, reduction of a carbonyl group, dehydration, and reduction of a double bond. These reactions occur over and over again until the sixteen-carbon palmitate molecule is created. Many of these reactions are reversed in β-oxidation.

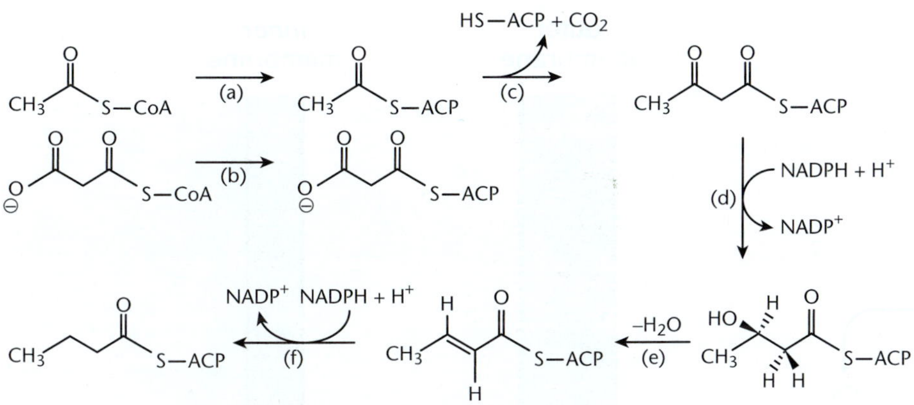

Figure 11.6 Action of Fatty Acid Synthase
Reactions include activation of the growing chain (a) and malonyl-CoA (b) with ACP, bond formation between these activated molecules (c), reduction of a carbonyl to a hydroxyl group (d), dehydration (e), and reduction to a saturated fatty acid (f).

Triacylglycerol (Triglyceride) Synthesis

Triacylglycerols, the storage form of fatty acids, are formed by attaching three fatty acids (as fatty acyl-CoA) to glycerol. Triacylglycerol formation from fatty acids and *glycerol 3-phosphate* occurs primarily in the liver and somewhat in adipose tissue, with a small contribution directly from the diet, as well. In the liver, triacylglycerols are packaged and sent to adipose tissue as very-low-density lipoproteins (VLDL), leaving only a small amount of stored triacylglycerols.

KEY CONCEPT

Fatty acid synthesis and β-oxidation are reverse processes. Both involve transport across the mitochondrial membrane, followed by a series of redox reactions, but always in the opposite direction of one another. Understanding one process will enable you to answer questions about both pathways.

Oxidation

Most fatty acid catabolism proceeds via **β-oxidation** that occurs in the mitochondria; however, peroxisomal β-oxidation also occurs. Branched-chain fatty acids may also undergo α-oxidation, depending on the branch points, while ω-oxidation in the endoplasmic reticulum produces dicarboxylic acids. You should be aware that these processes exist; however, the mechanisms are beyond the scope of the MCAT. We will take an in-depth look at β-oxidation, which will be much more heavily tested. Insulin indirectly inhibits β-oxidation while glucagon stimulates this process.

Activation

When fatty acids are metabolized, they first become activated by attachment to CoA, which is catalyzed by ***fatty-acyl-CoA synthetase***. The product is generically referred to as a fatty acyl-CoA or acyl-CoA. Specific examples would be acetyl-CoA containing a 2-carbon acyl group, or palmitoyl-CoA with a 16-carbon acyl group.

Fatty Acid Entry into Mitochondria

Short-chain fatty acids (2 to 4 carbons) and medium-chain fatty acids (6 to 12 carbons) diffuse freely into mitochondria, where they are oxidized. In contrast, while long-chain fatty acids (14 to 20 carbons) are also oxidized in the mitochondria, they require transport via a carnitine shuttle, as shown in Figure 11.7. ***Carnitine acyltransferase I*** is the rate-limiting enzyme of fatty acid oxidation. Very long chain fatty acids (over 20 carbons) are oxidized elsewhere in the cell.

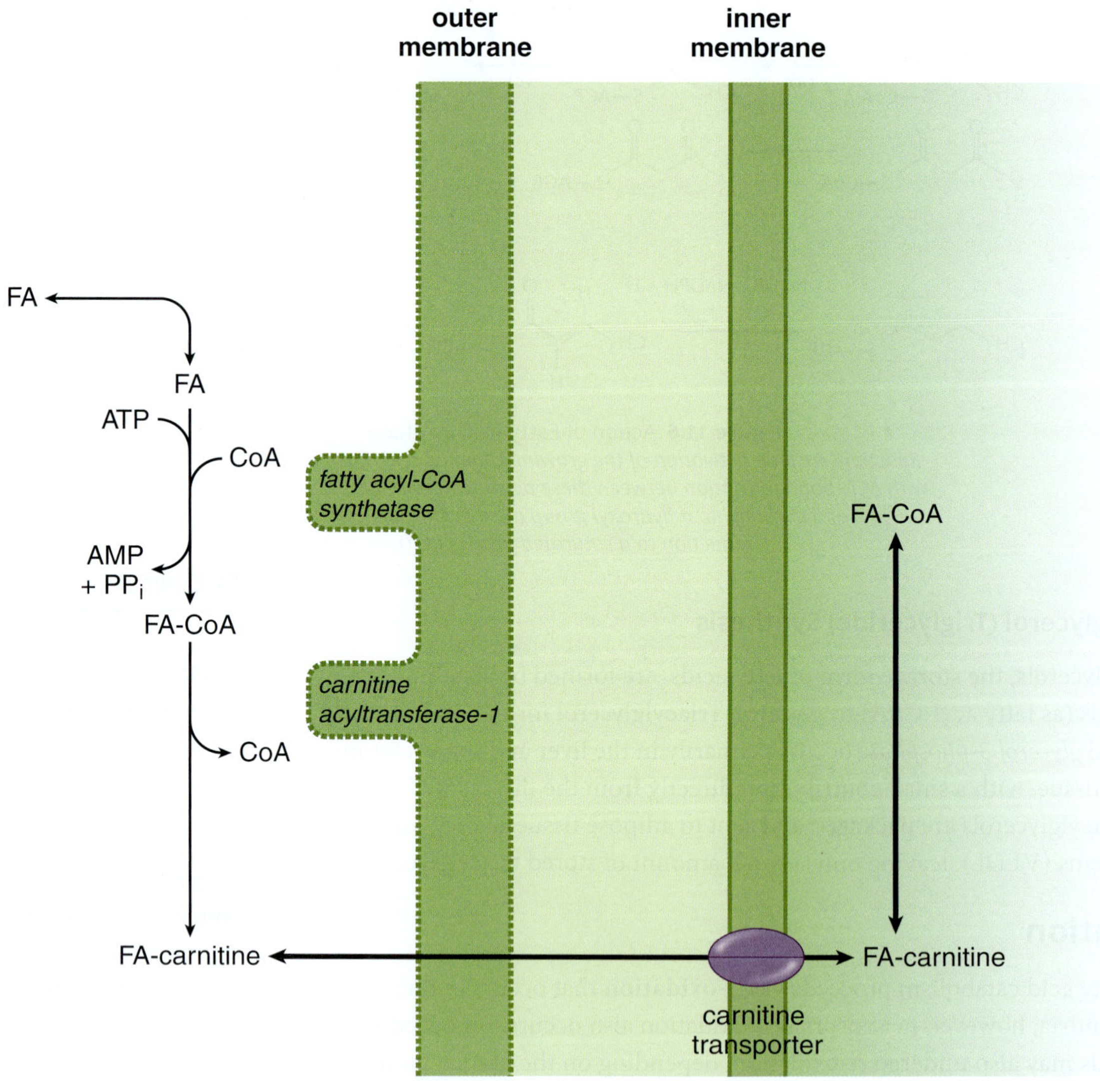

Figure 11.7 Fatty Acid Activation and Transport

β-Oxidation in Mitochondria

β-Oxidation reverses the process of fatty acid synthesis by oxidizing and releasing (rather than reducing and linking) molecules of acetyl-CoA. The pathway is a repetition of four steps; each four-step cycle releases one acetyl-CoA and reduces NAD^+ and FAD (producing NADH and $FADH_2$). The $FADH_2$ and NADH are oxidized in the electron transport chain, producing ATP. In muscle and adipose tissue, acetyl-CoA enters the citric acid cycle. In the liver, acetyl-CoA, which cannot be converted to glucose, stimulates gluconeogenesis by activating *pyruvate carboxylase*. In a fasting state, the liver produces more acetyl-CoA from β-oxidation than is used in the citric acid cycle. Much of the acetyl-CoA is used to synthesize ketone bodies (essentially two acetyl-CoA molecules linked together) that are released into the bloodstream and transported to other tissues.

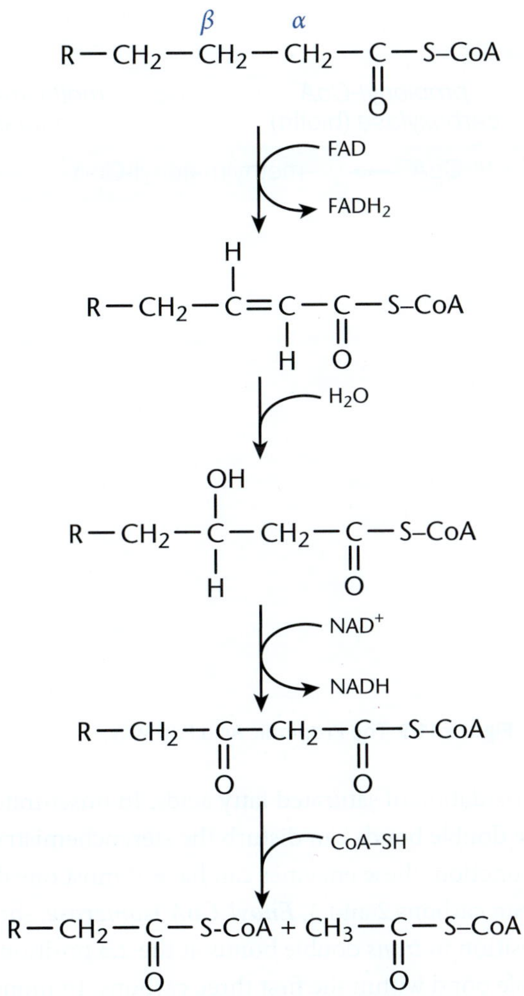

Figure 11.8 β-Oxidation

The four steps of β-oxidation, illustrated in Figure 11.8, are:

1. Oxidation of the fatty acid to form a double bond
2. Hydration of the double bond to form a hydroxyl group
3. Oxidation of the hydroxyl group to form a carbonyl (β-ketoacid)
4. Splitting of the β-ketoacid into a shorter acyl-CoA and acetyl-CoA

This process then continues until the chain has been shortened to two carbons, creating a final acetyl-CoA.

Fatty acids with an odd number of carbon atoms undergo β-oxidation in the same manner as even-numbered carbon fatty acids for the most part. The only difference is observed during the final cycle, where even-numbered fatty acids for the most part yield two acetyl-CoA molecules (from the four-carbon remaining fragment) and odd-numbered fatty acids yield one acetyl-CoA and one *propionyl-CoA* (from the five-carbon remaining fragment), as shown in Figure 11.9. Propionyl-CoA is converted to *methylmalonyl-CoA* by ***propionyl-CoA carboxylase***, which requires biotin (vitamin B_7). Methylmalonyl-CoA is then converted into *succinyl-CoA* by ***methylmalonyl-CoA mutase***, which requires cobalamin (vitamin B_{12}). Succinyl-CoA is a citric acid cycle intermediate and can also be converted to malate to enter the gluconeogenic pathway in the cytosol. Odd-carbon fatty acids thus represent an exception to the rule that fatty acids cannot be converted to glucose in humans.

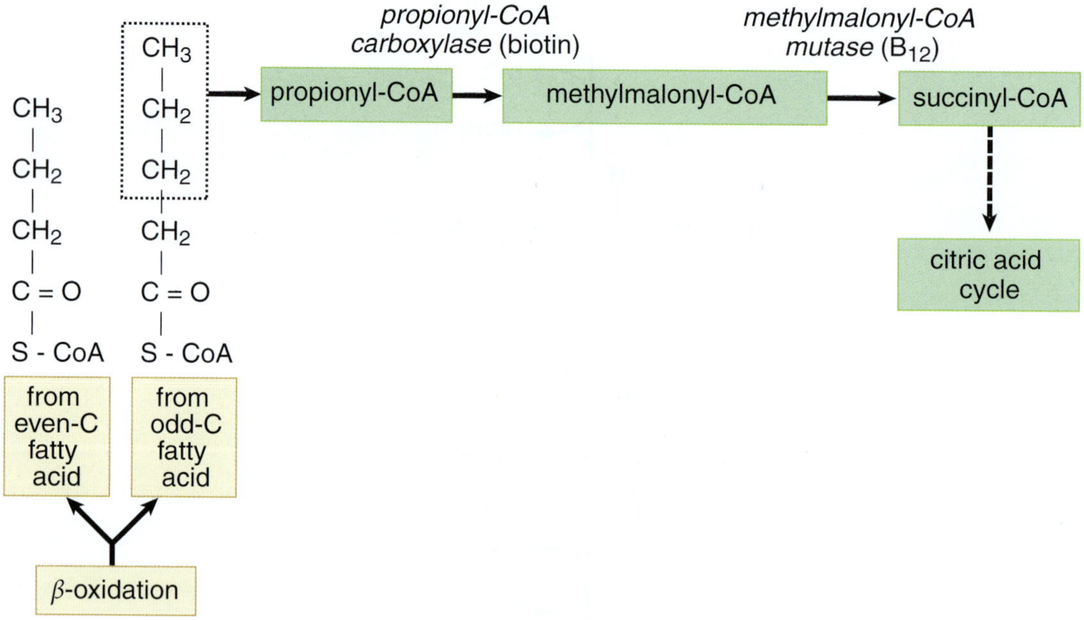

Figure 11.9 The Propionic Acid Pathway

Until now we've been discussing the oxidation of saturated fatty acids. In unsaturated fatty acids, two additional enzymes are necessary because double bonds can disturb the stereochemistry needed for oxidative enzymes to act on the fatty acid. To function, these enzymes can have at most one double bond in their active site; this bond must be located between carbons 2 and 3. ***Enoyl-CoA isomerase***, shown in Figure 11.10, rearranges *cis* double bonds at the 3,4 position to *trans* double bonds at the 2,3 position once enough acetyl-CoA has been liberated to isolate the double bond within the first three carbons. In monounsaturated fatty acids this single step permits β-oxidation to proceed.

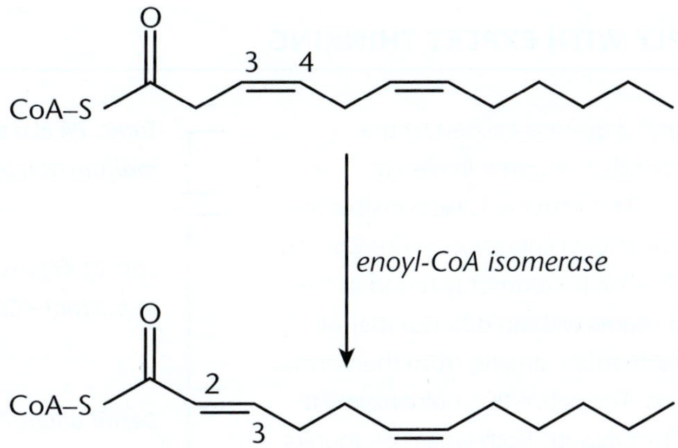

Figure 11.10 Reaction of Enoyl-CoA Isomerase

In polyunsaturated fatty acids, a further reduction is required using ***2,4-dienoyl-CoA reductase*** to convert two conjugated double bonds to just one double bond at the 3,4 position, where it will then undergo the same rearrangement as monounsaturated fatty acids (as shown in Figure 11.11) to form a *trans* 2,3 double bond.

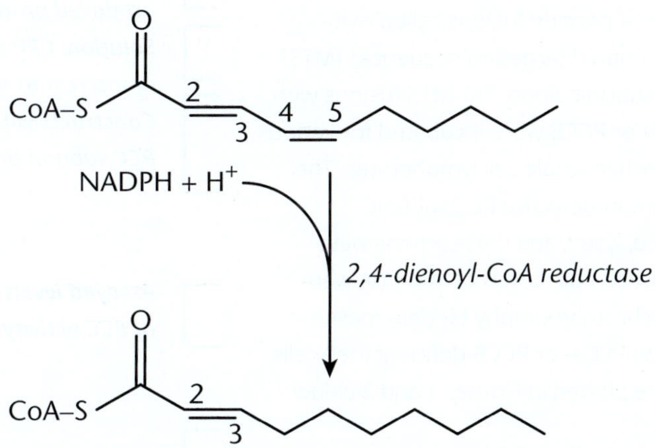

Figure 11.11 Reaction of 2,4-Dienoyl-CoA Reductase

Table 11.2 contrasts fatty acid synthesis and β-oxidation.

	Fatty Acid Synthesis	β-Oxidation
Location	Cytosol	Mitochondria
Carrier	Acyl Carrier Protein (ACP)	Coenzyme A (CoA)
Cofactor	NADPH (Reductant)	NAD^+, FAD (Oxidants)
Process	Adds 2-carbon units	Removes 2-carbon units

Table 11.2 Fatty Acid Synthesis vs. β-Oxidation

BIOCHEMISTRY GUIDED EXAMPLE WITH EXPERT THINKING

Propionic acidemia (PA) is a life-threatening disease caused by the deficiency of a mitochondrial biotin-dependent enzyme known as propionyl coenzyme-A carboxylase (PCC). This enzyme is responsible for degrading the metabolic intermediate propionyl coenzyme-A (PP-CoA) to create methylmalonyl-CoA (MM-CoA). PP-CoA is commonly found as the end product to β-oxidation of fatty acid chains with an odd number of carbons. PP-CoA is also a metabolic intermediate arising from the normal turnover of several essential amino acids. The native PCC holoenzyme is composed of six α (PCCA) and six β (PCCB) subunits. Both types of subunits must be functional for the enzyme to be operative. Deficiency in either or both PCC subunits and the consequent accumulation of PP-CoA leads to the pathogenesis of PA.

Topic: PA is a disease caused by malfunction of enzyme PCC

Lots of details here describing how important PCC is to metabolism

Detail about PCC structure: 6 α and 6 β; need both subunits to work

Enzyme replacement therapy is an approach that aims to restore the activity of an enzyme in cases of deficiency or abnormal production. To overcome the challenge of delivery and targeting proteins to the mitochondria of living cells, two groups of peptide fusions called twin-arginine translocation (TAT) and mitochondrial targeting sequences (MTS) were employed. Purified constructs of subunit alone, TAT-MTS fusions with PCCA or PCCB, or TAT fusions with PCCA or PCCB were incubated for various time periods with PCCA- and PCCB-defective whole cell lymphocytes. The lymphocytes endogenously express the non-defective PCC subunit. Mitochondria were subsequently isolated, lysed, and the reactions were terminated by the addition of trichloroacetic acid. Levels of MM-CoA were assayed using ultra performance liquid chromatography tandem mass spectrometry (UPLC-MS/MS). Normal and PCCA- or PCCB-deficient (def) cells were included as controls. The results are plotted in Figures 1 and 2 below.

Experimental technique used in passage tries to restore activity of deficient PCC

Issue: difficult to target externally produced proteins to mitochondria

Solution: CPP and MTS are fused to protein of interest to get them into mitochondria

Constructs with different combination of PCC subunit and peptide fusions

Assayed levels of MM-CoA as a measure of PCC activity

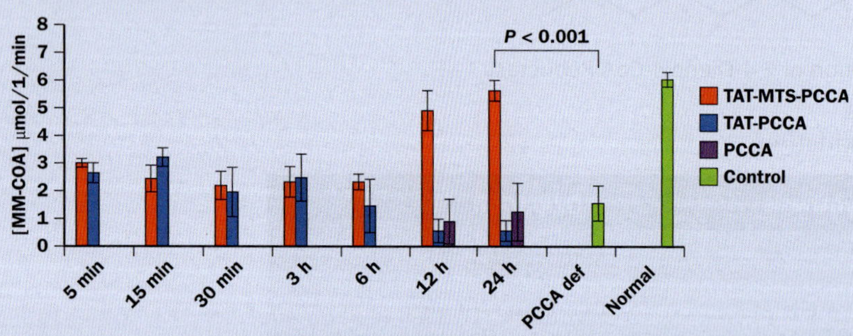

Figure 1

IVs: time assayed, type of construct

DV: levels of MM-CoA

Trend: significant difference in MM-CoA levels 24 hours after TAT-MTS-PCCA added compared to absence of PCCA

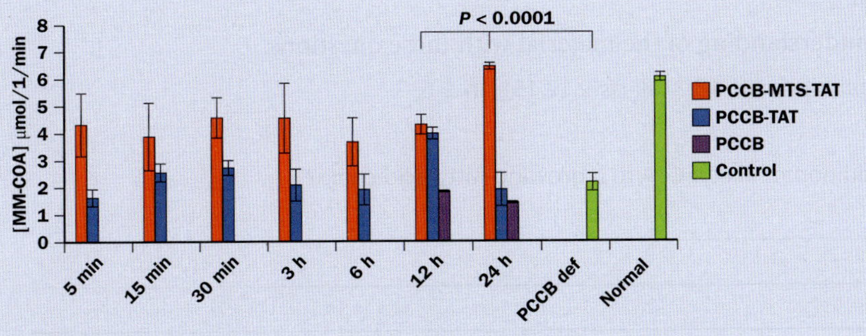

IVs: time assayed, type of construct

DV: levels of MM-CoA

Trend: significant difference in MM-CoA levels 12 and 24 hours after PCCB-MTS-TAT added compared to absence of PCCB

Figure 2

Adapted from Darvish-Damavandi, M., Ho, H.K., & Kang, T.S. (2016) Towards the development of an enzyme replacement therapy for the metabolic disorder propionic acidemia. *Molecular Genetics and Metabolism Reports*, 8, 51–60. doi:10.1016/j.ymgmr.2016.06.009.

According to the data, are MTS-TAT-PCC constructs able to successfully rescue PCC activity in deficient mitochondria?

This question begins with "according to the data", meaning it will require us to understand and analyze the data presented in the context of the experiment described in the passage. Given we have multiple, complex figures, it's important to get some context on the experiments and what the data represent first. The researchers are exploring treatment options for a disease caused by deficient PCC, which is an important metabolic enzyme in the mitochondria. We're told that PCC requires both types of subunits in order to function properly. Common methods of restoring protein activity in cells are at the transcriptional/translational level within the cell, but the method employed in this study produces the required protein outside of the cell, then adds the protein back into the cell. We should know from our content background that proteins are generally polar, so the challenge is getting the protein past the lipid bilayers of both the cellular and the mitochondrial membranes. The researcher's solution to this problem is to fuse PCC subunits to peptides that not only get PCC through the membranes, but also target the mitochondria. Also, note that the cell lines still express the non-deficient subunit: the cell lines in Figure 1 still express functional PCCB, so PCCA must be added and delivered to the mitochondria for there to be PCC activity; the opposite is true for the cell lines in Figure 2.

Diving into the data, the experimental layout and the results are similar for both PCCA and PCCB fusions. When the PCC-subunit is fused to TAT alone, or in the absence of fusion, the levels of MM-CoA are similar. However, when the PCC-subunit is fused to both MTS and TAT, we see significantly higher levels of MM-CoA. The first paragraph tells us that PCC will catalyze PP-CoA to produce MM-CoA, the product being measured in the experiment, so high levels of MM-CoA correlate to PCC activity.

Therefore, these results indicate that PCC activity can be rescued by exogenously expressing PCC-subunits and fusing them to both mitochondrial-targeting and cell-permeating proteins.

MCAT CONCEPT CHECK 11.5

Before you move on, assess your understanding of the material with these questions.

1. Draw the following fatty acids: palmitic acid, 18:3 (all-*cis*-9,12,15), an ω-6.

2. What are the five steps in the addition of acetyl-CoA to a growing fatty acid chain?
   1. ______
   2. ______
   3. ______
   4. ______
   5. ______

3. How does β-oxidation of unsaturated fatty acids differ from that of saturated fatty acids?

   ______

4. True or False: Fatty acids are synthesized in the cytoplasm and modified by enzymes in the smooth endoplasmic reticulum.

11.6 Ketone Bodies

LEARNING OBJECTIVES

After Chapter 11.6, you will be able to:

- Predict when fatty acids would be used to create ketone bodies rather than glucose
- Recall the conditions that favor ketogenesis and ketolysis

In the fasting state, the liver converts excess acetyl-CoA from β-oxidation of fatty acids into the **ketone bodies *acetoacetate*, *3-hydroxybutyrate*** (**β*-hydroxybutyrate***), and ***acetone,*** which can be used for energy in various tissues. Cardiac and skeletal muscle and the renal cortex can metabolize acetoacetate and 3-hydroxybutyrate to acetyl-CoA. During fasting periods, muscle will metabolize ketones as rapidly as the liver releases them, preventing accumulation in the bloodstream. After a week of fasting, ketones reach a concentration in the blood that is high enough for the brain to begin metabolizing them. The processes of ketogenesis and ketolysis are shown in Figure 11.12.

KEY CONCEPT

Ketone bodies are essentially transportable forms of acetyl-CoA. They are produced by the liver and used by other tissues during prolonged starvation.

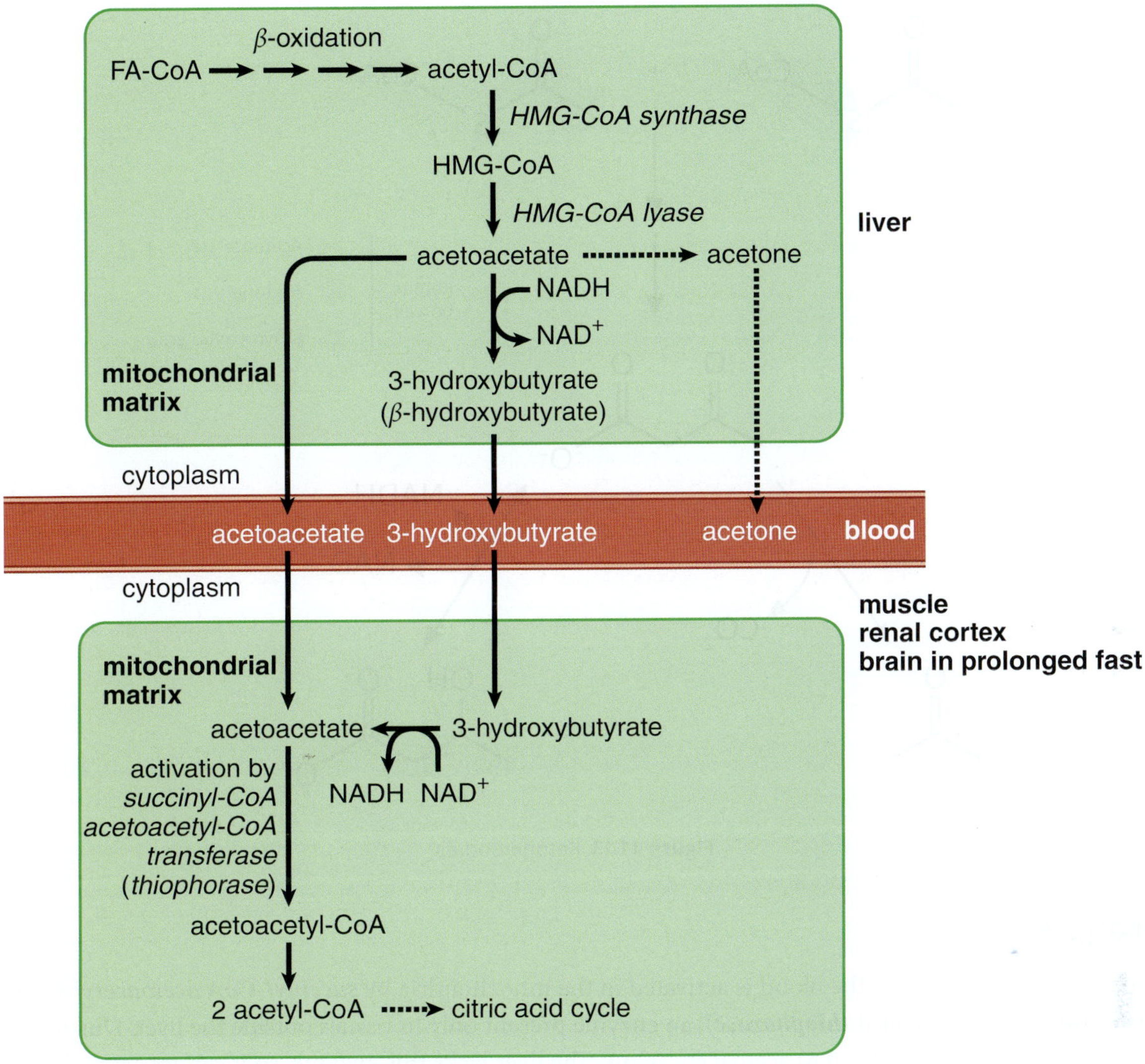

Figure 11.12 Ketogenesis and Ketolysis

Ketogenesis

Ketogenesis occurs in the mitochondria of liver cells when excess acetyl-CoA accumulates in the fasting state. ***HMG-CoA synthase*** forms HMG-CoA, and ***HMG-CoA lyase*** breaks down HMG-CoA into acetoacetate, which can subsequently be reduced to 3-hydroxybutyrate. Acetone is a minor side product that cannot be directly turned into acetyl-CoA, but can be converted into lactate and pyruvate. Figure 11.13 shows the creation of acetoacetate, β-hydroxybutyrate (3-hydroxybutyrate), and acetone from acetyl-CoA.

REAL WORLD

A significant increase in ketone levels in the blood can lead to ketoacidosis, a potentially dangerous medical condition. This occurs most often with fatty acid breakdown in type 1 (insulin-dependent) diabetes mellitus.

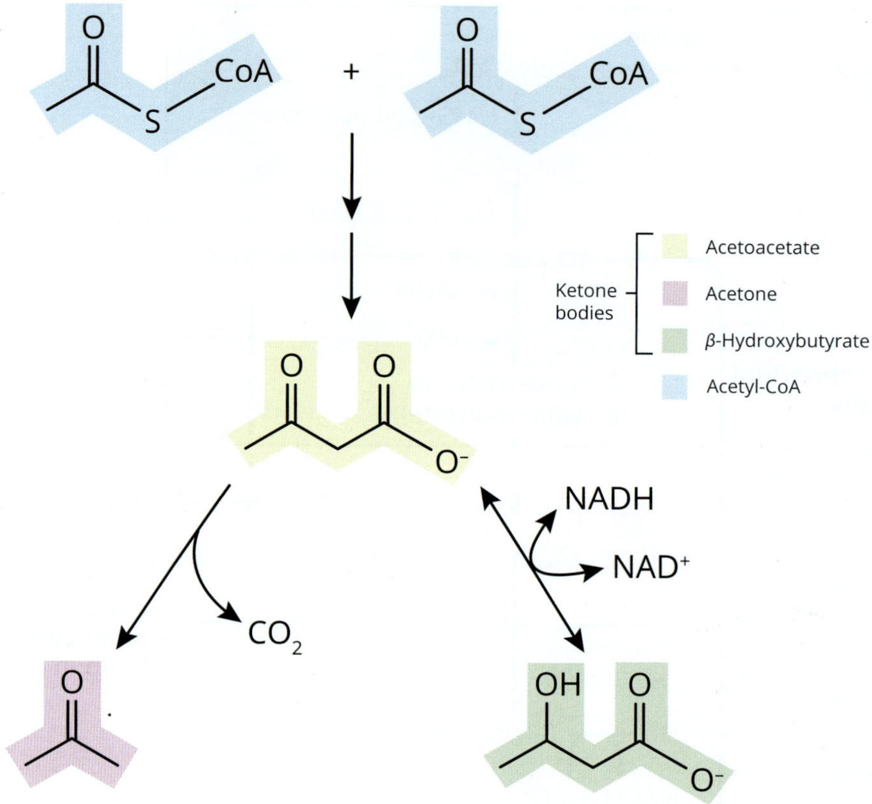

Figure 11.13 Ketone Bodies

Ketolysis

Acetoacetate picked up from the blood is activated in the mitochondria by ***succinyl-CoA acetoacetyl-CoA transferase*** (commonly called ***thiophorase***), an enzyme present only in tissues outside the liver. During this reaction, acetoacetate is oxidized to acetoacetyl-CoA. The liver lacks this enzyme, so it cannot catabolize the ketone bodies that it produces.

Ketolysis in the Brain

During a prolonged fast (longer than one week), the brain begins to derive up to two-thirds of its energy from ketone bodies. In the brain, when ketones are metabolized to acetyl-CoA, pyruvate dehydrogenase is inhibited. Glycolysis and glucose uptake in the brain decreases. This important switch spares essential protein in the body, which otherwise would be catabolized to form glucose by gluconeogenesis in the liver, and allows the brain to indirectly metabolize fatty acids as ketone bodies.

MCAT CONCEPT CHECK 11.6

Before you move on, assess your understanding of the material with these questions.

1. Why are fatty acids used to create ketone bodies instead of creating glucose?

____

2. What conditions and tissues favor ketogenesis? Ketolysis?

   - Ketogenesis:

____

   - Ketolysis:

____

11.7 Protein Catabolism

LEARNING OBJECTIVES

After Chapter 11.7, you will be able to:

- Identify common sources for acetyl-CoA used in lipid synthesis
- Recall the location(s) associated with large amounts of protein digestion
- Predict what will happen to the carbon skeleton, amino groups, and side chains of proteins that have been broken down

Protein is very rarely used as an energy source because it is so important for other functions; routinely breaking down protein would result in serious illness. However, under conditions of extreme energy deprivation, proteins can be used for energy. In order to provide a reservoir of amino acids for protein building by the cell, proteins must be digested and absorbed.

Proteolysis (the breakdown of proteins) begins in the stomach with ***pepsin*** and continues with the pancreatic proteases ***trypsin***, ***chymotrypsin***, and ***carboxypeptidases A*** and ***B***, all of which are secreted as zymogens. Protein digestion is completed by the small intestinal brush-border enzymes ***dipeptidase*** and ***aminopeptidase***. The main end products of protein digestion are amino acids, dipeptides, and tripeptides. Absorption of amino acids and small peptides through the luminal membrane is accomplished by secondary active transport linked to sodium. At the basal membrane, simple and facilitated diffusion transports amino acids into the bloodstream. Figure 11.14 illustrates the major transport mechanisms involved in moving amino acids across the luminal and basal membranes of intestinal cells.

KEY CONCEPT

Metabolism is directed toward conserving tissues to the greatest extent possible, especially the brain and heart. Digestion of protein compromises muscle—potentially that of the heart—so it is unlikely to occur under normal conditions.

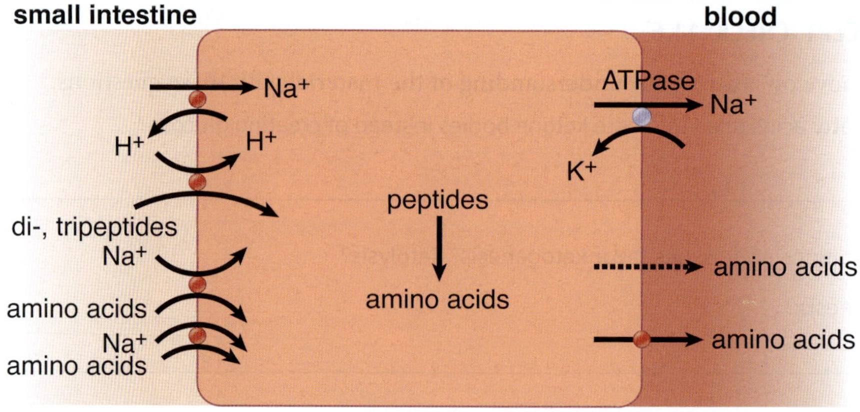

Figure 11.14 Absorption of Amino Acids and Peptides in the Intestine

Protein obtained from the diet or from the body (during prolonged fasting or starvation) may be used as an energy source. Body protein is catabolized primarily in muscle and liver. Amino acids released from proteins usually lose their amino group through **transamination** or **deamination**. The remaining carbon skeleton can be used for energy. Amino acids are classified by their ability to turn into specific metabolic intermediates: **glucogenic** amino acids (all but leucine and lysine) can be converted into glucose through gluconeogenesis; **ketogenic** amino acids (leucine and lysine, as well as isoleucine, phenylalanine, threonine, tryptophan, and tyrosine, which are also glucogenic as well) can be converted into acetyl-CoA and ketone bodies.

The amino groups removed by transamination or deamination constitute a potential toxin to the body in the form of ammonia, and must be excreted safely. The **urea cycle**, shown in Figure 11.15, occurs in the liver and is the body's primary way of removing excess nitrogen from the body. The MCAT is highly unlikely to test on the steps and intermediates of the urea cycle directly, but it is provided here as a point of reference.

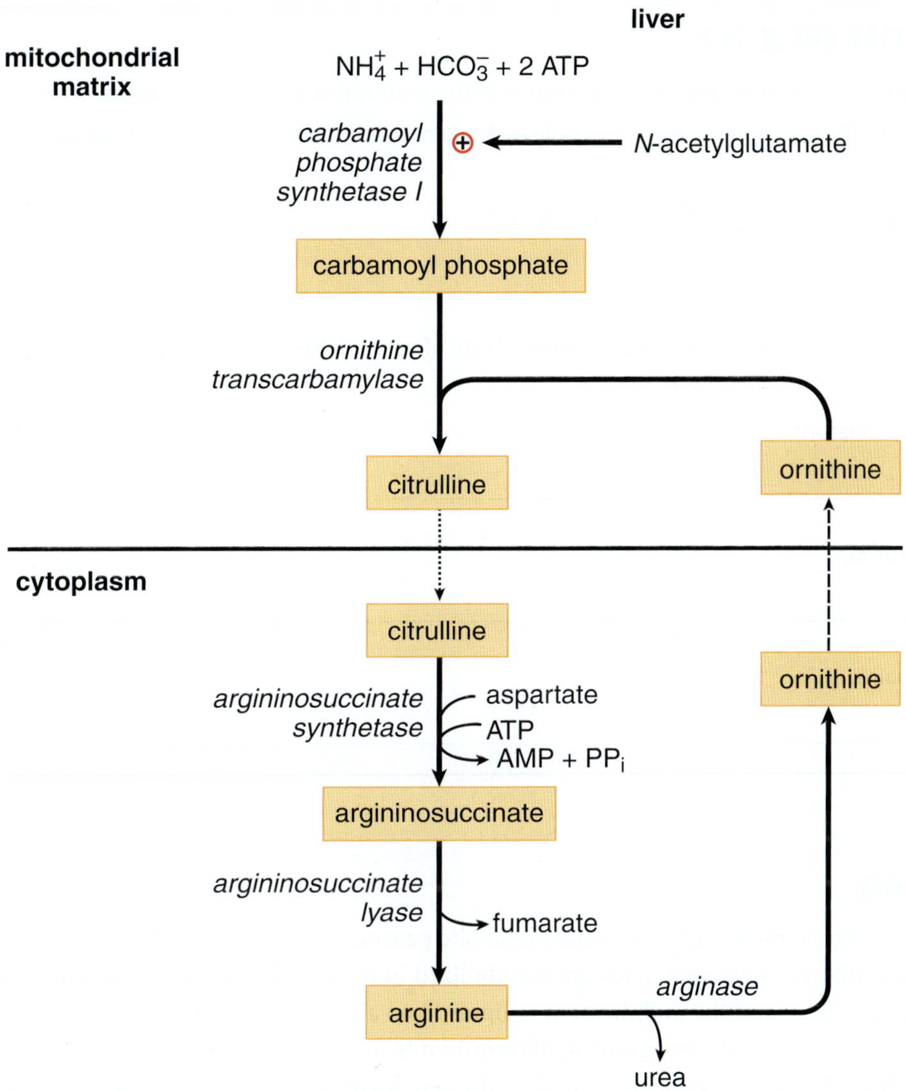

Figure 11.15 The Urea Cycle

The fate of the side chain from each amino acid depends on its chemistry. Basic amino acid side chains feed into the urea cycle, while the other side chains act like the carbon skeleton and produce energy through gluconeogenesis or ketone production.

MCAT CONCEPT CHECK 11.7

Before you move on, assess your understanding of the material with these questions.

1. True or False: Bodily proteins will commonly be broken down to provide acetyl-CoA for lipid synthesis.

2. Where does the bulk of protein digestion occur?

____

3. During protein processing, what is the eventual fate of each of the following components: carbon skeleton, amino group, and side chains?

    - Carbon skeleton:

    ____

    - Amino group:

    ____

    - Side chains:

    ____

Conclusion

At this point, we have examined all of the vital metabolic processes of the cell. In this chapter, we reviewed dietary lipids and different ways that lipids are metabolized in the cell. We also covered lipid transport in blood and lymphatic fluid and the mobilization of lipids from adipocytes. In addition, we went over the structure, synthesis, and breakdown of fatty acids required to address the energy needs of the cell. The importance of ketone bodies and how they are utilized by the cell during periods of starvation were also reviewed. Finally, we went over digestion and metabolism of proteins and amino acids.

Metabolism of the different macromolecules does not occur in isolation, as you've already seen: the acetyl-CoA produced in fatty acid oxidation regulates the pyruvate dehydrogenase complex and pyruvate carboxylase to create a shift in carbohydrate metabolism from glycolysis and the citric acid cycle to gluconeogenesis. In the next chapter, we'll dive into how the different pathways fit together and will integrate the metabolic knowledge that you've compiled in Chapters 9, 10, and 11 of *MCAT Biochemistry Review*.

▶ GO ONLINE

You've reviewed the content, now test your knowledge and critical thinking skills by completing a test-like passage set in your online resources!

CONCEPT SUMMARY

Lipid Digestion and Absorption

- Mechanical digestion of lipids occurs primarily in the mouth and stomach.
- Chemical digestion of lipids occurs in the small intestine and is facilitated by **bile**, **pancreatic lipase**, **colipase**, and **cholesterol esterase**.
- Digested lipids may form **micelles** for absorption or be absorbed directly.
- Short-chain fatty acids are absorbed across the intestine into the blood.
- Long-chain fatty acids are absorbed as micelles and assembled into **chylomicrons** for release into the lymphatic system.

Lipid Mobilization

- Lipids are mobilized from adipocytes by **hormone-sensitive lipase**.
- Lipids are mobilized from lipoproteins by **lipoprotein lipase**.

Lipid Transport

- **Chylomicrons** are the transport mechanism for dietary triacylglycerol molecules and are transported via the lymphatic system.
- **VLDL** transports newly synthesized triacylglycerol molecules from the liver to peripheral tissues in the bloodstream.
- **IDL** is a **VLDL remnant** in transition between triacylglycerol and cholesterol transport; it picks up cholesteryl esters from HDL.
- **LDL** primarily transports cholesterol for use by tissues.
- **HDL** is involved in the reverse transport of cholesterol.
- **Apoproteins** control interactions between lipoproteins.

Cholesterol Metabolism

- Cholesterol may be obtained through dietary sources or through *de novo* synthesis in the liver.
- The key enzyme in cholesterol biosynthesis is **HMG-CoA reductase**.
- **LCAT** catalyzes the formation of cholesteryl esters for transport with HDL.
- **CETP** catalyzes the transition of IDL to LDL by transferring cholesteryl esters from HDL.

Fatty Acids and Triacylglycerols

- Fatty acids are carboxylic acids, typically with a single long chain, although they can be branched.
- **Saturated fatty acids** have no double bonds between carbons. **Unsaturated fatty acids** have one or more double bonds.
- Fatty acids are synthesized in the cytoplasm from acetyl-CoA transported out of the mitochondria.
  - Synthesis includes five steps: activation, bond formation, reduction, dehydration, and a second reduction.
  - These steps are repeated eight times to form **palmitic acid**, the only fatty acid that humans can synthesize.
- Fatty acid oxidation occurs in the mitochondria following transport by the carnitine shuttle.
  - **β-Oxidation** uses cycles of oxidation, hydration, oxidation, and cleavage.
  - Branched and unsaturated fatty acids require special enzymes.
  - Unsaturated fatty acids use an **isomerase** and an additional **reductase** during cleavage.

Ketone Bodies

- Ketone bodies form (**ketogenesis**) during a prolonged starvation state due to excess acetyl-CoA in the liver.
- **Ketolysis** regenerates acetyl-CoA for use as an energy source in peripheral tissues.
- The brain can derive up to two-thirds of its energy from ketone bodies during prolonged starvation.

Protein Catabolism

- Protein digestion occurs primarily in the small intestine.
- Catabolism of cellular proteins occurs only under conditions of starvation.
- Carbon skeletons of amino acids are used for energy, either through gluconeogenesis or ketone body formation. Amino groups are fed into the **urea cycle** for excretion. The fate of a side chain depends on its chemistry.

ANSWERS TO CONCEPT CHECKS

11.1

1. Physical digestion is accomplished in the mouth and the stomach, reducing the particle size. Beginning in the small intestine, pancreatic lipase, colipase, cholesterol esterase, and bile assist in the chemical digestion of lipids. In the more distal portion of the small intestine, absorption occurs.
2. False. Small free fatty acids enter the circulation directly.
3. Micelles are collections of lipids with their hydrophobic ends oriented toward the center and their charged ends oriented toward the aqueous environment. Micelles collect lipids within their hydrophobic centers.

11.2

1. An increase in insulin levels will increase lipid storage and decrease lipid mobilization from adipocytes, leading to weight gain in patients who have diabetes and begin insulin injections.
2. The ratio of free fatty acids to glycerol is 3:1. A triacylglycerol molecule is composed of glycerol and three fatty acids.

11.3

1. Free fatty acids remain in the blood, bonded to albumin and other carrier proteins. A much smaller amount will remain unbonded.
2. With respect to protein content, HDL > LDL > IDL > VLDL > chylomicrons. VLDL and chylomicrons are the primary triacylglycerol transporters. HDL and LDL are mostly involved in cholesterol transport.
3. Lipoproteins are synthesized primarily by the intestine and liver.
4. As mentioned in the chapter, HDL is often considered "good" cholesterol because it picks up excess cholesterol from blood vessels for excretion. Because of this crucial role, HDL values are checked for being over a minimum value.

11.4

1. HMG-CoA reductase is most active in the absence of cholesterol and when stimulated by insulin. Cholesterol reduces the activity of HMG-CoA reductase, which is located in the smooth endoplasmic reticulum.
2. LCAT catalyzes the esterification of cholesterol to form cholesteryl esters. CETP promotes the transfer of cholesteryl esters from HDL to IDL, forming LDL.

11.5

1. Palmitic acid (16:0):

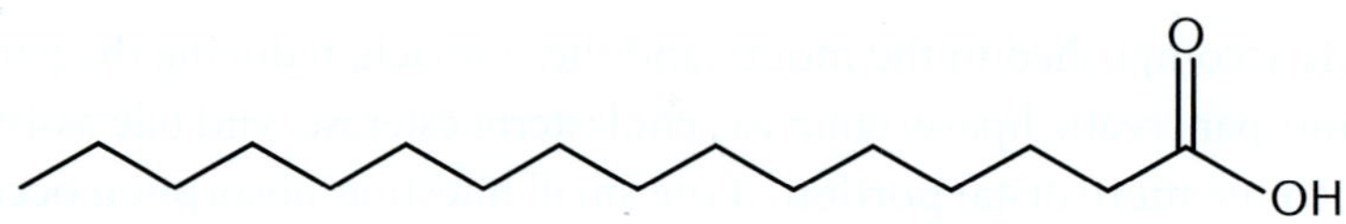

α-Linolenic acid (18:3 all-*cis*-9,12,15), an ω-3 fatty acid:

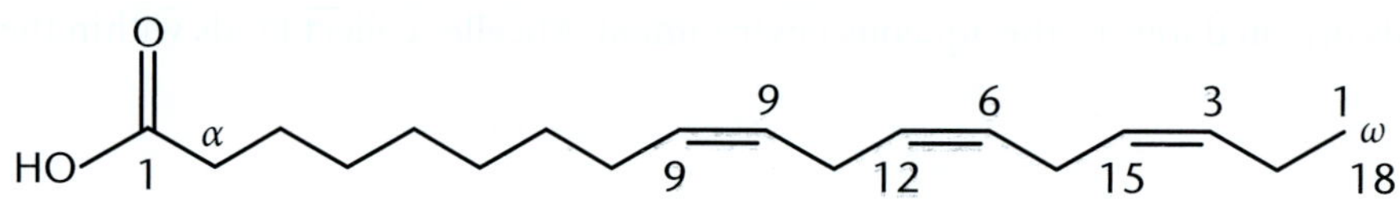

Linoleic acid (18:2 *cis,cis*-9,12), an ω-6 fatty acid:

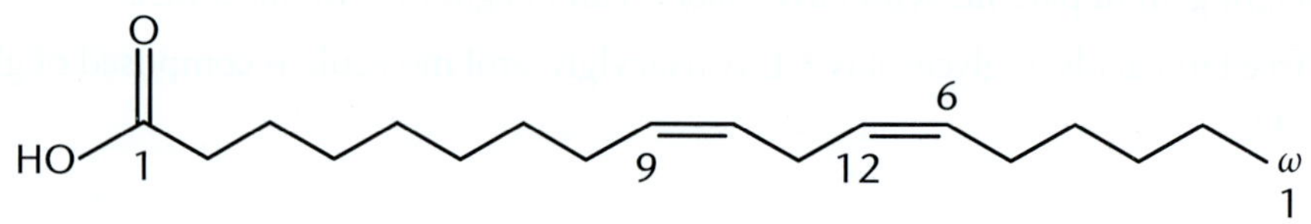

Note: As long as the last double bond is in the same position relative to the end of the chain, many answers are possible for the ω-6 fatty acid.

2. The steps in the attachment of acetyl-CoA to a fatty acid chain are attachment to acyl carrier protein, bond formation between molecules, reduction of a carbonyl group, dehydration, and reduction of a double bond. These steps are shown in Figure 11.6.
3. There is an additional isomerase and an additional reductase for the β-oxidation of unsaturated fatty acids, which provide the stereochemistry necessary for further oxidation.
4. True.

11.6

1. Fatty acid degradation results in large amounts of acetyl-CoA, which cannot enter the gluconeogenic pathway to produce glucose. Only odd-numbered fatty acids can act as a source of carbon for gluconeogenesis; even then, only the final malonyl-CoA molecule can be used. Energy is packaged into ketone bodies for consumption by the brain and muscles.
2. Ketogenesis is favored by a prolonged fast and occurs in the liver. It is stimulated by increasing concentrations of acetyl-CoA. Ketolysis is also favored during a prolonged fast, but is stimulated by a low-energy state in muscle and brain tissues and does not occur in the liver.

11.7

1. False. Proteins are more valuable to the cell than lipids, thus they will not commonly be broken down for lipid synthesis.
2. The bulk of protein digestion occurs in the small intestine.
3. The carbon skeleton is transported to the liver for processing into glucose or ketone bodies. The amino group will feed into the urea cycle for excretion. Side chains are processed depending on their composition. Basic side chains will be processed like amino groups, while other functional groups will be treated like the carbon skeleton.

SCIENCE MASTERY ASSESSMENT EXPLANATIONS

1. **B**

This question asks for the hormone that does not directly regulate the activity of hormone-sensitive lipase (HSL). Hormone sensitive lipase is an enzyme that cleaves fatty acids from their glycerol backbones, releasing these free fatty acids for use in energy production. HSL is directly activated by epinephrine and cortisol, so **(C)** and **(D)** can be eliminated. Regarding insulin vs. glucagon, observe that free fatty acid mobilization, and therefore HSL activity, is generally associated with low blood sugar, which is also associated with elevated glucagon levels. However, glucagon does not directly regulate the activity of HSL. Rather, HSL is activated by a drop in insulin levels. For this reason, insulin does directly regulate HSL activity, and therefore **(A)** can be eliminated. Only glucagon, **(B)**, does not directly influence HSL activity. Therefore **(B)** is the correct answer.

2. **A**

Short-chain fatty acids are soluble in the intestinal lumen, and thus do not interact with micelles as longer fatty acid chains do. The long-chain fatty acids are taken up by the intestinal cells and packaged into triacylglycerols for transport as chylomicrons. Chylomicrons exit the intestine through lacteals that feed into the lymphatic system, which joins with the bloodstream in the base of the neck through the thoracic duct.

3. **C**

During fatty acid mobilization, there is a breakdown of triacylglycerols in adipocytes by hormone-sensitive lipase (HSL). This breakdown results in the release of three fatty acids and a glycerol molecule. The glycerol may be used by the liver for gluconeogenesis, but adipocytes do not have the ability to carry out gluconeogenesis.

4. **B**

Chylomicrons and VLDL are very similar. Both contain apolipoproteins and primarily transport triacylglycerols, eliminating **(A)** and **(C)**. The only major difference between them is the tissue of origin. Chylomicrons transport dietary triacylglycerol and originate in the small intestine, while VLDL transport newly synthesized triacylglycerols and originate in the liver.

5. **D**

While the transport and lipid binding functions of most lipoproteins are independent of the apolipoprotein component, the interaction of these lipoproteins with the environment is controlled almost exclusively by apolipoproteins. Lipoproteins cannot exit or enter cells without apolipoproteins, and are unable to transfer lipids without specialized apolipoproteins or cholesterol-specific enzymes.

6. **A**

Statins are drugs that are prescribed to treat high cholesterol and act as competitive inhibitors of HMG-CoA reductase. HMG-CoA reductase is the rate-limiting enzyme of *de novo* cholesterol synthesis; inhibition of this enzyme lowers production of cholesterol, thus lowering overall levels of cholesterol.

7. **A**

LCAT adds a fatty acid to cholesterol, producing cholesteryl esters, which dissolve in the core of HDL, allowing HDL to transport cholesterol from the periphery to the liver.

8. **B**

Humans can only synthesize one fatty acid, palmitic acid. Palmitic acid is fully saturated and therefore does not contain any double bonds. Palmitic acid has 16 carbons, and is synthesized from eight molecules of acetyl-CoA. In shorthand notation, palmitic acid is written as 16:0 (16 carbons, no double bonds).

9. **C**

The steps in fatty acid synthesis are activation (attachment to acyl carrier protein), bond formation (between malonyl-CoA and the growing fatty acid chain), reduction (of a carboxyl group), dehydration, and reduction (of a double bond).

10. **C**

Ketone bodies are produced in the mitochondria of liver cells as acetyl-CoA accumulates during fasting, consistent with **(C)**. On the other hand, to eliminate **(B)**, observe that while acetyl-CoA is indeed converted to acetoacetate, 3-hydroxybutyrate, or acetone, the acetone that is produced is only a byproduct and is not used for energy, which conflicts with the assertion in **(B)** that "all of which are used for energy." Muscle cells will begin using ketone bodies for energy before the brain. The brain will only start using ketone bodies once they have accumulated to higher concentrations in the blood, eliminating choice **(D)**.

11. **D**

The liver is the major metabolic organ in the body and is responsible for much of the synthesis and interconversion of fuel sources. Most of the triacylglycerols that are synthesized in the liver are transported as VLDL to adipose tissue for storage. Both the adipocytes, **(A)**, and dietary intake, **(B)**, constitute a minor source of triacylglycerols.

12. **C**

In order for the enzymes of fatty acid oxidation to operate, there can be, at most, one double bond in the area of enzyme activity, and it must be oriented between carbons 2 and 3. In order to accomplish this in monounsaturated fatty acids, an isomerase is employed. When there are multiple double bonds that fall within the enzymatic binding site, both an isomerase and 2,4-dienoyl-CoA reductase are required for the oxidative enzymes to act on the fatty acid. For this question, simply recognizing that *dienoyl* refers to having multiple double bonds is sufficient to arrive at the answer.

13. **C**

Ketolysis is the breakdown of ketone bodies to acetyl-CoA for energy. This process occurs in the brain and muscle tissues, but cannot occur in the liver, which lacks an enzyme necessary for ketone body breakdown. Ketolysis is not associated with an increase in glucose metabolism because it most often occurs under conditions of starvation.

14. **D**

The energy contribution of an amino acid depends on its ability to be turned into glucose through gluconeogenesis (glucogenic amino acids), ketone bodies (ketogenic amino acids), or both. All of the amino acids listed in the answer choices are glucogenic; isoleucine is also ketogenic. The energy acquired from an amino acid will also depend on the number of carbons it can donate to these energy-creating processes, which depends on the size of its side chain. Isoleucine has the largest side chain of the answer choices, and will thus contribute the most energy per molecule.

15. **A**

The degradation of protein and processing by the liver implies a prolonged starvation state; protein will not be used for energy unless absolutely necessary. Thus, gluconeogenesis is the most likely process. When gluconeogenesis is not possible, easily metabolized molecules, such as ketone bodies, are synthesized. Fatty acid production occurs when energy is being stored; proteins would not be broken down to store energy in fatty acids.

GO ONLINE

Consult your online resources for additional practice.

SHARED CONCEPTS

Biochemistry Chapter 1
Amino Acids, Peptides, and Proteins

Biochemistry Chapter 5
Lipid Structure and Function

Biochemistry Chapter 8
Biological Membranes

Biochemistry Chapter 12
Bioenergetics and Regulation of Metabolism

Biology Chapter 9
The Digestive System

Biology Chapter 10
Homeostasis

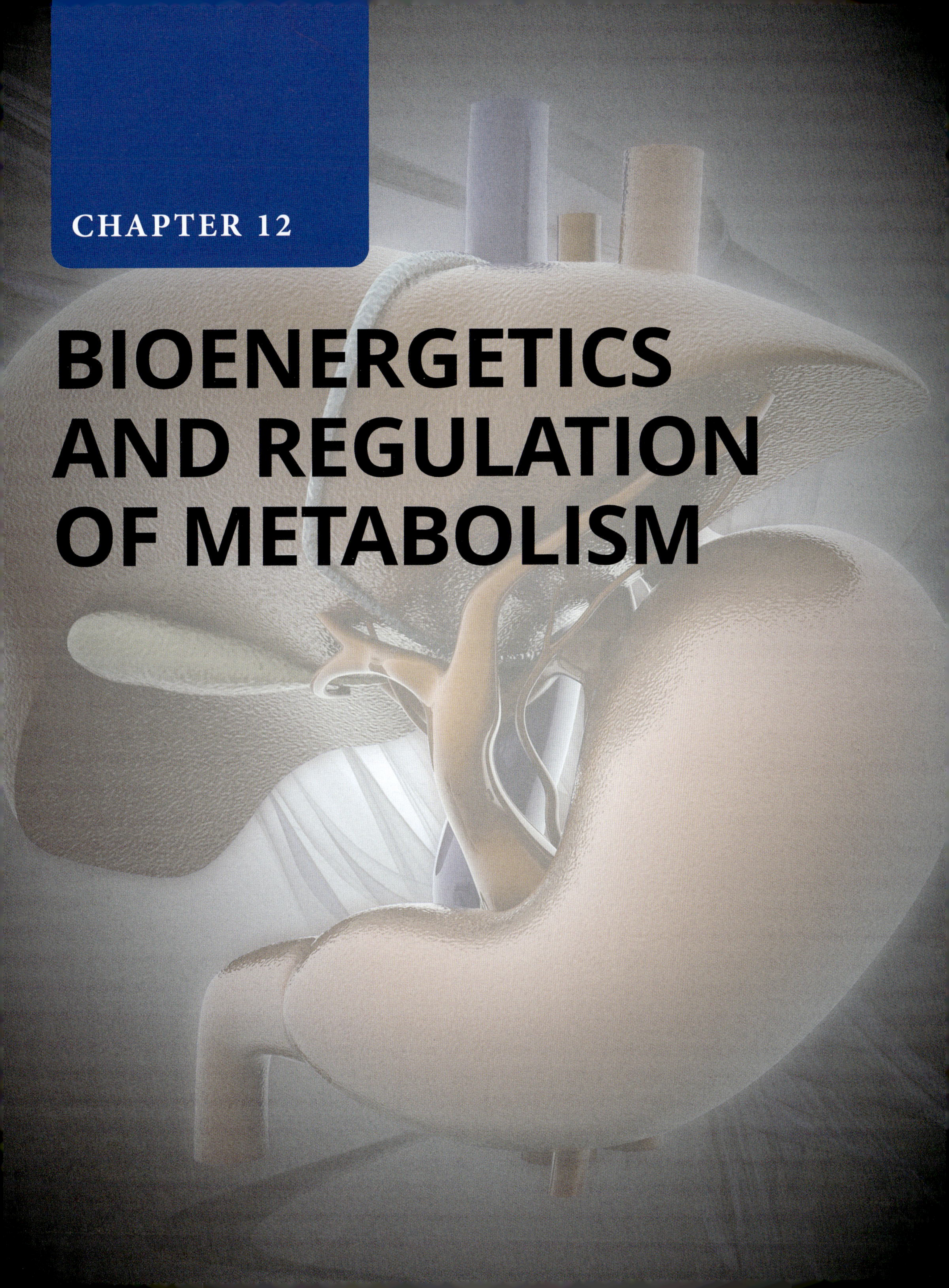

CHAPTER 12

BIOENERGETICS AND REGULATION OF METABOLISM

SCIENCE MASTERY ASSESSMENT

Every pre-med knows this feeling: there is so much content I have to know for the MCAT! How do I know what to do first or what's important?

While the high-yield badges throughout this book will help you identify the most important topics, this Science Mastery Assessment is another tool in your MCAT prep arsenal. This quiz (which can also be taken in your online resources) and the guidance below will help ensure that you are spending the appropriate amount of time on this chapter based on your personal strengths and weaknesses. Don't worry though—skipping something now does not mean you'll never study it. Later on in your prep, as you complete full-length tests, you'll uncover specific pieces of content that you need to review and can come back to these chapters as appropriate.

How to Use This Assessment

If you answer 0–7 questions correctly:

Spend about 1 hour to read this chapter in full and take limited notes throughout. Follow up by reviewing **all** quiz questions to ensure that you now understand how to solve each one.

If you answer 8–11 questions correctly:

Spend 20–40 minutes reviewing the quiz questions. Beginning with the questions you missed, read and take notes on the corresponding subchapters. For questions you answered correctly, ensure your thinking matches that of the explanation and you understand why each choice was correct or incorrect.

If you answer 12–15 questions correctly:

Spend less than 20 minutes reviewing all questions from the quiz. If you missed any, then include a quick read-through of the corresponding subchapters, or even just the relevant content within a subchapter, as part of your question review. For questions you got correct, ensure your thinking matches that of the explanation and review the Concept Summary at the end of the chapter.

1. Adding heat to a closed biological system will do all of the following EXCEPT:
   - **A.** increase the internal energy of the system.
   - **B.** increase the average of the vibrational, rotational, and translational energies.
   - **C.** cause the system to do work to maintain a fixed internal energy.
   - **D.** increase the enthalpy of the system.

2. At 25°C the $\Delta G°$ for a certain reaction $A \rightleftharpoons B + 2\ C$ is 0. If the concentration of A, B, and C in the cell at 25°C are all 10 mM, how does the ΔG compare to the measurement taken with 1 M concentrations?
   - **A.** ΔG is greater than $\Delta G°$, thus the reaction is spontaneous.
   - **B.** ΔG is less than $\Delta G°$, thus the reaction is spontaneous.
   - **C.** ΔG is greater than $\Delta G°$, thus the reaction is nonspontaneous.
   - **D.** ΔG is less than $\Delta G°$, thus the reaction is nonspontaneous.

3. Which of the following statements is true about the hydrolysis of ATP?
   - **A.** The free energy of ATP hydrolysis is independent of pH.
   - **B.** One mole of creatine phosphate can phosphorylate two moles of ADP.
   - **C.** The free energy of hydrolysis of ATP is nearly the same as for ADP.
   - **D.** ATP yields cyclic AMP after two hydrolysis reactions.

4. The reduction half-reaction in the last step of the electron transport chain is:
   - **A.** $O_2 + 4\ e^- + 4\ H^+ \rightarrow 2\ H_2O$
   - **B.** $NADPH \rightarrow NADP^+ + e^- + H^+$
   - **C.** $NADP^+ + e^- + H^+ \rightarrow NADPH$
   - **D.** Ubiquinone (Q) $\rightarrow$ Ubiquinol (QH_2)

5. The ability to exist in both an oxidized and a reduced state is characteristic of:
   - **A.** adenosine triphosphate (ATP).
   - **B.** electron carriers.
   - **C.** regulatory enzymes.
   - **D.** peptide hormones.

6. What energy state was described in the introduction to this chapter?
   - **A.** Absorptive
   - **B.** Postabsorptive
   - **C.** Starvation
   - **D.** Vegetative

7. Which of the following correctly pairs a tissue with its preferred energy source in the well fed state?
   - **A.** Liver - ketone bodies
   - **B.** Adipose tissue - fatty acids
   - **C.** Brain - amino acids
   - **D.** Cardiac muscle - fatty acids

8. How do hormonal controls of glycogen metabolism differ from allosteric controls?
   - **A.** Hormonal control is systemic and covalent.
   - **B.** Hormonal control is local and covalent.
   - **C.** Hormonal control is systemic and noncovalent.
   - **D.** Hormonal control is local and noncovalent.

9. Which of the following tissues is most dependent on insulin?

A. Active skeletal muscle
B. Resting skeletal muscle
C. Cardiac muscle
D. Smooth muscle

10. Glucocorticoids have been implicated in stress-related weight gain because:

A. they increase appetite and decrease satiety signals.
B. they increase the activity of catabolic hormones.
C. they increase glucose levels, which causes insulin secretion.
D. they interfere with activity of the leptin receptor.

11. In the absence of oxygen, which tissue will experience damage most rapidly?

A. Skin
B. Brain
C. Red blood cells
D. Liver

12. A respiratory quotient approaching 0.7 indicates metabolism primarily of which macromolecule?

A. Carbohydrates
B. Lipids
C. Nucleic acids
D. Amino acids

13. Which of the following side effects would be anticipated in someone taking leptin to promote weight loss?

A. Drowsiness
B. Increased appetite
C. Irritability
D. Fever

14. Which of the following statements is FALSE?

A. Growth hormone participates in glucose counterregulation.
B. T_4 acts more slowly than T_3.
C. ATP stores are turned over more than 10,000 times daily.
D. Catecholamines stimulate the sympathetic nervous system.

15. Which process is expected to begin earliest in a prolonged fast?

A. Ketone bodies are used by the brain.
B. Glycogen storage is halted.
C. Proteins are broken down.
D. Enzyme phosphorylation and dephosphorylation.

Answer Key

1. **C** (See section 12.1)
2. **B** (See section 12.1)
3. **C** (See section 12.2)
4. **A** (See section 12.3)
5. **B** (See section 12.3)
6. **B** (See section 12.4)
7. **D** (See section 12.6)
8. **A** (See section 12.5)
9. **B** (See section 12.5)
10. **C** (See section 12.5)
11. **B** (See section 12.6)
12. **B** (See section 12.7)
13. **A** (See section 12.7)
14. **C** (See section 12.2)
15. **D** (See section 12.4)

The relevant section of the chapter to review for each question is given in parentheses after the correct answer. Detailed explanations can be found at the end of the chapter.

CHAPTER 12

BIOENERGETICS AND REGULATION OF METABOLISM

In This Chapter

CHAPTER PROFILE

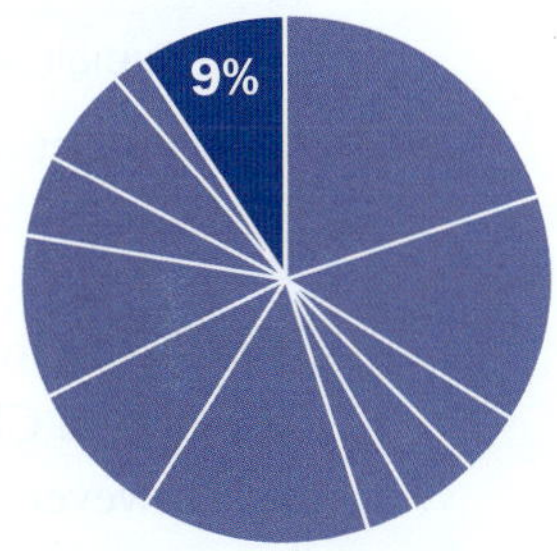

The content in this chapter should be relevant to about 9% of all questions about biochemistry on the MCAT.

This chapter covers material from the following AAMC content categories:

1D: Principles of bioenergetics and fuel molecule metabolism

5E: Principles of chemical thermodynamics and kinetics

Introduction

You got up this morning with a really ambitious plan: study for the MCAT! The day started with a big breakfast, and then you dove into *MCAT Biochemistry Review*. A few chapters in you noticed your stomach growling, but you were having so much fun that you ignored it. A little while later, your body realized it wasn't getting any more food for a while, but it still needed energy. Where does it come from?

The human body is an incredible system. When we skip lunch on a study day, we produce hormones that help raise the level of certain energy molecules in the bloodstream, mainly glucose. This is a good thing because the brain relies solely on glucose for most of its metabolism, and we always want to be thinking at our peak. Glucose in the blood comes from either our diet, such as when we eat a big breakfast, or from our fuel stores, through the processes of gluconeogenesis and glycogenolysis. These processes, just like the formation and consumption of ATP, are highly regulated.

In this chapter, we'll highlight the basic principles of bioenergetics, including thermodynamics: the sources of energy and the reactions that play a key role in moving that energy around. Then we'll examine the different energy states of the body before taking a look at the intimate relationship of hormones with metabolism. We'll spend some time examining the regulation of metabolism, regulatory enzymes for some common pathways, and how specific tissues preferentially metabolize particular macronutrients. By the end of this chapter, you'll be able to tell where and how your food is being used, and you probably won't choose to skip lunch again—no matter how much fun you're having!

12.1 Thermodynamics and Bioenergetics High Yield

LEARNING OBJECTIVES

After Chapter 12.1, you will be able to:

- Describe the relationship between $\Delta G°$ and $\Delta G°'$
- Explain why heat can be used as a measure of internal energy for biological systems
- Predict the spontaneity of a reaction given the signs of ΔH and ΔS

If we take a look back at what we learned about thermodynamics in Chapter 3 of *MCAT Physics and Math Review* and Chapter 7 of *MCAT General Chemistry Review*, it becomes evident that we already know quite a bit. However, most of the data that we've seen so far has been obtained under standard-state conditions (25°C, 1 atm pressure, and 1 M concentrations). These assumptions work in a chemistry lab, but must be adjusted for application in the human body.

Biological Systems

Biological systems are often considered **open systems** because they can exchange both energy and matter with the environment. Energy is exchanged in the form of mechanical work when something is moved over a distance, or as heat energy. Matter is exchanged through food consumption and elimination, as well as respiration. Most biochemical studies are performed on the cellular or subcellular level rather than in an entire organism. These systems can be considered **closed** because there is no exchange of matter with the environment. In such a system, we can make useful simplifications about the internal energy, U. **Internal energy** is the sum of all of the different interactions between and within atoms in a system; vibration, rotation, linear motion, and stored chemical energies all contribute.

Because the system is closed, the change in internal energy can come only in the form of work or heat. This can be represented mathematically through the First Law of Thermodynamics, $\Delta U = Q - W$. Work in thermodynamics refers to changes in pressure and volume. These are constant in most living systems, so the only quantity of interest in determining internal energy is heat.

MCAT EXPERTISE

The energy of chemical reactions is described as part of general chemistry, while work is generally associated with physics. Be aware that on Test Day, you will see crossover that allows you to draw on knowledge of the other subjects and to use that background information to your advantage.

Enthalpy, Entropy, and Free Energy

Bioenergetics is the term used to describe energy states in biological systems. Changes in **free energy** (ΔG) provide information about chemical reactions and can predict whether a chemical reaction is favorable and will occur. In biological systems, ATP plays a crucial role in transferring energy from energy-releasing catabolic processes to energy-requiring anabolic processes.

Whether a chemical reaction proceeds is determined by the degree to which enthalpy and entropy change during a chemical reaction. **Enthalpy** measures the overall change in heat of a system during a reaction. At constant pressure and volume, enthalpy (ΔH) and thermodynamic heat exchange (Q) are equal. Changes in **entropy** (ΔS) measure the degree of disorder or energy dispersion in a system. While the MCAT will not test on the level of statistical thermodynamics, this conceptual understanding of entropy (ΔS) will be helpful. Entropy carries the units $\frac{\text{J}}{\text{K}}$.

When combined together mathematically, along with temperature (T), these quantities can be related through the Gibbs free energy equation:

$$\Delta G = \Delta H - T\Delta S$$

Equation 12.1

which predicts the direction in which a chemical reaction proceeds spontaneously. Spontaneous reactions proceed in the forward direction, exhibit a net loss of free energy, and therefore have a negative ΔG. In contrast, nonspontaneous reactions, which would be spontaneous in the reverse direction, exhibit a net gain of energy and have a positive ΔG. Free energy approaches zero as the reaction proceeds to equilibrium and there is no net change in concentration of reactants or products.

BRIDGE

Enthalpy, entropy, and free energy are discussed more thoroughly in Chapter 7 of *MCAT General Chemistry Review.*

Physiological Conditions

The change in free energy (ΔG) that we have been discussing up to this point predicts changes occurring at any concentration of products and reactants and at any temperature. In contrast, standard free energy (ΔG°) is the energy change that occurs at standard concentrations of 1 M, pressure of 1 atm, and temperature of 25°C. These can be related by the equation:

$$\Delta G = \Delta G^\circ + RT\ln(Q)$$

Equation 12.2

where R is the universal gas constant, T is the temperature, and Q is the reaction quotient. Biochemical analysis works well under all standard conditions except one: pH. A 1 M concentration of protons would correspond to a pH of 0, which is far too acidic for most biochemical reactions. Therefore, in the **modified standard state**, $[\text{H}^+] = 10^{-7}$ M and the pH is 7. With this additional condition, ΔG° is given the special symbol $\Delta G^{\circ\prime}$, indicating that it is standardized to the neutral buffers used in biochemistry. Note that if the concentrations of other reactants and products differ from 1 M, these must still be adjusted for in the equation above.

The shift in ΔG as a result of changing concentration is not universally toward or away from spontaneity. There is a general trend that reactions with more products than reactants have a more negative ΔG, while reactions with more reactants than products have a more positive ΔG. While this trend is useful for making quick assessments, always double check with numbers on Test Day.

MCAT CONCEPT CHECK 12.1

Before you move on, assess your understanding of the material with these questions.

1. What conditions does $\Delta G^{\circ\prime}$ adjust for that are not considered with ΔG°?

____

2. Why can heat be used as a measure of internal energy in living systems?

____

____

3. Complete the following table relating the change in entropy and enthalpy of a reaction with whether the reaction is spontaneous.

	$+\Delta H$	$-\Delta H$
$+\Delta S$		
$-\Delta S$		

12.2 The Role of ATP High Yield

LEARNING OBJECTIVES

After Chapter 12.2, you will be able to:

- Predict the impact of ATP coupling on the energetics of a reaction
- Calculate free energy change for an overall reaction given energetic data for component reactions
- Relate the structure of ATP to its role as an energy carrier

The human body can make use of different energy sources with roughly the same efficiency, but all nutrient molecules are not created equally. For example, fats are much more energy-rich than carbohydrates, proteins, or ketones. Complete combustion of fat results in 9 $\frac{\text{kcal}}{\text{g}}$ of energy, compared with only 4 $\frac{\text{kcal}}{\text{g}}$ derived from carbohydrates, proteins, or ketones. Because fats are so much more energy-dense than other biomolecules, they are preferred for long-term energy storage. Think of the difference between fats and carbohydrates like the difference between a 16-GB and an 8-GB storage drive. The storage drive with a greater capacity occupies the same amount of physical space, but holds twice as much data. While different energy sources provide greater or lesser caloric values, the end goal is to have energy in a readily available form. For the cell, this is **adenosine triphosphate** (**ATP**), shown in Figure 12.1.

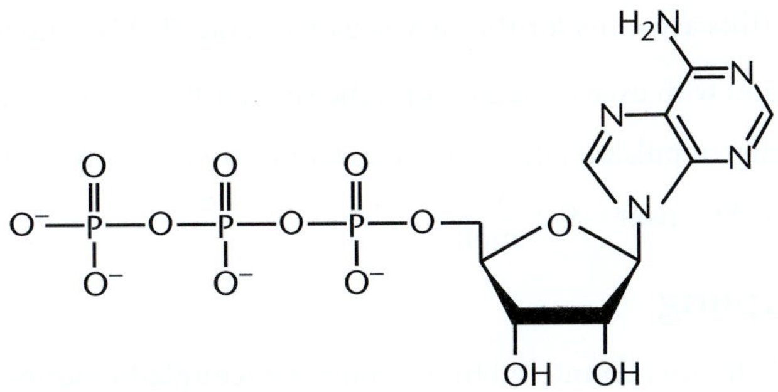

Figure 12.1 Adenosine Triphosphate (ATP)

ATP as an Energy Carrier

ATP is the major energy currency in the body. It is a mid-level energy carrier, as seen in Table 12.1, and is formed from **substrate-level phosphorylation**, as well as **oxidative phosphorylation**. Why do we want ATP to be a mid-level carrier and not a higher-level one? Think about your wallet. If you never had the ability to get change back after a purchase, what type of bill would you want in abundance? One dollar bills! Similarly, ATP cannot get back the "leftover" free energy after a reaction, so it's best to use a carrier with a smaller free energy. ATP provides about 30 $\frac{\text{kJ}}{\text{mol}}$ of energy under physiological conditions. If a reaction only requires 10 $\frac{\text{kJ}}{\text{mol}}$ to overcome a positive ΔG value, then 20 $\frac{\text{kJ}}{\text{mol}}$ have been wasted. The waste would be even higher with a higher-energy compound like creatine phosphate.

Compound	$\Delta G^{\circ\prime}\frac{\text{kj}}{\text{mol}}$	Function
cAMP	−50.4	Second messenger
Creatine phosphate	−43.3	Direct phosphorylation in muscle
ATP	−30.5	Energy turnover in all cell types
Glucose 6-phosphate	−13.9	Intermediate of glycolysis and gluconeogenesis
AMP	−9.2	ATP synthesis

Table 12.1 Free Energy of Hydrolysis for Key Metabolic Phosphate Compounds

Remember that most of the ATP in a cell is produced by mitochondrial *ATP synthase*, as described in Chapter 10 of *MCAT Biochemistry Review*, but some ATP is produced during glycolysis and (indirectly from GTP) in the citric acid cycle. ATP consists of an adenosine molecule attached to three phosphate groups, and is generated from ADP and P_i with energy input from an exergonic reaction or electrochemical gradient. ATP is consumed either through hydrolysis or the transfer of a phosphate group to another molecule. If one phosphate group is removed, **adenosine diphosphate** (**ADP**) is produced; if two phosphate groups are removed, **adenosine monophosphate** (**AMP**) is the result. In a single day, an average-sized person uses about 90 percent of body weight in ATP but only has about 50 grams of ATP available at any given time. Continuous recycling of ATP, ADP, and P_i more than 1000 times per day accounts for this discrepancy.

What makes ATP such a good energy carrier is its high-energy phosphate bonds. The negative charges on the phosphate groups experience repulsive forces with one another, and the ADP and P_i molecules that form after hydrolysis are stabilized by resonance. While ATP doesn't rapidly break down on its own in the cell, it is much more stable after hydrolysis. This accounts for the very negative value of ΔG. Under standard conditions ΔG° is about $-55\ \frac{\text{kJ}}{\text{mol}}$. At pH 7 and with excess magnesium, the standard free energy change is still $-30.5\ \frac{\text{kJ}}{\text{mol}}$. ADP, which also displays charge repulsion and resonance stabilization after hydrolysis, has similar ΔG values, but AMP has a much smaller ΔG° near $-9.2\ \frac{\text{kJ}}{\text{mol}}$.

Hydrolysis and Coupling

ATP hydrolysis is most likely to be encountered in the context of **coupled reactions**. Many coupled reactions use ATP as an energy source. For example, the movement of sodium and potassium against their electrochemical gradients requires energy, which is harnessed from the hydrolysis of ATP.

ATP cleavage is the transfer of a high-energy phosphate group from ATP to another molecule. Generally, this activates or inactivates the target molecule. With these **phosphoryl group transfers**, the overall free energy of the reaction will be determined by taking the sum of the free energies of the individual reactions.

KEY CONCEPT

ATP is used to fuel energetically unfavorable reactions or to activate or inactivate other molecules.

Phosphoryl Group Transfers

ATP can provide a phosphate group as a reactant. For example, in the phosphorylation of glucose in the early stages of glycolysis, ATP donates a phosphate group to glucose to form glucose 6-phosphate. The information in Table 12.1 indicates the free energy of hydrolysis, which can be conceptualized as the transfer of the phosphate group to water. To determine the free energy of phosphoryl group transfer to another biological molecule, one could use Hess's law and calculate the difference in free energy between the reactants and products:

BRIDGE

Hess's law, discussed in Chapter 7 of *MCAT General Chemistry Review*, applies for all of the state functions, including pressure, density, temperature, volume, enthalpy, internal energy, free energy, and entropy.

$$\text{creatine phosphate} + H_2O \rightarrow \text{creatine} + P_i \qquad \Delta G^{\circ\prime} = -43.3\ \frac{\text{kJ}}{\text{mol}}$$

$$ADP + P_i \rightarrow ATP + H_2O \qquad \Delta G^{\circ\prime} = 30.5\ \frac{\text{kJ}}{\text{mol}} \text{ (reverse reaction from Table 12.1)}$$

$$\text{creatine phosphate} + ADP \rightarrow \text{creatine} + ATP \qquad \Delta G^{\circ\prime} = -12.8\ \frac{\text{kJ}}{\text{mol}}$$

MCAT CONCEPT CHECK 12.2

Before you move on, assess your understanding of the material with these questions.

1. How does coupling with ATP hydrolysis alter the energetics of a reaction?

____

2. Explain why ATP is an inefficient molecule for long-term energy storage.

____

3. Using Table 12.1, calculate the free energy change for the synthesis of ATP from cAMP and inorganic phosphate. Note: cAMP is hydrolyzed to AMP, and the free energy of hydrolysis for ATP and ADP is approximately equal.

____

12.3 Biological Oxidation and Reduction

High Yield

LEARNING OBJECTIVES

After Chapter 12.3, you will be able to:

- Explain the benefits of analyzing half reactions for biological oxidation–reduction reactions
- Recall soluble electron carriers, such as NADH and CoQ, and the pathways they are paired with

Many key enzymes in ATP synthesis and other biochemical pathways have oxidoreductase activity.

Half-Reactions

Just as you practiced with general chemistry, an important skill in biochemistry is to be able to divide oxidation–reduction reactions into their half-reaction components to determine the number of electrons being transferred. For example, in lactic acid fermentation, pyruvate and NADH are converted to lactate and NAD^+ by *lactate dehydrogenase*. This reaction can be broken down into half-reactions as follows:

Overall reaction	$C_3H_4O_3 + NADH + H^+ \rightarrow C_3H_6O_3 + NAD^+$
Reduction	$C_3H_4O_3 + 2\,H^+ + 2\,e^- \rightarrow C_3H_6O_3$
Oxidation	$NADH \rightarrow NAD^+ + H^+ + 2\,e^-$

Remember that spontaneous oxidation–reduction reactions have a negative value of ΔG and a positive value of E (electromotive force).

Electron Carriers

In the cytoplasm, there are several molecules that act as **high-energy electron carriers**. These are all soluble and include NADH, NADPH, $FADH_2$, ubiquinone, cytochromes, and glutathione. Some of these electron carriers are used by the mitochondrial electron transport chain, which leads to the oxidative phosphorylation of ADP to ATP. As electrons are passed down the electron transport chain, they give up their free energy to form the proton-motive force across the inner mitochondrial membrane. The oxidized and reduced forms of NADH and $FADH_2$ are shown in Figure 12.2. In addition to soluble electron carriers, there are membrane-bound electron carriers embedded within the inner mitochondrial membrane. One such carrier is flavin mononucleotide (FMN), which is bonded to complex I of the electron transport chain and can also act as a soluble electron carrier. In general, proteins with prosthetic groups containing iron–sulfur clusters are particularly well suited for the transport of electrons.

BRIDGE

Oxidation–reduction reactions, discussed in Chapter 11 of *MCAT General Chemistry Review* and Chapter 4 of *MCAT Organic Chemistry Review*, are a staple of general chemistry and are characteristic of oxidoreductase enzymes. Take a moment to identify the oxidizing and reducing agents in the reaction catalyzed by lactate dehydrogenase.

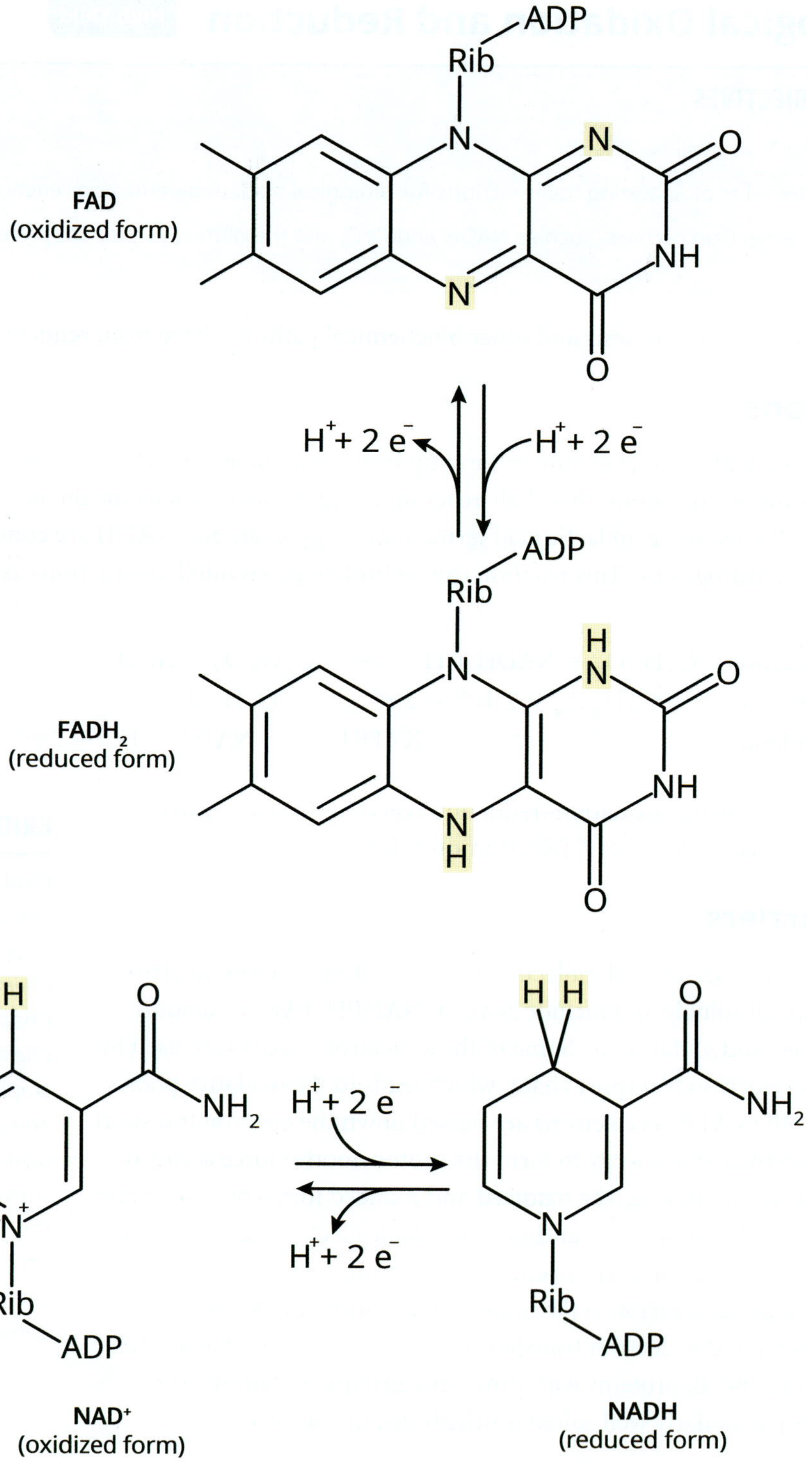

Figure 12.2 Oxidized and Reduced Forms of NADH and $FADH_2$

Flavoproteins

Flavoproteins contain a modified vitamin B_2, or ***riboflavin***. They are nucleic acid derivatives, generally either ***flavin adenine dinucleotide*** (**FAD**) or ***flavin mononucleotide*** (**FMN**). Flavoproteins are most notable for their presence in the mitochondria and chloroplasts as electron carriers. Flavoproteins are also involved in the modification of other B vitamins to active forms. Finally, flavoproteins function as coenzymes for enzymes in the oxidation of fatty acids, the decarboxylation of pyruvate, and the reduction of glutathione. The structure of FAD is shown in Figure 12.3 in comparison to the structure of NAD^+.

REAL WORLD

Deficiency of riboflavin, a key component of flavoproteins, leads to a lack of growth, failure to thrive, and eventual death in experimental models. In humans, riboflavin deficiency is very rare, but may occur in severely malnourished individuals.

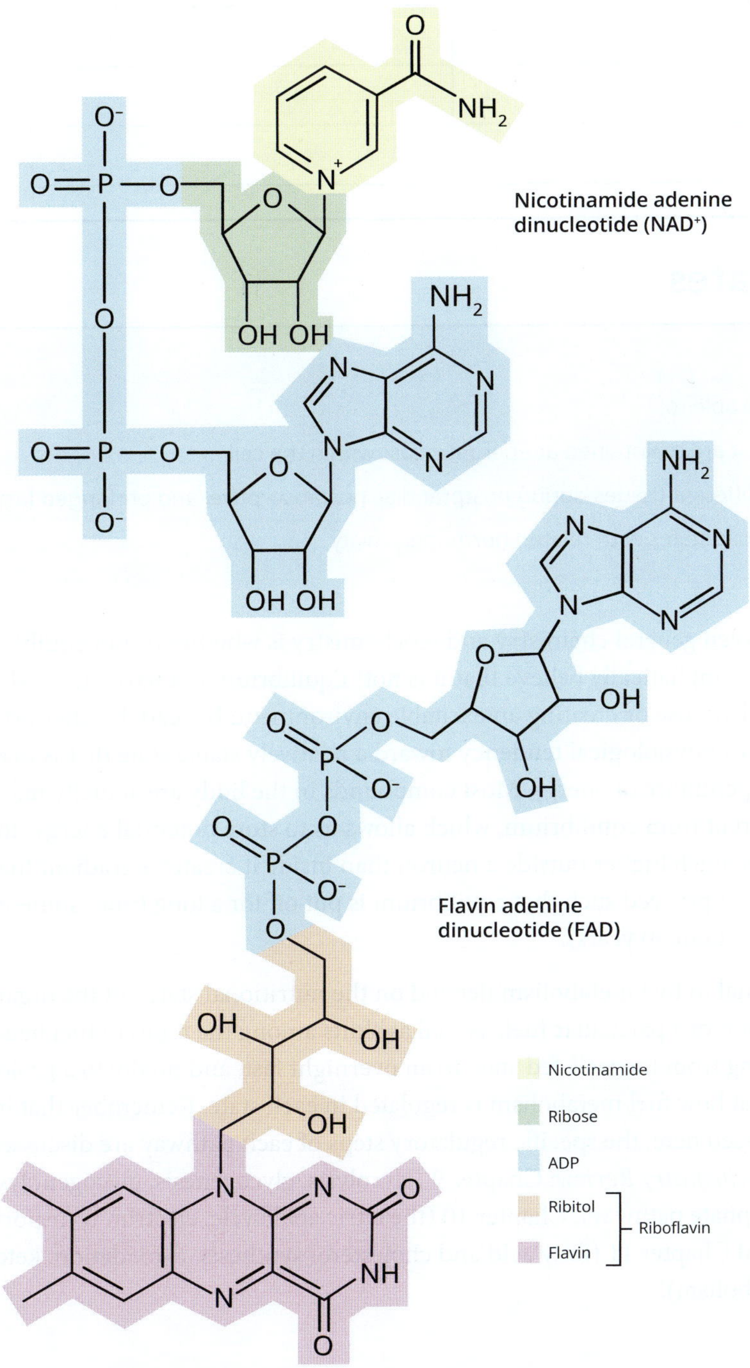

Figure 12.3 Structure of NAD^+ and FAD

MCAT CONCEPT CHECK 12.3

Before you move on, assess your understanding of the material with these questions.

1. What is an advantage of analyzing the half-reactions in biological oxidation and reduction reactions?

2. Name three soluble electron carriers and their relevant metabolic pathways in the cell.

Electron Carrier	Metabolic Pathway(s)

12.4 Metabolic States

LEARNING OBJECTIVES

After Chapter 12.4, you will be able to:

- Identify disequilibriums that are maintained at energetic cost within the cell
- Compare the behavior of different tissues during postprandial, postabsorptive, and prolonged fasting states
- Associate the three metabolic states with related hormone activity

One of the key differences between general chemistry and biochemistry is whether or not equilibrium is seen as a desirable state. Biochemists emphatically believe that it is not! Equilibrium is a fixed state, which prevents us from storing any energy for later use or creating an excitable environment. Instead, biochemists seek a state of homeostasis. **Homeostasis** is a physiological tendency toward a relatively stable state that is maintained and adjusted, often with the expenditure of energy. Most compounds in the body are actually maintained at a homeostatic level that is different from equilibrium, which allows us to store potential energy; for example, keeping sodium concentrations much higher outside a neuron than inside it creates a gradient that stores energy. In this state, reactions can proceed such that equilibrium is put off for a long time (someone born today can delay equilibrium for about 80 years).

The pathways that are operational in fuel metabolism depend on the nutritional status of the organism. Shifts between storage and mobilization of a particular fuel, as well as shifts among the types of fuel being used, are very pronounced when going from the well-fed state to an overnight fast, and finally to a prolonged state of starvation. We'll take a look at how fuel metabolism is regulated in each state. Remember that in addition to the "big-picture view" discussed here, the specific regulatory steps of each pathway are discussed in the previous chapters of *MCAT Biochemistry Review*: Chapter 9 (glycolysis, glycogenesis, glycogenolysis, gluconeogenesis, and the pentose phosphate pathway), Chapter 10 (the citric acid cycle, electron transport chain, and oxidative phosphorylation), and Chapter 11 (fatty acid and cholesterol synthesis, β-oxidation, ketogenesis and ketolysis, and amino acid metabolism).

Postprandial (Absorptive) State

The **postprandial state**, also called the **absorptive** or **well-fed state**, occurs shortly after eating. This state is marked by greater **anabolism** (synthesis of biomolecules) and fuel storage than **catabolism** (breakdown of biomolecules for energy). Nutrients flood in from the gut and make their way via the hepatic portal vein to the liver, where they can be stored or distributed to other tissues of the body. The postprandial state generally lasts three to five hours after eating a meal.

Just after eating, blood glucose levels rise and stimulate the release of insulin. The three major target tissues for insulin are the liver, muscle, and adipose tissue, as shown in Figure 12.4. Insulin promotes glycogen synthesis in liver and muscle. After the glycogen stores are filled, the liver converts excess glucose to fatty acids and triacylglycerols. Insulin promotes triacylglycerol synthesis in adipose tissue and protein synthesis in muscle, as well as glucose entry into both tissues. After a meal, most of the energy needs of the liver are met by the oxidation of excess amino acids.

Two types of cells—nervous tissue and red blood cells—are notably insensitive to insulin. Nervous tissue derives energy from oxidizing glucose to CO_2 and water in both the well-fed and normal fasting states. Only in prolonged fasting does this situation change. Red blood cells can only use glucose anaerobically for all their energy needs, regardless of the individual's metabolic state.

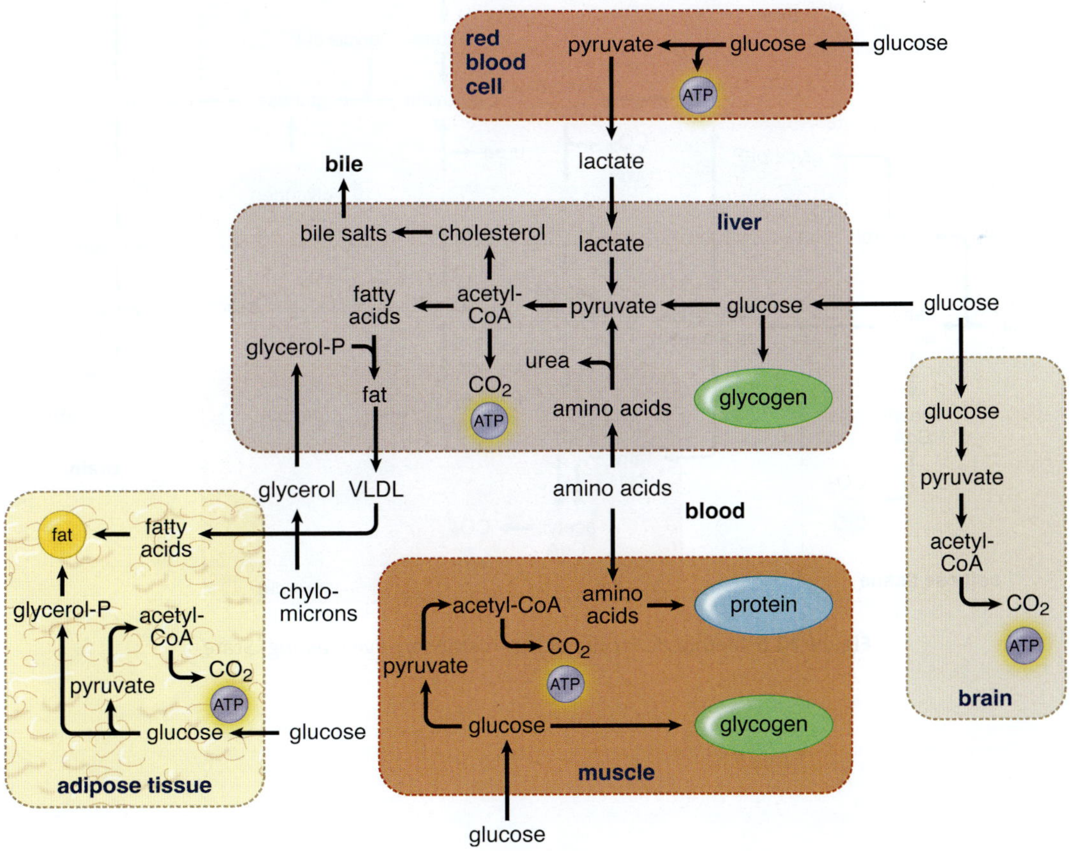

Figure 12.4 Metabolic Profile of the Postprandial (Absorptive) State

Postabsorptive (Fasting) State

Glucagon, cortisol, epinephrine, norepinephrine, and growth hormone oppose the actions of insulin. These hormones are sometimes termed **counterregulatory hormones** because of their effects on skeletal muscle, adipose tissue, and the liver, which are opposite to the actions of insulin. In the liver, glycogen degradation and the release of glucose into the blood are stimulated, as shown in Figure 12.5. Hepatic gluconeogenesis is also stimulated by glucagon, but the response is slower than that of glycogenolysis. Whereas glycogenolysis begins almost immediately at the beginning of the postabsorptive state, gluconeogenesis takes about 12 hours to hit maximum velocity.

The release of amino acids from skeletal muscle and fatty acids from adipose tissue are both stimulated by the decrease in insulin and by an increase in levels of epinephrine. Once carried into the liver, amino acids and fatty acids can provide the necessary carbon skeletons and energy required for gluconeogenesis.

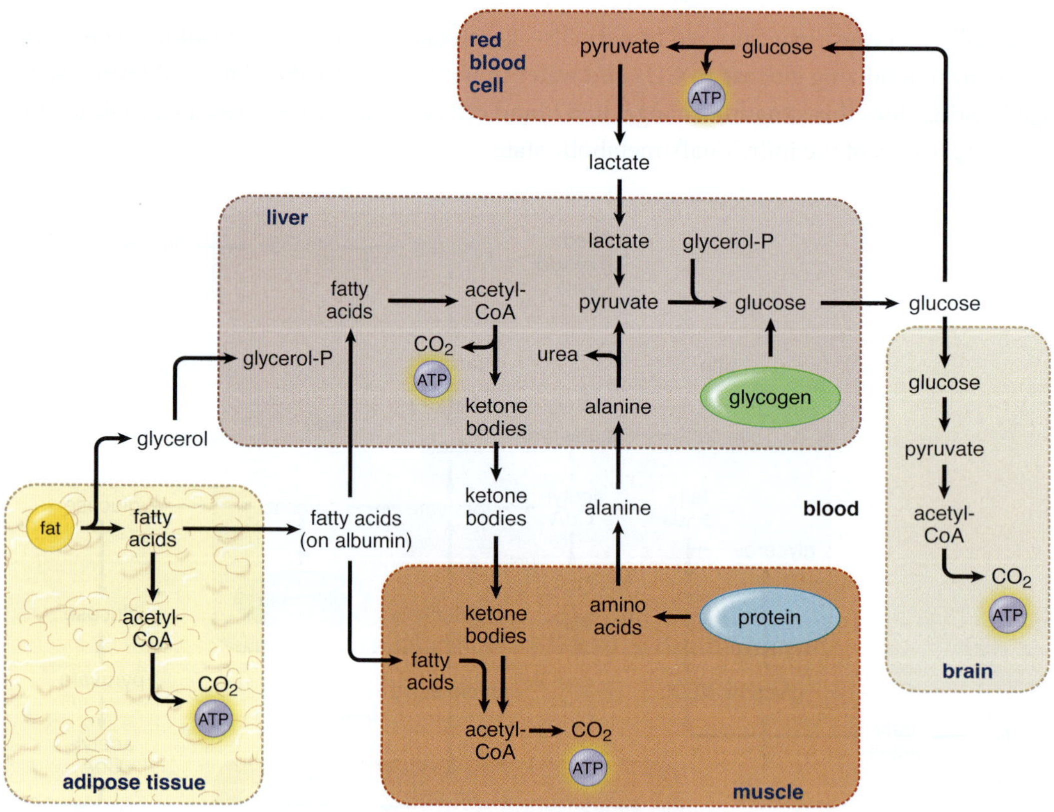

Figure 12.5 Metabolic Profile of the Postabsorptive (Fasting) State

Prolonged Fasting (Starvation)

Levels of glucagon and epinephrine are markedly elevated during starvation. Increased levels of glucagon relative to insulin result in rapid degradation of glycogen stores in the liver. As liver glycogen stores are depleted, gluconeogenic activity continues and plays an important role in maintaining blood glucose levels during prolonged fasting; after about 24 hours, gluconeogenesis is the predominant source of glucose for the body. Lipolysis is rapid, resulting in excess acetyl-CoA that is used in the synthesis of ketone bodies. Once levels of fatty acids and ketones are high enough in the blood, muscle tissue will utilize fatty acids as its major fuel source and the brain will adapt to using ketones for energy. After several weeks of fasting, the brain derives approximately two-thirds of its energy from ketones and one-third from glucose. The shift from glucose to ketones as the major fuel reduces the quantity of amino acids that must be degraded to support gluconeogenesis, which spares proteins that are vital for other functions. Cells that have few, if any, mitochondria, like red blood cells, continue to be dependent on glucose for their energy.

MCAT CONCEPT CHECK 12.4

Before you move on, assess your understanding of the material with these questions.

1. Provide an example of disequilibrium that is maintained at the expense of cellular energy.

___

2. What tissue is least able to change its fuel source in periods of prolonged starvation?

___

3. During what stage is there the greatest decrease in the circulating concentration of insulin?

___

12.5 Hormonal Regulation of Metabolism

LEARNING OBJECTIVES

After Chapter 12.5, you will be able to:

- Describe the impact of key metabolic hormones, such as insulin, glucagon, and thyroid hormones, on metabolic function
- Apply knowledge of the metabolic hormones to a given disease state
- Recall the general structures and traits of metabolic hormones:

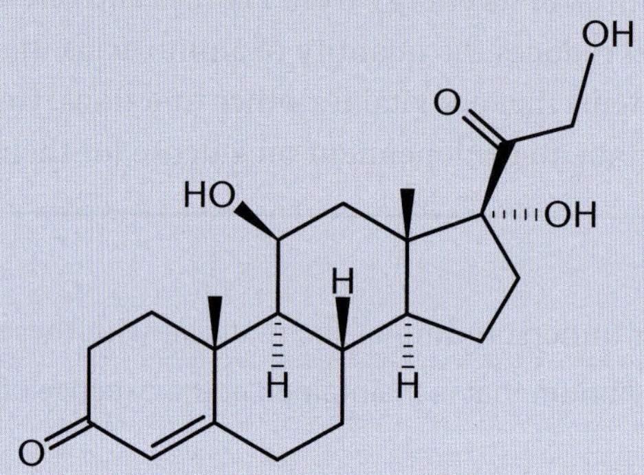

If each cell were acting independently of one another, metabolism would be a random process that could not be coordinated with outside events like meals or exertion. In order to make the most efficient use of the resources available, metabolism must be regulated across the entire organism. This regulation is accomplished best through hormonal means. Water-soluble **peptide hormones**, like insulin, are able to rapidly adjust the metabolic processes of cells via second messenger cascades, while certain fat-soluble **amino acid–derivative hormones**, like thyroid hormones, and **steroid hormones**, like cortisol, enact longer-range effects by exerting regulatory actions at the transcriptional level. Hormone levels are regulated by feedback loops with other endocrine structures, such as the hypothalamic–pituitary axis, or by the biomolecule upon which they act; for example, insulin causes a decrease in blood glucose, which removes the trigger for continued insulin release. Next, we'll examine the specific actions of several hormones involved in the regulation of metabolism and in maintaining homeostasis, including insulin and glucagon, epinephrine, glucocorticoids, and thyroid hormones.

Insulin and Glucagon

Insulin

Insulin is a peptide hormone secreted by the **β-cells** of the pancreatic islets of Langerhans, as shown in Figure 12.6. It is a key player in the uptake and storage of glucose. Glucose is absorbed by peripheral tissues via facilitated transport mechanisms that utilize glucose transporters located in the cell membrane. The tissues that require insulin for effective uptake of glucose are adipose tissue and resting skeletal muscle. Tissues in which glucose uptake is not affected by insulin include:

- Nervous tissue
- Kidney tubules
- Intestinal mucosa
- Red blood cells (erythrocytes)
- β-cells of the pancreas

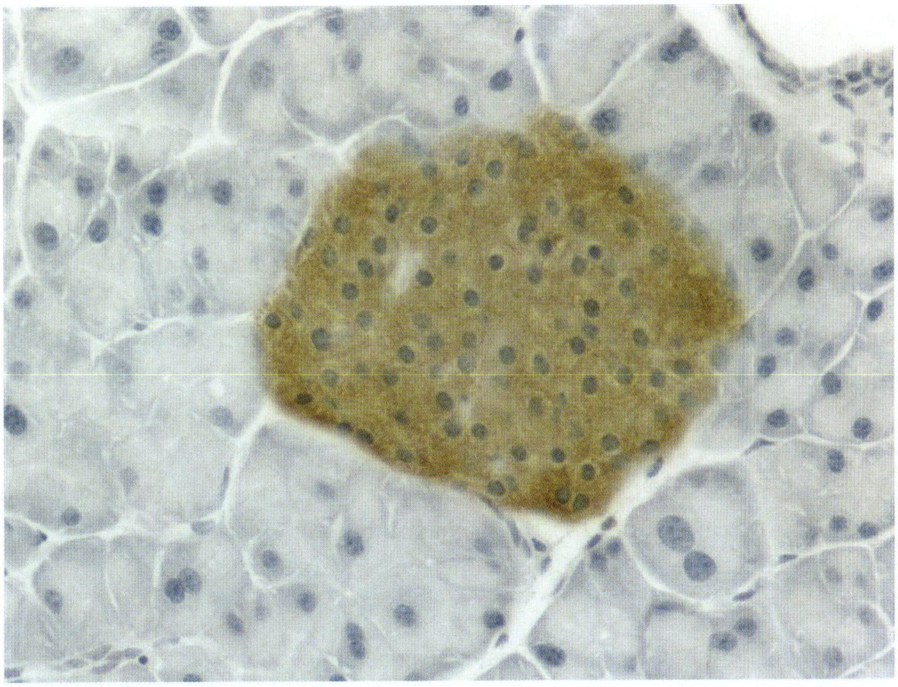

Figure 12.6 Insulin (Light Brown) in Pancreatic β-Cells

Take note of the differences between these types of tissues. Some tissues that require insulin actively store glucose when it is present in high concentrations, while other tissues that do not require insulin must still be able to absorb glucose even when the glucose concentration is low.

Insulin impacts the metabolism of the different nutrient classes in different ways. For carbohydrates, insulin increases the uptake of glucose and increases carbohydrate metabolism in muscle and fat. Increased glucose in muscle can be used as additional fuel to burn during exercise, or can be stored as glycogen. Insulin also increases glycogen synthesis in the liver by increasing the activity of *glucokinase* and *glycogen synthase*, while decreasing the activity of enzymes that promote glycogen breakdown (*glycogen phosphorylase* and *glucose-6-phosphatase*).

While the primary effects of insulin are on carbohydrate metabolism, it also changes the way that the body processes other macromolecules. For instance, insulin increases amino acid uptake by muscle cells, thereby increasing levels of protein synthesis and decreasing breakdown of essential proteins. Insulin also exhibits a significant impact on the metabolism of fats, especially in the liver and adipocytes. The effects of insulin on the metabolism of fats are described below.

Insulin increases:

- Glucose and triacylglycerol uptake by fat cells
- *Lipoprotein lipase* activity, which clears VLDL and chylomicrons from the blood
- Triacylglycerol synthesis (lipogenesis) in adipose tissue and the liver from acetyl-CoA

Insulin decreases:

- Triacylglycerol breakdown (lipolysis) in adipose tissue
- Formation of ketone bodies by the liver

The most important controller of insulin secretion is plasma glucose. Above a threshold of 100 $\frac{\text{mg}}{\text{dL}}$, or about 5.6 mM glucose, insulin secretion is directly proportional to plasma glucose. For glucose to promote insulin secretion, it must not only enter the β-cell but also be metabolized, increasing intracellular ATP concentration. Increased ATP leads to calcium release in the cell, which promotes exocytosis of preformed insulin from intracellular vesicles. Insulin secretion is also affected by signaling initiated by other hormones, such as glucagon and somatostatin.

Glucagon

Glucagon is a peptide hormone secreted by the **α-cells** of the pancreatic islets of Langerhans, as shown in Figure 12.7. The primary target for glucagon action is the hepatocyte. Glucagon acts through second messengers to cause the following effects:

- Increased liver glycogenolysis. Glucagon activates glycogen phosphorylase and inactivates glycogen synthase.
- Increased liver gluconeogenesis. Glucagon promotes the conversion of pyruvate to phosphoenolpyruvate by *pyruvate carboxylase* and *phosphoenolpyruvate carboxykinase* (PEPCK). Glucagon increases the conversion of fructose 1,6-bisphosphate to fructose 6-phosphate by *fructose-1,6-bisphosphatase.*
- Increased liver ketogenesis and decreased lipogenesis.
- Increased lipolysis in the liver. Glucagon activates *hormone-sensitive lipase* in the liver. Because the action is on the liver and not the adipocyte, glucagon is not considered a major fat-mobilizing hormone.

REAL WORLD

Patients with type 1 diabetes mellitus are incapable of synthesizing insulin, but still synthesize glucagon. This combination increases blood sugar much more than if an individual were to lose all pancreatic function or to develop insulin insensitivity.

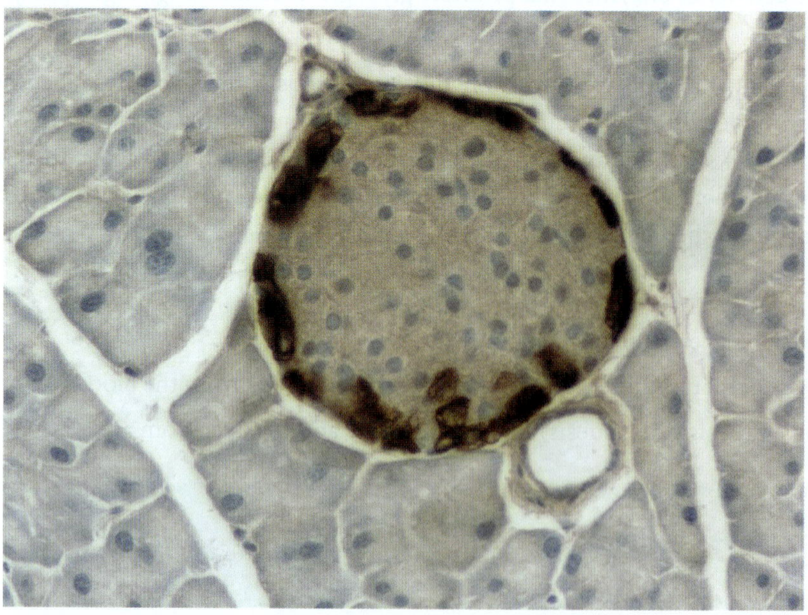

Figure 12.7 Glucagon (Dark Brown) in Pancreatic α-Cells

Low plasma glucose (hypoglycemia) is the most important physiological promoter of glucagon secretion, and elevated plasma glucose (hyperglycemia) is the most important inhibitor. Amino acids, especially basic amino acids (arginine, lysine, histidine), also promote the secretion of glucagon. Thus, glucagon is secreted in response to the ingestion of a meal rich in proteins.

Functional Relationship of Glucagon and Insulin

Insulin, associated with a well-fed, absorptive metabolic state, and glucagon, associated with a postabsorptive metabolic state, usually oppose each other with respect to pathways of energy metabolism. Enzymes that are phosphorylated by glucagon are generally dephosphorylated by insulin; enzymes that are phosphorylated by insulin are generally dephosphorylated by glucagon. Figure 12.8 displays a feedback diagram of the interaction of insulin and glucagon on plasma glucose concentration, as well as fat and protein metabolism.

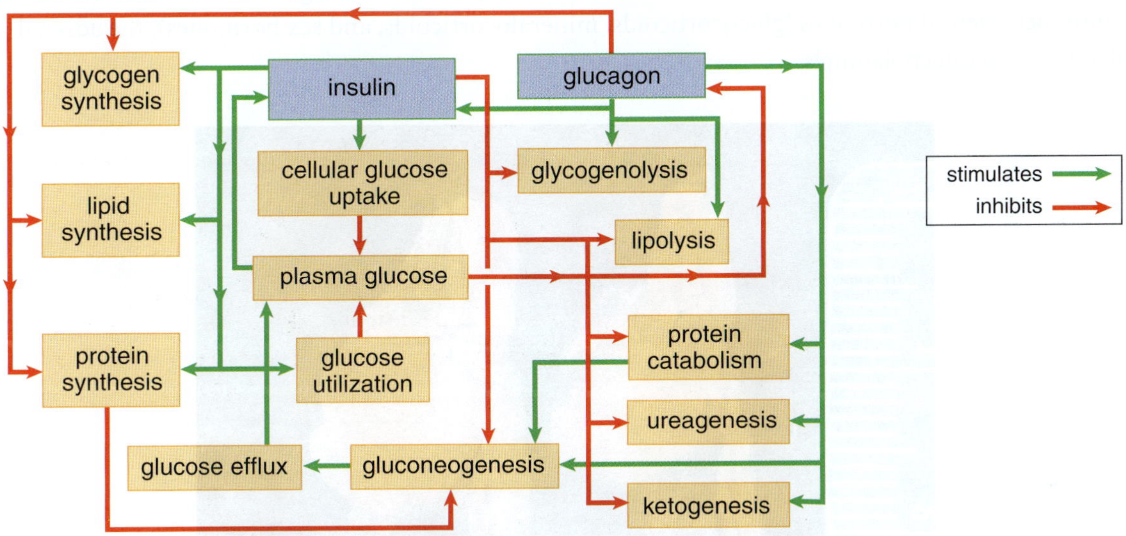

Figure 12.8 Relationship of Glucagon and Insulin in Metabolism

Glucocorticoids

Glucocorticoids from the adrenal cortex are responsible for part of the stress response. In order to make a getaway in the "fight-or-flight" response, glucose must be rapidly mobilized from the liver in order to fuel actively contracting muscle cells while fatty acids are released from adipocytes. Glucocorticoids, especially **cortisol**, are secreted with many forms of stress, including exercise, cold, and emotional stress. Cortisol, shown in Figure 12.9, is a steroid hormone that promotes the mobilization of energy stores through the degradation and increased delivery of amino acids and increased lipolysis. Cortisol also elevates blood glucose levels, increasing glucose availability for nervous tissue through two mechanisms. First, cortisol inhibits glucose uptake in most tissues (muscle, lymphoid, and fat) and increases hepatic output of glucose via gluconeogenesis, particularly from amino acids. Second, cortisol has a permissive function that enhances the activity of glucagon, epinephrine, and other catecholamines. Long-term exposure to glucocorticoids may be required clinically, but causes persistent hyperglycemia, which stimulates insulin. This actually promotes fat storage in the adipose tissue, rather than lipolysis.

BRIDGE

The endocrine system, discussed in Chapter 5 of *MCAT Biology Review*, is a major regulator of homeostasis. Like the glucocorticoids and catecholamines, mineralocorticoids and sex hormones are also synthesized by the adrenal glands and play a more minor role in metabolism.

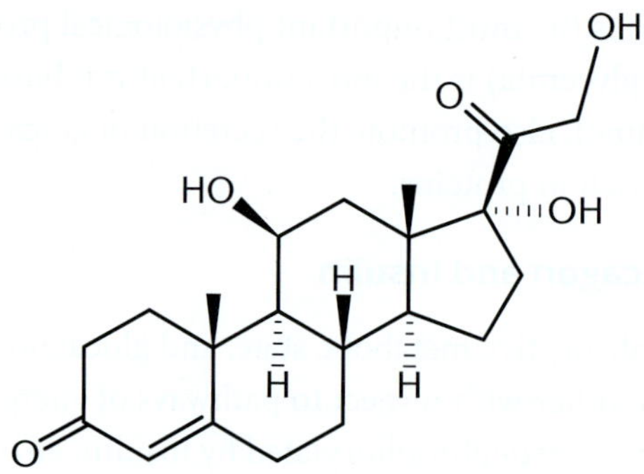

Figure 12.9 Structure of Cortisol

An enlarged adrenal gland (with a tumor of the adrenal cortex) is shown in Figure 12.10. While the adrenal cortex produces steroid hormones (glucocorticoids, mineralocorticoids, and sex hormones), the adrenal medulla produces catecholamines.

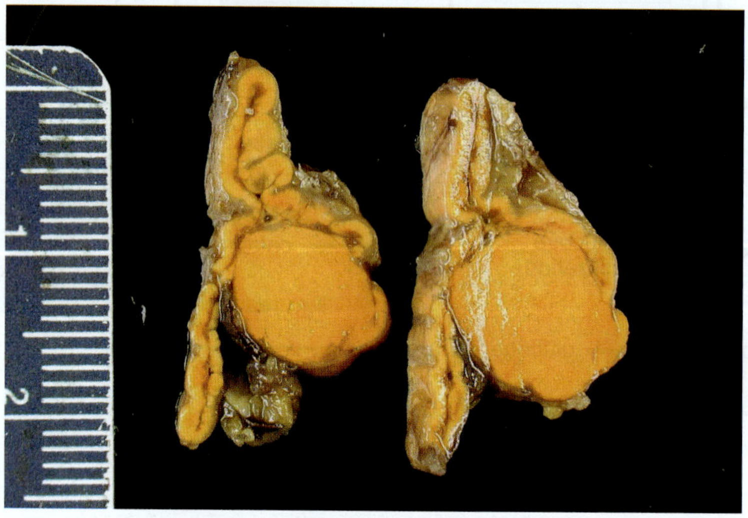

Figure 12.10 Adrenal Gland (Enlarged)
The adrenal cortex (yellow) and adrenal medulla (brown interior) are visible on both slices.

Catecholamines

Catecholamines are secreted by the adrenal medulla and include **epinephrine** and **norepinephrine**, also known as **adrenaline** and **noradrenaline**. The structures of these hormones are shown in Figure 12.11. Catecholamines increase the activity of liver and muscle glycogen phosphorylase, thus promoting glycogenolysis. This increases glucose output by the liver. Glycogenolysis also increases in skeletal muscle, but because muscle lacks glucose-6-phosphatase, glucose cannot be released by skeletal muscle into the bloodstream; instead, it is metabolized by the muscle tissue itself. Catecholamines act on adipose tissue to increase lipolysis by increasing the activity of hormone-sensitive lipase. Glycerol from triacylglycerol breakdown is a minor substrate for gluconeogenesis. Epinephrine also acts directly on target organs like the heart to increase the basal metabolic rate through the sympathetic nervous system. This increase in metabolic function is often associated with an *adrenaline rush*.

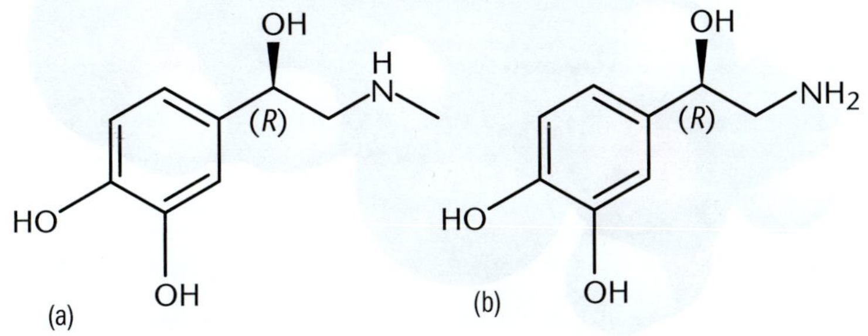

Figure 12.11 Structures of Adrenal Catecholamines
(a) Epinephrine; (b) Norepinephrine

Thyroid Hormones

Thyroid hormone activity is largely permissive. In other words, thyroid hormone levels are kept more or less constant, rather than undulating with changes in metabolic state. Thyroid hormones increase the basal metabolic rate, as evidenced by increased O_2 consumption and heat production when they are secreted. The increase in metabolic rate produced by a dose of ***thyroxine*** (T_4) occurs after a latency of several hours but may last for several days, while ***triiodothyronine*** (T_3) produces a more rapid increase in metabolic rate and has a shorter duration of activity. The subscript numbers refer to the number of iodine atoms in the hormone; iodine atoms are represented by purple spheres in the structures shown in Figure 12.12. T_4 can be thought of as the precursor to T_3; *deiodonases* (enzymes that remove iodine from a molecule) are located in target tissues and convert T_4 to T_3. Thyroid hormones have their primary effects in lipid and carbohydrate metabolism. They accelerate cholesterol clearance from the plasma and increase the rate of glucose absorption from the small intestine. Epinephrine requires thyroid hormones to have a significant metabolic effect.

REAL WORLD

While thyroid hormones are not responsible for day-to-day adjustments in metabolism, insufficient thyroid hormone levels (hypothyroidism) can cause symptoms including cold intolerance, fatigue, weight gain, and depression as metabolism suffers. Excessive thyroid hormone levels (hyperthyroidism) can cause rapid weight loss, anxiety, jitteriness, and fever.

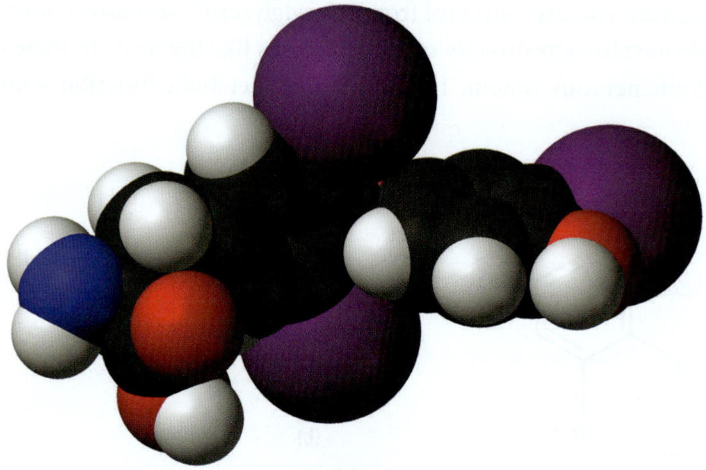

(a)

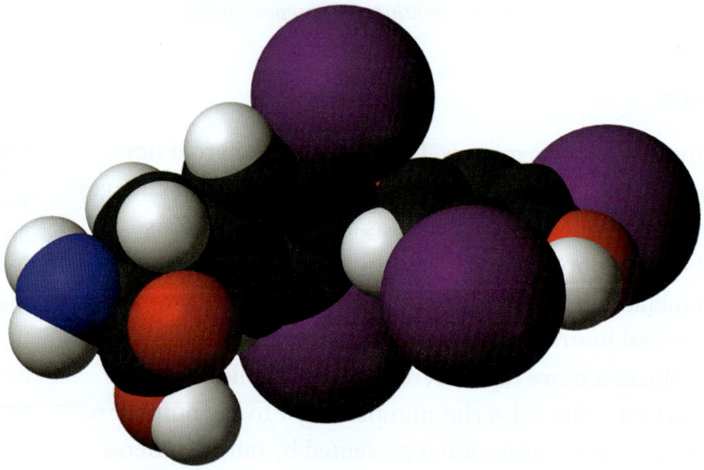

(b)

Figure 12.12 Structures of Thyroid Hormones
(a) Triiodothyronine (T_3); (b) Thyroxine (T_4)

MCAT CONCEPT CHECK 12.5

Before you move on, assess your understanding of the material with these questions.

1. Describe the primary metabolic function of each of the following hormones:
   - Insulin:

   ___

   - Glucagon:

   ___

   - Cortisol:

   ___

   - Catecholamines:

   ___

   - Thyroid hormones (T_3/T_4):

   ___

2. Thyroid storm is a potentially lethal state of extreme hyperthyroidism in which T_3 and T_4 levels are significantly above normal limits. What vital sign abnormalities might be expected in a patient with thyroid storm?

   ___

12.6 Tissue-Specific Metabolism

LEARNING OBJECTIVES

After Chapter 12.6, you will be able to:

- Identify the preferred fuel sources and fuel quantities for different tissue types, including skeletal muscle and the brain
- Recall the metabolic functions of the liver

Tissues have evolved so that their metabolic needs are met in a way corresponding to their form and function. The major sites of metabolic activity in the body are the liver, skeletal and cardiac muscles, brain, and adipocytes. Connective tissue and epithelial cells do not make major contributions to the consumption of energy. Remember though, that epithelial cells are the primary secretory cells, so they are involved in the regulation of metabolism. We have already discussed how the body operates under different nutritional conditions. The organ-specific patterns of fuel utilization in the well-fed and fasting states are summarized in Table 12.2.

Organ	Well-Fed	Fasting
Liver	Glucose and amino acids	Fatty acids
Resting skeletal muscle	Glucose	Fatty acids, ketones
Cardiac muscle	Fatty acids	Fatty acids, ketones
Adipose tissue	Glucose	Fatty acids
Brain	Glucose	Glucose (ketones in prolonged fast)
Red blood cells	Glucose	Glucose

Table 12.2 Preferred Fuels in the Well-Fed and Fasting States

Liver

Two major roles of the liver in fuel metabolism are to maintain a constant level of blood glucose under a wide range of conditions and to synthesize ketones when excess fatty acids are being oxidized. After a meal, glucose concentration in the portal blood is elevated. The liver extracts excess glucose and uses it to replenish its glycogen stores. Any glucose remaining in the liver is then converted to acetyl-CoA and used for fatty acid synthesis. The increase in insulin after a meal stimulates both glycogen synthesis and fatty acid synthesis in the liver. The fatty acids are converted to triacylglycerols and released into the blood as **very-low-density lipoproteins (VLDL)**. In the well-fed state, the liver derives most of its energy from the oxidation of excess amino acids. Between meals and during prolonged fasts, the liver releases glucose into the blood. The increase in glucagon during fasting promotes both glycogen degradation and gluconeogenesis. Lactate from anaerobic metabolism, glycerol from triacylglycerols, and amino acids provide carbon skeletons for glucose synthesis.

Adipose Tissue

After a meal, elevated insulin levels stimulate glucose uptake by adipose tissue. Insulin also triggers fatty acid release from VLDL and **chylomicrons** (which carry triacylglycerols absorbed from the gut). Lipoprotein lipase, an enzyme found in the capillary bed of adipose tissue, is also induced by insulin. The fatty acids that are released from lipoproteins are taken up by adipose tissue and re-esterified to triacylglycerols for storage. The glycerol phosphate required for triacylglycerol synthesis comes from glucose that is metabolized in adipocytes as an alternative product of glycolysis. Insulin can also effectively suppress the release of fatty acids from adipose tissue. During the fasting state, decreased levels of insulin and increased epinephrine activate **hormone-sensitive lipase** in fat cells, allowing fatty acids to be released into circulation.

Skeletal Muscle

Resting Muscle

The major fuels of skeletal muscle are glucose and fatty acids. Because of its enormous bulk, skeletal muscle is the body's major consumer of fuel. After a meal, insulin promotes glucose uptake in skeletal muscle, which replenishes glycogen stores and amino acids used for protein synthesis. Both excess glucose and amino acids can also be oxidized for energy. In the fasting state, resting muscle uses fatty acids derived from free fatty acids circulating in the bloodstream. Ketone bodies may also be used if the fasting state is prolonged.

Active Muscle

The primary fuel used to support muscle contraction depends on the magnitude and duration of exercise as well as the major fibers involved. A very short-lived source of energy (2–7 seconds) comes from **creatine phosphate**, which transfers a phosphate group to ADP to form ATP. Skeletal muscle has stores of both glycogen and some triacylglycerols. Blood glucose and free fatty acids may also be used. Short bursts of high-intensity exercise are also supported by anaerobic glycolysis drawing on stored muscle glycogen. During moderately high-intensity, continuous exercise, oxidation of glucose and fatty acids are both important, but after 1 to 3 hours of continuous exercise at this level, muscle glycogen stores become depleted, and the intensity of exercise declines to a rate that can be supported by oxidation of fatty acids.

BRIDGE

Fast-twitch muscle fibers have a high capacity for anaerobic glycolysis but are quick to fatigue. They are involved primarily in short-term, high-intensity exercise. Slow-twitch muscle fibers in arm and leg muscles are well vascularized and primarily oxidative. They are used during prolonged, low-to-moderate intensity exercise and resist fatigue. Slow-twitch fibers and the number of their mitochondria increase dramatically in trained endurance athletes. The musculoskeletal system is discussed in Chapter 11 of *MCAT Biology Review.*

Cardiac Muscle

Unlike other tissues of the body, cardiac myocytes prefer fatty acids as their major fuel, even in the well-fed state. When ketones are present during prolonged fasting, they can also be used. Thus, not surprisingly, cardiac myocytes most closely parallel skeletal muscle during extended periods of exercise. In patients with cardiac hypertrophy (thickening of the heart muscle), this situation reverses to some extent. In a failing heart, glucose oxidation increases and β-oxidation falls.

Brain

Although the brain represents only 2 percent of total body weight, it obtains 15 percent of the cardiac output, uses 20 percent of the total O_2, and consumes 25 percent of the total glucose, the brain's primary fuel. Blood glucose levels are tightly regulated to maintain a sufficient glucose supply for the brain (and sufficient concentration while studying). Normal function depends on a continuous glucose supply from the bloodstream. In hypoglycemic conditions $\left(< 70\ \frac{\text{mg}}{\text{dL}}\right)$, hypothalamic centers in the brain sense a fall in blood glucose level, and the release of glucagon and epinephrine is triggered. Fatty acids cannot cross the blood–brain barrier and are therefore not used at all as an energy source. Between meals, the brain relies on blood glucose supplied by either hepatic glycogenolysis or gluconeogenesis. Only during prolonged fasting does the brain gain the capacity to use ketone bodies for energy, and even then, the ketone bodies only supply approximately two-thirds of the fuel; the remainder is glucose.

BIOCHEMISTRY GUIDED EXAMPLE WITH EXPERT THINKING

A diet high in fat, low in carbohydrates, and sufficient in protein will automatically shift energy production in the body from being primarily dependent on glucose to primarily driven by ketone bodies. This dietary approach, termed a "ketogenic diet," was developed nearly 100 years ago as a metabolic therapy to mimic the metabolic changes that occur during fasting after observing that, upon halting food intake, seizures would stop in epileptic patients. Metabolic dysfunction is increasingly appreciated as a fundamental pathology across disease states, including neurodegenerative diseases, brain cancer, and treatment or reversal of type II diabetes and metabolic syndrome. Furthermore, implementing a ketogenic diet has shown improvement in these diseases. However, to date, there is no confirmation of any fundamental metabolic mechanism(s) that could explain the diverse beneficial effects seen across these numerous diseases.

Ketogenic diet (KD) = high fat, low carbs

KD known to help with epilepsy

A number of diseases are improved with KD

Researchers don't know how KD works to help so many different diseases

One possible avenue is exploring differential cellular energy production, which depends on the metabolic coenzyme nicotinamide adenine dinucleotide (NAD^+), a marker for mitochondrial and cellular health. Furthermore, NAD^+ activates downstream signaling pathways (such as the sirtuin enzymes) associated with major benefits such as longevity and reduced inflammation; thus, increasing NAD^+ is a coveted therapeutic endpoint. The Diagram 1 below outlines the usage of NAD^+ during the metabolism of glucose and ketone bodies (β-hydroxybutyrate and acetoacetate).

Possible mechanism: may depend on the role of NAD^+ in energy production

NAD^+ is a good candidate because it has overall broad health benefits

β-hydroxybutyrate and acetoacetate are both ketone bodies

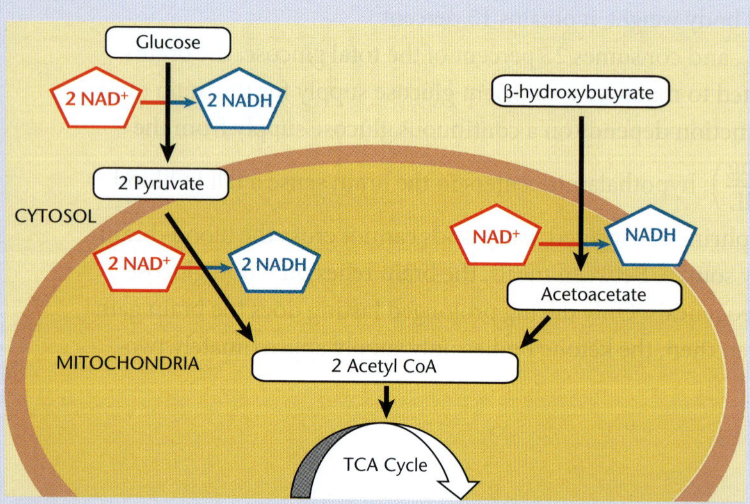

Glucose uses 4 NAD^+ to get to 2 acetyl-CoA;
β-hydroxybutyrate uses 1 NAD^+ to get to 2 acetyl-CoA

Diagram 1

Adapted from Elamin, M., Ruskin, D. N., Masino, S. A., & Sacchetti, P. (2017). Ketone-based metabolic therapy: is increased NAD^+ a primary mechanism? *Frontiers in Molecular Neuroscience*, 10, 377. doi:10.3389/fnmol.2017.00377

Given the information in the passage, if the researchers were to assay mice that were fed a ketogenic diet versus normal chow, how would the NAD^+/NADH ratio in ketogenic mice compare to that of normal mice? Why would the researchers likely be more interested in measuring NAD^+/NADH ratios specifically in the brain?

The first question asks us to compare the NAD^+/NADH ratio in KD mice to that of mice that were fed a normal diet, which means we should be combining our content background with the information in the passage to generate an answer. We know normal diets tend to be high in carbohydrates, whereas a ketogenic diet will be high in ketone bodies. Diagram 1 demonstrates that the metabolism of glucose and the metabolism of β-hydroxybutyrate each produce two acetyl-CoA molecules. However, the metabolism of glucose converts four NAD^+ molecules to NADH, while the metabolism of β-hydroxybutyrate only converts one NAD^+ molecule to NADH. This difference generates a higher NAD^+/NADH ratio in those mice that are subsisting on a KD diet, as NADH levels are relatively constant (due to its production from other sources in the body) but NAD^+ availability has increased.

The answer to the second question is superficially answered in the first paragraph—many of the diseases mentioned are focused on the brain (epilepsy, neurodegenerative diseases, brain cancer). However, if we dig a little deeper into our content background, we know that the brain can use only glucose or ketone bodies as its source of energy and there are no energy storage molecules, like glycogen or adipose cells, present in the brain. So, even in the early days of a ketogenic diet, while other tissues are still using alternative energy sources such as fatty acids, the brain is already shifting to utilizing a higher proportion of ketone bodies. Thus, an increased NAD^+/NADH ratio, as well as its potential associated benefits, will occur in the brain sooner and to a greater extent than anywhere else in the body. The passage states that NAD^+ activates pathways involving sirtuin enzymes, which reduce inflammation and fight the aging process. Such physiological changes also indirectly explain why a ketogenic diet could potentially help in so many brain-based diseases.

In short, mice on ketogenic diets would likely have a higher NAD^+/NADH ratio compared to mice on a normal diet, and NAD^+ levels in the brain would likely be more susceptible to diet changes because the brain only relies on plasma glucose and ketone bodies for energy.

MCAT CONCEPT CHECK 12.6

Before you move on, assess your understanding of the material with these questions.

1. What is the preferred fuel for most cells in the well-fed state? What is the exception and its preferred fuel?
   - Preferred fuel: ______________
   - Exception: ______________ Preferred fuel: ______________

2. What organ consumes the greatest amount of glucose relative to its percentage of body mass?

____

3. Describe the major metabolic functions of the liver.

____

____

____

12.7 Integrative Metabolism

LEARNING OBJECTIVES

After Chapter 12.7, you will be able to:

- Predict changes to respiratory quotient with changes in activity
- Explain the role of leptin, ghrelin, and orexin in regulating body mass
- Apply knowledge of measurement methods for metabolism to analytical approaches in a lab setting

Analysis of Metabolism

There are several methods of analyzing metabolic control of an organism. In humans, levels of glucose, thyroid hormones and thyroid-stimulating hormone, insulin, glucagon, oxygen, and carbon dioxide can all be measured in the blood. Because these hormones and substrates have a predictable effect on metabolism, they can be used as indicators of metabolic function. They can also be used as indicators of disorders, as in the case of blood glucose or thyroid-stimulating hormone.

MCAT EXPERTISE

The MCAT does not expect you to know what levels are healthy for any of these indicators, but can easily pose data interpretation questions related to them.

Respirometry allows accurate measurement of the respiratory quotient, which differs depending on the fuels being used by the organism. The **respiratory quotient (RQ)** can be measured experimentally, and can be calculated as:

$$RQ = \frac{CO_2 \text{ produced}}{O_2 \text{ consumed}}$$

Equation 12.3

for the complete combustion of a given fuel source. The respiratory quotient for carbohydrates is around 1.0, while the respiratory quotient for lipids is around 0.7. In resting individuals, the respiratory quotient is generally around 0.8, indicating that both fat and glucose are consumed. The respiratory quotient changes under conditions of high stress, starvation, and exercise as predicted by the actions of different hormones.

Calorimeters can measure **basal metabolic rate (BMR)** based on heat exchange with the environment. Human calorimetry makes use of large insulated chambers with specialized heat sinks to determine energy expenditure. Because of the isolationist nature of testing and the expense of creating a calorimetry chamber, other measures of BMR are preferred. Because of previous experimentation, BMR can be estimated based on age, weight, height, and phenotypical sex.

Regulation of Body Mass

Until now, we've been discussing metabolism on a very small scale, but metabolic controls are also involved in maintaining body mass (weight loss or gain). Body mass is determined by several factors, including water, carbohydrates, proteins, and lipids, while nucleic acids do not contribute significantly to its maintenance. The overall mass of carbohydrates and proteins tends to be stable over time, although it can be modified slightly by periods of prolonged starvation or by significant muscle-building activities. Water is very quickly adjusted by the endocrine system and the kidneys; therefore, it does not factor into our discussion of obesity and weight regulation. Water is the primary source of frequent minor weight fluctuations because it is subject to rapid adjustment. Therefore, lipids, stored in adipocytes, are the primary factor in the gradual change of body mass over time.

An individual who is maintaining body weight consumes the same amount of energy that is spent on average each day. If energy consumed is greater than energy expenditure over a significant period of time, then fat stores begin to accumulate. The opposite is also seen. If an energy deficit exists where calories consumed are less than calories burned, then a decrease in weight is observed. As individuals increase in mass, basal metabolic rate (the amount of energy required for one sedentary day) also increases. Thus, a caloric excess will cause an increase in body mass until equilibrium is reached between the new basal metabolic rate and the existing intake. In weight loss the reverse trend is seen.

This effect does have a threshold that differs between individuals. Small adjustments in intake, even over a prolonged period of time, are partially or fully compensated by changes in energy expenditure. Similarly, a small increase or decrease in activity level will be compensated by changes in hunger. Deliberate alterations of body mass require alterations above this threshold level, which is larger in negative energy balance than in positive energy balance—in other words, larger changes must be made to lose weight than to gain it.

BRIDGE

Motivation, a psychological concept discussed in Chapter 5 of *MCAT Behavioral Sciences Review*, is often linked with physiological drives and signaling pathways. The hypothalamus, which produces orexin and responds to leptin and ghrelin, is responsible for regulating hunger, thirst, and libido.

Diet (energy intake) and exercise (energy expenditure), genetics, socioeconomic status, and geography all play key roles in weight control. As described earlier, hormonal control by thyroid hormones, cortisol, epinephrine, glucagon, and insulin is critical to the integration of metabolism. In addition, there are hormones that control hunger and satiety, including *ghrelin*, *orexin*, and *leptin*. Have you ever wondered why, even if you don't feel hungry, when you walk into your favorite restaurant you're suddenly ravenous? This is the job of ghrelin and orexin. **Ghrelin** is secreted by the stomach in response to signals of an impending meal. Sight, sound, taste, and especially smell all act as signals for its release. Ghrelin increases appetite and also stimulates secretion of orexin. **Orexin** further increases appetite, and is also involved in alertness and the sleep–wake cycle. Hypoglycemia is also a trigger for orexin release. **Leptin** is a hormone secreted by fat cells that decreases appetite by suppressing orexin production. Leptin acts in a way that is complementary to ghrelin, as seen in Figure 12.13.

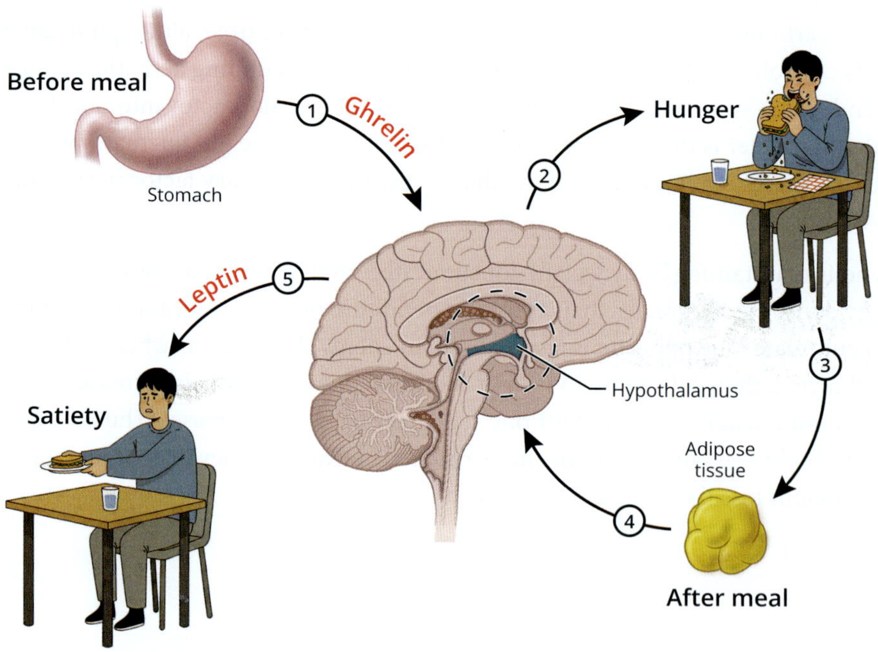

Figure 12.13 Ghrelin vs. Leptin

Genetic variations in the leptin molecule and its receptors have been implicated in obesity; a knockout mouse unable to produce leptin is shown on the left in Figure 12.14. These messengers and receptors are the target of current research; for now, questions regarding body mass modifications on the MCAT mostly come down to diet and exercise.

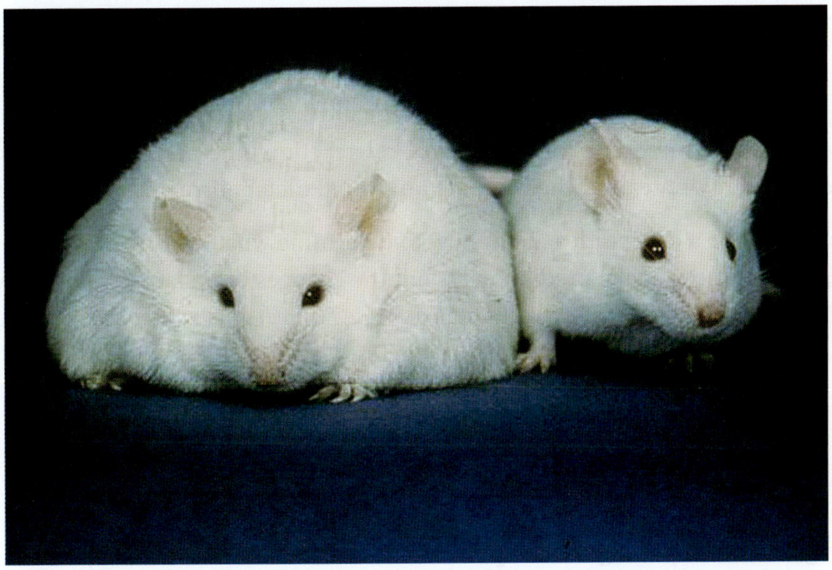

Figure 12.14 Leptin Knockout Mouse (left) Compared to Normal Mouse (right)

Body mass can be measured and tracked using the **body mass index (BMI)**, which is given by:

$$\text{BMI} = \frac{\text{mass}}{\text{height}^2}$$

Equation 12.4

where mass is measured in kilograms and height is measured in meters. A normal BMI is considered to be between 18.5 and 25; values lower than this are considered underweight. A BMI between 25 and 30 is considered overweight, whereas a BMI over 30 is considered **obese**.

MCAT CONCEPT CHECK 12.7

Before you move on, assess your understanding of the material with these questions.

1. How is the respiratory quotient expected to change when a person transitions from resting to brief exercise?

___

2. True or False: Body mass can be predicted by the leptin receptor phenotype and caloric intake alone.

3. True or False: It is easier to gain weight than to lose weight.

4. If you were designing a study to assess metabolism, which measurement method would you choose? Defend your answer.

___

Conclusion

In this chapter, we reviewed the principles of thermodynamics and thermochemistry that were introduced in general chemistry and physics and their applications to biological systems. We looked at the specific energy molecules of human metabolism, sources of energy, and key reaction types in ATP synthesis and hydrolysis. We compared different energy states and their impact on overall metabolism and tissue-specific metabolism.

At this point you should have a decent idea about how to determine what energy sources are being used from experimental data, and be able to make predictions about the changes in metabolism under varying conditions. Congratulations, because this is the last chapter of *MCAT Biochemistry Review* and you're just about ready to tackle any of the challenges that you will face on Test Day. Continue practicing, and try not to skip lunch!

GO ONLINE

You've reviewed the content, now test your knowledge and critical thinking skills by completing a test-like passage set in your online resources!

CONCEPT SUMMARY

Thermodynamics and Bioenergetics

- Biological systems are considered:
  - **Open**, wherein matter and energy can be exchanged with the environment, or
  - **Closed**, wherein only energy can be exchanged with the environment.
  - This determination is made based on the examination of the entire organism or an isolated process.
- Changes in **enthalpy** in a closed biological system are equal to changes in **internal energy**, which is equal to **heat exchange** within the environment.
- No work is performed in a closed biological system because pressure and volume remain constant.
- **Entropy** is a measure of energy dispersion in a system.
- Physiological concentrations are usually much less than standard concentrations.
- Free energy calculations must be adjusted for pH ($\Delta G^{\circ\prime}$), temperature (37°C = 98.6°F = 310 K), and concentrations.

The Role of ATP

- ATP is a mid-level energy molecule.
- ATP contains high-energy phosphate bonds that are stabilized upon hydrolysis by resonance, ionization, and loss of charge repulsion.
- ATP provides energy through **hydrolysis** and **coupling** to energetically unfavorable reactions.
- ATP can also participate in **phosphoryl group transfers** as a phosphate donor.

Biological Oxidation and Reduction

- Biological **oxidation** and **reduction** reactions can be broken down into component **half-reactions**.
- Half-reactions provide useful information about stoichiometry and thermodynamics.
- Many oxidation–reduction reactions involve an electron carrier to transport high-energy electrons.
- **Electron carriers** may be soluble or membrane-bound.
  - **Flavoproteins** are one subclass of electron carriers that are derived from riboflavin (vitamin B_2).

Metabolic States

- **Equilibrium** is an undesirable state for most biochemical reactions because organisms need to harness free energy to survive.
- In the **postprandial/well-fed** (**absorptive**) state, insulin secretion is high and anabolic metabolism prevails.
- In the **postabsorptive** (**fasting**) state, insulin secretion decreases while glucagon and catecholamine secretion increases.
  - This state is observed in short-term fasting (overnight).
  - There is a transition to catabolic metabolism.

- Prolonged fasting (**starvation**) dramatically increases glucagon and catecholamine secretion.
  - Most tissues rely on fatty acids.
  - At maximum, $\frac{2}{3}$ of the brain's energy can be derived from ketone bodies.

Hormonal Regulation of Metabolism

- **Insulin** and **glucagon** have opposing activities during most aspects of metabolism.
  - Insulin causes a decrease in blood glucose levels by increasing cellular uptake.
  - Insulin increases the rate of anabolic metabolism.
  - Insulin secretion by pancreatic β-cells is regulated by blood glucose levels.
  - Glucagon increases blood glucose levels by promoting gluconeogenesis and glycogenolysis in the liver.
  - Glucagon secretion by pancreatic α-cells is stimulated by both low glucose and high amino acid levels.
- **Glucocorticoids** increase blood glucose in response to stress by mobilizing fat stores and inhibiting glucose uptake.
  - Glucocorticoids increase the impact of glucagon and catecholamines.
- **Catecholamines** promote glycogenolysis and increase basal metabolic rate through their sympathetic nervous system activity.
- **Thyroid hormones** modulate the impact of other metabolic hormones and have a direct impact on basal metabolic rate.
  - T_3 is more potent than T_4, but has a shorter half-life and is available in lower concentrations in the blood.
  - T_4 is converted to T_3 at the tissues.

Tissue-Specific Metabolism

- The liver is the most metabolically diverse tissue.
  - Hepatocytes are responsible for the maintenance of blood glucose levels by glycogenolysis and gluconeogenesis in response to pancreatic hormone stimulation.
  - The liver also participates in the processing of lipids and cholesterol, bile, urea, and toxins.
- Adipose tissue stores lipids under the influence of insulin and releases them under the influence of epinephrine.
- Skeletal muscle metabolism differs based on the current activity level and fiber type.
  - Resting muscle conserves carbohydrates in glycogen stores and uses free fatty acids from the bloodstream.
  - Active muscle may use anaerobic metabolism, oxidative phosphorylation of glucose, direct phosphorylation from creatine phosphate, or fatty acid oxidation, depending on fiber type and exercise duration.
- Cardiac muscle uses fatty acid oxidation in both the well-fed and fasting states.
- The brain and other nervous tissues consume glucose in all metabolic states, except for prolonged fasts, where up to $\frac{2}{3}$ of the brain's fuel may come from ketone bodies.

Integrative Metabolism

- Metabolic rates can be measured using **calorimetry**, **respirometry**, consumption tracking, or measurement of blood concentrations of substrates and hormones.
- Composition of fuel that is actively consumed by the body is estimated by the **respiratory quotient (RQ)**.
- Body mass regulation is multifactorial with consumption and activity as modifiable factors.
  - The hormones **leptin**, **ghrelin**, and **orexin**, as well as their receptors, play a role in body mass.
  - Long-term changes in body mass result from changes in lipid storage.
  - Changes in consumption or activity must surpass a **threshold** to cause weight change. The threshold is lower for weight gain than for weight loss.
  - Body mass can be measured and tracked using the **body mass index (BMI)**.

ANSWERS TO CONCEPT CHECKS

12.1

1. $\Delta G^{\circ\prime}$ adjusts only for the pH of the environment by fixing it at 7. Temperature and concentrations of all other reagents are still fixed at their values from standard conditions and must be adjusted for if they are not 1 M.
2. The cellular environment has a relatively fixed volume and pressure, which eliminates work from our calculations of internal energy; if $\Delta U = Q - W$ and $W = 0$, $\Delta U = Q$.
3.

	$+\Delta H$	$-\Delta H$
$+\Delta S$	Spontaneous at high temperatures	Spontaneous
$-\Delta S$	Nonspontaneous	Spontaneous at low temperatures

12.2

1. ATP hydrolysis yields about 30 $\frac{\text{kJ}}{\text{mol}}$ of energy, which can be harnessed to drive other reactions forward. This may either allow a nonspontaneous reaction to occur or increase the rate of a spontaneous reaction.
2. ATP is an intermediate-energy storage molecule and is not energetically dense. The high-energy bonds in ATP and the presence of a significant charge make it an inefficient molecule to pack into a small space. Long-term storage molecules are characterized by energy density and stable, nonrepulsive bonds, primarily seen in lipids.
3.

$$\begin{aligned} &\text{cAMP} + H_2O \rightarrow \text{AMP} && \Delta G^{\circ\prime} = -50.4\ \tfrac{\text{kJ}}{\text{mol}} \\ &\text{AMP} + P_i \rightarrow \text{ADP} + H_2O && \Delta G^{\circ\prime} = 30.5\ \tfrac{\text{kJ}}{\text{mol}} \\ &\text{ADP} + P_i \rightarrow \text{ATP} + H_2O && \Delta G^{\circ\prime} = 30.5\ \tfrac{\text{kJ}}{\text{mol}} \\ \hline &\text{cAMP} + 2\,P_i \rightarrow \text{ATP} + H_2O && \Delta G^{\circ\prime} = 10.6\ \tfrac{\text{kJ}}{\text{mol}} \end{aligned}$$

12.3

1. Analyzing half-reactions can help to determine the number of electrons being transferred. This type of analysis also facilitates balancing equations and the determination of electrochemical potential if reduction potentials are provided.
2.

Electron Carrier	Metabolic Pathway(s)
NADH	Glycolysis, fermentation, citric acid cycle, electron transport chain
NADPH	Pentose phosphate pathway, lipid biosynthesis, bleach formation, oxidative stress, photosynthesis
Ubiquinone (CoQ)	Electron transport chain
Cytochromes	Electron transport chain
Glutathione	Oxidative stress

12.4

1. Any excitable cell is maintained in a state of disequilibrium. Classic examples include muscle tissue and neurons. In addition, cell volume and membrane transport are regulated by the action of the sodium–potassium pump, which can maintain a stable disequilibrium state in most tissues.
2. Cells that rely solely on anaerobic respiration are the least adaptable to different energy sources. Therefore, red blood cells are the least flexible during periods of prolonged starvation and stay reliant on glucose.
3. During the postabsorptive state, there is the greatest decrease in insulin levels. The concentrations of the counterregulatory hormones (glucagon, cortisol, epinephrine, norepinephrine, and growth hormone) begin to rise.

12.5

1. Insulin promotes glucose uptake by adipose tissue and muscle, glucose utilization in muscle cells, and macromolecule storage (glycogenesis, lipogenesis). Glucagon increases blood glucose levels by promoting glycogenolysis, gluconeogenesis, lipolysis, and ketogenesis. Cortisol increases lipolysis and amino acid mobilization, while decreasing glucose uptake in certain tissues and enhancing the activity of other counterregulatory hormones. Catecholamines increase glycogenolysis in muscle and liver and lipolysis in adipose tissue. Thyroid hormones increase basic metabolic rate and potentiate the activity of other hormones.
2. Thyroid storm presents with hyperthermia (high temperature), tachycardia (fast heart rate), hypertension (high blood pressure), and tachypnea (high respiratory rate).

12.6

1. The preferred fuel for most cells in the well-fed state is glucose; the exception is cardiac muscle, which prefers fatty acids.
2. The brain consumes the greatest amount of glucose relative to its percentage of body mass.
3. The liver is responsible for maintaining a steady-state concentration of glucose in the blood through glucose uptake and storage, glycogenolysis, and gluconeogenesis. The liver also participates in cholesterol and fat metabolism, the urea cycle, bile synthesis, and the detoxification of foreign substances.

12.7

1. As a person begins to exercise, the proportion of energy derived from glucose increases. This transition to almost exclusively carbohydrate metabolism will cause the respiratory quotient to approach 1.
2. False; energy expenditure, genetics, socioeconomic status, geography, and other hormones also play a role in body mass regulation.
3. True; the threshold is lower for uncompensated weight gain than it is for uncompensated weight loss. Therefore, it is easier to surpass this threshold and gain weight than to lose weight.
4. The methods described in the text include chemical analysis, which is objective and can quantify specific metabolic substrates, products, and enzymes; calorimetry, which is most accurate for basal metabolic rate but also most expensive; respirometry, which provides basic information about fuel sources; and caloric analysis at constant weight (food and exercise logs), which is the least invasive. Any of these answers could be defended.

SCIENCE MASTERY ASSESSMENT EXPLANATIONS

1. **C**

In a closed biological system, enthalpy, heat, and internal energy are all directly related because there is no change in pressure or volume. Because pressure and volume are fixed, work cannot be done, thus **(C)** is correct.

2. **B**

To solve this question, we can use the equation $\Delta G = \Delta G^{\circ} + RT \ln Q$. Q, the reaction quotient, is $\frac{[B][C]^2}{[A]}$ for this reaction. Plugging in the variables, we get:

$$\Delta G = 0 + RT \ln \frac{[10 \times 10^{-3}][10 \times 10^{-3}]^2}{[10 \times 10^{-3}]}$$
$$= RT \ln 10^{-4} = -4\ RT \ln 10.$$

Because both R and T are positive, and natural log values being greater than 0, we know that ΔG must be negative and therefore lower than the original value. A negative ΔG corresponds to a spontaneous reaction.

3. **C**

The hydrolysis of ATP is energetically favorable because there are repulsive negative charges that are relieved when hydrolyzed, and the new compounds are stabilized by resonance. This is true of both ATP and ADP. Some of the other answer choices are tempting, though. In **(A)**, ATP hydrolysis relies on pH because a protonated ATP molecule contains less negative charge and therefore experiences less repulsive force. For **(B)**, the energy released by one mole of creatine phosphate upon hydrolysis is not sufficient to phosphorylate two moles of ADP according to Table 12.1; creatine phosphate donates one phosphate group to a molecule of ADP, so one mole of creatine phosphate will phosphorylate one mole of ADP. For **(D)**, the removal of two phosphate groups from ATP yields AMP, not cyclic AMP.

4. **A**

Reduction is a gain of electrons, which eliminates **(B)** because it is an oxidation reaction. NADPH, **(C)**, is a product of the pentose phosphate pathway. Ubiquinone, **(D)**, transfers electrons during the course of the electron transport chain, but is not the final electron acceptor. This title belongs to oxygen.

5. **B**

In order to transport electrons, electron carriers like flavoproteins must be able to exist in a stable oxidized state and a stable reduced form. ATP can be dephosphorylated but is generally not oxidized or reduced. Regulatory enzymes may also be phosphorylated or dephosphorylated but are not generally oxidized or reduced.

6. **B**

Skipping a single meal is not a prolonged fast. However, the increase in hormones that promote gluconeogenesis and glycogenolysis indicates that the absorptive phase has ended.

7. **D**

In the well-fed state, the liver runs off of glucose and amino acids, the brain and adipose tissue run off of glucose, and cardiac muscle runs off of fatty acids. Only **(D)** correctly pairs the tissue with its energy source.

8. **A**

Hormonal controls are coordinated to regulate the metabolic activity of the entire organism, while allosteric controls can be local or systemic. The modification of the enzymes of glycogen metabolism by insulin and glucagon is either through phosphorylation or dephosphorylation, both of which modify covalent bonds.

9. **B**

Adipose tissue and resting skeletal muscle require insulin for glucose uptake. Active skeletal muscle, **(A)**, uses creatine phosphate and glycogen (regulated by epinephrine and AMP) to maintain its energy requirements.

10. **C**

Short-term glucocorticoid exposure causes a release of glucose and the hydrolysis of fats from adipocytes. However, if this glucose is not used for metabolism, it causes an increase in glucose level which promotes fat storage. The net result is the release of glucose from the liver to be converted into lipids in the adipose tissue under insulin stimulation.

11. **B**

The brain uses aerobic metabolism of glucose exclusively and therefore is very sensitive to oxygen levels. The extremely high oxygen requirement of the brain (20% of the body's oxygen content) relative to its size (2% of total body weight) implies that brain is the most sensitive organ to oxygen deprivation.

12. **B**

The respiratory quotient (RQ) gives an indication of the primary fuel being utilized. An RQ around 0.7 indicates lipid metabolism, 0.8–0.9 indicates amino acid metabolism, **(D)**, and 1.0 indicates carbohydrate metabolism, **(A)**. Nucleic acids do not contribute significantly to the respiratory quotient.

13. **A**

Leptin acts to decrease appetite by inhibiting the production of orexin. Orexin is also associated with alertness, so decreasing the level of orexin in the body is expected to cause drowsiness. Even without this information, the answer should be apparent because the body tends to maintain an energy balance. If consumption decreases, energy expenditures are expected to decrease as well.

14. **C**

ATP stores are turned over about 1,000 times per day, not 10,000.

15. **D**

A prolonged fast is characterized by an increase in glucagon, which accomplishes its cellular activity by phosphorylating and dephosphorylating metabolic enzymes. Glycogen storage, **(B)**, is then halted, but this requires enzyme regulation by glucagon to occur. Later in the postabsorptive state, protein breakdown, **(C)**, begins. Eventually, in starvation, ketone bodies, **(A)**, are used by the brain for its main energy source.

GO ONLINE

Consult your online resources for additional practice.

EQUATIONS TO REMEMBER

(12.1) **Gibbs free energy:** $\Delta G = \Delta H - T\Delta S$

(12.2) **Modified standard state:** $\Delta G = \Delta G^{\circ} + RT\ln(Q)$

(12.3) **Respiratory quotient:** $\text{RQ} = \dfrac{\text{CO}_2 \text{ produced}}{\text{O}_2 \text{ consumed}}$

(12.4) **Body mass index:** $\text{BMI} = \dfrac{\text{mass}}{\text{height}^2}$

SHARED CONCEPTS

Biochemistry Chapter 9
Carbohydrate Metabolism I

Biochemistry Chapter 10
Carbohydrate Metabolism II

Biochemistry Chapter 11
Lipid and Amino Acid Metabolism

Biology Chapter 5
The Endocrine System

General Chemistry Chapter 11
Oxidation–Reduction Reactions

Physics and Math Chapter 3
Thermodynamics

GLOSSARY

Absolute configuration–The nomenclature system used for the three-dimensional arrangement of atoms in isomers; the most common systems are D/L and (*R*)/(*S*).

Acetal–A carbon atom bonded to an alkyl group, two $-$OR groups, and a hydrogen.

Acetyl-CoA–An important metabolic intermediate that links glycolysis and β-oxidation to the citric acid cycle; can also be converted into ketone bodies.

Activation–The conversion of a biomolecule to its active or usable form, such as activation of tRNA with an amino acid or activation of a fatty acid with CoA to form fatty acyl-CoA.

Activation energy–The energy required to change the state of a molecule or group of molecules to the transition state; the energy required for a reaction to occur.

Active site–The catalytically active portion of an enzyme.

Active transport–The movement of a molecule against its concentration gradient with energy investment; primary active transport uses ATP, whereas secondary active transport uses a favorable transport gradient of a different molecule.

Activity–The measure of the catalytic activity of an enzyme, also called the velocity or rate. It is often measured as a V_{max} and may be analyzed after protein isolation.

Activity analysis–The determination of the enzymatic activity of an isolated protein by interaction with a substrate; usually colorimetric in nature.

Adenosine triphosphate (ATP)–The primary energy molecule of the body; it releases energy by breaking the bond with the terminal phosphate to form ADP and inorganic phosphate.

Adipocyte–A cell specializing in fat storage.

Aerobic respiration–A collection of energy-producing metabolic processes that require oxygen, including the citric acid cycle, electron transport chain, and oxidative phosphorylation.

Agglutination–Clumping of particles caused by the binding of antibody to target antigen.

Aldose–A sugar in which the highest-order functional group is an aldehyde; can be categorized by number of carbons (triose, tetrose, pentose, hexose, etc.).

Allosteric enzymes–Enzymes that experience changes in their conformation as a result of interactions at sites other than the active site, called allosteric sites; conformational changes may increase or decrease enzyme activity.

α-Helix–An element of secondary structure, marked by clockwise coiling of amino acids around a central axis.

Alternative splicing–The production of multiple different but related mRNA molecules from a single primary transcript of hnRNA.

Amino acid–A dipolar compound containing an amino group ($-NH_2$) and a carboxyl group ($-$COOH).

Amphipathic–Having both hydrophilic and hydrophobic regions.

Amphoteric–The ability to act as an acid or base.

Amplification–Increased transcription (and translation) of a gene in response to hormones, growth factors, and other intracellular conditions.

Anabolism–The series of metabolic processes that result in the consumption of energy and the synthesis of molecules.

Anaerobic respiration–The series of energy-producing metabolic processes that do not require oxygen, including glycolysis and fermentation.

Anomers–A subtype of epimers in which the chiral carbon with inverted configuration was the carbonyl carbon (anomeric carbon).

Antibody–A specialized protein molecule produced by lymphocytes for interaction with antigens; antibodies consist of two heavy and two light chains that have constant and variable regions. Antibodies, also called immunoglobulins, are mediators of the immune response.

Anticodon–A three-nucleotide sequence on a tRNA molecule that pairs with a corresponding mRNA codon during translation.

Antigen–The region of a molecule that interacts with an antibody; in most cases, antigens are proteins.

Apoenzyme–An enzyme devoid of the prosthetic group, coenzyme, or cofactor necessary for normal activity.

Apolipoproteins–Protein molecules responsible for the interaction of lipoproteins with cells and the transfer of lipid molecules between lipoproteins; also called apoproteins.

Aromaticity–The ability of a molecule to delocalize π electrons around a conjugated ring, creating exceptional stability.

Autoradiography–A technique used to detect radioactive substances by exposing a sample to film or a digital detector, creating an image based on the emitted radiation.

Basal metabolic rate–The amount of energy consumed in a given period of time by a resting organism.

β-mercaptoethanol (βME)–A reducing agent often used in reducing PAGE to break disulfide bonds.

β-Oxidation–The catabolism of fatty acids to acetyl-CoA.

β-Pleated sheet–An element of secondary structure, marked by peptide chains lying alongside one another, forming rows or strands.

Bile–A mixture of salts, pigments, and cholesterol that acts to emulsify lipids in the small intestine.

Binding proteins–Proteins that transport or sequester molecules by binding to them. Binding proteins have affinity curves for their molecules of interest.

Bioenergetics–Biochemistry of the energy involved in bond interactions in biological organisms.

Biosignaling–The process by which cells receive and act on messages.

Blotting–A technique for transferring molecules (DNA, RNA, or protein) from a gel to a thin membrane, allowing for detection and semi-quantitative analysis.

Bradford protein assay–A colorimetric method of determining the concentration of protein in an isolate against a protein standard; relies on a transition of absorption between bound and unbound Coomassie Brilliant Blue dye.

C-terminus–The free carboxyl end of a polypeptide.

Cahn–Ingold–Prelog system–The system used to name isomers ((*E*) *vs.* (*Z*); (*R*) *vs.* (*S*)), based on the atomic numbers of their substituents and their orientation in three-dimensional space.

Calorimeter–A device for measuring the heat change during the course of a reaction.

Carboxylation–The addition of carboxylic acid groups to a molecule.

Carotenoids–A group of molecules that are tetraterpenes (made of eight isoprene units).

Catabolism–The series of metabolic processes that result in the release of energy and the breakdown of molecules.

Catalyst–A substance or enzyme that increases the rate of a reaction by lowering activation energy. Catalysts are not consumed during the catalyzed reaction.

Catalytic efficiency–The ratio of k_{cat}/K_m. Catalytic efficiency is directly related to efficiency of enzyme function.

Catecholamines–Mediators of the sympathetic nervous system and adrenal gland; include epinephrine and norepinephrine.

Cell adhesion molecules–Specialized structural proteins that are involved in cell–cell junctions as well as transient cellular interactions; common cell adhesion molecules are cadherins, integrins, and selectins.

Cellulose–A homopolysaccharide of glucose, and the main structural component of plants. Cellulose is indigestible for humans.

Central dogma of molecular biology–The major steps in the transfer of genetic information, from transcription of DNA to RNA to translation of that RNA to protein.

Centrifugation–The process of separating components on the basis of their density and resistance to flow by spinning a sample at very high speeds; the highest density materials form a solid pellet and the lowest density materials remain in the supernatant (liquid portion).

Centromere–The area of a chromosome where sister chromatids are joined; it is also the point of attachment to the spindle fiber during mitosis and meiosis.

Ceramide–The simplest sphingolipid, with a single hydrogen as its head group.

Cerebroside–A sphingolipid containing a carbohydrate as a head group.

Chaperones–Proteins that assist in protein folding during posttranslational processing.

Chargaff's rule–DNA from any source should have a 1:1 ratio of pyrimidine to purine bases, with adenine equal to thymine and cytosine equal to guanine.

Chemiosmotic coupling–The utilization of the proton-motive force generated by the electron transport chain to drive ATP synthesis in oxidative phosphorylation.

Chiral–Describes a molecule with a nonsuperimposable mirror image.

Chiral center–A carbon atom bonded to four different substituents; a chiral compound must have at least one chiral center.

Cholesterol–A molecule containing four linked aromatic rings; cholesterol provides both fluidity and stability to cell membranes and is the precursor for steroid hormones.

Chromatid–Each of the two chromosomal strands formed by DNA replication in the S phase of the cell cycle, held together by the centromere. Identical pairs of chromatids are referred to as sister chromatids.

Chromatography–The process of separating molecules by their interactions with a stationary phase and a mobile phase; most chromatographic methods rely on the chemical similarity of molecules, with the exception of size-exclusion chromatography.

Chromosome–A filamentous body found within the nucleus of a eukaryotic cell or nucleoid region of a prokaryotic cell, composed of DNA.

Citric acid cycle–A metabolic pathway that produces GTP, energy carriers, and carbon dioxide as it burns acetyl-CoA; also called the Krebs cycle or tricarboxylic acid (TCA) cycle; can share intermediates with many other metabolic processes including fatty acid and cholesterol synthesis, gluconeogenesis, amino acid metabolism, and others.

Closed system–A system capable of exchanging energy, but not matter, with the environment.

Coding strand–The strand of DNA that is not used as a template during transcription; also called the sense strand.

Codon–A three-nucleotide sequence in an mRNA molecule that pairs with an appropriate tRNA anticodon during translation.

Coenzyme–An organic molecule that helps an enzyme carry out its function.

Cofactor–An inorganic molecule or ion that helps an enzyme carry out its function.

Colligative properties–Physical properties that change according to the concentration of solutes, but not their identity. Colligative properties include vapor pressure depression, boiling point elevation, freezing point depression, and osmotic pressure.

Colloid–A mixture composed of large molecules of one substance suspended within another substance.

Competitive inhibition–A decrease in enzyme activity that results from the interaction of an inhibitor with the active site of an enzyme; competitive inhibition can be overcome by addition of excess substrate.

Condensation reaction–A reaction in which the removal of a water molecule accompanies the formation of a bond; also called a dehydration reaction.

Conformational coupling–A less-accepted mechanism of ATP synthase activity in which the protons cause a conformational change that releases ATP from ATP synthase.

Conjugated protein–A protein that derives part of its function from covalently attached molecules (prosthetic groups).

Cooperativity–The interaction between subunits of a multi-subunit protein in which binding of substrate to one subunit increases the affinity of other subunits for the substrate; unbinding of substrate from one unit decreases the affinity of other subunits for the substrate.

Corepressor–A species that binds with a repressor, allowing the complex to bind to the operator region of an operon, stopping transcription of the relevant gene.

Cori cycle–A metabolic pathway in which lactate produced by anaerobic glycolysis in muscles is transported to the liver, converted to glucose via gluconeogenesis, and then returned to the muscles.

Cristae–The infoldings of the inner mitochondrial membrane that increase the surface area available for electron transport chain complexes.

Dalton (Da)–Molar mass unit used for protein molecular weight. One amino acid weighs approximately 100 Da, or 100 $\frac{g}{mol}$.

Degeneracy–A characteristic of the genetic code, in which more than one codon can specify a single amino acid.

Denaturation–The loss of secondary, tertiary, or quaternary structure in a protein, leading to loss of function. Also the name of the first step of the polymerase chain reaction (PCR) technique, in which two DNA strands are separated by heat.

Deoxyribonucleic acid (DNA)–A nucleic acid found exclusively in the nucleus that codes for all of the genes necessary for life; transcribed to mRNA and always read 5′ to 3′.

Desmosomes–Cell–cell junctions that anchor layers of epithelial cells to one another.

Diastereomers–Compounds with at least one—but not all—chiral carbons in inverted configurations; differ in physical properties.

Dideoxynucleotides (ddNTPs)–Modified nucleotides lacking a hydroxyl group at the 3' carbon of the ribose sugar. Their incorporation into a growing DNA strand terminates chain elongation, a key feature in Sanger sequencing.

Diprotic–Containing two hydrogens (acid), or being able to pick up two hydrogens (base).

Disulfide bond–A covalent interaction between the –SH groups of two cysteine residues; an element of tertiary and quaternary structure.

Dithiothreitol (DTT)–A reducing agent commonly used in reducing PAGE to break disulfide bonds.

Double-displacement (ping-pong) reaction–An enzyme-catalyzed reaction in which one substrate binds and is converted to product, resulting in a modified enzyme intermediate before the second substrate binds.

Edman degradation–A stepwise process for determining the amino acid sequence in an isolated protein.

Electrochemical gradient–An uneven separation of ions across a biological membrane, resulting in potential energy.

Electrophoresis–The process of separating compounds on the basis of size and charge using a porous gel and an electric field; protein electrophoresis generally uses polyacrylamide, while nucleic acid electrophoresis generally uses agarose.

Elongation (PCR)–The third step of the polymerase chain reaction (PCR) technique, in which a heat-stable DNA polymerase synthesizes new complementary DNA strands starting from the primers.

Elongation (transcription)–The stage of transcription in which RNA polymerase moves along the template strand of DNA, synthesizing mRNA in the 5′ to 3′ direction.

Elongation (translation)–The three-step cycle that is repeated for each amino acid being added to a protein during translation.

Emulsification–The mixing of two normally immiscible liquids.

Enantiomers–Compounds that are nonsuperimposable mirror images; have the same physical and chemical properties except for rotation of plane-polarized light and interaction with a chiral environment.

Endocytosis–The transport of molecules into a cell through the invagination of cell membrane and the formation of a vesicle; phagocytosis is the endocytosis of solid, pinocytosis is the endocytosis of liquid.

Endothermic reaction–A reaction that requires heat (positive ΔH).

Enhancer–A collection of several response elements that allow for the control of one gene's expression by multiple signals.

Enthalpy–The overall change in heat of a system during a reaction.

Entropy–The disorder of a system; systems in which entropy is increased are generally favored.

Enzyme–A biological molecule with catalytic activity; includes many proteins and some RNA molecules. Enzymes are specified for target substrate molecules.

Enzyme activity–A measure of the rate at which an enzyme catalyzes a specific biochemical reaction, expressing the amount of substrate converted to product per unit of time.

Enzyme-linked receptor–A transmembrane protein that displays catalytic activity in response to ligand binding.

Epimers–A subtype of diastereomers that differ in absolute configuration at exactly one chiral carbon.

Euchromatin–The looser, less-dense collections of DNA that appear light colored under a microscope; transcriptionally active.

Exocytosis–The transport of molecules out of a cell by release from a transport vesicle; the vesicle fuses to the cell membrane during secretion.

Exon–A portion of hnRNA that is spliced with other exons to form mature mRNA.

Exothermic reaction–A reaction that releases heat (negative ΔH).

Facilitated diffusion–The movement of solute molecules across the cell membrane down their concentration gradients through a transport protein or channel; used for ions and large or polar molecules.

Fatty acid–A monocarboxylic acid without additional substituents; fatty acids may be saturated (all single bonds) or unsaturated (contain at least one double bond); natural fatty acids are in the *cis* conformation.

Feedback inhibition–The inhibition of an enzyme by its product (or a product further down a metabolic pathway); used to maintain homeostasis.

Feed-forward activation–The stimulation of an enzyme by an intermediate that precedes the enzyme in a metabolic pathway.

Fermentation–The conversion of pyruvate to either ethanol and carbon dioxide (yeast) or lactic acid (animal cells); does not require oxygen.

Fibrous protein–A protein composed of long sheets or strands, such as collagen.

Fischer projection–A method of drawing organic molecules in which horizontal lines are coming out of the page (wedges) and vertical lines are going into the page (dashes).

Flavin adenine dinucleotide (FAD)–An energy carrier that accepts electrons and feeds them into the electron transport chain.

Flavoprotein–A protein bonded to FAD.

Fluid mosaic model–The representation of the plasma membrane as a dynamic phospholipid bilayer with interactions of cholesterol, proteins, and carbohydrates.

Fluorescent tag–A fluorescent molecule attached to a non-fluorescent molecule to enable detection using light.

Frameshift mutation–A change in DNA in which the reading frame of the codons in mRNA is shifted due to the insertion or deletion of nucleotides (other than in multiples of three).

Fructose–A monosaccharide found predominantly in fruit and honey.

Furan–A five-membered aromatic ring containing one oxygen atom and four carbon atoms.

Furanose–A five-membered ring sugar.

G protein-coupled receptors–A special class of membrane receptors with an associated GTP-binding protein; activation of a G protein-coupled receptor involves dissociation and GTP hydrolysis.

Galactose–A monosaccharide found predominantly in dairy.

Ganglioside–A sphingolipid with a head group containing an oligosaccharide and one or more *N*-acetylneuraminic acid (NANA) molecules.

Gap junctions–Cell–cell junctions that allow for the passage of small molecules between adjacent cells.

Gene–A unit of DNA that encodes a specific protein or RNA molecule.

Globoside–A sphingolipid with multiple carbohydrate groups attached as a head group.

Globular protein–A protein with a roughly spherical structure, such as myoglobin.

Glucagon–A mediator of glucose release that is secreted by pancreatic α-cells; rises in response to low blood glucose.

Glucogenic–Describes amino acids that can be converted into intermediates that feed into gluconeogenesis; all except leucine and lysine.

Gluconeogenesis–The production of glucose from other biomolecules; carried out by the liver and kidney.

Glucose–The primary monosaccharide used for fuel by all cells of the body, with the formula $C_6H_{12}O_6$.

Glycerol–A three-carbon alcohol that serves as the backbone for glycerophospholipids, sphingolipids, and triacylglycerols.

Glycerophospholipid–Also referred to as a phosphoglyceride; a lipid containing a glycerol backbone with a phosphate group, bonded by ester linkages to two fatty acids.

Glycogen–A branched polymer of glucose that represents a storage form of glucose.

Glycogenesis–The synthesis of glycogen granules.

Glycogenolysis–The breakdown of glycogen granules.

Glycolysis–The breakdown of glucose to two molecules of pyruvate, with the formation of energy carriers (NADH); occurs under both aerobic and anaerobic conditions.

Glycosidic linkage–The bond between the anomeric carbon of a sugar and another molecule.

Glycosphingolipid–A sphingolipid with a head group composed of sugars; includes cerebrosides and globosides.

Glycosylation–The addition of sugars to a molecule.

Haworth projection–A method for depicting cyclic sugars as planar rings with $-OH$ groups sticking up or down from the plane of the sugar.

Hemiacetal–A carbon atom bonded to an alkyl group, an $-OR$ group, an $-OH$ group, and a hydrogen.

Hemiketal–A carbon atom bonded to two alkyl groups, an $-OR$ group, and an $-OH$ group.

Hess's law–A relationship that states that the total change in any state function is the same regardless of the path taken or the number of steps, and is equal to the difference between initial and final values of that state function.

Heterochromatin–The tightly coiled DNA that appears dark colored under a microscope; transcriptionally inactive.

Heterocycle–A ringed structure that contains at least two different elements in the ring.

Heterotrimer–A protein complex formed by three different protein subunits; a *homotrimer* would contain three of the same subunits.

Heterogeneous nuclear RNA (hnRNA)–The precursor to processed mRNA; converted to mRNA by adding a poly-A tail and 5′ cap and splicing out introns.

Hill's coefficient–A quantitative measure of cooperative binding effects in enzymes.

Histone–A lysine- and arginine-rich structural protein about which DNA is coiled in eukaryotic cells. Histone association with DNA can be altered by acetylation of histone proteins or methylation of the DNA strand.

Histone acetyltransferase–An enzyme that transfers an acetyl group to lysine residues on histones, neutralizing their positive charge.

Histone deacetylases (HDACs)–Enzymes that remove acetyl groups from lysine residues on histones, restoring their positive charge.

Histone methyltransferases–Enzymes that add methyl groups to lysine and arginine residues on histones.

Holoenzyme–An enzyme that has already bound a required prosthetic group, coenzyme, or cofactor.

Homeostasis–The stable internal state of an organism; homeostasis is not synonymous with equilibrium.

Homodimer–A protein complex formed by two identical protein subunits; a *heterodimer* would contain two different subunits.

Homogenization–The process of breaking cell membranes and creating a uniform mixture of cell components for further separation; may be accomplished chemically or physically.

Hormone-sensitive lipase–The enzyme responsible for the mobilization of fatty acids from adipocytes; responds to a decrease in insulin levels.

Hückel's rule–One condition for aromaticity, which states the compound must have $4n + 2$ (where n is any integer) π electrons.

Hybridization–In research techniques involving DNA, the joining of complementary base pair sequences.

Hydrolase–An enzyme that catalyzes the cleavage of a molecule with the addition of water.

Hydrolysis–Breaking a covalent bond with the assistance of a water molecule.

Hydrophilic–Being attracted to water; describes polar and charged compounds and those that can participate in hydrogen bonding.

Hydrophobic–Being repelled by water; describes nonpolar, uncharged compounds (usually lipids or certain R groups of amino acids).

Hypertonic–A solution that has a greater concentration than the one to which it is being compared.

Hypotonic–A solution that has a lower concentration than the one to which it is being compared.

Indole–A double-ring heterocyclic system containing a nitrogen atom, found in the amino acid tryptophan.

Induced fit model–The best-supported of the most prominent theories of enzyme specificity; states that the enzyme and substrate experience a change in conformation during binding to increase complementarity. Usually contrasted with the lock and key theory.

Inducible system–An operon that requires an inducer to remove a repressor protein from the operator site to begin transcription of the relevant gene.

Initiation (transcription)–The stage of transcription in which RNA polymerase, with the help of transcription factors, binds to the promoter region of DNA, unwinds the DNA double helix, and begins RNA synthesis.

Initiation (translation)–The start of translation, in which the small subunit of the ribosome binds to the mRNA molecule, and the first tRNA (methionine or *N*-formylmethionine) is bound to the start codon (AUG).

Insulin–The primary mediator of carbohydrate metabolism that is secreted by pancreatic β-cells; rises in response to high blood glucose.

Intercalator–A molecule that inserts itself between the stacked bases of DNA, often used for visualization or to disrupt DNA replication and transcription. Ethidium bromide is a common example used to visualize DNA in gel electrophoresis.

Internal energy–The sum of all of the different interactions between and within atoms in a system; vibration, rotation, linear motion, and stored chemical energies all contribute.

Intron–A portion of hnRNA that is spliced out to form mRNA; remains in the nucleus during processing.

Ion channels–Proteins that form a pore through the membrane in which they are embedded.

Irreversible inhibition–A decrease in enzyme activity that results from the interaction of an inhibitor that binds permanently at either the active site or an allosteric site; in laboratory settings, irreversible inhibitors are sometimes called suicide substrates.

Isoelectric focusing–A specialized method of separating proteins by their isoelectric point using electrophoresis; the gel is modified to possess a pH gradient.

Isoelectric point (pI)–The pH at which an amino acid is predominantly in zwitterionic form.

Isoform–A slightly different version of the same protein, often specific to a given tissue.

Isomerase–An enzyme that catalyzes the constitutional or stereochemical rearrangement of a molecule.

Isotonic–A solution that has the same concentration as the one to which it is being compared.

Jacob–Monod model–The description of the structure and function of operons in prokaryotes, in which operons have structural genes, an operator site, a promoter site, and a regulator gene.

k_{cat}–Rate of catalytic conversion of substrate. This value gives the number of substrate molecules turned over per enzyme molecule per second.

Ketal–A carbon atom bonded to two alkyl groups and two —OR groups.

Ketogenesis–The synthesis of ketone bodies from the metabolic products of β-oxidation or amino acid metabolism; occurs under conditions of starvation.

Ketogenic–Describes amino acids that can be converted into ketone bodies.

Ketolysis–The breakdown of ketone bodies for use as acetyl-CoA.

Ketose–A sugar in which the highest-order functional group is a ketone; can be categorized by number of carbons (triose, tetrose, pentose, hexose, and so on).

Kinase–A specific transferase protein that catalyzes the movement of a phosphate group, generally from ATP, to a molecule of interest.

Knockdown–A technique using siRNA to temporarily reduce the expression of a specific gene and its corresponding protein by promoting mRNA degradation before translation can occur.

Knockout–A genetic modification that permanently inactivates or deletes a gene, preventing its expression.

K_m–The concentration of substrate at which an enzyme runs at half its maximal velocity; a measure of enzyme affinity (the higher the K_m, the lower the affinity).

Lactose–A disaccharide composed of glucose and galactose.

Lariat–The lasso-shaped structure formed during the removal of introns in mRNA processing.

Ligase–An enzyme that catalyzes the synthesis of large polymeric biomolecules, most commonly nucleic acids.

Lipid–A molecule that is insoluble in water and soluble in nonpolar organic solvents.

Lipoprotein–The transport mechanism for lipids within the circulatory and lymphatic systems; includes chylomicrons and VLDL, which transport triacylglycerols; and HDL, IDL, and LDL, which transport cholesterol and cholesteryl esters.

Loading controls–Proteins used in western blots (or molecules used in other assays) to ensure equal amounts of sample have been loaded in each lane.

Lock and key theory–One of the two most prominent theories of enzyme specificity; states that the enzyme and the substrate have a static but complementary state. Less supported than the induced fit model.

Lyase–An enzyme that catalyzes the cleavage or synthesis of a molecule without the addition or loss of water.

Maltose–A disaccharide composed of two glucose molecules.

Matrix–The contents of the inner mitochondrial membrane; includes soluble enzymes of the electron transport chain and mitochondrial DNA.

Melting point (T_m)–The midpoint of a thermal denaturation curve, indicating the temperature at which 50% of a protein is unfolded.

Membrane–In cell biology, a double layer of phospholipids and proteins that forms the boundaries of cells and organelles within cells.

Membrane receptors–Transmembrane protein molecules that act enzymatically or as ion channels to participate in signal transduction.

Messenger RNA (mRNA)–The strand of RNA formed after transcription of DNA; transfers to the cytoplasm to be translated.

Micelle–A collection of fatty acid or phospholipid molecules oriented to minimize free energy through hydrophobic and hydrophilic interactions; generally a sphere with a hydrophobic core and hydrophilic exterior.

Midpoint concentration (C_m)–The midpoint of a chemical denaturation curve, representing the concentration of a denaturant at which 50% of a protein is unfolded.

Migration velocity–the velocity at which a compound moves through a gel during electrophoresis.

Missense mutation–A mutation in which one amino acid is substituted for by a different amino acid.

Mitochondria–The organelle responsible for aerobic respiration, generating ATP from the breakdown products of other biomolecules and energy carriers reduced in various metabolic pathways; contains an inner and outer membrane.

Mixed inhibition–A decrease in enzyme activity that results from the interaction of an inhibitor with an allosteric site; mixed inhibitors bind to free enzyme and to substrate-bound enzyme with different affinities. They cannot be overcome by addition of substrate and impact both K_m and V_{max}.

Molecular cloning–A technique used to isolate a gene sequence and insert it into a vector for amplification.

Molten globules–Intermediate states in the folding of a protein.

Monocistronic–The coding pattern of eukaryotes in which one mRNA molecule codes for only one protein.

Monoprotic–Containing only one hydrogen (acid), or being able to pick up only one hydrogen (base).

Monosaccharide–A single sugar monomer; common examples are glucose, galactose, and fructose.

Motor proteins–Proteins that are involved in cell motility through interactions with structural proteins; motor proteins have ATPase activity and include myosin, kinesin, and dynein.

Multiple cloning site (MCS)–A short DNA region within a vector containing multiple restriction enzyme recognition sites, facilitating the insertion of foreign DNA; also known as a polylinker.

Mutagenesis–The process of deliberately introducing mutations into a DNA sequence in order to produce a mutant gene or protein.

Mutarotation–The rapid interconversion between different anomers of a sugar.

Mutation–A genetic variation that is below 1% of allele frequency in a population.

N-terminus–The free amino end of a polypeptide.

Negative control–In prokaryotic genetics, an operon that requires the binding of a protein to decrease transcription.

Nicotinamide adenine dinucleotide (NAD^+)–An energy carrier that accepts electrons and feeds them into the electron transport chain.

Nicotinamide adenine dinucleotide phosphate ($NADP^+$)–An electron donor produced in the pentose phosphate pathway that is involved in biosynthesis, oxidative stress, and immune function.

NMR spectroscopy–A method of determining molecular structure that uses the relative position of carbons and hydrogens determined by the relative shielding and spins of electrons observed when molecule is exposed to a magnetic field.

Noncompetitive inhibition–A decrease in enzyme activity that results from the interaction of an inhibitor with an allosteric site; noncompetitive inhibitors bind equally well to free enzyme and to substrate-bound enzyme. They cannot be overcome by addition of substrate.

Nonsense mutation–A mutation in which a coding codon is changed to a stop codon. Also called a truncation mutation.

Nontemplate synthesis–The method of *de novo* synthesis of lipids and carbohydrates that relies on gene expression and enzyme specificity rather than the genetic template of DNA or RNA.

Northern blot–A technique used to detect specific RNA sequences in a sample. RNA fragments are separated by gel electrophoresis, transferred to a membrane, and then probed with labeled complementary nucleotide sequences.

Nuclear pore–A hole in the nuclear envelope that permits the entrance and exit of substrates.

Nucleoside–Molecule composed of a pentose bound to a nitrogenous base at the C-1′ position of the sugar.

Nucleotide–Molecule composed of one or more phosphate groups bound to the C-5′ position of a nucleoside.

Nucleotide excision repair–Method for removing thymine dimers from DNA strands via a cut-and-patch process.

Okazaki fragments–Small strands formed on the lagging strand during DNA synthesis due to the unidirectional nature of DNA synthesis.

Oncogenes–Mutated genes that cause cancer.

Open system–A system capable of exchanging both matter and energy with the environment.

Operator site–A component of the operon in prokaryotes; a nontranscribable region of DNA that is capable of binding a repressor protein.

Operon–In prokaryotes, a cluster of genes transcribed as a single mRNA that can be regulated by repressors or inducers, depending on the system.

Opsonization–The marking of a pathogen by an antibody for later destruction.

Ordered sequential reaction–An enzyme-catalyzed reaction in which substrates bind to the enzyme in a specific order.

Origins of replication–Sites at which DNA unwinds to allow replication of new DNA. Generation of new DNA in both directions occurs at origins of replication, resulting in replication forks.

Osmosis–The simple diffusion of water.

Osmotic pressure–The pressure necessary to counteract the effect of an osmotic gradient against pure water; one of the colligative properties.

Oxidative phosphorylation–The transfer of a phosphate group, generally to ATP that is powered by a gradient formed by oxidation–reduction reactions; occurs in the mitochondria.

Oxidoreductase–An enzyme that catalyzes an oxidation–reduction reaction, often using an electron carrier as a cofactor.

Pancreatic lipase–The primary enzyme involved in the digestion of lipids.

Pancreatic proteases–The enzymes that are primarily responsible for the digestion of proteins in the small intestine; they include trypsin, chymotrypsin, and carboxypeptidases A and B, and are secreted as zymogens.

Paracellular transport–The transport of materials through the interstitial space without interactions with the cytoplasm or cell membrane.

Passive transport–The movement of a molecule down its concentration gradient without energy investment; includes simple and facilitated diffusion and osmosis.

Pentose phosphate pathway–A metabolic process that produces NADPH and ribose 5-phosphate for nucleotide synthesis.

Peptide–A molecule composed of more than one amino acid residue; can be subdivided into dipeptides (two amino acids), tripeptides (3), oligopeptides (up to 20), and polypeptides (more than 20).

Peptide bond–An amide bond between the carboxyl group of one amino acid and the amino group of another amino acid.

Phospholipid–A lipid containing a phosphate and alcohol (glycerol or sphingosine) joined to hydrophobic fatty acid tails.

Phosphorylation–The placement of a phosphate group onto a compound.

Pi stacking–A non-covalent attractive interaction between two aromatic rings, often observed in nucleotides, in which partially-negative carbon atoms align with partially-positive hydrogen atoms on the rings.

Pi-teeing–A type of pi stacking in which one aromatic ring is perpendicular to the other, forming a "T" shape to align partially negative carbon atoms with partially positive hydrogen atoms; also known as T-shaped.

Plasmid–A small, circular DNA molecule often used as a vector in molecular cloning.

pK_a–The pH at which half of the of the molecules of a given acid are deprotonated; $[HA] = [A^-]$.

Point mutation–The substitution of one nucleotide for another in DNA.

Polarity–An uneven sharing of electrons in a molecule, creating a slightly positive side and a slightly negative side.

Polycistronic–The coding pattern of prokaryotes, in which one mRNA may code for multiple proteins.

Polymerase chain reaction–An automated process to produce copies of a DNA sequence without use of bacteria for amplification.

Polymorphism–A genetic variation with an allele frequency greater than 1% in a population.

Polyprotic–Containing more than one hydrogen (acid), or being able to pick up more than one hydrogen (base).

Polysaccharide–A long chain of monosaccharides linked by glycosidic bonds; can be divided into homopolysaccharides (only one type of monosaccharide is used) and heteropolysaccharides (more than one type of monosaccharide is used).

Positive control–In prokaryotic genetics, an operon that requires the binding of a protein to increase transcription.

Postprandial state–State shortly after eating characterized by increased anabolism and fuel storage. Also referred to as the absorptive or well-fed state.

Prenylation–The addition of lipid groups to a molecule.

Primary antibody–An antibody that specifically binds directly to an antigen of interest.

Primary structure–The linear sequence of amino acids in a polypeptide.

Primer annealing–The second step of the polymerase chain reaction (PCR) technique, in which the reaction mixture is cooled to allow primers to bind to complementary sequences flanking the target DNA region.

Promoter region–The portion of DNA upstream from a gene; contains the TATA box, which is the site where RNA polymerase II binds to start transcription.

Prostaglandin–A group of 20-carbon molecules that are unsaturated carboxylic acids derived from arachidonic acid; act as paracrine or autocrine hormones.

Prosthetic group–A cofactor or coenzyme that is covalently bonded to a protein to permit its function. Proteins with lipid, carbohydrate, and nucleic acid prosthetic groups are referred to as lipoproteins, glycoproteins, and nucleoproteins, respectively.

Protein–A molecule made up of at least one chain of amino acids joined by peptide bonds.

Proteinogenic–The ability of certain (20) amino acids to be integrated into proteins.

Proton-motive force–The proton concentration gradient across the inner mitochondrial membrane that is created in the electron transport chain and used in oxidative phosphorylation.

Purification yield–A measure of the efficiency of a purification procedure, expressed as the percentage of total enzyme activity retained throughout a purification process.

Purine–Nitrogen-containing base found in nucleotides possessing a two-ring structure. The purines are adenine and guanine.

Pyranose–A six-membered ring sugar.

Pyridine–A heterocyclic aromatic compound with the chemical formula C_5H_5N, similar in structure to benzene with one carbon replaced by a nitrogen atom.

Pyrimidine–Nitrogen-containing base found in nucleotides possessing a one-ring structure. The three pyrimidines are cytosine, thymine, and uracil.

Pyrrole–A five-membered heterocyclic aromatic compound containing nitrogen, which serves as a key structural component of heme, the iron-containing prosthetic group in hemoglobin responsible for oxygen transport.

Pyruvate–An important metabolic intermediate that can feed into the citric acid cycle, fermentation, or gluconeogenesis.

Q cycle–The shuttling of electrons between ubiquinol and ubiquinone in the inner mitochondrial membrane as a part of Complex III's function.

Quaternary structure–The interaction between different subunits of a multi-subunit protein; stabilized by R group interactions.

Radiolabeling–The process of incorporating radioactive isotopes into molecules for tracking and detection purposes.

Random sequential reaction–An enzyme-catalyzed reaction in which substrates can bind to the enzyme in any order.

Reaction coupling–The tendency of unfavorable biological reactions to occur concurrently with favorable reactions, often catalyzed by a single enzyme.

Reading frame–In translation, the three nucleotides that make up a codon.

Receptor tyrosine kinase (RTK)–A class of enzyme-linked membrane receptors, composed of monomers that dimerize upon ligand binding, which activates their intracellular catalytic domains to phosphorylate themselves (via autophosphorylation) and downstream target proteins.

Recombinant DNA–DNA that has been formed by combining genetic material from multiple sources in a laboratory.

Recombinant vector–A vector backbone, such as a plasmid, containing a foreign DNA insert.

Reducing PAGE–A type of polyacrylamide gel electrophoresis that uses a reducing agent to break disulfide bonds in proteins, disrupting tertiary and quaternary structure while preserving non-covalent interactions.

Reducing sugar–A sugar that can reduce other compounds and can be detected by Tollens' or Benedict's reagent.

Regulator gene–In an operon, the gene that codes for the repressor protein.

Release factor–The protein that binds to the stop codon during termination of translation.

Renaturation–The regaining of the correct secondary, tertiary, and quaternary structure after denaturation of a protein.

Replisome–Set of specialized proteins that assist DNA polymerase during replication.

Repressible system–An operon that requires a repressor to bind to a corepressor before binding to the operator site to stop transcription of the relevant gene.

Repressor–For enzymes, an inhibitor of enzyme action; for operons, a species that binds to the operator region to stop transcription of the relevant gene.

Respiratory control–The coordinated regulation of the different aerobic metabolic processes.

Respiratory quotient–A numerical representation that can be used to determine the most prevalent type of biomolecule being used in metabolism; the ratio of carbon dioxide produced to oxygen consumed.

Respirometry–A method of measuring metabolism through the consumption of oxygen.

Resting membrane potential–The electrical potential that results from the unequal distribution of charge around the cell membrane; resting membrane potential characterizes a cell that has not been stimulated.

Restriction enzyme–Enzymes that recognize palindromic double-stranded DNA sequences and cut through the backbone of the double helix at those locations.

Restriction site–A specific palindromic DNA sequence recognized and cut by a restriction enzyme.

Reverse transcriptase–An RNA-dependent DNA polymerase that synthesizes a complementary DNA strand from an RNA template.

Reverse transcription polymerase chain reaction (RT-PCR)–A technique that converts RNA into complementary DNA (cDNA) using reverse transcriptase, followed by amplification of the cDNA using PCR. This method is often used to measure gene expression levels.

Ribonucleic acid (RNA)–A nucleic acid found in both the nucleus and cytoplasm and most closely linked with transcription and translation, as well as some gene regulation.

Ribosomal RNA (rRNA)–The structural and enzymatic RNA found in ribosomes that takes part in translation.

Ribosome–Organelle composed of RNA and protein; it translates mRNA during protein synthesis.

Ribozyme–An RNA molecule with enzymatic activity.

RNA-induced silencing complex (RISC)–A multi-protein complex that incorporates siRNA and guides it to the target mRNA for degradation, leading to post-transcriptional gene silencing.

Salt bridge–An interaction formed through a combination of hydrogen bonding and ionic interaction between amino acids with charged R groups.

Sanger sequencing–A DNA sequencing method that utilizes dideoxynucleotides (ddNTPs) to terminate DNA strand elongation at specific bases, allowing for the determination of the DNA sequence.

Saponification–The reaction between a fatty acid and a strong base, resulting in a negatively charged fatty acid anion bound to a metal ion; creates soap.

Saturation–The presence or absence of double bonds in a fatty acid; saturated fatty acids have only single bonds, whereas unsaturated fatty acids have at least one double bond.

SDS-PAGE–A type of polyacrylamide gel electrophoresis, in which sodium dodecyl sulfate (SDS) denatures proteins and imparts a uniform negative charge, causing them to separate based only on mass.

Secondary antibody–An antibody that binds to a primary antibody, usually at the Fc site. Typically used for detection and signal amplification.

Secondary structure–The local structure of neighboring amino acids; most common are α-helices and β-pleated sheets.

Sequencing–Determining the order of amino acids in a polypeptide, or of nucleotides in a nucleic acid.

Shine–Dalgarno sequence–The site of initiation of translation in prokaryotes.

Shuttle mechanism–A method of functionally transferring a compound across a membrane without the actual molecule crossing; common examples are the glycerol 3-phosphate shuttle and malate–aspartate shuttle.

Sialic acid–The common name of *N*-acetylneuraminic acid (NANA), which is the terminal portion of the head group in a ganglioside.

Side chain–The variable component of an amino acid that gives the amino acid its identity and chemical properties; also called an R group.

Silent mutation–A mutation in the wobble position of a codon or noncoding DNA that leads to no change in the protein produced during translation.

Simple diffusion–The movement of solute molecules through the cell membrane down their concentration gradients without a transport protein; used for small, nonpolar, lipophilic molecules and water.

Single-stranded DNA-binding protein–Proteins that bind to unraveled DNA strands to prevent reassociation of DNA or degradation of DNA during replication events.

Site-directed mutagenesis–A method that introduces specific mutations into DNA using mutated primers.

Small nuclear ribonucleoproteins (snRNPs)–The protein portion of the spliceosome complex.

Small interfering RNA (siRNA)–Double-stranded RNA molecules that interfere with post-transcriptional gene expression by targeting and degrading specific mRNA sequences, leading to decreased protein production; also called silencing RNA.

Small nuclear RNA (snRNA)–The RNA portion of the spliceosome complex.

Sodium-potassium pump–An ATPase that exchanges three sodium cations for two potassium cations; responsible for maintaining cell volume and the resting membrane potential.

Solvation layer–The layer of solvent particles that interacts directly with the surface of a dissolved species.

Southern blot–A technique used to detect specific DNA sequences in a sample. DNA fragments are separated by gel electrophoresis, transferred to a membrane, and then probed with labeled complementary nucleotide sequences.

Specific activity–A measure of enzyme purity that expresses the amount of enzyme activity per unit mass of total protein in a sample, calculated by dividing enzyme activity by the total protein concentration.

Sphingolipid–A lipid containing a sphingosine or sphingoid backbone, bonded to fatty acid tails; include ceramide, sphingomyelins, glycosphingolipids, and gangliosides.

Sphingomyelin–A sphingophospholipid containing a sphingosine backbone and a phosphate head group.

Spliceosome–The apparatus used for splicing out introns and bringing exons together during mRNA processing.

Staggered stacking–A type of pi stacking in which the aromatic rings are parallel but offset, with partially negative carbon atoms positioned above partially positive hydrogen atoms of the adjacent ring; also known as parallel displaced.

Starch–A branched polymer of glucose used for energy storage in plants; common examples are amylose and amylopectin.

Start codon–The first codon in an mRNA molecule that codes for an amino acid (AUG for methionine or *N*-formylmethionine).

Stereoisomers–Compounds that have the same chemical formula and backbone, differing only in their spatial orientation; also called optical isomers.

Steroid–A derivative of cholesterol.

Stop codon–The last codon of translation (UAA, UGA, or UAG); release factor binds here, terminating translation.

Structural gene–Within an operon, the region that codes for the protein of interest.

Structural proteins–Proteins that are involved in the cytoskeleton and extracellular matrix; they are generally fibrous in nature and include collagen, elastin, keratin, actin, and tubulin.

Substrate–The molecule upon which an enzyme acts.

Substrate-level phosphorylation–The transfer of a phosphate group from a high-energy compound to ATP or another compound; occurs in glycolysis.

Sucrose–A disaccharide composed of glucose and fructose.

Supercoiling–Wrapping of DNA on itself during replication, characterized by torsional stress and potential for strand breakage.

Surfactant–A compound that lowers the surface tension between two solutions, acting as a detergent or emulsifier.

TATA box–The site of binding for RNA polymerase II during transcription; named for its high concentration of thymine and adenine bases.

Tautomerization–The rearrangement of bonds within a compound, usually by moving a hydrogen and forming a double bond.

Telomere–Repeating unit at the end of DNA that protects against the loss of information with repeated DNA replication.

Template strand–The strand of DNA that is transcribed to form mRNA; also called the antisense strand.

Termination (transcription)–The stage of transcription in which RNA polymerase reaches a termination sequence, ending transcription and releasing the newly synthesized hnRNA (pre-mRNA).

Termination (translation)–The end of translation, in which the ribosome finds a stop codon and release factor binds it, allowing the peptide to be freed from the ribosome.

Terpene–A class of lipids built from isoprene moieties; have carbon groups in multiples of five.

Terpenoid–A terpene derivative that has undergone oxygenation or rearrangement of the carbon skeleton.

Tertiary structure–The three-dimensional shape of a polypeptide, stabilized by numerous interactions between R groups.

Thyroid hormones–The primary permissive metabolic hormones involved in the regulation of the basal metabolic rate.

Tight junctions–Cell–cell junctions that prevent the paracellular transport of materials; tight junctions form a collar around cells and link cells within a single layer.

Titration–A laboratory technique in which a solution of unknown concentration is mixed with a solution of known concentration to determine the unknown concentration.

Transcellular transport–The transport of materials through the cell; requires interaction with the cytoplasm and may require transport proteins.

Transcription–The production of an mRNA molecule from a strand of DNA.

Transcription factors–Proteins that help RNA polymerase II locate and bind to the promoter region of DNA.

Transfer RNA (tRNA)–A folded strand of RNA that contains a three-nucleotide anticodon that pairs with an appropriate mRNA codon during translation and is charged with the corresponding amino acid.

Transferase–An enzyme that catalyzes the transfer of a functional group.

Translation–The production of a protein from an mRNA molecule.

Translocase–An enzyme that catalyzes the transport of molecules across a cell membrane.

Triacylglycerol–A glycerol molecule esterified to three fatty acid molecules; the most common form of fat storage within the body.

Turn–A secondary structural motif that leads to a change in direction in a polypeptide chain, often including a main chain hydrogen bond between nearby residues.

Uncompetitive inhibition–A decrease in enzyme activity that results from the interaction with an inhibitor at the allosteric site; uncompetitive inhibitors bind only to the substrate-bound enzyme and cannot be overcome by addition of substrate.

UV spectroscopy–A method of determining the concentration of protein in an isolate by comparison against a protein standard; relies on the presence of aromatic amino acids. It can also be used with nucleic acids and other compounds.

van't Hoff factor–The number of particles obtained from a molecule when dissociated in solution.

Vector backbone–A DNA molecule (often a plasmid) used as a carrier for foreign DNA fragments in molecular cloning.

Vitamin–An organic essential coenzyme that assists an enzyme in carrying out its action.

V_{max}–Maximum velocity for a given quantity of enzyme. V_{max} occurs when the enzyme is fully saturated.

Watson-Crick model–This model proposed the structure of DNA as a double stranded helix.

Wax–A high-melting point lipid composed of a very long chain alcohol and a very long chain fatty acid.

Western blot–A technique used to detect specific proteins in a sample. Proteins are separated by gel electrophoresis, transferred to a membrane, and then probed with antibodies.

Wobble–The third nucleotide of a codon that often plays no role in specifying an amino acid; an evolutionary development designed to protect against mutations.

X-ray crystallography–A method of determining molecular structure using apparent bond angles and diffraction and refraction of X-rays.

Zwitterion–A molecule that contains charges, but is neutral overall. Most often used to describe amino acids.

Zymogen–An enzyme that is secreted in an inactive form and must be activated by cleavage; common examples are digestive enzymes.

INDEX

Symbols

A

F

G

H

N

O

P

T

U

ART CREDITS

Chapter 1 Cover—Image credited to Yikrazuul. From Wikimedia Commons.

Figure 1.28(a)—Image credited to ibreakstock. Modified from original. From Shutterstock.

Chapter 3 Cover—Image credited to Heiti Paves. From Shutterstock.

Figure 3.16—Image credited to ggw. From Shutterstock.

Figure 3.21—Image credited to User: Dcrjsr. From Wikimedia Commons. Copyright © 1971. Used under license: CC-BY-3.0.

Chapter 4 Cover—Image credited to Sea Wave. From Shutterstock.

Chapter 5 Cover—Image credited to Captain Yeo. From Shutterstock.

Figure 5.5—Image credited to User: Alex Hindemith. From Wikimedia Commons.

Chapter 6 Cover—Image credited to: anyaivanova. From Shutterstock.

Figure 6.21—Image credited to Madeline Price Ball. From Wikimedia Commons. Copyright © 2011.

Figure 6.33—Imaged credited to Nickle and Barrett-Ng/*DNA Analysis—Blotting and Hybridization*/CC BY-SA 3.0/ Modified (original—J.Locke).

Figure 6.35—Imaged credited to Mnolf/Wikimedia Commons/CC BY-SA 3.0.

Chapter 7 Cover—Image credited to Mopic. From Shutterstock.

Chapter 8 Cover—Image credited to somersault1824. From Shutterstock.

Figure 8.12—Image credited to Holly Fischer. From Wikimedia Commons. Copyright © 2013. Used under license: CC-BY-3.0.

Image in Concept Check 8.2—Image credited to ellepigrafica. From Shutterstock.

Chapter 9 Cover—Image credited to Christian Bertrand. From Shutterstock.

Chapter 10 Cover—Image credited to RAJ CREATIONZS. From Shutterstock.

Chapter 11 Cover—Image credited to Bernd Juergens. From Shutterstock.

Chapter 12 Cover—Image credited to O2 creationz. From Shutterstock.

Figure 12.10—Image credited to Michael Feldman, MD, PhD. From Wikimedia Commons. Copyright © 2005. Used under license: CC-BY-2.0.

Notes